WOMEN'S GYNECOLOGIC HEALTH

Kerri Durnell Schuiling,
PhD, WHCNP, CNM, FACNM
Professor and Associate Dean of Nursing Education
Northern Michigan University School of Nursing
Marquette, Michigan

Frances E. Likis,
MSN, FNP, CNM, WHCNP
Women's Health Course Coordinator
Frontier School of Midwifery and
    Family Nursing
Hyden, Kentucky

JONES AND BARTLETT PUBLISHERS
Sudbury, Massachusetts
BOSTON   TORONTO   LONDON   SINGAPORE

World Headquarters
Jones and Bartlett Publishers
40 Tall Pine Drive
Sudbury, MA 01776
978-443-5000

Jones and Bartlett Publishers Canada
2406 Nikanna Road
Mississauga, ON L5C 2W6
CANADA

Jones and Bartlett Publishers International
Barb House, Barb Mews
London W6 7PA
UK

Jones and Bartlett's books and products are available through most bookstores and online booksellers. To contact Jones and Bartlett Publishers directly, call 800-832-0034, fax 978-443-8000, or visit our website at www.jbpub.com.

Substantial discounts on bulk quantities of Jones and Bartlett's publications are available to corporations, professional associations, and other qualified organizations. For details and specific discount information, contact the special sales department at Jones and Bartlett via the above contact information or send an email to specialsales@jbpub.com.

Copyright © 2006 by Jones and Bartlett Publishers, Inc.

The symbol on the cover is adapted from *The Changer* by K Robins and is used with the permission of K Robins Designs: www.krobinsdesigns.com.

Library of Congress Cataloging-in-Publication Data
Women's gynecologic health / [edited] by Kerri Durnell Schuiling, Frances E. Likis.
   p. ; cm.
  ISBN 0-7637-4717-3
  1. Generative organs, Female—Diseases. 2. Gynecology. 3. Reproductive health. 4. Women—Health and hygiene.
  [DNLM: 1. Genital Diseases, Female. 2. Reproduction. 3. Women's Health. WP 140 W872 2006] I. Schuiling, Kerri Durnell. II. Likis, Frances E.
  RG101.W773 2006
  618.1—dc22

                                                        2005005144

Production Credits
Acquisitions Editor: Kevin Sullivan
Production Director: Amy Rose
Production Assistant: Alison Meier
Associate Editor: Amy Sibley
Marketing Manager: Emily Ekle
Manufacturing Buyer: Amy Bacus
Cover Design: Kristin E. Ohlin
Composition: Northeast Compositors
Printing and Binding: Malloy Inc.
Cover Printing: Malloy Inc.

Printed in the United States of America
09 08 07 06 05   10 9 8 7 6 5 4 3 2 1

10/12/05

Dedication

To our best teachers: our students and the women for whom we have provided care.
—*Kerri and Francie*

To:
My mom and stepfather, Marie and Don Hall, who always believe in me;
My children, Mary, Sean, and Sarah, who sustain me;
My husband, Judd, whose endless patience supports my work;
Dr. Earl Williams for always encouraging me; and,
The memory of my beloved father, Frank E. Durnell, DO.
—*Kerri*

To:
My parents and stepparents, Kenny, Katey, Lori, and Ron, who steadfastly support me;
My sister, Mary, who encourages me and helps me take life less seriously;
My brothers and nieces, James, Ben, Katherine, and Elizabeth, who bring great joy to my life;
Tekoa, who is an exceptional mentor and friend;
And last, but certainly not least, Zan, the one who never lets go.
—*Francie*

Contents

SECTION III WOMEN'S GYNECOLOGIC HEALTH CARE MANAGEMENT   291

12 INTIMATE PARTNER VIOLENCE AND SEXUAL ASSAULT   293
Daniel J. Sheridan
Linda A. Fernandes
Alida D. Alden
Dawn M. Van Pelt
Jacquelyn C. Campbell

17 GYNECOLOGIC INFECTIONS 403
Catherine Ingram Fogel

24 URINARY INCONTINENCE   635

Sandra H. Hines
Janis M. Miller

Preface

Historically, women's health was framed within a biomedical model by clinicians. Textbooks typically used a biomedical framework to present women's health content. Although this approach can be useful on many levels, it also has limitations that can have significant negative effects on women's health, particularly gynecologic health. A biomedical model is disease-oriented and focuses on curing illness. This approach risks pathologizing normal aspects of female physiology. When a biomedical lens is used to assess women's health, there is risk of essentializing women and reducing them to biologic parts. An example of this proclivity is that for many years women's health meant reproductive health, regardless of whether or not the woman planned to bear children. This reductionism transfers to practice where a woman's *parts* become the focus of diagnosis and treatment. The meaning of the diagnosis to the woman, as well as the impact that the diagnosis has on her, her significant others, and the work she does, is not addressed.

Recently, feminists have developed theories about women's growth and development that provide a different perspective from earlier male-oriented models. These feminist models include women's lived experiences and the importance of relationships to women. Women's agency is supported by recognizing each woman as an expert knower. The focus is holistic, and health is assessed within the context of each woman's life.

It is important for our readers to know that we, as the editors of this book, are experienced women's health clinicians whose practice philosophy is grounded in caring for the whole woman within her lived experience. As teachers, we were repeatedly frustrated at the inability to locate a gynecologic book that we felt was suitable for our course. Many of the books that were available were written primarily from a biomedical perspective and did not, in our opinion, provide sufficient content about the normalcy of women's reproductive physiology. Books such as those authored by the Boston Women's Health Book Collective were extremely helpful with ideas about health and holism but lacked the necessary content to educate student clinicians. Other books did not provide the health-oriented perspective that is vital to the philosophy of care espoused by nursing and midwifery, in which we both strongly believe. Additional books provided elements of both biomedical and health-oriented views and had very useful decision trees or categorization of concerns or problems. We felt, however, that these books would not encourage students and practicing clinicians to think critically and to appreciate the importance of making decisions based on the most recent evidence.

For these myriad reasons we embarked on producing a book that presents women's gynecologic health from a feminist and holistic viewpoint. Our goal was to create a book that emphasizes the importance of respecting the normalcy of female physiology, and provides medical content appropriate for assessment, diagnosis, and treatment of pathology. We believe this book embodies these perspectives and underlines the importance of collaboration among health care clinicians.

Some aspects of this feminist approach will be very obvious to our readers, while others may be more subtle. For example, illustrations of whole women, rather than pictures of only breasts or genitalia, are used when possible. Women are not referred to by a condition, but as a woman who has a specific concern. For example, we speak of the woman who is experiencing menopause, as opposed to the menopausal woman. We used the term birth as opposed to delivery because it situates the power to give birth within the woman versus transferring it to the clinician as in "being delivered." We purposefully used "women's" rather than "gynecologic" as the first word of the book title. The goal is to help readers to keep first in their mind that they are treating a whole woman, not her body parts, and not just a condition. We hope this emphasizes the importance of treating women holistically within their lived experiences.

We were fortunate to have many excellent contributors to this book. Some are nationally known, and others might be new to many of you. The common thread among all of our contributors is their expertise in their respective areas and their recognition of the importance of evidence-based practice. Many of our contributors are expert clinicians and others are expert scientists. Frequently co-authored chapters represent a clinician and researcher team, whose collaboration provides readers with a real-world view that is grounded in evidence.

This book encompasses both health promotion and management of gynecologic conditions that women experience. All of the content is evidence-based. The first section of the book introduces the feminist framework of the book and provides readers with a context for evaluating evidence and determining best practice. The second section of the book provides a foundation for assessment and promotion of women's gynecologic health. The third and final section addresses the evaluation and management of clinical conditions frequently encountered in gynecologic health care.

This is a first edition book, and we welcome feedback from our readers that will help us in future revisions! Please contact us at womensgynhealth@earthlink.net.

Kerri Durnell Schuiling, PhD, WHCNP, CNM, FACNM
Frances E. Likis, MSN, FNP, CNM, WHCNP

Acknowledgments

We quickly discovered that publishing a book is a huge undertaking that definitely requires some risk taking. Therefore, we thank Kitty Ernst, DSc (Hon), MPH, CNM, FACNM, for teaching us about the importance of being risk takers, and Susan Stone, DNSc, CNM, FACNM, for showing us how to be successful at risk taking.

Thank you to the many talented and dedicated contributors. You were all wonderful to work with and taught us so much. We are deeply indebted to each of you and believe women's gynecologic health will be better because you were willing to share your expertise.

We appreciate the many people at Jones and Bartlett who made the publication of this book possible. We particularly thank Amy Sibley, Amy Rose, and Alison Meier, who always had the answers to our questions and provided support whenever it was needed. The book was published on time because of the invaluable assistance of these women. We also thank Emily Ekle for her marketing expertise.

We are very grateful to K Robins for graciously allowing us to adapt her design *The Changer* for our book's cover. We encourage readers to visit www.krobinsdesigns.com, where *The Changer* and other symbols are available as pendants.

We thank all of you who were instrumental in some way to the publication of this book. There are too many to mention each of you by name, but you know that we know who you are. We truly appreciate the support you provided.

—*Kerri and Francie*

Mentors are critical to success. The mentors who most shaped my professional (and at times my personal) life and to whom I am forever indebted are Carolyn Sampselle, PhD, RN, FAAN; Judith Fullerton, PhD, CNM, FACNM; Katherine Camacho Carr, PhD, ARNP, CNM, FACNM; and Maureen Chrzanowski, MSN, CNM, FNP. These women mentored me in my clinical and academic worlds, and I know that my success and passion for my work are, in many ways, directly attributable to their support of my growth and development.

I could not have worked on this book without the constant support of my dean, Cameron Howes, PhD, who provided me with both time and understanding (and even some cheerleading at times).

Thanks also to my wonderful secretaries, Pat Woods and Terry Johnson, and our work-study student Ryan, who were all still smiling as they copied yet another draft or were willing to make "just one more run" to the post office.

I work with an extremely creative and talented faculty in the School of Nursing at Northern Michigan University. They all have been supportive in some way during the writing of this book. Some have taken on additional tasks because I was pushing a book-related deadline, while others provided their expertise as contributors to the book. Thank you to all of you for being so supportive of my professional development.

As our book explains, the relationships women have are critically important to our lives. Friends are important. I am blessed with some very special and extremely talented friends. My dear friend and colleague, Cyndy Perkins, MSN, ANP, CNM, gave me many ideas for this book when she and I co-taught a course about women's health. Her humor and positive attitude always provide a smile when needed. Lisa Kane Low, PhD, CNM, FACNM, and Julia Seng, PhD, CNM (who brought me up to really "get it" when we talked late into the night walking across the campus at the University of Michigan) are two of my dearest friends and colleagues. Both sustained me with laughter, encouragement, and a bit of realism as the book project wore on. Lisa graciously (and eloquently, as you will read) contributed to two of the chapters of this book and helped Francie and me understand some of the complexities of more current feminist thought. Joani Slager, MSN, CNM, who has been a very dear friend for many years, is a pragmatic wonder and reminds me of the importance of keeping a busy life balanced. Donovan Royal, PsyD, is my one true confidante and, at times, my greatest supporter or muse, depending on how he sees it. Nonetheless, he loves me always, and I count on his friendship to see me through.

And finally (although far from least), thank you to my dear friend and colleague Francie Likis, who completely understands me and continues to work with me anyway.

—Kerri

My colleagues at the Frontier School of Midwifery and Family Nursing, many of whom were my midwifery teachers, have been integral to my professional endeavors. I am fortunate to be part of a community of such wise and strong women. Our work would not be possible without the wonderful staff in Kentucky and Michigan. Thank you also to the Multimedia Team at Frontier, all of whom have been extremely patient and generous with their technical support, and especially to the men who have probably learned far more about women's health than they ever wanted to know.

David Grimes, MD, inspired me long before we met, and he is now an invaluable mentor and friend. Heidi Schumacher Dahlborg, LM, is an exemplary midwife, and she has taught me a great deal about how to be a truly holistic clinician. Some would say that my career path is genetic because Howard A. Kelly, MD, was my great-great-grandfather. He was one of the four founding physicians of Johns Hopkins School of Medicine, contributed significantly to the establishment of gynecology as a specialty, and was an innovative clinician and prolific writer. I hope that I am continuing his legacy in a way that would make him proud.

I am blessed with a wonderful family. Thank you to my grandparents, aunts, uncles, cousins, and favorite brother-in-law for your love and support. My life would not be the same without Sander and Niki Blue in it, and I am grateful to be a member of their family.

My friends are an important part of who I am. Virginia Spradlin, Missy Reynolds, Carrie Comer, Katie Cocks, and Bo Harmon have stood by me through good and bad for many years. Lory Warren knows me very well, and she still always manages to see the best in me. Ruth Stewart must have been my sister in another life, and she is a friend in the truest sense of the word. Emily Bobrow has been an endless source of support during my doctoral studies and the writing of this book. I will always owe her for staying up all night with me to make sure the manuscript got to Jones and Bartlett on time. Clint Hobbs influenced my life beyond words, and not a day passes that I don't miss him.

There are few tasks that can test a friendship to the extent that writing a book together does. I am grateful to have shared the journey of bringing this book to fruition with Kerri, and for the fact that we remain friends!

—Francie

Contributors

Alida D. Alden, RN, BSN, FNE-A, SANE-A
Graduate Student, CNS Forensic Focus
Johns Hopkins University School of Nursing
Baltimore, Maryland

Ivy M. Alexander, PhD, C-ANP
Associate Professor
Yale University School of Nursing
Adult Nurse Practitioner, Primary Care Clinician
Yale University Health Services, Department of Internal Medicine
New Haven, Connecticut

Heather M. Aliotta, MSN, RNC
Nurse Practitioner
Gillette Center for Women's Cancers
Massachusetts General Hospital
Boston, Massachusetts

Christine L. Anderson, MSN, WHCNP, ANP
Planned Parenthood of the Rochester/Syracuse Region
Rochester, New York

Linda C. Andrist, PhD, WHNP, RNC
Associate Professor
Coordinator Adult/Women's Health NP Specialty
Graduate Program in Nursing
MGH Institute of Health Professions
Boston, Massachusetts

Linda A. Bernhard, PhD, RN
Associate Dean for Academic Affairs
College of Nursing
Associate Professor, Nursing and Women's Studies
Ohio State University
Columbus, Ohio

Jacquelyn C. Campbell, PhD, RN, FAAN
Associate Dean for Faculty Practice/Professor
Johns Hopkins University School of Nursing
Baltimore, Maryland

Katherine Camacho Carr, PhD, ARNP, CNM, FACNM
Associate Professor
Seattle University College of Nursing
Nurse-Midwife
Highline Midwifery and Women's Health
Seattle, Washington

Susan Chasson, MSN, JD, CNM, APRN, BC
Lecturer
Brigham Young University
Provo, Utah

Linell Dehlin, MSN, RNC, WHNP
Nurse Educator
Bay de Noc Community College
Escanaba, Michigan

Mary Ann Faucher, CNM, PhD
Assistant Professor
Louise Herrington School of Nursing
Baylor University
Dallas, Texas

Linda A. Fernandes, BSN, RN, FNE-A
Graduate Student, CNS Forensic Focus
Johns Hopkins University School of Nursing
Baltimore, Maryland

Catherine Ingram Fogel, PhD, RNC (WHCNP), FAAN
Professor and Women's Health Practice Area Coordinator
School of Nursing
University of North Carolina at Chapel Hill
Chapel Hill, North Carolina

Sandra H. Hines, MS, RNC, WHCNP
Research Investigator
University of Michigan
School of Nursing
Ann Arbor, MI

Nancy J. Hughes, LTC, AN, CNM
Nursing Director OB/GYN, Pediatrics, Family Medicine Product Lines
Tripler Army Medical Center
Honolulu, Hawaii

Holly Powell Kennedy, PhD, CNM, FNP, FACNM
Assistant Professor
University of California, San Francisco
San Francisco, California

Suzanne M. Leclaire, MSN, MHS, RN
Head Nurse/Care Manager ENT Clinic
Tripler Army Medical Center
Honolulu, Hawaii

Lisa Kane Low, PhD, CNM, FACNM
Assistant Research Scientist
School of Nursing
Lecturer III
Program in Women's Studies
University of Michigan
Ann Arbor, Michigan

Janis M. Miller, PhD, APRN
Assistant Research Scientist
School of Medicine, Department of Obstetrics and Gynecology
School of Nursing
University of Michigan
Ann Arbor, Michigan

Katherine Morgan, MS, WHNP, ANP
Assistant Professor (Clinical)
University of Utah, College of Nursing
Salt Lake City, Utah

Patricia Aikins Murphy, CNM, DrPH, FACNM
Associate Professor
Annette Poulson Cumming Presidential Endowed Chair in Women's and Reproductive Health
University of Utah
Salt Lake City, Utah

Deborah Narrigan, CNM, MSN
Department of Internal Medicine
Meharry Medical College
Nashville, Tennessee

Ellen Olshansky, DNSc, RNC, FAAN
Professor and Chair
Department of Health and Community Systems
University of Pittsburgh School of Nursing
Pittsburgh, Pennsylvania

Kathryn Osborne, MSN, CNM
Academic Faculty
Frontier School of Midwifery and Family Nursing
Hyden, Kentucky

Anna Sanford, MSN, APRN, BC, AOCN
Associate Professor
School of Nursing
Northern Michigan University
Marquette, Michigan

Nancy J. Schaeffer, MSN, APRN, BC
Nurse Practitioner
Massachusetts General Hospital
Gillette Center for Women's Cancers
Boston, Massachusetts

Beth A. Collins Sharp, PhD, RN
Health Scientist Administrator
Center for Outcomes and Evidence
Agency for Healthcare Research and Quality
Rockville, Maryland

Daniel J. Sheridan, PhD, RN, FAAN
Assistant Professor
Johns Hopkins University School of Nursing
Baltimore, Maryland

Katherine Simmonds, MSN, RNC, MPH
Clinical Instructor
MGH Institute of Health Professions
Director
The Reproductive Options Education Consortium
Boston, Massachusetts

Nancy M. Steele, PhD, RNC, CNS, WHNP
Nurse Manager/Antepartum-Gynecology Unit
Tripler Army Medical Center
Honolulu, Hawaii

Diana Taylor, RN, NP, PhD, FAAN
Professor Emeritus, School of Nursing
Adjunct Professor, Center for Reproductive Health Policy
University of California-San Francisco
San Francisco, California

Dawn M. Van Pelt, RN, BSN
Graduate Student, CNS Forensic Focus
Johns Hopkins University School of Nursing
Baltimore, Maryland

Carol A. Verga, CNM, ARNP
Center for Women's Health at Evergreen
Kirkland, Washington
Clinical Instructor
University of Washington
Seattle, Washington

Mary Wallace, RN, MSN, CFNP
Professor and Coordinator Family Nurse Practitioner Program
Department of Nursing
Northern Michigan University
Marquette, Michigan

SECTION I

INTRODUCTION TO WOMEN'S GYNECOLOGIC HEALTH

WOMEN'S HEALTH FROM A FEMINIST PERSPECTIVE

LISA KANE LOW
KERRI DURNELL SCHUILING

What does gender have to do with women's health? The most obvious answer is that women's health is about women and their health; therefore gender is an issue. However, gender is an issue only because the focus is women. The true challenge to answering the question accurately is gaining an understanding that the answers all depend on definitions. For example, if we were only speaking about gender as if it was synonymous with sex, then the stated answer "women's health is about women; therefore gender is an issue" would be correct, but gender is *not* synonymous with sex. Gender is defined as a person's self-representation as man or woman or how social institutions based on the individual's gender presentation respond to that person. Gender is used when referring to social and cultural influences based on sex (Pinn, 2003a). It is rooted in biology and shaped by the environment and experience (Pinn, 2003b). This broader definition of gender makes the answer to the question "What does gender have to do with women's health?" much more complex.

There are three aspects to consider when answering the question "What does gender have to do with women's health?" The first is an aspect of comparison: exploring women's health as compared to men's health. The second aspect is context: exploring the context of gender and how it affects the process of providing health care services. The third aspect to consider is the social construction of gender and how it affects women's health. The significance of answering the question from each of these perspectives is that each one has implications for the manner in which women access, receive, and respond to health care. These three aspects provide opportunities for us to better understand women's health care experiences. They also assist in the identification of some of the underlying factors of health care disparities that women experience. The purpose of this chapter is to provide an overview of women's health using gender considerations as a lens for exploring women's health in general and gynecologic health in particular.

WOMEN'S HEALTH CARE AND GYNECOLOGIC HEALTH

The state of women's health care today is a direct reflection of women's status and position in society. There have been many health care advances made under the rubric of women's health; however, there is still a long way to go before all women receive comprehensive, compassionate health care services that address the complexity and diversity of how women live their lives and experience health and disease.

This textbook is based on a feminist framework in an effort to advance health care provided to women in today's society. The authors attempt to acknowledge the complexity of women's health by paying particular attention to women's status in society and their unequal access to opportunity, while focusing on women's gynecologic health and well-being.

FEMINISM

What is feminism? Feminism is not a singular "what." There are multiple definitions of feminism. One definition that is well suited for addressing the context in which women experience health and wellness is that offered by bell hooks. hooks (2000) defines feminism as a perspective that acknowledges the oppression of women within a patriarchal society, and struggles toward the elimination of sexist oppression and domination for all human beings. Acknowledging the oppression of women is increasingly more difficult within many Western societies. Affluence and an increase in opportunity within some sectors of employment or education are often construed as equal access or equity in opportunity for all women. However, oppression is defined as "not having a choice." When this definition is used, many more individuals are able to recognize constraints in their personal experiences, and acknowledgment of oppression in its various forms becomes possible. Examples include a range of extremes from forced marriage, forced sterilization, unfair labor practices, denial of access to pharmaceutical methods of contraception, to not being able to access desired health care providers. The ranges of extremes represent the vast breadth of experiences women may have within the context of a patriarchal society that denies equal access to power, resource, and opportunity for women.

Characteristics of a feminist perspective include the use of critical analysis to question assumptions about societal expectations and the value various roles have on both a political and individual level. The process of critical analysis is accomplished by rejecting conceptualizations of women as homogeneous. It acknowledges power imbalances, and uses the influence of gender as the foremost consideration in the analysis. Using a gender lens that is informed by feminism permits areas of disparity to be identified both between groups based on gender and within groups based on the recognition of heterogeneity among women.

TABLE 1-1   Components of a Feminist Perspective in Women's Health

- Works with women as opposed to for women
- Uses heterogeneity as an assumption, not homogeneity
- Minimizes or exposes power imbalances
- Rejects androcentric models as normative
- Challenges the medicalization and pathologizing of normal physiologic processes
- Seeks social and political change to address women's health issues

Feminism requires exploration of women's health within the context of how women live their lives collectively and individually within a patriarchal society. The social, environmental, and economic aspects become integral to understanding the context in which women are able to achieve health and well-being. Furthermore, feminism requires consideration of health, as influenced by the intersection of sexism, racism, class, nation, and gender, within a framework that acknowledges the role of oppression as it affects women and their health as individuals and as a group. Table 1–1 offers components of a feminist perspective when considering women's health issues or models of care, thus enabling you to reframe your view of women's health in a feminist perspective.

MODEL OF CARE BASED ON A FEMINIST PERSPECTIVE

A model of care that is based on a feminist perspective contrasts sharply with a biomedical model, particularly in areas of power and control. A feminist model supports egalitarian relationships and identifies the woman as the expert knower. The woman is the center of the health care model. The following discussion provides further insights into a feminist-based model of care:

1. The model of care must focus on being *with* women not *doing for* women. This frames the model of care as a partnership with women as opposed to one that is directed by others and then assigned to women through a process of authoritative knowledge being handed down on the assumption that it is correct.
2. Heterogeneity rather than homogeneity must be used as an assumption. Considerations of "all women" or offering grand theories regarding women or using broad gender-based assumptions serves to essentialize women rather than acknowledge the diversity within the larger group that comprises women. An assumption of heterogeneity considers women on an individual basis, tailoring health care and services to a woman's unique needs rather than treating all women as a group with the assumption of similarity across all considerations of health.
3. The model of care must seek to minimize or expose power imbalances that are inherent in most current health care models, especially those based on a biomedical model.

Power should be distributed equally within the health care interaction. The interaction should be based on a belief in a woman's right to self-determination. Therefore, the role of health care provider is that of providing support, information, and skillful knowledge as opposed to asserting authority over the decision-making ability of the individual.

4. A feminist framework rejects androcentric models of health and disease as normative. The pervasiveness of male-based models being extrapolated and applied to women on the assumption that a woman is merely a biologic variant of man serves to constrain a full consideration of women's health issues. This misapplication of androcentric models to women's health also serves to medicalize or pathologize normal physiologic processes of women such as menstruation, childbirth, and menopause (Lorber, 1997).

5. A feminist perspective challenges the process of medicalization and pathologizing by identifying and exploring women's unique health experiences and normalizing them. Medicalizing is a process of labeling conditions as diseases or disorders as a basis for providing medical treatment. The medicalization of many of women's biologic functions, such as menstruation and pregnancy, frequently has been cited to illustrate both the social construction of the disease and the general expansion of medical control into everyday life (Conrad, 1992; Zola, 1972).

6. A feminist framework acknowledges the broader context in which women live their lives and the subsequent challenges to their health as a result of living within a patriarchal society and argues for a process of social and political change that would eliminate gender bias and sexism and result in the betterment of all human beings.

THE SOCIAL CONSTRUCTION OF GENDER AND HEALTH

A discussion of the social construction of gender is provided as a basis for exploration of the value of a feminist framework in understanding women's health. This discussion is followed by strategies to analyze women's health issues from a feminist perspective. Lorber (1997) identifies that

> as a social phenomenon, illness has to be gendered because gender is one of the most important statuses in any society. Gender is also socially constructed. Girls and boys are taught their society's expectations of appropriate behavior; they grow up to enact their society's gendered social roles. Gender is a social institution that patterns interaction in everyday life and in major social organizations. (p. 5)

Gender influences health services that are offered, what health risks are identified for an individual, and which treatments are potentially offered at all levels of interaction. While many of these differences are arguably biologically based, a feminist perspective

TABLE 1–2   Definitions of Sex, Gender, and Biology

Sex	The classification of living things as man or woman according to their reproductive organs and functions assigned by chromosomal complement
Gender	A person's self-representation as man or woman or who that person is responded to by social institutions based on the individual's gender presentation. Gender is rooted in biology and shaped by the environment and experience.
Biology	The study of life and living organisms, including the genetic, molecular, biochemical, hormonal, cellular, physiological, behavioral, and psychosocial aspects of life

Source: Adapted from Wizemann and Pardue as cited in Pinn, 2003a.

argues that gender and sexism instead are the key components of these differences. Table 1–2 provides definitions of sex, gender, and biology so that the reader may gain an appreciation of the differences in the terms.

The significance of the social construction of gender is a critical consideration in the process of defining, providing, and receiving health care services. "The juxtaposition of gender and illness presents two major problems: sex differences versus gender differences and between group and within group differences" (Lorber, 1997, p. 5).

Social construction is a process by which societal expectations of behavior become interpreted or ascribed as innate characteristics that are biologically determined. Thus, attributes associated with femininity—attributes that are socially expected and thus performed in compliance with social expectations—become confused with innately determined behaviors rather than socially constructed behaviors. As a result, health risks, treatments, and approaches to care are not necessarily scientifically or biologically based aspects of women's health. Instead they are determined by social expectations that are based on assumptions about gender differences. In addition, diagnoses can be influenced by gendered assumptions regarding behavior or what is socially constructed as feminine behavior. There is significant documentation of such influences affecting the manner of diagnosis and treatment, particularly within the mental health arena (Tavris, 1992) and in the misdiagnosis of women's cardiovascular risk (Healy, 1991).

What becomes evident when the considerations of gender are explored within the context of health is that gender interacts with many of the other variables that are considered factors affecting health outcomes. Women tend to ask more questions, receive more information about their health, and have a more partnership-building relationship with their health care providers than men (Xu & Borders, 2003). Yet, women are also more likely to be affected by financial barriers than men. "In particular, women who had lower incomes were consistently less likely to have visited a physician while men were more deterred by nonfinancial barriers to health care such as the length of time in a waiting room" (Xu & Borders, p. 1077). Women as a group experience greater barriers to obtaining health care services.

Poor or low-income women and women who are members of disadvantaged racial or ethnic minorities often obtain fewer or receive different health services than do women that are more affluent. Women from disadvantaged backgrounds often experience different risks to their health and have worse health statuses than their wealthier counterparts (Weisman, 1998). In fact, low income predicts who receives health care. Low socioeconomic status is the single most powerful contributor to illness and premature death (Lantz, House, Lepkowski, Williams, Mero, & Chen, 1998). Therefore, while understanding gender differences in the utilization of health care services is important, treating women as a homogeneous group has limitations, particularly when socioeconomic status and racial or ethnic identity are considered.

Nearly 40 million of the 140 million American women alive today are members of racial and ethnic minority groups (Satcher, 2001). Women of racial and ethnic minority groups experience many of the same health concerns as do white women; however, as a group they are "in poorer health, use fewer health services, and continue to suffer disproportionately from premature death, disease, and disabilities" (Weisman, 1998, p. 11). Racial and ethnic health disparities have been explained by locating the differences in health outcomes in biologic explanations that presume homogeneity among racial and ethnic groups. Biologic explanations focus on biologic solutions rather than exploring the context in which health disparities occur. Today the use of race as a marker for capturing biologic divisions within the population has been challenged scientifically (Williams, 2002).

> Our racial categories are more alike than different in terms of biologic characteristics and genetics, and they do not capture patterns of genetic variation well. Thus it is not biologically plausible for genetic differences alone to play a major role in racial or ethnic differences in health. (Williams, p. 590)

It is not sufficient to explore differences in health issues simply by ethnic or racial identity or simply by gender. Gender interacts with many social causes of health and illness: age, socioeconomic status, race, and ethnicity (Weisman, 1998). As previously stated, socioeconomic status is a significant contributor to poor health outcomes, but gender further increases that risk. It is also evident that women from an ethnic minority receive lower-quality health care and less health care overall than wealthier, better-educated, higher-status white women (Davis & Huber, 2004). What is missing from consideration is how socioeconomic status is often used as a proxy to explain racial and ethnic health differences in women's health outcomes. When specific health conditions such as hypertension are explored, socioeconomic status is found to be strongly associated with its prevalence. There are also significant differences in the incidence of hypertension between black and white women. The differences in the incidence of hypertension in black and white women is about as large as the difference in the incidence of hypertension found in poor black women compared to black women of higher incomes. According to public health expert David Williams (2002), examples such as these demonstrate the complexity of trying to understand health disparities that are based solely on race or solely on ethnic identity. The intersection of these various factors creates complexity when trying to research women's health issues such as health disparities. Williams argues for consideration of the social embeddedness of women's health and a need to attend to additional factors such as types of medical care, geographic location, migration, acculturation and racism, exposure to stress, and access to resources when exploring disparities in women's health. Only by including consideration of these factors can we fully and accurately identify the health disparities women experience.

Access to quality and culturally appropriate health care services is further limited by age and gendered assumptions. Social role differences between men and women are thought to affect health primarily by influencing access to health-producing resources such as nutrition, shelter, education, paid employment, supportive social networks, health care insurance, and health care services (Weisman, 1998). The manner in which women negotiate the health care system is also founded upon gendered assumptions that promote differential access to resources resulting in power imbalances as opposed to promoting equally open and accessible health care across genders.

Gender has important health consequences that are intertwined with cultural values and considerations. An estimated 94 million girls and women are "missing" worldwide as a result of discriminatory treatment that ultimately increases mortality (Klasen & Wink, 2002). To the extent that social and economic resources are differentially allocated by gender, or that gender conceptions vary by subcultural context, specific subgroups of women may have health experiences that are quite different from those of other women (Weisman, 1998). Gender-based cultural rituals or social role expectations can create undue burdens for women and may subsequently lead to increased health risks. For example, being denied access to contraceptive options may create reproductive health risks for some women. The practice of female circumcision carries significant health risk and long-lasting health implications for some young women (see Chapter 6). Being denied access to education by virtue of gender can decrease economic opportunities and thus limit life choices for women. Extensive cultural preoccupation with dieting and thinness create unsafe dieting practices and may precipitate eating disorders. When various health conditions are explored, there are a number of examples of disease states that are prominent for women without a clear biologic explanation, such as anorexia and bulimia. Another example of a gender-based health risk is the disproportionate amount of gender-based violence women experience. Gender-based violence was defined by the United Nations General Assembly in 1993 as:

> Any action of gender-based violence that results in or is likely to result in physical, sexual, or psychological harm or suffering to women, including threats of such acts, coercion, or arbitrary deprivations of liberty, whether occurring in public or private life. (Velzeboer, Ellsberg, Arcas, Garcia-Moreno, 2003)

The multiple health consequences of gender-based violence reveal the long-lasting layers of health consequences associated with a gender-based health risk. (Refer to Chapter 12 for further discussion of this topic.) "Gender-based violence is the most widespread human rights abuse and public health problem in the world today, affecting as many of one out of every three women" (Velzeboer, et al., 2003, p. xi).

A HUMAN RIGHTS PERSPECTIVE FOR WOMEN'S HEALTH

The preceding examples provide evidence of the manner in which the social construction of gender creates undue health risks for women. This burden of risk that women endure has been the basis of addressing women's health disparities from a human rights perspective. A human rights framework acknowledges a basic set of rights, regardless of gender, that members of a society should have access to or be guaranteed.

> Basic human rights generally refer to respect as a person of worth/value (human dignity), safety or security of one's person, food and nutrition, shelter, privacy, freedom from any form of discrimination, a right to information and education. . . and the right to health and equitable access to health and illness services of high quality. (Thompson, 2004, p. 177)

A feminist perspective is in concert with a human rights framework but would argue that human rights are disproportionately denied to women.

While human rights have been defined within the World Health Organization (WHO) for many years, in the last 20 years, reproductive rights were added to the basic human rights framework. More recently, a human rights framework has been advocated within the context of addressing maternal morbidity and mortality on a global level (Starrs, 1997; Thompson, 2004). Gender equity issues are a more recent consideration (Velzeboer et al., 2003). The goal of using a human rights framework is to

> characterize women's multiple disempowerments not just during pregnancy and childbirth but from their own births as a cumulative injustice that societies are obligated to remedy. The re-characterization of maternal mortality from a health disadvantage to a social injustice places governments under a legal obligation to remedy the injustice. (Starrs, p. 9)

Table 1–3 lists the four categories of basic human rights relating to safe motherhood.

TABLE 1-3   Human Rights Framework for Safe Motherhood

- Rights relating to life, liberty, and security of the person
- Rights relating to the foundation of families and of family life
- Rights relating to the highest attainable standard of health and the benefits of scientific progress, including health information and education
- Rights relating to equality and nondiscrimination on grounds such as sex, marital status, race, age, and class

---

DEFINITION OF HEALTH: SOCIAL MODEL VERSUS BIOMEDICAL MODEL

As the discussion of the social construction of gender and its relationship to health has unfolded, it becomes evident that a broader model of health must be employed to address the health consequences of gender bias and sexism and the implications for the overall health and well-being of women. While the use of a human rights framework is congruent with the components of a feminist framework, again the acknowledgment of gender equity has been limited and less transparent in its application to models of health. Furthermore, the ability to hold governments accountable for a human rights framework is in its infancy of application regarding the health rights of women (Starrs, 1997; Thompson, 2004; Velzeboer et al., 2003). A feminist framework encourages grassroots activism to promote acknowledgment of women's need for greater access to human rights and thus provides opportunity for an increase in awareness related to health disparities that are gender-based.

The first step in broadening the model of health requires redefining health. Health is biomedically defined as the absence of disease. This narrow definition does not address the context in which the absence of disease may occur. As feminist health advocates note, "No single or singular view of women's health will adequately reflect the complexities of women's lives, although dominant biomedical models are often taken to represent 'all of women's health' " (Ruzek, Olsen, & Clark, 1997, p. 12). It is argued that the dominance of the medical model must be challenged in an effort to broaden the opportunities to understand this complexity within the health care system, health research, and the experiences of health within the individual and the collective community. The biomedical model does not address health beyond an individual perspective.

An alternative to the biomedical definition of health is the definition developed in 1946 by WHO: "health is a state of complete physical, mental, and social well-being and not merely the absence of disease or infirmity." This broader definition of health is based on some assumptions of what must be present to secure health for individuals and the community in which they live. There are prerequisites that must be in place before health can occur, and they include the following:

- Freedom from the fear of war
- Equal opportunity for all
- Satisfaction of basic needs for food, water and sanitation, education, and decent housing
- Secure work
- Useful role in society
- Political will
- Public support (Ruzek et al., 1997, p. 14)

Germaine to this definition is WHO's commitment to address social injustice, equity, economic development and opportunity, and accessibility of health care services as a basic human right for all individuals in any society (Tejada de Rivero, 2003). The WHO definition of health requires that the community and environment in which women live their lives must also be considered in the same context as a new medical procedure. The constraints of an individualistic, disease-only focused biomedical model of health are apparent when WHO's broader context and definition of health are considered.

An alternative to the biomedical model and more congruent with a feminist perspective is a social model of health. The social model of health places the focus of health on the community rather than the individual. There is then an opportunity to focus on health disparities that are rooted in social and cultural forces that affect how women live their lives. "Developing more inclusive models of health requires recognizing and dealing with complexities and differences in women's lives. Educational levels, income, culture, ethnicity, race and a host of other identities and experiences shape women's lives" (Ruzek et al., 1997, p. 20).

The interconnectedness of working and living conditions, environmental conditions, and access to community-based health care services becomes a focus when health and well-being are framed within a community context. Questions about health and well-being for an individual are focused on these factors as well as lifestyle decisions and health habits. The prevention of health problems becomes both a social and an individual responsibility. This forces greater consideration of the social factors that can create or destroy an individual's health (Ruzek et al., 1997).

A social model of health also requires asking questions about the health effects of socially situated factors such as racism, sexism, and other forms of oppression. Consideration of women as central to the health model rather than marginal to it is a requirement of a feminist social model of health care. The broader social models do not ignore biologic or genetic components of health nor is the significance of individual lifestyle health habits denied. However, the broader social model frames these issues as important to health, as are women's experiences within everyday life, their access to health care services, their socioeconomic status, racial and ethnic identity, and their membership within a community (Schiebinger, 2003).

The health risks associated with the social construction of gender and the inequities associated with gender-based assumptions are essential components of a feminist social model of health. As the links are made between human rights, social models of health, women's health disparities, and opportunities to address those disparities, a feminist perspective offers new strategies and ways of thinking or asking questions that can promote expanded approaches to women's health issues.

WOMEN'S HEALTH FROM A FEMINIST PERSPECTIVE

There are several aspects of analysis that are important when considering women's health from a feminist perspective. The following strategies of analysis of women's health from a feminist framework are adapted from Franz and Stewart's (1994) strategies for conducting feminist research. Each of the strategies listed in Table 1–4 can be used as a question to

TABLE 1–4   Strategies for Analysis of Women's Health from a Feminist Perspective

Strategies	Questions
Look for what has been left out or what we do not know.	• What do we know, how do we know it, and who knows it? • Why don't we know? What do we want to know and why? • Who determines what is left out or who has access to what we want to know?
Analyze your own role or relationship to the issue or topic.	• Is it personal? Is it political? • Are you objective and removed, or engaged and subjective? • Are you invested in the outcome or topic or not? • Why do you care about the issue?
Identify women's agency in the midst of social constraint and the biomedical paradigm.	• Are woman really victims or are they acting with agency? • Are individuals making choices despite positions of powerlessness? Are the choices allowing individuals to remain in control or do they allow for some form of power in the context of the situation?
Consider the social construction of gender and how its assumptions may limit options or presume choices made within the context of health. This includes the social construction of health itself.	• What is defined as a health problem or concern? • Explore assumptions about the value of anatomy such as breasts or facial appearance. • Ask the question: "Would this health issue be defined or explored in the same manner if it primarily affected men or women?"
Explore the precise ways in which gender defines or affects power relationships and the implications of those power dynamics in terms of health.	• Doctor/nurse • Parent/child • Doctor/patient • Father/daughter • Parent/adolescent • Married woman/single woman • Husband/wife • Lesbian/heterosexual
Identify other significant aspects of an individual's or group's social position, and explore the implications of that position as it relates to health issues.	• Consider examples such as an adolescent who is seeking reproductive health care services or a same sex couple seeking fertility services. • Ask who has access to what forms of health care services and resources and who does not. • Consider the intersections of race, class, gender, sexuality, and socioeconomic status. • Who has a choice, what constitutes a choice, and who is able to exercise their right to choices within the context of health?
Consider the risks and benefits of generalizations and speaking in terms of groups versus individuals.	• Who are "we" or "all women"? Are "all women" the same? • When is coherence or consistency the goal compared to diversity in the health care consideration or experience? Which reflects reality most accurately? • When "grouping" occurs, who is missing from the group or who might not be reflected in the group process?

Source: Adapted from Franz & Stewart, 1994.

ask about women's health issues. The strategies provide a feminist lens and allow for new considerations as health issues are reframed. The following discussion highlights the manner in which some of the strategies can be applied.

LOOK FOR WHAT HAS BEEN LEFT OUT OR WHAT WE DO NOT KNOW

This strategy is particularly applicable to the scientific basis of women's health. Much of what we know about women's health needs, outside of reproductive health, is historically based on androcentric models of men's health considerations (Rosser, 1994; Tavris, 1992). Almost all medical research (until recently) that was not gynecologic related used male subjects (human and animal) and generalized the findings to women. Large-scale investigations focusing on health promotion have been based primarily on study populations composed of only men. This practice continued well into the 1990s (Schiebinger, 2003). According to feminist scientist Londa Schiebinger's analysis, many common health promotion measures have been assumed to be true for both men and women despite the limitation that the study populations were composed of only men. Examples of these studies include The Physician's Health Study on the use of aspirin to prevent health disease and the Multiple Risk Factor Intervention Trial that evaluated correlations between blood pressure, smoking, cholesterol, and health disease. The research populations in these studies were composed of only men. In fact, one of the first studies to investigate the use of estrogen for heart disease was conducted on a study population of only men (Schiebinger)!

Research agendas reflect a societal bias that favors powerful, white, middle- to upper-class men in the United States (Rosser, 1994). Similarly, most large-scale research trials focused on or recruited primarily from this population for their research participants, yet most of the scientific members of the team would arguably claim lack of awareness of the inherent sexism in these study designs (Schiebinger, 1999). "Reforming certain aspects of how medical research is conducted with respect to females required new judgments of social worth and a new political will." (Schiebinger, p. 973)

The lack of representation of women in research trials extended through 1988 when clinical trials of new drugs were routinely conducted predominately on men even though women consume approximately 80% of pharmaceuticals in the United States (Schiebinger, 2003; Wood, 2001). What was left out? Considerations of women's biologic variations in processing drugs! We now know that acetaminophen is eliminated in women at 60% of the rate it is eliminated in men. This finding obviously has gender-related influences to consider when prescribing dosage regimens (Schiebinger, 2003).

Examples abound of the problematic manner in which the scientific base for women's health, beyond that of reproductive health, was initially developed. Even when positive study examples are cited, often limitations are present in the design of the study. Many key women's health studies, such as the Framingham Heart Study and the Nurses Health Study I and II, were either observational or epidemiological investigations instead of randomized clinical trials, long considered the gold standard for investigative research

(Schiebinger, 2003). Clearly women were being left out of the scientific understanding of many health issues that directly affected them.

Consumer health advocates, women's health activists, and members of the scientific community have been instrumental in coming together to address the many limitations concerning women and scientific investigations of women's health issues. In 1993 the National Institutes of Health Revitalization Act required that

> women and minorities and their subpopulations be included in all NIH-supported biomedical and behavioral research, in phase III clinical trials in numbers adequate for valid analysis of differences, in intervention effects, and that cost not be the basis for exclusion, and that there needed to be support for outreach programs to recruit these individuals for clinical trials. (Schiebinger, 2003)

The next decade saw a significantly greater inclusion of women and minorities in research investigations as a result of this change. Asking "what had been left out" or "what was missing" provided an opportunity to alter what had been left out of women's health research. Even though much has been achieved, critics call for continued innovation in medical theories and practice in this field (Ruzek et al., 1997; Schiebinger, 2003).

There is an ongoing need to employ this strategy to expose blind spots in what is being presented under the rubric of women's health. An example of this is the current focus on heart disease in women. Heart disease is now the number one killer of women in the United States. It has been argued that from identification of symptoms to diagnosis, treatment, and referral, gender differences abound. Johnson, Karvonen, Phelps, Nader, and Sanborn (2003) reviewed the literature regarding cardiovascular disease and found 30 systematic reviews. The limitations identified in the studies focusing on women and cardiovascular disease gave rise to the conclusion that there were not enough large-scale clinical trials or meta-analyses concerning cardiovascular disease in women. The need to explore this disease process in women is clear when the question of "what has been left out of prior studies" is asked. The answers can help frame new ways to address this health condition. Rather than inappropriate misapplication of findings on women when the research was conducted with only men participants, there is a need to explore new avenues of research and ways of asking the research question.

ANALYZE YOUR OWN ROLE OR RELATIONSHIP TO THE ISSUE OR TOPIC

Traditionally the focus of women's health was relegated to "between the breasts and the knees." Pregnancy and childbirth were the focus as a means of securing survival of society. The value of women was based on their role in procreation and continuation of the citizenry. There are multiple examples in history of how a focus on reproductive health created opportunities to promote maternal and child health reforms in the public health arena. This was an example of women using the focus on reproductive health to advance an agenda that addressed maternal and child health. However, there were also risks of focusing solely on reproductive health. This focus enabled normal physiological reproductive processes to be medicalized within a biomedical context.

In response to the process of medicalizing aspects of women's health and traditional models of women's health care, consumer activism by women is directed at reframing women's health and calling for reforms at even the most basic levels. The strategy of analyzing your own role or relationship to the issue may help to reveal the role women play in relation to the process of rejecting medicalization of many of the normal healthy physiologic processes they experience. Over the years, various aspects of women's health have become topics of public debate and of organized social action; together these episodes could be considered waves in a women's health mega-movement (Weisman, 1998).

Recently there have been two waves in the women's health mega-movement. One wave coincided with social action movements such as the civil rights and women's rights movements. A key feature of this wave was that it was grassroots oriented with a key focus on access to information and expanded knowledge regarding health. One outcome of this movement was the creation of the Boston Women's Health Book Collective (BWHBC) and their publication of *Our Bodies Ourselves* for consumers in 1974. The BWHBC is composed of women who are health care consumers. They developed a consumer-oriented women's health textbook through a process of conducting individual research related to women's health. During this time, the primary access to health-related information was only through medical textbooks. It was an opportunity for women to reclaim control of women's health and to offer new definitions or ways of thinking about physiologic processes. A key aspect of this process includes demystifying health conditions and processes in an effort to empower women with knowledge so they can ask questions about their health and pose these questions to their health care providers. An outcome of this change supported women taking responsibility for health care decision making rather than the biomedical model of the 1960s and 1970s, which placed authority for decision making in the control of the health care provider.

This wave of reclaiming control of health care from health care providers and focusing on women's role and authority over their own health was initially promoted by well-educated women from middle- and upper-level income groups. A critique of this wave of the women's health movement reveals that it generalized women's health issues as a global consideration that included ethnic and cultural variation. In response, there were women's health groups that organized based on ethnic and cultural considerations related to women's health.

CONSIDER THE RISKS AND BENEFITS OF SPEAKING IN TERMS OF GROUPS VERSUS INDIVIDUALS

Using the strategy of 'considering the risks and benefits of speaking in terms of groups versus individuals' was an aspect of the 1960s and 1970s women's health movements that was problematic. In an effort to be inclusive, many advocates of the women's health movement during this period claimed to be speaking collectively for all women, yet the primary focus and emphasis was on women who were privileged in society and not women who were marginalized. Schiebinger (2003) summarizes the progress of the women's health movement by stating "Whereas the women's health movement of the

1970s sought to solidify sisterhood through the commonalities of female childbirth experiences, there is now an emphasis on the differing health needs of different racial and ethnic groups of women" (p. 974). Today, women's health activists represent greater diversity and focus on a wider range of issues affecting women's and their families' health. This also includes attention to ageism, which was inherent in much of the earlier waves of the women's health movement (Pohl & Boyd, 1993).

CONSIDER THE SOCIAL CONSTRUCTION OF GENDER AND HOW ITS ASSUMPTIONS MAY LIMIT OPTIONS OR PRESUME CHOICES THAT ARE MADE WITHIN THE CONTEXT OF HEALTH

Earlier discussions regarding the social construction of gender highlighted the implications of this strategy. An additional aspect to consider is the manner in which women's health issues are described. The language used for many of women's health concerns has been described by anthropologist Emily Martin (1992) as reflecting an androcentric bias, for example the image of menstruation in medical texts is that of "failed reproduction" (Martin, p. 92).

Another example includes referring to a woman who has experienced sexual assault as a victim rather than as a survivor of the process, implying inherent weakness rather than strength. Descriptions of childbirth usually invoke the term delivery or a woman "being delivered" rather than giving birth. The former terms focus on the actions of the health care provider and place the woman in a passive position rather than as the central figure: the one giving birth.

EXPLORE THE PRECISE WAYS IN WHICH GENDER DEFINES POWER RELATIONSHIPS AND THE IMPLICATIONS OF THOSE POWER DYNAMICS ON HEALTH

Creating health care from a feminist perspective requires the elimination of power differentials between the individuals who are consuming health care and those providing it. A partnership model more accurately reflects the manner in which health care interactions should occur. In this model, rather than invoking a level of authority by virtue of being a health care provider, the health care provider acknowledges the life experiences and knowledge that the individual brings to the interaction. What makes a practice feminist is not who is providing the health care, but how that care is provided, how the individual thinks about her work, and the populations with whom she works (Brown, 1994).

While hierarchical relationships and structures are common elements of the health care delivery system, feminist practice requires an active process of action to eliminate asymmetrical relationships. Simple actions, such as not having a woman undress prior to meeting her clinician, allow the woman to greet the health care provider as an equal rather than from a vulnerable position, undressed and in an ill-fitting paper gown. Having a woman check her own weight and urine as opposed to having someone else do this for her places some accountability for health on the woman's shoulders. It gives the message that she can control aspects of her health. Although these are simple changes that can be made in the health care office setting, each demonstrates power sharing rather than placing the woman in a dependent position in relation to aspects of her health care that she should rightly control.

Each of the strategies discussed provides an opportunity to consider the details as well as the global aspects of women's health care and women's health issues. The strategies can be applied individually and collectively. They are not meant to be an exhaustive checklist to determine if something is being considered from a feminist perspective, but instead they are meant to offer guidelines and considerations that allow for the identification of blind spots in how we are able to think about women's health issues when we are potentially constrained by the limitations of the biomedical model. Through the use of these strategies, health care providers, policy makers, and women themselves are able to reframe expectations, approaches, and the focus of women's health research, health care delivery, and even the receipt of health care services.

WHY A TEXTBOOK ON GYNECOLOGY?

Taking the same feminist strategies we use for analyzing women's health and applying them to this textbook on gynecologic aspects of women's health raises opportunities as well. Why, when a feminist perspective is being presented and the limitations of only considering women's health as reproductive health, would a textbook purportedly using a feminist framework focus only on gynecologic aspects of women's health? The reason is that gynecologic health is still important. Focusing on gynecology for health care professionals is important because reframing and expanding considerations of gynecologic health from a feminist perspective may more accurately reflect the experience for women in their everyday lives. By offering a feminist perspective throughout the chapters, we seek to dispel myths that pathologize normal gynecologic functioning, and we seek to support normality as opposed to medicalizing it. Rather than ignoring gynecologic health and allowing it to remain within the biomedical domain, this textbook seeks to reframe aspects of gynecologic health issues within a feminist framework. It is hoped this will expand opportunities for understanding gynecologic health from within a wellness-oriented, women-centered framework that encourages providers to look beyond the medical model and support normalcy instead of "manage" it.

REFERENCES

Boston Women's Health Book Collective. (1974). *Our bodies, ourselves.* New York: Simon & Schuster.

Brown, L. (1994). *Subversive dialogues.* New York: BasicBooks.

Conrad, P. (1992). Medicalization and social control. *Annual Review of Sociology, 18,* 209–232.

Davis, R., & Huber, K. (2004). Class, ethnicity, age, physical status, and sexual orientation: Implications for health and healthcare. In M. Condon (Ed.),

Women's health (pp. 21–41). Upper Saddle River, NJ: Prentice Hall.

Franz, C., & Stewart, A. (Eds.). (1994). *Women creating lives: Identities, resilience, and resistance.* Boulder, CO: Westview Press.

Healy, B. (1991). The Yentil syndrome. *New England Journal of Medicine, 325,* 274–276.

hooks, bell (2000). *Feminism is for everybody.* Cambridge, MA: South End Press.

Johnson, S. M., Karvonen, C. A., Phelps, C. L., Nader, S., & Sanborn, B. M. (2003). Assessment of analysis by gender in the Cochrane reviews as related to treatment of cardiovascular disease. *Journal of Women's Health, 12*(5), 449–457.

Klasen, S., & Wink, C. (2002). A turning point in gender bias in mortality? An update on the number of missing women. *Population and Development Review, 28*, 285–312.

Lantz, P., House, J., Lepkowski, J., Williams, D., Mero, R., & Chen, J. (1998). Socioeconomic factors, health behaviors, and mortality: Results from a nationally representative prospective study of US adults. *Journal of the American Medical Association, 279*(21), 1703–1708.

Lorber, J. (1997). *Gender and the social construction of illness.* Thousand Oaks, CA: Sage.

Martin, E. (1992). *The woman in the body: A cultural analysis of reproduction.* Boston: Beacon Press.

Pinn, V. (2003a). Sex and gender factors in medical studies: Implications for health and clinical practice. *Journal of the American Medical Association, 289*(4), 397–400.

Pinn, V. (2003b). Expanding the frontiers of women's health research—US style. *The Medical Journal of Australia 178*(16), 598–599.

Pohl, J., & Boyd, C. (1993). Ageism within feminism. *Image, 25*, 200–203.

Rosser, S. V. (1994). Gender bias in clinical research: The difference it makes. In A. Dan (Ed.), *Reframing women's health* (pp. 253–265). Thousand Oaks, CA: Sage.

Ruzek, S., Olsen, V., & Clark, A. (1997). Social, biomedical and feminist models of women's health. In S. Ruzek, V. Olsen, & A. Clark, (Eds.), *Women's health: Complexities and differences.* Columbus, OH: Ohio State University Press.

Satcher, D. (2001). American women and health disparities. *Journal of the American Medical Women's Association, 56*(4), 131–133.

Schiebinger, L. (1999). *Has feminism changed science?* (pp. 107–125). Cambridge, MA: Harvard University Press.

Schiebinger, L. (2003). Women's health and clinical trials. *The Journal of Clinical Investigation, 112*(7), 973–977.

Starrs, A. (1997). *The Safe Motherhood Action Agenda: Report on the safe motherhood technical consultation.* Sri Lanka: Family Care International.

Tavris, C. (1992). *The mismeasure of women.* New York: Simon & Schuster.

Tejada de Rivero, D. (2003). Alma-Ata revisited. *Perspectives in Health Magazine, 8*(2), 2–7.

Thompson, J. (2004) A human rights framework for midwifery care. *Journal of Midwifery and Women's Health. 49*(3), 175–181.

Velzeboer, M., Ellsberg, M., Arcas, C. C., & Garcia-Moreno, C. (2003). *Violence against women: The health sector responds.* Washington, DC: Pan American Health Organization.

Weisman, C. S. (1998). *Women's health care.* Baltimore: The John's Hopkins University Press.

Williams, D. (2002). Racial/ethnic variations in women's health: The social embeddedness of health. *American Journal of Public Health, 92*(4), 588–597.

Wizeman, T. M., & Pardue, M. L. (Eds.). (2001). *Exploring the biological contributions to human health: Does sex matter?* Washington, DC: National Academies Press.

Wood, S. (2001). Office of women's health, food and drug administration: Future directions for women's health. *The Journal of American Medical Women's Association, 56*(4), 197–198.

Xu, K.T., & Borders, T. (2003). Gender health and physician visits among adults in the United States. *American Journal of Public Health, 93*(7), 1076–1078.

Zola, I. (1972). Medicine as an institution of social control. *Sociological Review, 20*, 487–504.

WOMEN'S GROWTH AND DEVELOPMENT ACROSS THE LIFE SPAN

KERRI DURNELL SCHUILING
LISA KANE LOW

Clinical textbooks typically describe what is considered normal growth and development; this description frames the upcoming chapters of the textbook's discussion of variations from what is considered normative. Although this approach may seem comprehensive, the dilemma is that the initial discussion of women's growth and development is often from a biomedical perspective. This representation deconstructs women's bodies into biologic parts and physiologic processes. While this enables quantification of growth, it is known that qualitative aspects of women's lives also impact their growth.

The biomedical model of health is individualist and disease oriented. In Chapter 1, this model is contrasted with a feminist and social model of health. The latter model acknowledges the influence of the culture women live in, their economic status, the social interactions they experience, and the context in which they access and receive health care. The feminist model acknowledges the many other factors beyond the physiologic functioning of women and the genetic inheritance that affect their growth and development. As a result, even the manner in which we understand and explain what normative growth and development includes changes in the expanded framework of a feminist perspective, thus allowing for a clearer understanding of the complexity inherent in women's growth and development.

As a first step in considering women's development (cognitive, psychosocial, and functional behaviors), it is important to acknowledge that the traditional models that are used were developed from research about men. For example, psychoanalyst Erick Erikson (1950) expanded developmental theory beyond the years of adolescence to offer a grand theory of human development (Table 2–1). He identified eight general stages of development that included several within adulthood. The eight virtues that are the goals of the stages are: trust, autonomy, initiative, industry, identity, intimacy, generativity, and integrity.

TABLE 2-1   Erikson's Eigenetic Model

Age period for crisis	Stages							
	1	2	3	4	5	6	7	8
Infancy	Trust vs. Mistrust							
Early childhood		Autonomy vs. Shame and Doubt						
Play age			Initiative vs. Guilt					
School age				Industry vs. Inferiority				
Adolescence					Identity vs. Identity Diffusion			
Young Adult						Intimacy vs. Isolation		
Adulthood							Generativity vs. Self-absorption	
Mature age								Integrity vs. Disgust
Despair								

Source: Low, 2001

Through a process of resolving eight developmental crises that are sequentially confronted, Erikson's theory offers a comprehensive account of individual development throughout the life span that until recently was applied to both males and females. It is important to understand that Erikson's Stages of Psychosocial Development are based on studies of white, middle-class males (Erikson, 1968), and yet the model is universally applied to women with some gendered assumptions. The underlying gendered assumptions within Erickson's grand theory of development must be recognized because within this theory individuals are treated as a monolith with minimal attention to gender, socioeconomic, or ethnic variability (Gilligan, 1982; Taylor, 1994). Some of the gender-based assumptions include a normative linear pattern of identity, followed by marriage (intimacy), and then childbearing (generativity) in adulthood. Erikson's theory assumes the need for a female to first develop an intimate relationship with another before she can complete her sense of self as an individual. Interestingly, males (according to this theory) do not have the same requirement. So while the larger context of the theory assumes the desirability of autonomy and distancing from your family of origin, for females, autonomy is defined as being dependent on another within the context of a relationship with a primary focus on caretaking by females.

Other examples of grand theories that are misapplied to women are those of Kohlberg (1981) and Perry (1968). Kohlberg's levels of moral development are based on interviews with only men, and Perry actually discarded interviews he had with women, using only data from interviews with men to formulate his model of intellectual development. The difficulty that occurs when these scales are used to assess a woman's developmental level is that they assume universality in development and, again, treat all women as a monolith, not acknowledging the multiple variables that can affect progress through the stages (Belenky, Clinchy, Goldberger, & Tarule, 1986; Low, 2001). Tavris (1992) observes that "because of the (mis)measures we use, women fail to measure up to having the right body and fail to measure up to having the right life" (p. 36). The use of these androcentric models constrains the manner in which women's development is framed, and women's development is presented as an aberration in comparison to white male development, which is held as the standard.

This chapter discusses growth and development by contrasting traditional male-biased theoretical constructs with newer feminist theories that challenge some of the basic assumptions about women's growth and development. Alternative theories of female development were offered by feminist psychologists and researchers beginning in the 1970s (Taylor, 1994). Although there is substantial variation in the emphasis of feminist scholars, a primary focus is on the self-in-relation to others or in connection with others (family and peers) as a means of further development. Feminist theories of development emphasize the quality and nature of individual women's experiences. Women's development is construed as broader than the traditional process of individualization and includes the value of maintaining connection and continuity within relationships (Gilchrist, 1997). The definition of relationships within this model contains not just the self-in-relation to others but also inner constructions of relationships that form the sense of self of the female (Kaplan, Gleason, & Klein, 1991). These relationships progressively contain conflict, and it is through resolution of conflict that the relationships become more complex, requiring flexibility that allows connections and relationships to be maintained (Baker Miller, 1991). This is in opposition to traditional theories of development that emphasize conflict resolution as entailing greater disconnection and the development of distinct boundaries around identity formation or the process of "becoming one's own man" (Baker Miller).

Feminist theories are primarily offered in contrast to Erikson's theory of psychosocial development. Gilligan (1982) and other feminist scholars have critiqued his work as being descriptive not only of male development in general but as descriptive of primarily white, privileged male development. Black-feminist scholarship has furthered this critique beyond that of the traditional male-based model to include limitations in contrasting models offered by early feminist theorists.

The limitation of early feminist models is that they were developed by white middle-class Euro-American women who interpret relationships and connection as being similar across all women regardless of ethnic identity or the influence of racism (Collins, 2000). Thus much of early feminist scholarship was still limited by a lack of understanding of the role of ethnic identity and socioeconomic level on development.

The intention of newer feminist models is not to replace male generalist models of development with feminist generalist models of development, but to offer alternatives to the constrained models that were previously misapplied to all women. This chapter will provide an overview of growth and development within the linear stages of adolescence through older age using a feminist perspective. Emphasis is placed on contrasting models of development outside of the traditional biomedical focus.

It should be noted that subscription to a model that delineates gender differences versus one that identifies gender similarities and provides an explanation for differences based on gender is a key philosophical dilemma for developmental theorists. The emphasis on difference rather than similarity evokes a debate about the risk of essentializing women's development. The difficulty is that gender differences described by these theories are ascribed as biologic or innate characteristics rather than considering the social and cultural context that can create these differences. Thus the differences described are consistent with social constructs of femininity rather than being biologically determined, but they are wrongly assumed to be biologic (Gilligan, 1982; Martin, 1992). While noting the work of Gilligan and other early feminist theorists who argue that women have a "different voice" through which they develop and speak, several feminist psychologists and theorists offer the critique that in recent developmental theories, what feminist theorists have described as being uniquely female is instead likely to be based in the social construction of gender roles and has been inadequately explored (Hare-Mustin & Marecek, 1998; Riger, 1998). This results in differing expectations at different times based on gender. This perspective is consistent with that of Erikson (1950). He argues that the particular developmental crisis is not necessarily chronologically driven but is driven by social expectations for behavior. Thus expectations for caregiving and consideration by females of themselves in relation to others may have more to do with socially prescribed gender roles of femininity rather than with biologically differing pathways for development. More similarities than difference between males and females may become evident when gender boundaries are broken down and males have a greater level of participation in caretaking for others rather than primarily for themselves. Until that time, however, contrasting developmental models with an emphasis on differences that are primarily socially constructed have prevailed and thus will inform the perspectives presented in this chapter.

ADOLESCENCE

The adolescent years are generally described biologically as beginning with the onset of puberty and extending 8 to 10 years beyond (Murray & Zentner, 1997). These years chronologically encompass the ages of 11 to 21 (Condon, 2004). Often this period is described as the "stormy" years because of the stress of puberty and the accompanying bodily changes. However, for most adolescents, the transition is quite smooth in spite of the physical, developmental, emotional, and cognitive changes that occur during this time (Lewis & Bernstein, 1996). Stages of adolescence are commonly categorized into early adolescence (ages 11–13 years), mid-adolescence (ages 14–17 years), and late adolescence (ages 17–21 years) (Lewis & Bernstein, 1996; Slap, 1986). Although changes are discussed in the contexts of biology and physiology, it is important to remember from a health care standpoint that qualitative aspects must be considered. For example, an adolescent woman's sense of body image may be tied to her weight as much as it is to her past experiences (Leight, 2003).

BIOLOGY AND PHYSIOLOGY

Significant physical changes occur during a young woman's adolescence. Adult height and weight are usually attained during this time, and probably most significant to the adolescent female are changes due to the development of secondary sex characteristics. The usual sequence of female pubertal events begins with a growth spurt that occurs around the ages of 11–12. The growth spurt is followed by thelarche (breast development), adrenarche (growth of pubic hair due to androgen stimulation), and menarche (Skillman-Hull, 2003; Woods, 1995). Peak height usually occurs about two years after breast budding and about one year prior to menarche (Speroff & Fritz, 2005). On average, the growth spurt in girls begins around age 10, reaches its maximum rate at age 12, and subsides around age 16 (Bassey, Sayer, & Cooper, 2002).

Girls reach puberty earlier than boys. The timing of puberty and onset of menses is controlled primarily by the neuroendocrine system (Lewis & Bernstein, 1996) and genetic inheritance, although it is also believed to be affected by external factors such as general health and nutrition, race, geographic location, amount of exposure to light, and psychological makeup (Skillman-Hull, 2003). Girls who perceive themselves to be "on time" for puberty tend to have a better self-image and are more likely to view themselves as attractive than girls who believe themselves to be early or late for puberty (Woods, 1995). Although the pubertal changes provoke perceptions about puberty, these perceptions are also shaped by the dominant culture (Woods). Lee (1998) observes that women say their bodies become problematic at menarche; their breasts are too big or too small, and their hips are an enemy because fat accumulates there.

The onset of puberty depends on a changing body accumulation of adipose tissue and thus creates the beginning of a tension between biologic development and the social context in which it occurs. Our culture today demands perfection, and as a result, many young women suffer great anxiety about their bodies. The challenges that present for young women vary based on ethnicity, self-esteem, the social environment, and the contrast between the individual adolescent's sense of herself and how that compares to what is perceived as the societal standard for beauty. It is particularly important to note that many of the changes of puberty are framed within the social context of sexual development. As the physical sexual characteristics develop, many young women are challenged by a potential mismatch between their socially perceived sexual development and their interpersonal level of maturity and development. Clinicians can become an important source of support and information during what is often framed culturally as a tumultuous phase of development.

A commonly used scale for staging sexual maturity is the Tanner Scale, which relies on development of the breasts and growth of pubic hair. The Tanner model divides sexual physical maturity into five stages that extend from preadolescence to the adult (Figures 2–1 through 2–3). The Tanner model, although widely accepted for staging sexual maturity, is not appropriate to use for determining chronological age (Rosenbloom & Tanner, 1998). Additionally, Rosenbloom and Tanner note that because of the variability in timing of stages and of pubic hair growth, both which are important elements of Tanner staging, the scale should not be used for staging individuals of Asian ethnicity.

Probably the most anticipated, feared, and socially misconstrued aspect of female adolescent development and puberty is menarche, or the onset of menses. The menarche is an important milestone in a young girl's life. The median age for the onset of menstruation for adolescent girls in the United States is 12.8 years with a range of ages 9–17 (Speroff & Fritz, 2005). The events of puberty trigger the onset of menses when a positive feedback of estrogen on the pituitary and hypothalamus stimulates a surge of luteinizing hormone at midcycle, which is critical to ovulation (Speroff & Fritz). The first several menstrual cycles usually do not result in ovulation, and often a girl's first-year experience of menstruating is characterized by irregular anovulatory cycles, along with heavy bleeding (Speroff & Fritz).

The menarche is integrally linked to many layers of social meaning for girls and women. It is an event that symbolizes reproduction and sexual potential (Lee, 1998). Menarche is important as a physiological happening, albeit framed by biomedical metaphors of scientific knowledge, and because it is the social and cultural juncture at which girls become women and gender relations are reproduced (Lee). These relations are about power and its absence, about women's agency, and the ability to move through the world with credibility and respect (Lee).

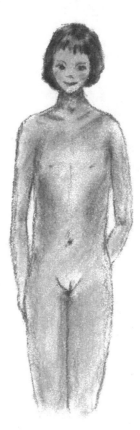

FIGURE 2–1   Tanner Stage 1: Preadolescent (ages 10–14): Breasts have elevation of nipple only. There is no pubic hair except for vellus hair, which is fine body hair like that noted on abdomen. *Illustrator: Marie Hall.*

PSYCHOSOCIAL DEVELOPMENT

Adolescence, as previously described, focuses on changes associated with puberty in combination with preparation for the future (Goldharber, 1986). The traditional developmental task of adolescence is to develop a sense of identity and autonomy before progressing toward adulthood. There is a tendency to "try on" various roles as adolescents struggle with who they want to be and how they want to live (Crain, 1980). The role of peers becomes critical in this process, and traditionally a distancing from parents and other adults has been described (Goldharber). Within almost all cultures there is an acknowledgment that failure to successfully negotiate the developmental tasks of adolescence limits an individual's ability to function productively as an adult (Musick, 1993). The interaction between an adolescent's behavior and role performance promotes or confuses his or her sense of identity depending upon the social context in which it occurs.

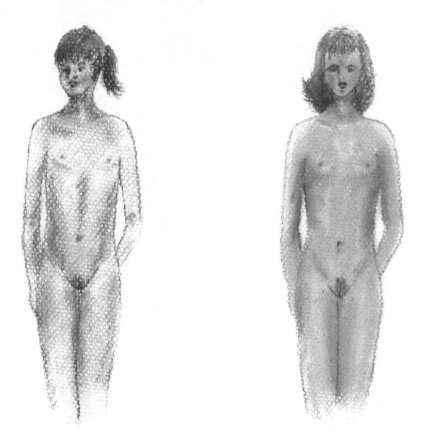

FIGURE 2–2 Tanner Stages 2 & 3: Tanner Stage 2 (left) is referred to as the breast bud stage. There is an elevation of the breast and nipple and the areola widens. Pubic hair growth is sparse, long, and only slightly curly. It is observed mainly on the labia. Tanner Stage 3 (right) (ages 12–14 or middle adolescence): The breast and areola are enlarged further with increased elevation of the breast and nipple; however, there is no separation of their contours. The pubic hair growth begins to occur over the mons pubis, and hair is now darker, coarser, and curlier. *Illustrator: Marie Hall.*

Through a process of trial and experimentation, individuals develop their own set of values and beliefs as well as a sense of themselves as they formalize or commit to their own identity. Initiation of sexual activity, pregnancy, childbearing, and parenting are all gendered roles and experiences that differ in their impact on any one individual adolescent based on the social, cultural, and historical definition that is associated with these behaviors and roles, as well as their peers' and family's perceptions of these events.

In contrast, a feminist perspective of female adolescent development emphasizes the young girl's relationship with others instead of distancing from others in the process of

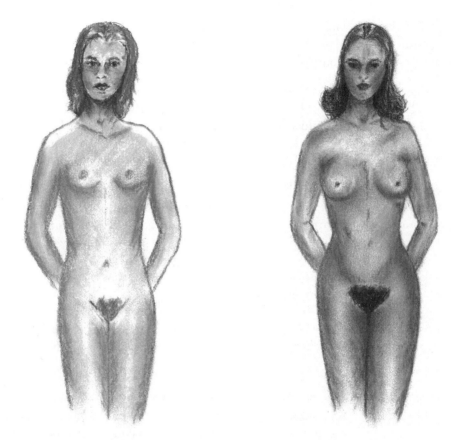

FIGURE 2-3 Tanner Stages 4 and 5: Tanner Stage 4 (left) reveals breasts with areola and nipple forming a secondary mound with projection of the nipple. Pubic hair is adult type but is observed over a smaller area and none is noted on thigh. Tanner Stage 5 (right) (ages 14–16 late adolescence): Breasts are fully mature and only the nipple protrudes as the areola is usually flush with the breast contour. However, a normal variation is for the areola to continue as a secondary mound. The pubic hair is normal adult type: thick, coarse, and curly, and spreads onto the medial surfaces of the thighs. Adult female hair pattern (inverted triangle) is observed. *Illustrator: Marie Hall.*

individuation as described by Erikson (1950). Current theorists argue that the hallmark of healthy identity development is development of a sense of connection to others with a primary task being the ability to participate in mutual relationships in which the individual feels both active, effective, and is not "lost within" the relationship (Kaplan et al., 1991). The self-in-relation model of adolescent development proposed by Baker Miller and her colleagues at the Wellesley College Stone Center (1991) defines a woman's sense of self as emerging out of experience with a relational process that begins in infancy. From initial interactions with caregivers through the process of becoming a care-taker, the self-in-relation theory argues that women are socialized to care more and more about the development of relationships.

> Beginning with the earliest mother–daughter interactions, this relational sense of self develops out of women's involvement in progressively complex relationships, characterized by mutual identifications, attention to interplay between each other's emotions, and caring about the process and activity of relationship. (Kaplan et al., 1991, p. 123)

Development is delayed if the young girl's relationships are suppressive or oppressive (Woods, 1995), and unfortunately, too often this is the case for many young women. The predominate culture in the United States discourages a young girl from acting with a sense of self when she is in a relationship; acting as an autonomous agent is discouraged (Woods), and dependence is traditionally encouraged.

Girls usually interact closely with their mothers and because of this are more apt to learn and appreciate the importance of empathy. Woods (1995) points out that this may strengthen girls' sense of connection and being emotionally understood, which in turn provides an advantage to girls growing up in Western cultures because they will be carriers of aspects of human experience, including emotionality, vulnerability, and growth fostering.

Reasoning changes as a child grows to adolescence. Instead of just understanding a general rule governing the immediate and concrete, the thinking of the adolescent involves using symbols and moving to a world of possibilities (Strauss & Clark, 1996). This type of thinking influences and explains the risk-taking behaviors of adolescents. Strauss and Clark point out that the adolescent girl might not be able to appreciate logical sequencing of events, such as pregnancy following an act of intercourse. Maturation in thinking behavior is supported by understanding family members, an emotionally stable environment, parental discipline, and positive life experiences.

CLINICAL APPLICATION

The health of adolescents is critically important to their health in later years (Woods, 1995). Almost from birth, females are socialized to be highly oriented to others, so it is not surprising that risk behaviors and conditions, such as depression or early sexual activity, are more likely influenced by the nature of an adolescent female's relational experiences with significant others, family, peers, and others (Baker Miller, 1991). In fact, the major health problems of adolescents relate to their risk-taking behaviors, and in contrast to males, these behaviors in females are more influenced by a desire to maintain important relationships than a desire to "take on" adult behaviors. Female adolescent morbidity is most likely to include pregnancy, sexually transmitted infections, running away, and suicide (Lee, 1998). Risk taking can also be a result of the young girl's environment or may be an expression of symptoms of depression.

Finally, expanding on the developmental self-in-relation model offered by feminist scholars, this model can be extended into the health care visit. Trust is a key component of any therapeutic relationship and cannot be emphasized enough for providers caring for adolescents. Additional time is often needed to establish a trusting relationship with an adolescent.

Sherwin (1998) suggests a relational approach when providing adolescent females' health care services. The relational approach takes into consideration the full range of influential human relations that influence how adolescent females define their health (Sherwin). For example, asking an adolescent to "Tell me about your friends or who you hang out with" and "How would you describe yourself in relation to your friends?" are the types of questions that can be asked in a health care visit to assess who influences the adolescent and how she sees herself in relationship to others. The goal is not to isolate the behavior from the relational context in which it occurs but to acknowledge the health implications of behaviors. This enables a more affective approach to risk reduction because the behavior is addressed along with the context in which it occurs. This relational model can be extended as a woman progresses in her health care needs across the life span.

EARLY ADULTHOOD

Young adulthood is generally accepted as spanning the time from late adolescence (age 18) to the beginning of the perimenopausal years (ages 35–50). Commonly this period is referred to as the "reproductive years," reflecting a societal value of women primarily for their reproductive capacities (Olshansky, 1996). Health care during the young adulthood years traditionally focuses on health promotion and maintenance with primary emphasis on reproductive capacity rather than a broader, comprehensive focus on health promotion throughout the life span.

BIOLOGY AND PHYSIOLOGY

The years between 18 and 35 are biomedically considered optimal for reproduction. Generally, most women experience regular menstrual cycles that are ovulatory, providing opportunity for pregnancy if unprotected intercourse occurs. The biologic changes that accompany a pregnancy and that impact motherhood and aging also have a psychological impact in our youth-oriented culture (Blakenship, 2003). Contraception is an important health consideration for heterosexual couples during these years.

Physical health in young adulthood is promoted by adequate diet and exercise and monitoring overall well-being. Health promotion and maintenance are best met when a woman lives within a social context that is conducive to health (Olshansky, 1996). Optimal health is more achievable when a woman does not have to confront racism, sexism, or classism but instead has access to health care, economic stability, and other resources

(Olshansky). However, most women have lives that are confronted by multiple and competing demands related to work, economics, childbearing, and childrearing.

Women's changing roles from traditional homemaker to working outside the home have come at a cost to their health, probably because women working outside the home continue to have significant responsibilities within the home. Balancing the competing demands increases the stress level of many women (Condon, 2004). As stress increases, many women have coped by developing unhealthy behaviors such as smoking, lack of exercise, and poor nutrition. As a result, women's health risks for some diseases are now similar to that of men's. For example, cardiac disease is now the number one killer of women in the United States, whereas two decades ago the primary cause of illness and health risk for women was related to reproduction. Common health problems that occur during this stage of life include cardiac disease, arthritis, occupational injury and related illnesses, cancer, infections (sexually transmitted and otherwise), and reproductive disorders (Olshansky, 1996). Chapters 4 and 7 discuss health promotion and health maintenance in more specific detail.

PSYCHOSOCIAL DEVELOPMENT

Erikson's (1968) model identifies two crises that occur during early adulthood. The first is the development of intimacy versus isolation: the process of entering into a life partnership with another individual. It is in this developmental phase that gender assumptions about behavior become more typically defined. As previously noted, women are assumed to require intimacy as a prerequisite for the completion of their identity development, while males may progress into this phase without any prior development related to their ability to participate in relationships. It is this contrast of what is described as normative for both males and females that challenged Franz and White (1985) to offer an expansion of Erikson's theory of development. Using a feminist lens, Franz and White discourage the use of a single pathway of development that primarily focuses on individuation and instead encourage the consideration of a two-pathway process that includes both individuation and a process of attachment. They argue that Erikson does *not* conceptualize being female as somehow inferior or lacking in purpose, nor simply as a vehicle for childbearing and caretaking (Franz & White). Instead they describe his work as not attending to the process by which attachment occurs through intimacy and relationships with others. Franz and White argue that Erickson does not provide adequate opportunity in his traditional framework for male development of the capacity for intimacy and attachment. Thus the expansion Franz and White propose includes two processes of development: individuation combined with an attachment pathway in a double helix model. The double helix model allows for these two separate strands to be interconnected, thus representing the relationship between psychological individuation and attachment as ascending in a spiral that represents the human life span (Franz & White). The strand representing individuation is essentially the same as it is in Erikson's model, but the attachment strand addresses the neglected relational dimension of human development. Table 2–2 represents

TABLE 2-2   Franz & White's Adaptation of Erikson's Theory of Development to a Two-Path Model

	Infancy	Early childhood	Play age	School age	Adolescence	Young adulthood	Adulthood	Old age
Individuation Pathway	Trust vs. mistrust	Autonomy vs. shame and doubt	Initiative vs. guilt	Industry vs. inferiority	Identity vs. identity diffusion	Career, lifestyle exploration vs. drifting	Lifestyle consolidation vs. emptiness	Integrity vs. despair
Attachment Pathway	Trust vs. mistrust	Object & self-constancy vs. loneliness and helplessness	Playfulness vs. passivity or aggression	Empathy & collaboration vs. excessive caution or power	Mutuality interdependence vs. alienation	Intimacy vs. isolation	Generativity vs. self-absorption	Integrity vs. despair

Source: Low, 2001.

the individuation and attachment "strands" as described by Franz and White. The authors argue:

> With changing times and mores, if attachment processes were to undergo fuller development in men and individuation processes were to undergo fuller development in women, sex differences might become more elusive than ever, but individuation and attachment would retain their power as psychological variables associated with psychological value in important nomological nets. (Franz & White, 1985, p.166)

The second crisis of early adulthood is acquiring the ability to become generative versus stagnation. Here "generative" is defined as acting on one's concern for the welfare of the next generation. Reproduction and parenting may accomplish this as can service to others. Stagnation occurs when the person is unable to step outside her or himself and be generative. As stated earlier, Erikson's work is based on men and may not be an accurate model for assessing women's development. Newer models of women's development emphasize the relational aspects of women's lives. Understanding women's lives within their individual social context provides a women-oriented perspective for conceptualizing the degree to which a woman reaches a particular level of psychosocial development (Olshansky, 1996).

During the young adulthood years, women's psychosocial development may involve a variety of factors such as accepting responsibilities (parenting, caring for others), creating a career, forming enduring relationships, caring for elderly parents, and deciding whether or not to become a parent. All of these factors impact a woman's psychosocial development, but they cannot be understood in generalities that are applied to all women, nor should each be assessed in isolation. Instead, each woman's relation to these factors, to herself and others, the social context of her life, and her lived experience provides insight into her level of psychosocial development.

CLINICAL APPLICATION

A woman goes through many transitional periods from age 18 to 35. For women at risk of pregnancy, contraceptive decisions are of paramount importance, and it is critical to have access to and receive information and education about contraceptive options. Decisions related to childbearing (or not) are also prominent and frame much of the health care services that women traditionally receive during this phase of their lives. Many lifestyle-related health problems may become apparent during this time. Substance abuse, intimate partner violence, and stress related to her life or those she cares for can negatively impact a woman's health. Some psychiatric illnesses that may become apparent during these years include bipolar disorder, schizophrenia, and psychosis, which may or may not be related to childbearing.

Although young adult women are primarily healthy, it is evident there are many opportunities for life events to negatively impact their health. Health promotion and maintenance during this period are critical to optimal health in later years.

MIDLIFE

Midlife for women encompasses the perimenopausal years (ages 35–50) to menopause (ages 50–65) (Davis & Huber, 2004; Fogel & Woods, 1995). Midlife is actually a transition more than a phase of the human life cycle, and during this time many women experience a recognition that their lives are changing irrevocably. Some women will pursue goals and dreams they may have deferred as a result of the greater life demands they faced in younger adulthood. If they were parenting during their earlier adulthood, then transitions into other aspects of their lives may be prompted by their children leaving home. Still others may be in the active phases of parenting as more and more women delay childbearing decisions until later into the early phases of midlife. During this phase of the life span, Erikson (1950) would continue to identify the phases of generativity versus stagnation as a continuing process.

BIOLOGY AND PHYSIOLOGY

Perimenopause and menopause are biologic markers of the transition from young adult to midlife. Neither of these is a syndrome or disease, but instead demonstrates a natural maturing of the reproductive system. Social constructions of perimenopause and menopause abound. Martin (1992) encourages us to reframe perimenopause and menopause so that our ideas of a "single purpose" for the menstrual cycle can be reconstructed into images of healthy transitions.

During the perimenopausal years women may experience physical changes associated with decreasing estrogen levels such as the vasomotor symptoms of hot flashes and flushes. Other changes associated with aging include a decrease in the size of genitalia, changes in breast structure, and a decrease in skin elasticity. These changes are more fully described in Chapter 11.

Although for many years it was believed a preponderance of midlife women suffered mood changes caused by a deficiency of estrogen during this time of life, more recent studies suggest that psychosocial factors have a much greater effect on a midlife woman's mood than do the physiologic transitions of menopause. In fact, mood changes reported by women experiencing menopause may be caused by myriad factors including hormonal changes, normal aging processes, psychological transitions, and cultural beliefs and expectations (Fogel & Woods, 1995).

PSYCHOSOCIAL DEVELOPMENT

Midlife is a dynamic period of development during which many complex changes occur (Fogel & Woods, 1995). Women during this time often experience a burst of new energy, termed "menopausal zest" by anthropologist Margaret Mead (Davis & Huber, 2004) and pursue new interests, acquire new skills, and enjoy more time with friends and family (Boston Women's Health Collective, 1998). Conversely, Gilligan (1982) argues that midlife may be a time of risk for women precisely because of their embeddedness in relationships, orientation to interdependence, ability to subordinate achievement to care, and conflicts over competitive success. Women face midlife by making sense out of their experiences based on their relationships (Fogel & Woods, 1995).

CLINICAL APPLICATION

A common myth is that women lose their interest in sex when they reach middle age. Although aging decreases vaginal lubrication, use of vaginal lubricants aid comfortable intercourse. Women who engage in sexual intercourse with men and who are perimenopausal should be provided with information about contraception if they want to avoid pregnancy.

Some women experience changes in memory and cognition as they enter midlife. Research is sparse on this subject, and although some studies implicate decreasing estrogen as a possible cause (Phillips & Sherwin, 1992), others contradict these findings (Buckwalter, Crooks, Robins, & Petitti, 2004; Kang, Weuve, & Grodstein, 2004)

Ageism and bias due to age are common in Western society. As a health care provider, it is important to provide supportive care throughout a woman's life span and not assume a woman's health concerns are entirely related to her age.

OLDER WOMEN

The term "older women" refers to women who have completed menopause. The population of older adults in the United States is primarily female (Davis & Huber, 2004). Many of these women live in poverty and have health problems because they have outlived their support systems (Davis & Huber). Medicare reimbursement is either poor or nonexistent for many of the health care services needed by this population. Health care issues related to aging are primarily women's issues, because older women significantly outnumber older men (Davis & Huber).

BIOLOGY AND PHYSIOLOGY

Aging changes are due to decrease or loss of functioning at the cellular and/or tissue level, diminished capacity of an organ or system, and a reduction in body capabilities (Pfister & Dougherty, 1996). Several theories abound about the cause of aging and the biologic and physiologic impacts of aging. However, more research is needed to produce definitive findings. Specifically, gender-related distinctions need more study.

Loss of lean muscle mass, diminished immune functioning, an increase in cardiovascular problems (coronary heart disease and hypertension), and osteoporosis and bone loss are all observed with advanced age (Dimond, 1995; Pfister & Dougherty, 1996).

PSYCHOSOCIAL DEVELOPMENT

Older women are often caregivers for ailing spouses and also often live alone (because they outlive their male partners), but they continue to maintain a connectedness to other family members (Dimond, 1995). Cognitive abilities involve a range of capacities including motivation, short- and long-term memory, intelligence, learning and retention, and many factors that either facilitate or impede cognitive functioning (Dimond). It is not possible to definitively attribute changes in cognitive functioning to aging because there are so few studies that have been done that include repeated measures over time with the same subjects (Dimond). Theories suggest that as we age we begin to disengage from society, that we make adjustments based on our lifelong patterns, likes, and dislikes. However, there are not enough studies to support these hypotheses.

CLINICAL APPLICATION

Health issues of older women are substantial. The elderly are commonly viewed as frail and vulnerable persons who consume a significant amount of health care time, space, and dollars (Pfister & Dougherty, 1996). Ageism, or stereotyping and discrimination of a person based on age, is even more common at this stage of life. Elderly women not only contend with ageism, but also with sexism. Youth and beauty are highly valued in the United States and while older men may be viewed as attractive, the older woman is often pressured to ward off aging (Pfister & Dougherty). Pohl and Boyd (1993) suggest that a key area in which clinicians might begin to link feminist theory with aging women is in health policies and the inequities inherent in them. To promote health and wellness in older women, clinicians must provide them with adequate information about their health status, risks, and ways of improving health through diet and exercise commensurate with their age and capabilities.

CONCLUSION

The remainder of the chapters within this textbook will present more detailed discussions of the clinical assessment and management of women's gynecologic health. Through the continued use of a feminist framework, an expanded model of gynecologic health is presented that includes great opportunity to both affect change and improve health outcomes for women.

REFERENCES

Baker Miller, J. (1991). The development of women's sense of self. In J. Jordan, A. Kaplan, J. Miller, I. Stiver, & J. Surrey (Eds.), *Women's growth in connection: Writings from the Stone Center* (pp. 11–34). New York: Guilford Press.

Bassey, J., Sayer, A., & Cooper, C. (2002). A life course approach to musculoskeletal aging: Muscle strength, osteoporosis, and osteoarthritis. In D. Kuh & R. Hardy (Eds.), *A life course approach to women's health* (pp. 141–160). Oxford: University Press.

Belenky, M., Clinchy, B., Goldberger, N., & Tarule, J. (1986). *Women's ways of knowing.* New York: Harper Collins.

Blakenship, V. (2003). Psychosocial development of women. In E. Breslin & V. Lucas (Eds.), *Women's health nursing: Toward evidence-based practice* (pp. 133–169). St. Louis, MO: Saunders.

Boston Women's Health Collective. (1998). *Our bodies, ourselves for the new century.* New York: Simon & Schuster.

Buckwalter, J., Crooks, V., Robins, S., & Petitti, D. (2004). Hormone use and cognitive performance in women of advanced age. *Journal of Advanced Geriatrics, 52,* 182–186.

Collins, P. (2000). *Black feminist thought: Knowledge, consciousness, and the politics of empowerment.* London: Harper Collins.

Condon, M. (Ed.). (2004). *Women's health.* New Jersey: Pearson Education.

Crain, W. (1980). *Theories of development: Concepts and application.* New Jersey: Prentice Hall.

Davis, R., & Huber, K. (2004). Class, ethnicity, age, physical status, and sexual orientation: Implications for health and healthcare. In M. Condon (Ed.), *Women's health* (pp. 21–40). Upper Saddle River, NJ: Prentice Hall.

Dimond, M. (1995). Older women's health. In C. Fogel & N. Woods (Eds.), *Women's health care* (pp. 101–110). London: Sage.

Erikson, E. (1950). *Childhood & society.* New York: W.W. Norton.

Erikson, E. (1968). *Identity, youth and crisis.* New York: W.W. Norton.

Fogel, C., & Woods, N. (1995). Midlife women's health. In N. Fogel (Ed.), *Women's health* (pp. 79–100). London: Sage.

Franz, C., & White, K. (1985). Individuation and attachment in personality development: Extending Erikson's theory. *Journal of Personality, 53*(2), 224–256.

Gilchrist, V. (1997). Psychosocial development of girls and women. In J. Rosenfeld (Ed.), *Women's health in primary care* (1st ed., pp. 21–28). Baltimore: Williams & Wilkins.

Gilligan, C. (1982). *In a different voice: Psychological theory and women's development.* Cambridge, MA: Harvard University Press.

Goldharber, D. (1986). *Lifespan and human development.* New York: Harcourt Brace Jovanovich, Inc.

Hare-Mustin, R. T., & Marecek, J. (1998). The meaning of difference: Gender theory, postmodernism and psychology. In B. McVicker Clinchy & J. K. Norem (Eds.), *The gender and psychology reader* (pp. 125–143). New York: New York University Press.

Kang, J., Weuve, J., & Grodstein, F. (2004). Postmenopausal hormone therapy and risks of cognitive decline in community-dwelling women. *Neurology, 63,* 101–107.

Kaplan, A., Gleason, N., & Klein, R. (1991). Women's self-development in late adolescence. In J. Jordan, A. Kaplan, J. Miller, I. Stiver, & J. Surrey (Eds.), *Women's growth in connection: Writings from the Stone Center* (pp. 122–140). New York: Guilford Press.

Kohlberg, L. (1981). *The philosophy of moral development.* San Francisco: Harper & Row.

Lee, J. (1998). Menarche and the (hetero) sexualization of the female body. In R. Weitz (Ed.), *The politics of women's bodies. Sexuality, appearance and behavior* (pp. 82–99). New York: Oxford University Press.

Leight, S. (2003). Health history. In E. Breslin & V. Lucas (Eds.), *Women's health nursing. Toward evidence-based practice* (pp. 251–274). Baltimore: Saunders.

Lewis, J., & Bernstein, J. (1996). *Women's health.* Boston: Jones & Bartlett.

Low, L. K. (2001). *Adolescents' experiences of childbirth: Nothing is simple.* Unpublished doctoral dissertation. University of Michigan, Ann Arbor, MI.

Martin, E. (1992). *The woman in the body.* Boston: Beacon Press.

Murray, R., & Zentner, J. (1997). *Nursing assessment and health promotion* (6th ed.). Upper Saddle River, NJ: Prentice Hall.

Musick, J. (1993). *Young, poor and pregnant: The psychology of teenage motherhood.* New Haven, CT: Yale University Press.

Olshansky, E. (1996). The reproductive years. In J. Lewis & J. Bernstein (Eds.), *Women's health* (pp. 105–143). Boston: Jones & Bartlett.

Perry, W. (1968). *Forms of intellectual and ethical development in the college years.* New York: Holt, Rinehart & Winston.

Pfister, S., & Dougherty, M. (1996). Growing older. In J. Lewis & J. Bernstein (Eds.), *Women's health: A relational perspective across the life cycle* (pp. 192–236). Boston: Jones & Bartlett.

Phillips, S., & Sherwin, B. (1992). Effects of estrogen on memory function in surgically menopausal women. *Psychoneuroendocrinology, 17,* 485–495.

Pohl, J., & Boyd, C. (1993). Ageism within feminism. *Image, 25,* 200–203.

Riger, S. (1998). Epistemological debates, feminist voices: Science, social values and the study of women. In B. McVicker Clinchy and J. K. Norem (Eds.), *The gender and psychology reader* (pp. 34–53). New York: New York University Press.

Rosenbloom, A., & Tanner, M. (1998). Misuse of Tanner scale [Letter to the editor]. *Pediatrics, 102,* 1494.

Sherwin, S. (1998). A relational approach to autonomy in health care. In S. Sherwin, F. Baylis, M. Bell, M. DeKonick, J. Downie, & A. Lippmann (Eds.), *The politics of women's health. Exploring agency and autonomy* (pp. 19–47). Philadelphia: Temple University.

Skillman-Hull, L. (2003). Adolescent women's health care. In E. Breslin & V. Lucas (Eds.), *Women's health nursing. Toward evidence-based practice* (pp. 432–552). Baltimore: Saunders.

Slap, G. (1986). Normal physiological and psychological growth in the adolescent. *Journal of Adolescent Health Care, 7,* 13S–23S.

Speroff, L., & Fritz, M. (2005). *Clinical gynecologic endocrinology and infertility* (7th ed.). Baltimore: Williams & Wilkins.

Strauss, S., & Clark, B. (1996). Adolescence. In J. Lewis & J. Bernstein (Eds.), *Women's health. A relational perspective across the lifespan* (pp. 65–106). Boston: Jones & Bartlett.

Taylor, C. (1994). Gender equity in research. *Journal of Women's Health, 3,* 143–153.

Tavris, C. (1992). *Mismeasure of women.* New York: Simon & Schuster.

Woods, N. (1995). Young women's health. In C. Fogel & N. Woods (Eds.), *Women's health care* (pp. 61–78). London: Sage.

Chapter 3

USING EVIDENCE TO SUPPORT CLINICAL PRACTICE

HOLLY POWELL KENNEDY
KATHERINE CAMACHO CARR

WHAT IS EVIDENCE-BASED PRACTICE?

Sackett, Strauss, and colleagues (2000) define the elements of evidence-based practice (EBP) or medicine as "the integration of the best research evidence with clinical expertise and patient values" (p. 1). EBP demands a high level of scientific evidence at all decision-making points in a woman's care (Eisenberg, 2001; Sackett Strauss, Richardson, Rosenberg, & Hayes, 2000). The influence of EBP is increasingly evident in clinical practice and in the education of health care clinicians (Eisenberg, 2001; Sackett et al., 2000; Guyatt & Drummond, 2001; Sackett, Hayes, Guyatt, & Tugwell, 2000; Wuff & Gotzsche, 2000).

EBP begins with a clinical question (or query about best practice) and proceeds to identifying and evaluating the best research available to find the answer. To comprehensively and accurately answer the question there must be integration of clinical experience and patient preferences with the research evidence. Every clinician is a researcher on some level. What this means is that each person in clinical practice must solve clinical problems. Sometimes we use evidence generated by other researchers and at other times we conduct research personally. For some clinicians conducting research may be a small study to develop a clinical protocol, while for others it may be supervising a clinical trial. Regardless of the scope of the research, the principles are the same. The focus of this chapter is to review research principles, methods, and critique techniques to assist clinicians to develop skills in practice-based research to provide care that is truly evidence-based.

PRINCIPLES OF EVIDENCE-BASED PRACTICE

- Provides foundation for practice guidelines, diagnostic testing, and changes in procedures or treatments
- Forms the evidence base for pathways of care and helps to standardize care or eliminate wide variations in care that may not be efficacious or may be superfluous
- Assists with the development of clinical benchmarking and process- or outcome-based performance measures
- Eliminates unnecessary processes or procedures
- Sorts through research findings to find therapies that are effective or control costs

A FEMINIST PERSPECTIVE ON RESEARCH

This book is founded on a feminist framework that recognizes that hierarchies are an oppressive reality in health care. These hierarchies are implicated in women's health disparities, as well as in the historical lack of research devoted to women's health issues (Doyal, 1995). Wuest (1994) notes that the major goal of feminist research is "seeing the world through the eyes of the other" (p. 578) to emancipate the world from systemic bias based on gender and class. By interpretatively studying social realities we can move critically to change bias in our culture (Holland, 1990). Most feminists would agree that science is not acontextual or ahistorical—it must understand the woman's history and context of her life. Campbell and Bunting (1991) provide a helpful guide to critiquing research from a feminist perspective that we believe should be considered in the design and evaluation of research:

1. Research should be based on women's experiences.
2. Artificial dichotomies should be scrutinized.
3. The context and relationships of phenomena, such as history and concurrent events, should be considered.
4. The questions asked are as important as the questions answered.
5. Research should address questions women want answered.
6. The researcher's point of view should be described as part of the data to place the researcher on a plane with the researched.
7. Research should be nonhierarchal; participants and researchers should be partners.
8. Interpretations of observations should be validated and shared with participants.

THE HISTORY OF EVIDENCE-BASED PRACTICE

Nursing science has a rich heritage of applying evidence to practice. Florence Nightingale (1957) outlined the basic principles of nursing science in her best known work

Notes on Nursing in 1859. The Nightingale method of nursing included rigorous monitoring of all treatments for their effectiveness, an early version of EBP. Authority for Nightingale's work in public health and hygiene was based on trial and error, intuition, clinical experience, as well as careful observation and discussion with patients (McDonald, 2004). She used statistical data to improve health, sanitation, administration of health services, and nursing education. Nightingale was not a romantic Victorian gentlewoman, but a bright, organized, tough feminist and mathematician. She applied statistics to the study of public health and mortality data and invented the polar diagram (pie chart) to display research findings (Holliday & Parker, 1997; McDonald, 2002). Her work and that of other nurse theorists, researchers, and clinicians provided the foundation for a long tradition in nursing that combines careful scientific observation with sensitivity to the individual's needs.

The initiation of the modern EBP movement in health care is attributed to a British epidemiologist, Dr. Archie Cochrane, who was concerned that clinicians often failed to evaluate the effectiveness of their own care and did not have widespread access to the scientific literature (Fullerton-Smith, 1995). His initial work in the 1970s led to the review of all randomized controlled trials in perinatal medicine and ultimately established the Cochrane Collaboration in 1992, which currently has a much wider scope covering reviews in many fields of health care. The Cochrane Database of Systematic Reviews (2004), an electronic database that is part of the Cochrane Library, remains one of the largest, most comprehensive reviews of evidence available.

The EBP movement is often described as a paradigm change in medicine, moving from reliance on expert opinion and experience to reliance on scientific evidence as the basis for practice (Eisenberg, 2001; Evidence-Based Medicine Working Group, 1992; Kuhn, 1970). The present paradigm shift to evidence-based care identifies the best drugs, clinical practices, and surgical procedures through rigorous study with randomized clinical trials, meta-analyses, and systematic reviews of the scientific literature forming the primary evidence base for patient care (Sackett, Strauss, et al., 2000). In response to this shift away from expert opinion, articles, books and Web sites instructing clinicians how to conduct, evaluate, interpret and apply the medical literature have proliferated over the last decade (Guyatt & Drummond, 2001; Oxman, Cook, & Guyatt, 1994; Sackett, Hayes, et al., 2000; Sackett, Strauss, et al., 2000; Wuff & Gotzsche, 2000). (See also Appendix 3–A) This compendium of resources on EBP supports a shift in the sort of evidence that is most valued for diagnosis, therapeutic decisions and interventions, and questions related to the patient's prognosis.

An examination of the state of the EBP movement, the philosophy of science, and the state of nursing science, however, suggests that the use of evidence is not a new or revolutionary paradigm shift and may explain only part of the science upon which the change is based (Sehon & Stanley, 2003). Quine (1952), another philosopher of science, describes the scientific worldview as a web of beliefs, like a spider web with an exterior edge or frame secured to an existing structure, and possessing an interconnecting interior of radii and connecting points. Using this metaphor, the web of scientific beliefs can comprise sensory information and new untested theories that now exist on the developing edge of the web. Foundational theories such as the laws of nature, logic, or mathematics form the center of the web. The interconnections between the center and the periphery are composed of well-proven hypotheses about health and clinical practice. According to the Quinian metaphor, we use a vast network or web of health care beliefs with logical and evidential relationships to determine best practices, including the findings of experimental research, primarily randomized clinical trials (RCTs), and intuition and experience (Quine).

The sciences of medicine and nursing are composed of a vast network of beliefs, scientific observations, practices, hypothetical relationships, and theories. For example, in practice we include observations (blood pressure), hypotheses (how the blood pressure may need to be repeated before we accept that it is an accurate measurement), and theories (the psychophysiology of blood pressure regulation). Quine also suggests that scientific observations must be contextually examined as part of a whole and not in isolation from the rest of scientific knowledge. The concept of a web of knowledge along with interconnected relationships between practices and underlying theories supports a multiple-method approach to examining phenomena. The complexity of the human condition and human psychophysiology also demands multiple approaches in order to identify best clinical practices, interventions, and medications, and to identify basic scientific knowledge or antecedent plausibility (Goodman, 1999a, 1999b).

Much of our existing science in medicine and nursing comes from a variety of sources and not all are evidence based. There is not always a best way to obtain scientific information about clinical practice, and we must remain open and creative about research methods that will give us the best answer or will help us better define the interconnected web of knowledge related to the phenomena of interest. Nursing science values multiple ways of knowing because clinical practice is a complex and multidimensional process and patients are unique human beings who each define health and illness differently (Mitchell, 1999).

RESEARCH AND CLINICAL DECISION MAKING

Research and practice are reciprocally linked in the web of health care knowledge (Lanuza, 1999). Clinical questions provide the basis for research, and research provides a way to evaluate the safety and efficacy of practice. In other words, practice and science are mutually informative (Barrett, 2002). We also know that in addition to research, knowledge needed for practice is also based on intuition, experience, tradition, and common sense (Ervin, 2002).

APPLICATIONS OF EVIDENCE-BASED PRACTICE

- Many types of evidence are used in a variety of clinical decision-making scenarios (e.g., assessments, diagnostic tests, therapies, and treatments).
- The evidence is scrutinized for validity and applicability to the circumstances and the individual patient (i.e., What works? When, where, and why does it work? For whom does it work?).
- Lack of evidence about efficacy is not the same as evidence that something is ineffective. (There will be missing evidence about some things.)
- EBP uses information technology to make evidence available when needed by the clinician.
- Clinicians need to have ready access to evidence to support clinical decision making in women's health care.
- While working toward a common goal of providing or receiving the highest-quality health care, clinicians and patients need information they can both understand.

The educational preparation of clinicians usually includes core content on the research process. This can range from actual participation in research studies to general discussions about how to apply research findings to practice. We have found, however, that the word research can engender anxiety in many clinicians who are years removed from their educational experience. Research, like any skill, must be used on a regular basis to be effective.

One basic premise that helps clinicians shed their tentativeness in either considering conducting research or in applying research to clinical practice is to reformulate how they think about the entire subject. Research follows the exact same principles that any good clinician follows in everyday clinical management. These are ongoing and often circular in nature. For example, one step usually leads to another, but can also raise new questions that take you either back to the beginning or in a new direction. Table 3–1 outlines the steps in the clinical management and research processes.

TYPES OF RESEARCH EVIDENCE

Research evidence comes in many forms. We prefer to call them 'types' of evidence, rather than 'levels' to dispel the notion that one is necessarily better than another, or to suggest linearity. As previously mentioned, clinical experience and patient preferences are two parts of the triad of clinical decision-making criteria. They are combined with an evaluation of current clinical research.

The RCT is often held as the gold standard in Western medicine. However, not all clinical problems lend themselves to this kind of research. The key point is that the

TABLE 3–1 Alignment of Clinical and Research Processes

The Clinical Management Process	The Research Process
Gathering the Data	
• Focused toward individual clinical scenario.	• Focused on a broader perspective of a health issue.
• Historical, physical, and laboratory data may be gathered.	• Historical data, review of literature, and pilot study may be involved.
Identifying the Problem	
• Assessment is made of the individual's clinical problem.	• A research question and/or hypothesis is generated.
Development of the Plan	
• An evidence-based clinical management plan is developed to meet the client's needs.	• A research design is constructed that will best answer the research question.
Implementation	
• The management plan is implemented.	• The research study is conducted.
Evaluation of the Results	
• Clinical follow-up is conducted to assess the effectiveness of the treatment plan.	• Data are analyzed to provide answers to the research questions.

research method used must serve the research question being asked, and the results should be evaluated in terms of the quality of the study and the potential benefit or harm to the patient. In the United States the US Preventive Services Task Force takes the lead on setting guidelines for evaluating health care research evidence (Harris et al., 2001). Table 3–2 presents this approach.

RESEARCH METHODS TO INFORM CLINICAL PRACTICE

The historically defined parameters of science, particularly in the Western tradition, can create tension among researchers as to what truly counts as scientific evidence. Both quantitative and qualitative research approaches use a variety of methods and techniques, and both aim to expand knowledge about a specific phenomenon. Attempting to pinpoint a defining difference between the two creates the possibility of oversimplifying the complexity of each. Our goal is to help you understand the differences, understand what is credible from both perspectives, and to decide what is applicable to your practice and research. It is not to debate whether one approach is better than another because that assumes one has more truth-value. Actually, both approaches help us to fill in the "open spaces in the web of knowledge" according to Quine (1952).

TABLE 3–2   Recommendations for Using Research Evidence in Clinical Practice

U.S. Preventive Services Task Force Ratings

Strength of Recommendations

The U.S. Preventive Services Task Force grades its recommendations about specific health services or treatments according to one of five classifications, which reflect the strength of evidence and magnitude of net benefit (benefits minus harms).

A   Strongly recommended—There is good evidence that the service or treatment improves important health outcomes and benefits substantially outweigh harms.

B   Recommended—There is at least fair evidence that the service or treatment improves important health outcomes and benefits outweigh harms.

C   No recommendation for or against provision of the service or treatment—There is at least fair evidence that the service or treatment can improve health outcomes, but the balance of benefits and harms is too close to justify a general recommendation.

D   Recommends against—There is at least fair evidence that the service or treatment is ineffective and harms outweigh benefits.

I   Insufficient to recommend for or against—Evidence that the service or treatment is effective is lacking, of poor quality, or conflicting, and the balance of benefits and harms cannot be determined.

	Net Benefit			
Quality of Evidence	**Substantial**	**Moderate**	**Small**	**Negative**
Good: Evidence includes consistent results from well-designed, well-conducted studies in representative populations that directly assess effects on health outcomes.	A	B	C	D
Fair: Evidence is sufficient to determine effects on health outcomes, but the strength of the evidence is limited by the number, quality, or consistency of the individual studies, generalizability to routine practice, or indirect nature of the evidence on health outcomes.	B	B	C	D
Poor: Evidence is insufficient to assess the effects on health outcomes because of limited number or power of studies, important flaws in their design or conduct, gaps in the chain of evidence, or lack of information on important health outcomes.		Poor = I		

TABLE 3-2 Recommendations for Using Research Evidence in Clinical Practice (continued)

Hierarchy of Research Designs

I	Evidence obtained from at least one properly conducted, randomized controlled trial.
II-1	Evidence obtained from well-designed controlled trials without randomization.
II-2	Evidence obtained from well-designed cohort or case-control analytic studies, preferably from more than one center or research group.
II-3	Evidence obtained from multiple time series with or without the intervention. Dramatic results in uncontrolled experiments (such as the introduction of penicillin treatment in the 1940s) could be regarded as this type of evidence.
III	Opinions of respected authorities, based on clinical experience, descriptive studies and case reports, or reports of expert committees.

Source: Adapted from Harris et al., 2001.

Research often begins with a clinical problem or question that needs an answer. The clinical problem or question usually arises from a broad topical area, and the first task of the researcher is to clearly define the problem. Research questions can arise from everyday practice or from other research studies, especially where discrepancies, inconsistencies, or remaining questions about patient care practices, interventions, or products used exist. Social issues, such as access to care, models of care, effects of racism or gender bias on health, health disparities, poverty, and violence can also give rise to research questions. These questions are then translated into research aims, or what the study proposes to do. Minimally the aims should meet two criteria: reveal a gap in our current knowledge and be significant (National Institutes of Health, 2001). This means your exploration of the literature must reveal prior research in this area that could specifically address your questions. It also means that the results of the study could make a difference in the health care delivery or outcomes for the population being studied.

QUANTITATIVE RESEARCH

Quantitative research methods identify cause and effect relationships. A hypothesis is developed that poses a relationship between variables (e.g., drug A will effectively treat disease X). In general, certain problems or questions are better suited for quantitative research methods. These include problems with well-developed concepts, a prior body of knowledge, and reliable methods of measurement for the variables under study. Many times quantitative research is designed to verify, extend, or clarify previous work (Polit & Beck, 2004).

Theories or conceptual relationships can be sources of quantitative research questions, although the researcher must make deductions from the theory for testing (Polit & Beck, 2004). Quantitative research can contribute to an improvement in practice by evaluating interventions, therapies, patient care protocols, practice guidelines, products, procedures, and medications used in patient care, as well as outcomes of care. Comparative analyses (benchmarking) of practices and outcomes across providers, settings, geographic regions, and other variables can also be accomplished through quantitative research (Lindsey, 1999).

Quantitative Research Design and Methods   Research studies using quantitative methods explore problems by deduction. They use scientific experiments to manipulate variables to explore their relationships with one another and attempt to control outside influences. The independent variable (researcher controlled) is often applied as an intervention (e.g., medication), and its effect is measured (dependent variable) as an outcome (e.g., resolution of a disease). Objective observations (often numerical) are gathered to measure the dependent variables (e.g., temperature or Likert scale results).

Quantitative research includes experimental, quasi-experimental, and nonexperimental designs (Polit & Beck, 2004). A true experimental design includes random assignment of subjects to the experimental or control group. The experimental group is exposed to the independent variable, and the control group either receives a placebo or no exposure. The effect is measured by the dependent variable. The best known example of experimental research design, the RCT, is considered to be the most powerful method available to clinicians to test cause-and-effect relationships and permits validation or rejection of hypotheses. It allows for the temporal ordering of the cause before the effect, shows an empirical relationship between the manipulated independent variable and the dependent variable, and most importantly eliminates confounding variables from interfering with the results (Polit & Beck, 2004). It is, however, sometimes impractical or unethical to conduct RCTs of medications or procedures, and other methods must be used to identify an effective practice.

Quasi-experimental design is similar to experimental design but does not include random assignment of subjects to an experimental or control group for practical, ethical, or other reasons. This weakness prohibits causal inference because it can no longer be assumed that the two groups are equal. The findings could possibly be explained by differences between the groups or some other factor. Most researchers try to establish some control over these extraneous variables by matching groups or by establishing group equivalency with a variety of quasi-experimental designs and statistical analyses (Polit & Beck, 2004). The strength of quasi-experimental design lies in its practicality and feasibility in the real world of health care and informed choice, where subjects often cannot be randomly assigned to groups.

Nonexperimental research answers questions that do not lend themselves to manipulation of a variable. For example, if we want to study the effects of the death of a child on the mother, the independent variable (the death of a child) is clearly not something that can be manipulated or controlled. Nevertheless, an experimental and control group could be identified and composed of those mothers who did not experience the death of a child, and those who did, as it naturally occurs. Psychological and physical well-being could still be described and measured and compared in both groups, but cause and effect cannot be determined. A vast array of human factors cannot be manipulated and therefore cannot be studied experimentally (Polit & Beck, 2004). They can, however, be described and interrelationships can be examined with nonexperimental research.

Meta-analyses and systematic reviews are considered to be highly reliable forms of evidence. Meta-analysis uses the single study as the unit of analysis and statistically combines the findings of several similarly designed studies on the same topic. The method provides a standardized way to compare findings across studies, adding together larger numbers to observe patterns and relationships that might not have otherwise been observed in a single study (Polit & Beck, 2004). A well-conducted meta-analysis allows for a more objective assessment of the evidence obtained in RCTs, especially where there is disagreement or uncertainty with findings from multiple studies. This might be important when testing a new drug, procedure, or intervention, which may have different effects in subgroups or varying results in different studies.

A systematic review is the method used to analyze a general body of scientific data using clearly defined criteria. Systematic reviews can include meta-analyses, appraisals of single trials, and other sources of evidence. Great care is taken to find all relevant published and unpublished studies, assess each study, synthesize the findings, present a balanced and unbiased summary of the findings, and consider any flaws that may be present in the evidence. Many high-quality systematic reviews are available in journals and online, most notably the Cochrane Library. The need for rigor in systematic review has led to a formal process for their conduct. Although meta-analysis always uses a quantitative statistical analysis of the findings, systematic review may include a quantitative meta-analytic combination of study results, or a more qualitative summary of the aggregated data (Davies & Crombie, 2001).

Rigor in Quantitative Research   Just as in clinical practice, quality research is dependent on adherence to standards to ensure it is conducted accurately and ethically. It is always important that the description of the research design is clear so the reader can fully assess what took place and could replicate the study if desired. Errors in any step of the process will invalidate the results. Error can be minimized by careful attention to accuracy of the instruments used for measurement, sample selection, and understanding how to apply the findings in the acceptance or rejection of the research hypotheses.

Variables must be well defined—you must be sure you understand what is being tested and measured. Validity tells how well the measurement actually measures the variable. For example, a sphygmomanometer must accurately reflect a blood pressure measurement. The reliability of the measure is how consistently it performs. Machines are operated by humans; therefore reliability includes how well the operator conducts the measurement (e.g., using the correct size cuff and positioning each time a measurement is obtained).

A research sample must reflect the population it is meant to represent. Error is minimized by sampling techniques and random assignment to study groups. For example, if you were measuring the reporting of menopausal symptoms, you might find a difference in prevalence if you obtained your sample from a women's clinic (where women might be seeking therapy), versus going to a local supermarket where there might be a more representative population. In addition, where that supermarket is located may also affect the outcome because of socioeconomic or cultural differences that may bias the results. These issues can potentially affect the generalizability of the study findings, or their ability to be applied to populations other than the sample group studied. The size of the sample reflects its "power" and also affects the research findings. A sample that is too small will not have enough power to detect a significant difference between study groups. Likewise, a sample too large may provide significant results related to size only and not to meaningful findings (Munro, 2001).

There are two commonly cited types of errors in research—Type I and Type II (Polit & Beck, 2004). A Type I error is made when the researcher concludes that a relationship exists—Drug A is effective in treating Disease X—when it actually does not (false positive in clinical terms). The differences observed between the groups are often due to a sampling error such as self-selection bias. Random assignment to groups controls for sampling error and associated Type I error. The level of significance, referred to as "alpha" or "α" and reported as a "p" value, will also influence a Type I error. The most frequently used levels of significance or alpha levels are .05 and .01. With a .05 alpha the researcher accepts the probability that out of 100 samples, a true hypothesis will be falsely rejected only five times, and in 95 out of 100 samples a true hypothesis will be correctly accepted. With a .01 alpha there is only 1 chance out of 100 that the true hypothesis will be falsely rejected, so this level of significance makes the incidence of Type I error lower. Usually, the minimal acceptable level of significance in quantitative research is .05.

A Type II error, also called "beta" or "β", is made when the researcher concludes that no relationship exists when it actually does (false negative in clinical terms). As the risk of a Type I error is lowered, the risk of committing a Type II error increases. Researchers try to avoid both Type I and Type II errors and frequently will conduct a power analysis to identify a sample size, while taking into account the desired level of significance (alpha level) and the probability of Type II error (beta). Random sampling, random assignment to groups to avoid selection bias, and adequate sample size are all measures to avoid these kinds of errors.

Confidence intervals provide more information than p values because they give a range of values and allow inference of the true placement of a parameter applied to the population (Munro, 2001). The range specifies where the parameter (e.g., the mean) is most likely to lie (Polit & Beck, 2004). Most are set at 95% and provide a statement of the level of confidence the researcher has about the findings.

QUALITATIVE RESEARCH

Qualitative research methods use different techniques and answer different questions than quantitative research methods. Guba and Lincoln (1998) propose that how we perceive reality provides the backdrop for how we conduct science. This sets the stage for understanding the nature between the knower (researcher) and what can be known, commonly called epistemology. Together they form the question about method—how does one choose a way to learn about the world? A person's view of the world shapes the answers to these questions and influences their entire approach to science. Denzin and Lincoln (1998) suggest that scientists who value qualitative research believe that reality is relative and never completely apprehended. They believe there are many ways to tell and hear a story. The richness and details of the individual story provide the data we need to extend our knowledge of the world. The individual's point of view within the constraints of everyday life can only be known from the specifics of each case and cannot be controlled. Scientists using qualitative methods believe the researcher cannot be fully removed from the researched and sometimes call it "naturalistic" because the testing usually takes place in a setting that is not controlled.

These are different perspectives from the more objectivist stance of traditional Western science where quantitative methods, particularly the RCT, are highly valued. However, it is simply a different language and a different perspective. Each has its place and role; each can inform the other. One induces why something happens, and the other deduces the reason or explanation of why it happens. A simple example is the development of a hypothesis from clinical observations and discussions with women that a specific method of contraception causes weight gain (qualitative findings). To support this hypothesis a study using quantitative methods can be designed to examine whether this actually does occur.

The research questions most appropriate for qualitative methods are often exploratory. Why do things happen? What does it feel like? What does it mean? How should I interpret this result? These are all examples of questions ripe for qualitative methods. The questions can arise from either clinical problems or specific gaps in clinical evidence.

There are a variety of "lenses" that comprise the traditions of qualitative research. The term "bricoleur" is often applied to a scientist who can navigate these traditions and lenses to answer the original research question and those that emerge as the study progresses. A bricoleur is characterized by his or her ability to "put together a complex array of data, derived from a variety of sources, and using a variety of methods" (Polit & Beck, 2004, p. 245). Skills required include astute observation, reflection, interpretation, and introspection.

Qualitative Research Design and Methods   Qualitative research explores a problem by induction and often moves toward hypothesis or theory development. Data are derived from multiple sources such as interviews, fieldwork, observations, videotapes, art, media, and other documents, but is usually textual in composition rather than numerical. The researcher is considered to be the "instrument" and his or her role is closely tied to the collection and interpretation of the data. Sometimes the researcher is also a participant, such as in fieldwork where observations of specific clinical practices are being conducted. This can lead to an increase in trust between those being observed and the researcher. Qualitative studies are descriptive from the perspective of those who have experienced a particular phenomenon; therefore, samples are not random, but are "purposive" (Speziale & Carpenter, 2003). This means specific research participants are sought who can shed the most light on the research problem. For example, if you wanted to learn about the experience of postpartum depression, it would be fruitless to interview people who had never been exposed to the phenomenon. To refine ideas based on emerging findings in the data analysis the researcher may "theoretically sample" to answer specific questions (Charmaz, 2000). Sample size is usually not predetermined and the power of samples in qualitative studies reflects the robust richness of the textual data. Data collection usually continues until the researcher observes saturation or redundancy, or until nothing new is coming to light or being observed. Data analysis is conducted in a variety of ways, but usually results with findings richly descriptive in textual or thematic language.

Choosing from among the many qualitative methods demands from the researcher an understanding of his or her disciplinary focus. Each has its own complexity and methodology beyond the scope of this chapter. For an easier understanding of some of the basic methods, they have been organized into general categories adapted from Polit & Beck (2004) to reflect the area of knowledge they explore.

Understanding the Experiences and Processes of Health and Illness   Many of our research questions address what it is like to go through a certain health event, for the purpose of helping us find ways to make the way better understood for others who have similar experiences. These approaches include understanding the basic experiences and processes of how a person moves through the event. The methods come from the traditions of philosophy and sociology.

Phenomenology is derived from a philosophical tradition that provides a "textual reflection on the lived experiences and practical actions of everyday life with the intent to increase one's thoughtfulness and practical resourcefulness or tact" (van Manen, 1990, p. 4). The focus is on understanding what it is like for this person to be in this experience within the context of his or her life. The work is interpretative or hermeneutical. The findings are often presented as paradigm cases or exemplars, creating "a dialogue between practical concerns and lived experience through engaged reasoning and imaginative dwelling in the immediacy of the participant's worlds" (Benner, 1994, p. 99). The results provide a vivid description that can help us to better understand the social, political, or historical context (Polit & Beck, 2004).

Asking questions from the tradition of sociology assists us in understanding how social structures and human interactions affect people's experience of health and illness (Polit & Beck, 2004; Speziale & Carpenter, 2003). These approaches can range from understanding how people make sense of their social interactions (symbolic interaction) to how social processes are structured and developed (grounded theory). Charon (1992) describes four central foci of symbolic interactionism: (1) the nature of the social interaction; (2) human action both causes and results from social interaction; (3) present rather than a past focus; and (4) actions of the person are unpredictable and active in his or her world. Grounded theory was developed by Glaser and Strauss in the 1960s as a research method that addresses both the chief concern or problem for people and the basic processes available to address that concern (Glaser, 1978, 1992; Strauss & Corbin, 1998). Its goal is to develop theory in a substantive area that is grounded directly from the data. Grounded theories "are likely to offer insight, enhance understanding, and provide a meaningful guide to action" (Strauss & Corbin, 1998, p. 12). One example is Quinn's work on the process women go through during perimenopause (1991).

Understanding Human Behavior   The tradition of psychology focuses specifically on how and why people act; its aim is to describe behavior. Studying human behavior can help us understand how behaviors are related to health and illness. Ethology examines the evolution of human behavior in its natural context (Polit & Beck, 2004). Observations of human behavior are used to expose structures essential to life. One example is the observation of attachment behaviors as necessary and instinctive to survival (Ardovini, 2002; Sable, 2004). This observational approach can also be used from an environmental perspective as in ecological psychology. Ecological models examine the relationship of environmental influences with specific human attributes (Humpel et al., 2004). For example, immigration status (acculturation into a new environment) has been demonstrated to be a risk factor for psychological distress and unhealthy eating behaviors (Skreblin & Sujoldzic, 2003).

Learning how people communicate is another approach to learning about human behavior. Human communication has many processes and forms. Scientists explore the construction of meaning in the nuances of these processes. The methods stem from both sociology and linguistics. Sociolinguistics is the examination of the forms and rules of conversation through discourse analysis (Polit & Beck, 2004). Mishler (1984) proposes that by examining the talk between providers and patients we can encourage the development of noncoercive discourse and humane clinical practice.

Understanding Cultural Traditions and Influences   One of the oldest qualitative traditions comes from the field of anthropology where scientists strive to understand cultural variations among the many peoples of the world. There are several approaches, but ethnography is the most common. An ethnographer's goal is to carefully describe a specific culture. Historically, grand ethnographies often explored indigenous peoples. In health-related research smaller specific subsets are often the focus of study. For example, Ka'opua & Mueller (2004) studied how cultural values and social support practices relate to adherence to highly active antiretroviral therapy for HIV among Native Hawaiians, a group with historic difficulty in using Western health care services because of cultural conflict.

Synthesizing Qualitative Research Findings   Metasynthesis is another qualitative method. This research method analyzes, synthesizes, and interprets a specified body of research and holds the potential to provide valuable insight and knowledge about the distinctive aspects of a phenomenon (Kennedy, Rousseau, & Kane Low, 2003). It has some commonalties with meta-analysis in quantitative research, but with some important differences. It provides an organized yet interpretive approach to a specific group of qualitative studies (Noblit & Hare, 1988). Sandelowski and her colleagues (1997) note that it is essential to systematically examine qualitative findings (about a specific phenomenon) to keep from repeating ourselves in order to have an impact on practice and policy making. The method involves identifying similar qualitative studies about a particular phenomenon, determining how they are related, and synthesizing the findings. This, however, is more than a systematic review and becomes an interpretative study itself.

Rigor in Qualitative Research   Just as in quantitative research, a clearly articulated study design is essential to understanding the purpose and results of any project. Because qualitative research uses textual rather than numerical data, relative terms such as "trustworthiness" or "dependability" are used to describe results, whereas an "error" corresponds to quantitative study results (Speziale & Carpenter, 2003). There are several terms that can help you assess whether the results of qualitative studies are valid and reliable. Credibility reflects how much confidence you can put into the study results (Polit & Beck, 2004). It is enhanced by complete descriptions of the sample and setting, the data collection, and analytic procedures, how decisions were made, and the researcher's role in the study. In qualitative research the researcher represents an "instrument" as he or she is often collecting and analyzing data. Preparation and experience with the methods and acknowledgment of preconceived ideas, sometimes called bracketing, are helpful in understanding the researcher's perspective and influence on the study. This is similar to evaluating whether a specific statistical test is appropriate in a quantitative study.

A qualitative study should provide enough documentation so that the results can be confirmed, sometimes called "confirmability" (Polit & Beck, 2004). This helps to assure that another researcher could follow the analysis and understand how decisions were made. The findings are enhanced when there is evidence of a team of researchers involved with peer debriefing and searches for negative cases (Polit & Beck). These procedures allow the research team to reflect on their analysis and to check for bias and interpretative errors. Another approach, called "member checking," is to have study participants read and react to the researchers' analytic decisions to see if their findings reflect their personal experience with the phenomenon.

The research findings should make conceptual sense. There should be enough thick, rich, description that the results clearly fit with the data provided. "Transferability" refers to how well the findings can be applied to another setting and is similar to generalizability in quantitative research (Polit & Beck, 2004). A study should provide enough evidence in the description of the study to help you assess whether the findings could apply to your setting.

MIXED RESEARCH METHODS

Sometimes the research questions beg for a mixed method approach, or a combination of quantitative and qualitative methods. There are multiple ways to combine methods with one method being more dominant than the other, or perhaps conducted sequentially

(Tashakkori & Teddlie, 1998). A helpful way to think about this is to consider how different lenses help you see different things. You might design a study that examines how a specific intervention affects a woman's perinatal outcomes and health behaviors (quantitative measures). Yet, within the same study you could also interview women (qualitative methods) about the experience of the intervention—how it affected their lives. Another term appropriate to this discussion is triangulation, which refers to the use of multiple referents to capture a more complete and contextualized picture of the phenomenon (Polit & Beck, 2004). This can involve the use of multiple sources of data, time collection points, sites, and samples, all providing different perspectives on the same research question.

MOVING FROM BEST EVIDENCE TO BEST PRACTICE

Research can improve practice by providing answers to clinical questions, evaluating the safety, effectiveness, or cost of therapeutics, refining practice guidelines, or testing theories relevant to practice (Lanuza, 1999). Increased access to research evidence that has been reviewed, compiled, and analyzed by a variety of credible resources enhances our ability to obtain research findings. These resources include the Cochrane Collaboration, professional organizations, and institutions of government. A comprehensive list of resources is included in Appendix 3–A. This information has been made available via the Internet for "just in time" or as needed information for the busy clinician. Yet a struggle remains with how to move the results of research to practice—how do you actually make it happen?

Clinicians must be able to use the computer and must be familiar with the EBP resources in all fields of health. We must also be cognizant of the criticisms and limitations of EBP, including an overreliance on the RCT and systematic reviews, an emphasis on the "routinization" of practice, and the daunting effort to stay current, as today's evidence may be tomorrow's inappropriate practice (Kim, 2000).

Clinicians must be able to critically appraise individual studies to determine how much faith should be put into the findings. The strengths and weaknesses of a study must be identifiable. Evidence hierarchies rank studies according to the strength of the evidence they provide (Polit & Beck, 2004). Most hierarchies put meta-analyses of RCTs at the top and opinions of experts at the bottom. There is some concern that using such hierarchies emphasizes a scientific and rational focus and assumes causation (the design of the tightly woven web structure) can be identified only by rigorous quantitative study. This approach fails to recognize the gaps in the web of knowledge and discounts qualitative research or naturalistic observations that focus on the understanding of the human experience. EBP attempts to escape this reductionist approach by integrating information from a variety of well-designed studies, clinical experience, existing resources, and the woman's preference. When developing clinical practice guidelines, protocols, or clinical pathways, all of these elements should be included (Camacho Carr, 2000). No single study or group of studies can provide an infallible answer to a clinical question.

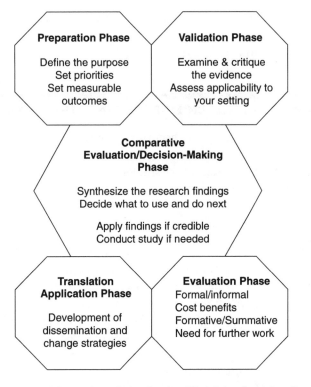

FIGURE 3-1   Conceptual Adaptation of the Stetler Model for Applying Research Findings into Clinical Practice

The Stetler (2001) model of research utilization was designed to help individual clinicians, as well as organizations, move the best evidence into the practice setting. Individual clinicians or organizations can use this model to critically analyze the research evidence and apply the findings to practice (see Figure 3–1).

There are five sequential phases in the current model. The preparation phase includes the identification of the purpose of the project, the searching, sorting, and selection of the research evidence. The validation phase involves a critique of the evidence. If the evidence is found to be sound, then the process continues to the comparative evaluation and decision-making stage. The evidence is synthesized and four criteria are used to assess the applicability of the evidence. The fit of the setting, feasibility, current practice, and the substantiating evidence are examined. Fit with the setting examines the similarity of the study's environment with the one in which the findings will be applied and compares the characteristics of the study population with the client population where the evidence will be applied. Feasibility implies that potential benefits outweigh any risk to patients, resources for implementation are available, and the involved persons are ready for change. Congruency with current practice philosophy and values must also be considered. Finally, the level of successful integration of the evidence into practice must be assessed. Using a model such as the one proposed by Stetler (2001) can make EBP more focused and acceptable to those clinicians who assert, "This is the way we've always done it." Integrating a methodical approach to applying evidence to practice can be effective in overcoming this too frequent mantra.

BARRIERS TO USING RESEARCH EVIDENCE IN CLINICAL PRACTICE

The two most common reasons we hear from clinicians (and students) about their lack of applying the latest research evidence are: (1) lack of confidence in critiquing research studies and (2) lack of time to find the studies. We empathize with both concerns and can offer some practical strategies.

CRITIQUING RESEARCH STUDIES

Critiquing research studies takes practice and some basic knowledge about how research is conducted. We suggest that all clinicians have a basic research text on their bookshelf to look up unfamiliar terms and statistics. We have used Polit & Beck's (2004) *Nursing Research. Principles and Methods* to provide some structure for this chapter and find it easy to read and practically written; however, there are many other good basic texts. The *Journal of the American Medical Association* has also compiled an extensive set of *Users' Guides to the Medical Literature* that are both instructive and illustrative (Giacomini, 2000a, 2000b; Guyatt & Drummond, 2001).

To assess applicability of any research findings to patient care, clinicians must evaluate the validity of the research, determine the practicality of implementing the findings, weigh any associated risks and benefits to the patient, and consider the ethical issues, available resources, and cost. Clinicians applying EBP guidelines must be able to recognize the limitations of the available databases, the limitations of scientific evidence, as well as know how to integrate clinical expertise, ethical considerations, patient individuality, and choice. Additional objectives of EBP can also include cost reduction, a desire to reduce wide variation in health care practices, and the desire to include clients as partners in their own care (Agency for Health Care Research & Quality, 2004; Gray, Hayes, Sackett, Cook, & Guyatt, 1997). None of these ideas are novel to practitioners. Table 3–3 provides a brief summary of important points to consider when evaluating the quality of a research study and whether you should apply the findings to your practice.

FINDING THE RELEVANT RESEARCH

Today's information-rich world places the most recent research virtually at your fingertips. It is important to realize, however, that published findings are dated the minute they hit the press. Journal articles can take one to two years from first submission to printed page, and textbooks take even longer. The Internet has substantially improved our ability to keep up with the most recently published research.

TABLE 3–3   Practical Points in Critiquing Research Studies

Title

Does the title of the article accurately describe the study? Is the language that is used in the title understandable and informative?

Abstract

Does the abstract accurately present the study? It should state the purpose of the study, the problems that were investigated, the research question or hypotheses, a description of the study design and the methodology used, the sample, instruments used, other data collection procedures, and the results or findings.

Research Questions and Purpose of the Study

What are the research questions? Are these questions researchable in the sense that they can be carried out by the investigators? What is the significance of the study in terms of practice, adding to the body of scientific knowledge, etc.? Are the research questions stated in a concise and precise manner?

Research Variables

Can you delineate the independent and dependent variables if it is a quantitative study? Is the phenomenon of study clear if it is a qualitative study?

Review of the Literature and Conceptual Frameworks/Model

Is the literature review relevant to the study? Does it include timely as well as classic articles that pertain to the study? Does the review provide adequate background information? Do the authors state how this review provides support for their study, i.e., give background information for the identified research problem/question?

Sample and Setting

Is there a description of how the sample was selected and the location of the study? What are the sources of bias, if any, that are associated with the sample selection process. Were power and effect size calculated for this study? In qualitative studies was the sample purposive, and when was sampling stopped?

Ethical Considerations

Do the authors address protection of human subjects? Did they obtain permission to conduct this study in the setting?

Method: The Design

Is the design appropriate for the research questions? Is it described? What extraneous variables are associated with the design, if any? Are they identified? Is the description adequate enough to allow replication of the entire study?

The Instrumentation and Data Collection Procedures

How are issues of scientific rigor addressed? Are validity and reliability of the instruments described? Was collection of data conducted in a standardized manner? In qualitative research, is the "researcher as instrument" described?

(continues)

TABLE 3-3   Practical Points in Critiquing Research Studies (continued)

Data Analysis

Are the analytic techniques supportive and appropriate for the research design? Does the article include supportive graphs, tables, or charts? Do these help to describe the results? Are they easily understood?

Results

Do the results follow logically from the design and method? Do the authors describe the results in a way that is understandable and clear? Do the results answer the research questions(s) or hypotheses?

Summary and Conclusions

What is your overall impression of the study? Does the author convince you about the conclusions that are drawn? Do the conclusions seem logical in light of the method and procedures, etc.?

Source: Adapted from lectures and presentations by Judith Fullerton, CNM, PhD, FACNM at the American College of Nurse-Midwives Annual Meeting 2002, Atlanta, GA.

Several excellent sources provide the best evidence in a succinct format for the busy clinician, including the Cochrane Database of Systematic Reviews from the Cochrane Collaboration, an organization that makes up-to-date, accurate information about the effects of health care readily available worldwide. It produces and disseminates systematic reviews of health care interventions and promotes the search for evidence in the form of clinical trials and other well-controlled studies (Cochrane Database of Systematic Reviews, 2004). MEDLINE (2004), the National Library of Medicine's database of over 4500 peer-reviewed biomedical journals published in the United States and over 70 other countries, provides another excellent source for research findings, although the reader must evaluate most of the studies for scientific merit and clinical applicability. The Agency for Health Research and Quality (2004) provides Evidence Reports and Technology Assessments, consisting of technical reviews on many clinical topics. The Database of Abstracts of Reviews of Effectiveness (2004) is another database, produced at the University of York in England. This database provides quality-assessed evidence reviews. Many other agencies and organizations prepare evidence-based guidelines and protocols, which can usually be accessed conveniently on the World Wide Web. Additional resources for EBP are included in Appendix 3-A.

CONCLUSION

It is helpful to look at what using evidence in practice actually means. Examples of applying evidence to clinical practice abound from choice of pharmaceutical versus alternative therapies for vaginitis to whether women need continuous electronic fetal monitoring during labor. Every clinical scenario faced will need to be addressed from your personal experience, the woman's desires, and the best evidence to support your recommendations. Your challenge is to blend them artfully in everyday practice.

If you walk away with anything from this chapter, it should be to question everything. Those questions need not immobilize you, but should set the stage for thinking critically about the causes of clinical problems and how to search for the best evidence available. Women will be your partners in this as they access the Internet and come to you with questions about different strategies in their health care. A recent study was described in the journal *Nature* in which Tilly and his colleagues (Johnson, Canning, Kaneko, Pru, & Tilly, 2004) surmise that the theory that we are born with a finite number of oocytes is questionable. If the results of their research on mice are extrapolated, they propose that we actually may use stem cells to continue reproducing oocytes, a finding that could significantly affect the way we look at fertility in the future. Dr. Allen Spradling of the Carnegie Institution in Washington was interviewed about this study on National Public Radio (Hamilton, 2004). His personal reaction to this rather stunning paradigm shift was chagrin with himself for never questioning the original theory of a finite set of oocytes: "I shouldn't have believed that. Why wasn't I more skeptical?" As clinicians and researchers, we should never be caught wondering, "Why didn't I ask the question?" We owe it to women and to ourselves to search for the best evidence to support our health care practices.

REFERENCES

Agency for Health Care Research & Quality. (2004). *National Guideline Clearinghouse Fact Sheet. Clinical Practice Guidelines.* Retrieved February 11, 2004, from http://www.ahcpr.gov/clinic/cpgsix.htm.

Agency for Research and Quality Evidence Reports and Technology Assessments. (2004). Retrieved February 11, 2004, from http://www.ahcpr.gov/clinic/.

Ardovini, C. (2002). Attachment theory, metacognitive functions and the therapeutic relationship in eating disorders. *Eating and Weight Disorders, 7*(4), 328–331.

Barrett, E. A. (2002). What is nursing science? *Nursing Science Quarterly, 15*(1), 51–60.

Benner, P. (1994). The tradition and skill of interpretive phenomenology in studying health, illness, and caring practices. In P. Benner (Ed.), *Interpretive phenomenology. embodiment, caring, and ethics in health and illness.* Thousand Oaks, CA: Sage.

Camacho Carr, K. (2000). Developing an evidence-based practice protocol: Implications for midwifery practice. *Journal of Midwifery & Women's Health, 45*(6), 544–551.

Campbell, J. C., & Bunting, S. (1991). Voices and paradigms: Perspectives on critical and feminist theory in nursing. *Advances in Nursing Science, 13*(3), 1–15.

Charmaz, K. (2000). Grounded theory. Objectivist and constructivist methods. In N. K. Denzin & Y. S. Lincoln (Eds.), *Handbook of Qualitative Research* (2nd ed., pp. 509–535). Thousand Oaks, CA: Sage.

Charon, J. M. (1992). *Symbolic interactionism: An introduction, an interpretation, an integration* (4th ed.). Englewood Cliffs, NJ: Prentice Hall.

Cochrane Database of Systematic Reviews. BMJ Publishing Group, London. Retrieved April 22, 2004, from http://www.update-software.com/cochrane/.

Database of Abstracts of Reviews of Effectiveness. (2004). Retrieved February 11, 2004, from http://agatha.york.ac.uk/darehp.htm.

Davies, H. T. O., & Crombie, I. K. (2001). *What is a systematic review?* Retrieved March 2, 2004, from http://www.evidence-based-medicine.co.uk.

Denzin, N. K., & Lincoln, Y. S. (Eds.) (1998). *The landscape of qualitative research. Theories and issues.* Thousand Oaks, CA: Sage.

Doyal, L. (1995). *What makes women sick? Gender and the political economy of health.* New Brunswick, NJ: Rutgers University Press.

Eisenberg, J. M. (2001). *Evidence-based medicine. Expert voices.* Washington, DC: Agency for Healthcare Research & Quality.

Ervin, C. E. (2002). Evidence-based nursing practice: Are we there yet? *Journal of the New York State Nurses Association, 33*(2), 11–16.

Evidence-Based Medicine Working Group. (1992). Evidence-based medicine. A new approach to teaching the practice of medicine. *Journal of the American Medical Association, 268*(17), 2420–2425.

Fullerton-Smith, I. (1995). How members of the Cochrane Collaboration prepare and maintain systematic reviews of the effects of health care. *Evidence-Based Medicine, 1*, 7–8.

Giacomini, M. K. (2000a). Users guide to the medical literature: XXIII. Qualitative research in health care. B. What are the results and how do they help me care for my patients? *Journal of the American Medical Association, 284*(4), 478–482.

Giacomini, M. K. (2000b). Users guide to the medical literature: XXIII. Qualitative research in health care. A. Are the results of the study valid? *Journal of the American Medical Association, 284*(3), 357–362.

Glaser, B. G. (1978). *Theoretical sensitivity.* Mill Valley, CA: The Sociology Press.

Glaser, B. G. (1992). *Basics of grounded theory analysis.* Mill Valley, CA: The Sociology Press.

Goodman, S. N. (1999a). Toward evidence-based medical statistics, 1. The *p* value fallacy. *Annals of Internal Medicine, 130*, 995–1004.

Goodman, S. N. (1999b). Toward evidence-based medical statistics, 2. The Bayes factor. *Annals of Internal Medicine, 130*, 1005–1013.

Gray J., Hayes, R. B., Sackett, D., Cook, D., & Guyatt, G. H. (1997). Transferring evidence from research into practice: 3. Developing evidence-based clinical policy. *American College of Physicians Journal Club, 126*(2), A14–A16.

Guba, E. G., & Lincoln, N. K. (1998). Competing paradigms in qualitative research. In N. K. Densin & Y. S. Lincoln (Eds.), *The landscape of qualitative research. Theories and issues* (pp. 195–220). Thousand Oaks, CA: Sage.

Guyatt, G. H., & Drummond. R. (Eds.). (2001). *Users' guide to the medical literature: A manual for evidence-based practice.* Chicago: American Medical Association.

Hamilton, J. [Interviewer]. (2004, March 11). *Study: Ovaries may replenish eggs.* [Morning Edition broadcast]. National Public Radio, Washington, DC. Available at http://www.npr.org/rundowns/rundown.php?prgId=3&prgDate=11-Mar-2004.

Harris, R. P., Helfand, M., Woolf, S. H., Lohr, K. N., Mulrow, C. D., Teutsch, S. M., et al. (2001). Current methods of the U.S. Preventive Services Task Force: A review of the process. *American Journal of Preventive Medicine, 20*(Suppl. 3), 21–35.

Holland, N. J. (1990). *Is women's philosophy possible?* Savage, MD: Rowman and Little.

Holliday, M. E., & Parker, D. L. (1997). Florence Nightingale, feminism and nursing. *Journal of Advanced Nursing, 26*, 483–488.

Humpel, N., Owen, N., Leslie, E., Marshall, A. L., Bauman, A. E., & Sallis, J. F. (2004). Associations of location and perceived environmental attributes with walking in neighborhoods. *American Journal of Health Promotion, 18*(3), 239–242.

Johnson, J., Canning, J., Kaneko, T., Pru, J. K., & Tilly, J. L. (2004). Germline stem cells and follicular renewal in the postnatal mammalian ovary. *Nature, 428*(6979), 145–150.

Ka'opua, L. S. I., & Mueller, C. W. (2004). Treatment adherence among native Hawaiians living with HIV. *Social Work, 49*(1), 55–63.

Kennedy, H. P., Rousseau, A. L., & Kane Low, L. (2003). An exploratory metasynthesis of midwifery care. *Midwifery, 19*(3), 203–214.

Kim, M. (2000). Evidence-based nursing: Connecting knowledge to practice. *Chart, 97*(9), 1, 4–6.

Kuhn, T. S. (1970). *The structure of scientific revolutions.* Chicago: University of Chicago Press.

Lanuza, D. M. (1999). Research and practice. In M. Mateo & Kirchoff (Eds.), *Using and conducting nursing research in the clinical setting* (2nd ed., pp. 2–12). Philadelphia: Saunders.

Lindsey, A. (1999). Integrating research and practice. In M. Mateo & K. Kirchoff (Eds.), *Using and conducting nursing research in the clinical setting* (2nd ed., pp. 42–55). Philadelphia: WB Saunders.

McDonald, L. (Ed.). (2002). *Collected works of Florence Nightingale: Vol. 1. Florence Nightingale: An introduction to her life and family.* Ontario, Canada: Wilfred Laurien University Press.

McDonald, L. (Ed.). (2004). *Florence Nightingale and the foundations of public health care, as seen through her collected works.* Retrieved February 6, 2004, from http://www.sociology.uoguelph.ca/ fnightingale/Public%20Health%20Care/.

Mishler, E. G. (1984). *The discourse of medicine. Dialectics of medical interviews.* Norwood, NJ: Ablex.

Mitchell, G. J. (1999). Evidence-based practice: Critique and alternative view. *Nursing Science Quarterly, 12*(1), 30–35.

Munro, B. H. (2001). *Statistical methods for health care research* (4th ed.). New York: Lippincott.

National Institutes of Health. (2001). *NIH Publication No. 02-5046. Qualitative Methods in Health Research.* Bethesda, MD: Office of Behavioral and Social Sciences Research, NIH.

Nightingale, F. (1957). *Notes on nursing: What it is and what it is not.* Philadelphia: Lippincott. (Originally published, 1859).

Noblit, D. W., & Hare, R. D. (1988). *Meta-ethnography: Synthesizing qualitative studies.* Newbury Park, CA: Sage.

Oxman, A. D., Cook, D. J., & Guyatt, G. H. (1994). Users' guides to the medical literature: VI. How to use an overview. *Journal of the American Medical Association, 272*(17), 1367–1371.

Polit, D. F., & Beck, C. T. (2004). *Nursing research. Principles and methods* (7th ed.). New York: Lippincott Williams & Wilkins.

Quine, W. V. (1952). *From a logical point of view* (2nd ed.). Cambridge, MA: Harvard University Press.

Quinn, A. A. (1991). A theoretical model of the perimenopausal process. *Journal of Nurse-Midwifery, 36*(1), 25–29.

Sable, P. (2004). Attachment, ethology and adult psychotherapy. *Attachment and Human Development, 6*(1), 3–19.

Sackett, D. L., Hayes, R. B., Guyatt, G. H., & Tugwell, P. (2000). *Clinical epidemiology and science for clinical medicine* (2nd ed.). Boston: Little Brown.

Sackett, D. L., Strauss, S. E., Richardson, W. S., Rosenberg, W., & Hayes, R. B. (2000). *Evidence-based medicine. How to practice and teach EBM.* New York: Churchill Livingstone.

Sandelowski, M., Docherty, S., & Emden, C. (1997). Qualitative metasynthesis: Issues and techniques. *Research in Nursing & Health, 20,* 365–371.

Sehon, S. R., & Stanley, D. E. (2003). A philosophical analysis of the evidence-based medicine debate. *BMC Health Services Research, 3*(14). Retrieved February 9, 2004, from http://www.biomedcentral.com/1472-6963/3/14.

Skreblin, L., & Sujoldzic, A. (2003). Acculturation process and its effect on dietary habits, nutrition behavior and body-image in adolescents. *Collegium antropologicum, 27*(2), 469–477.

Speziale, H. J. S., & Carpenter, D. R. (2003). *Qualitative research in nursing. Advancing the humanistic imperative* (3rd ed.). New York: Lippincott Williams & Wilkins.

Stetler, C. B. (2001). Updating the Stetler model of research utilization to facilitate evidence-based practice. *Nursing Outlook, 49,* 272–279.

Strauss, A., & Corbin, J. (1998). *Basics of qualitative research. Techniques and procedures for developing grounded theory* (2nd ed.). Thousand Oaks, CA: Sage.

Tashakkori, A., & Teddlie, C. (1998). *Mixed methodology. Combining qualitative and quantitative approaches.* Thousand Oaks, CA: Sage.

van Manen, M. (1990). *Researching lived experience. Human science for an action sensitive pedagogy.* Ontario, Canada: State University of New York Press.

Wuest, J. (1994). A feminist approach to concept analysis. *Western Journal of Nursing Research, 16*(5), 577–586.

Wuff, H. R., & Gotzsche, P. C. (2000). *Rational diagnosis and treatment: Evidence-based clinical decision-making* (3rd ed.). Boston: Blackwell.

SOURCES OF RESEARCH EVIDENCE

Agency for Research and Quality Evidence Reports and Technology Assessments
http://www.ahcpr.gov/clinic/

American College of Physicians, ACP Journal Club on CD-ROM
http://acponline.org

Best Evidence database (CD-ROM available through BMJ Publishing, BMA House, Tavistock Square, London WC1H9JR)
http://hiru.hirunet.mcmastet:ca/acpjc

Cochrane Database of Systematic Reviews
http://www.cochrane.org/index0.htm

Core Library for Evidence Based Practice. Comprehensive Web site that is a virtual library with many links to full-text documents on all aspects of evidence-based practice including texts, the *Users' Guides to the Medical Literature (Journal of the American Medical Association* articles), basic statistics for clinicians, systematic reviews from the *Annals of Internal Medicine,* and instructions for how to read various kinds of scientific papers series from *BMJ.*
http://www.shef.ac.uk/~scharr/ir/core.html

Database of Abstracts of Reviews of Effectiveness (DARE)
http://agatha.york.ac.uk/darehp.htm

MEDLINE. The peer-reviewed biomedical literature and review articles on the state of the science.
http://www.ncbi.nlm.nih.gov/entrez/query/static/overview.html

USEFUL WEB SITES FOR SYSTEMATIC REVIEWS

Bandolier
http://www.jr2.ox.ac.uk/bandolier/index.html

Center for Evidence-Based Medicine at Oxford
http://cebm.jr2.ox.ac.uk

Cochrane Collaboration
http://hiru.mcmaster.ca/cochrane/default.htm

NHS Centre for Reviews and Dissemination
http://www.york.ac.uk/inst/crd/welcome.htm

Systematic Reviews Training Unit
http://www.ich.ucl.ac.uk/srtu

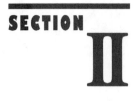

SECTION II

HEALTH ASSESSMENT AND PROMOTION

HEALTH PROMOTION

KATHRYN OSBORNE

The leading causes of death in the United States currently are related to modifiable, behavioral risk factors (Centers for Disease Control and Prevention [CDC], 2002; Mokdad, Marks, Stroup, & Gerberding, 2004; National Center for Health Statistics [NCHS] 2002a). Smoking-related illnesses kill an average of 178,311 women each year (CDC, 2002). An increasing number of women also experience morbidity and mortality as a result of being overweight or obese. Between 1999 and 2000, it was estimated that 62% of all American women were overweight, and that over half of these women were obese (NCHS, 2002b). In addition to causing premature death and disability, illnesses related to just these modifiable behavioral risk factors led to medical expenditures of over $150 billion in 1998 (CDC, 2002; Finkelstein, Fiebelkorn, & Wang, 2004). Health promotion and disease prevention must be priorities to improve the overall health of the nation and to reduce the spending of limited health care dollars on illnesses related to modifiable risk factors.

HEALTH PROMOTION: A NATIONAL INITIATIVE

The 1979 Surgeon General's report *Healthy People* set the stage for the development of a national initiative focusing on disease prevention. One year later *Promoting Health/Preventing Disease: Objectives for the Nation,* and *Healthy People 2000: National Health Promotion and Disease Prevention Objectives* established health objectives for use by state and local agencies, and private organizations, in the development of plans to move the population toward improved levels of wellness.

Healthy People 2010 expands the content found in these documents and establishes a set of health-related objectives for the nation to achieve in the new millennium. *Healthy*

People 2010 is a program built on scientific evidence and is designed to measure changes in health status over time. The primary goals of *Healthy People 2010* are to "increase quality and years of healthy life and to eliminate health disparities" (*Healthy People 2010,* 2004). The membership of the initiative is made up of private and public sector groups including the Department of Health and Human Services, state and local health departments, and hundreds of private sector groups and organizations. Members of the initiative periodically assess the health status of the nation and evaluate the effectiveness of specific interventions (*Healthy People, 2010*).

Ten leading health indicators were identified prior to the establishment of health goals. *Healthy People 2010* identifies multiple objectives that are associated with each of these indicators that reflect the major health concerns in the United States:

- Physical activity
- Overweight and obesity
- Tobacco use
- Substance abuse
- Responsible sexual behavior
- Mental health
- Injury and violence
- Environmental quality
- Immunization
- Access to health care (*Healthy People 2010,* 2004)

Healthy People 2010 also has 28 focus areas. These focus areas demonstrate the breadth of this document (Table 4–1). Health care providers are encouraged to utilize the objectives in establishing local programs focused on the improvement of the health of communities. More information about these objectives, specifically ways in which they may be applied to the delivery of women's health care, can be found at http://www.healthypeople.gov/.

As the United States begins to deal with the financial realities of health care, it is becoming increasingly clear to policy makers, health care clinicians, and insurance underwriters that there are benefits from allocating health care dollars for health promotion and disease prevention. The United States spent more money on health care than any other country in the world in the year 2000. The US spending on health care in 2000 reached $1.3 trillion, which was 13.2% of the Gross Domestic Product (National Information Center on Health Services Research & Health Care Technology, 2003; World Bank, 2004). An estimated 10–12% of total health care expenditures and 27% of the Medicare budget was spent on end-of-life care (Weiss, 1999). The most recent figures available indicate that only approximately 3% of the total health care budget is spent on preventive services (CDC, 1992). Changing from the traditional medical focus on the treatment of illness to health care (which includes health promotion and disease prevention) is an important step in the quest for cost containment (Shi & Singh, 2004).

The looming question is, "How does a health care delivery system that is illness centered undergo a paradigm shift to focus on wellness?" Health care providers are taking ini-

TABLE 4-1   *Healthy People 2010* Focus Areas

Access to quality health services	Injury and violence prevention
Arthritis, osteoporosis, and chronic back conditions	Maternal, infant, and child health
	Medical product safety
Cancer	Mental health and mental disorders
Chronic kidney disease	Nutrition/overweight
Diabetes	Occupational safety and health
Disability and secondary conditions	Oral health
Educational and community-based programs	Physical activity and fitness
Environmental health	Public health infrastructure
Family planning	Respiratory diseases
Food safety	Sexually transmitted infections
Health communication	Substance abuse
Heart disease and stroke	Tobacco use
HIV	Vision and hearing
Immunization and infectious diseases	

Source: *Healthy People 2010,* 2004.

tial steps by clarifying the definitions of "health" and "prevention." The multidisciplinary nature of health care delivery creates an opportunity for variations in these definitions.

DEFINING HEALTH

Many organizations and specialty groups have their own standard definition of health. Perhaps the broadest of these definitions was that established by the World Health Organization (WHO) in 1948 (2003): "Health is a state of complete physical, mental and social well-being and not merely the absence of disease or infirmity." To some, this definition may appear to make health unattainable; yet when health is viewed through a holistic lens, this definition begins to make sense. A holistic view of health includes its assessment in the context of physical, mental, and social well-being. Health, as defined in various contexts, can be achieved even in the presence of illness. For example, a young woman who has been HIV positive for five years may feel a sense of physical, mental, and social well-being if she is being cared for in a health care delivery system that addresses her health care needs in this holistic fashion. The presence of a disease state does not exclude her from being considered healthy according to the WHO definition of health.

The American Medical Association (2003) defines health as a "state of physical and mental well-being." The medical model's perspective of health has historically been from the clinician's point of view. However, as the practice of medicine evolves and focuses on cost-effectiveness and respect for patient autonomy, this perspective will necessarily shift and become patient oriented. Subjective information from the patient will determine his or her relative health, not just the clinician's viewpoint. Changing to a patient-oriented perspective of health will encourage physicians to shift from evaluating and assessing patient's bodies to assessing the complete lives of their patients (Sullivan, 2003).

Nursing is a discipline that focuses on health and wellness. Numerous nursing theorists have proposed definitions of health. Perhaps one of the most well known is that of Martha Rogers (1970), who theorized that the study of human beings would only yield meaningful theories and concepts when their wholeness is perceived. Rogers' definition of health was a springboard for the development of myriad nursing definitions of health, each of which used a holistic lens, viewing human beings as whole persons: mind, body, and spirit.

Madeleine Leininger, expanding on the earlier work of nurse theorists, provides a conceptual framework for nursing care. She proposes that *caring* is the essence of nursing and theorizes that while it may be expressed in different ways, caring is universal across cultures (Leininger, 1985). Supporting this theory are reports that the cultural beliefs of patients influence their perceptions of health, and that outcomes of care are improved when the patient's definition of health is considered and when that care is provided within the patient's cultural context (Kerns, Meehan, Carr, & Parks, 2003). Applying Leininger's theory of cross-cultural caring to earlier definitions of health, one could conclude that proper health care requires a consideration of the whole person and must include knowledge and appreciation for the cultural context of the individual. This view provides a definition of health that is patient specific and includes the individual patient's cultural perceptions of health. "Health promotion" then encompasses the delivery of a wide range of services that are delivered within the cultural context of the patient and that promote the general health and well-being of individuals and the communities in which they live.

DEFINING PREVENTION

The delivery of health care services aimed at the prevention of physical and mental illness and disease is defined on three levels:

- *Primary prevention*—Includes services that focus on preventing disease in susceptible populations (Shi & Singh, 2004). Examples of primary preventive efforts include health education and counseling, and targeted immunization.
- *Secondary prevention*—Services focus on the early detection of disease states and subsequent prompt treatment that will reduce the severity and limit the short- and long-term sequelae of the disease (Shi & Singh). Routine laboratory screening is an example of secondary prevention.
- *Tertiary prevention*—The delivery of services that limit disability and promote rehabilitation from clinical disease states (Shi & Singh).

The rest of this chapter focuses on primary preventive efforts in health care delivery.

COUNSELING AND EDUCATION AS PREVENTIVE STRATEGIES

Health care providers are in a prime position to offer information that provides the patient with tools for maintaining a healthy lifestyle and that assist in altering behaviors that may cause harm or illness. Patients often seek information during their yearly physical exam that can guide them in making lifestyle changes and confirm that their current practices are an effective means of maintaining health. However, episodic visits may offer more frequent opportunities for providing health promotion and disease prevention information. Statistics reveal that between 1992 and 2001, 46.6% of ambulatory health care visits were made for acute problems (including injuries), while 16.8% were made for preventive care (Cherry, Burt, & Woodwell, 2003).

The US Preventive Services Task Force (USPSTF or "Task Force") provides guidelines for clinicians regarding effective counseling interventions (see Chapter 7 for a detailed discussion of the USPSTF). USPSTF guidelines indicate that health care providers should utilize every patient interaction as an opportunity to participate in counseling and education.

EFFECTIVE INTERVENTIONS FOR HEALTHY, ASYMPTOMATIC WOMEN

DENTAL HEALTH

The USPSTF guidelines indicate that in combination with regular oral hygiene practices all women should be counseled to seek regular care from a dentist. Regular oral hygiene practices include daily brushing with fluoride-containing toothpaste and daily flossing between the teeth (USPSTF, 1996).

DIET AND EXERCISE

In the second edition of the *Guide to Clinical Preventive Services* the USPSTF (1996) recommends that all women be counseled to limit the amount of fat and cholesterol in their diet. Plans for diet and regular exercise should be designed so that caloric intake is balanced with energy expenditures. Women's diets should contain a variety of foods, particularly whole grains, fruits, and vegetables. In addition, efforts should be taken to limit saturated fats, trans-fatty acids, and cholesterol. Studies reviewed by the USPSTF reveal that individuals who follow these guidelines have lower rates of morbidity and mortality from coronary artery disease and certain forms of cancer (USPSTF).

Further recommendations are that all women consume the recommended daily allowance of calcium (1200–1500 mg/day for adolescents and young adults; 1000 mg/day for women aged 25–50 years, and 1000–1500 mg/day for postmenopausal women) and participate in regular physical activity to reduce both bone mineral loss and the risk of osteoporosis. In addition to slowing bone mineral loss, regular exercise reduces the risk of developing diabetes, obesity, heart disease, and hypertension. The Task Force recommends that clinicians encourage patients to implement exercise programs that gradually increase activity levels over time, and emphasizes the importance of regular physical activity rather than sporadic exercise practices (USPSTF, 1996).

During 2002 and 2003 the Task Force amended these recommendations after reviewing more recent research and concluded that there was insufficient evidence to advise either for or against routine dietary counseling or behavioral counseling to promote physical activity in the primary care setting. The evidence supports intensive dietary counseling provided by a clinician for adult women with hyperlipidemia or other known risk factors for cardiovascular or other diet-related chronic diseases. Health care providers who choose to provide dietary counseling to women who are not at increased risk should follow the recommendations published in the second edition of the *Guide to Clinical Preventive Services* as noted above (USPSTF, 2002, 2003).

INJURY PREVENTION

Motor vehicle accidents result in over 4 million emergency department visits and approximately 500,000 hospitalizations each year. Over 41,000 people in the United States die each year as a result of motor vehicle accidents and almost one-third of them are women (NCHS, 2003; NCIPC, 2004). Consequently, the Task Force recommends that all women be encouraged to use lap and shoulder restraints and that passengers in the cars they drive also use restraints (including age appropriate restraints for infants and young children). The guidelines also recommend urging the appropriate use of bicycle, all-terrain vehicle, and motorcycle helmets. All women should be counseled on the dangers of operating a motor vehicle while under the influence of alcohol or other drugs, as well as riding in the vehicle of an impaired driver. In particular, adolescents and young adults should be counseled on the importance of not combining driving and substance use, with an emphasis on making arrangements for alternative forms of transportation at times when alcohol and other drugs have been used (USPSTF, 1996).

HOUSEHOLD SAFETY

The Task Force recommends counseling women about several aspects of household safety. Smoke detectors should be installed in appropriate places in all homes and tested regularly for proper functioning. Infants and children should be dressed in flame resistant bedclothes for sleeping. Water heaters should be set at 120–130° Fahrenheit. All homes with children should have a 1-ounce bottle of syrup of ipecac, and easily accessible phone numbers to poison control centers and emergency departments (USPSTF, 1996). The American Association of Poison Control Centers (2004) advises that in the event of a poisoning, the first line of action should be to call the local poison control center. Individuals suspected of poisoning should not take anything by mouth or be forced to vomit unless directed by the poison control center. Medications and toxic substances should be placed out of the reach of children. Installing gates or barriers in front of stairways can prevent falls. A 4-foot enclosed fence should surround swimming pools, and swimming pool owners should be encouraged to learn to perform cardiopulmonary resuscitation. Window guards should be placed in buildings that pose a high risk for falls. Firearms should either be removed from the home or stored, unloaded, in locked compartments (USPSTF, 1996).

RECREATIONAL SAFETY

The Task Force recommends counseling women about recreational safety. The Task Force recommends wearing bright orange clothing when hunting, and following safe boating practices, including the wearing of approved flotation devices (USPSTF, 1996). Accidental injury is the leading cause of death for women ages 15–34 and the cause of death for over 15,000 women ages 15–65 each year (NCHS, 2002a). Although the number of these accidents that occur recreationally may be small, health care providers should counsel women about safety with regard to all aspects of their lives.

PREVENTION FOR ELDERLY WOMEN

The Task Force advises counseling older women about preventing falls. Counseling should include recommendations for exercise, learning safety-related skills and behaviors, reducing environmental hazards, and monitoring and adjusting medications under the direction of their care provider (USPSTF, 1996).

SEXUAL BEHAVIOR

The Task Force recommends that all women be advised of the risk factors for sexually transmitted infections (STIs) and counseled about effective measures to reduce the risk of infection. Counseling should be based on individual risk factors, which can be assessed during a careful drug and sexual history (see Chapters 6 and 18), as well as local information about the epidemiologic risks for STIs. Patients identified as being at increased risk for the acquisition of an STI need to receive information about risk factors and ways to reduce the likelihood of infection. Such measures include abstinence, maintaining a mutually monogamous sexual relationship with a partner who is not infected, regular use of latex condoms, and avoiding sexual interaction with individuals who are themselves at increased risk of infection (USPSTF, 1996).

Women who are at increased risk of infection should be advised to use a condom with every sexual encounter and to avoid anal intercourse. Those who use condoms should be advised to use them in accordance with product recommendations. Measures to reduce the chance of infection when a partner will not use a condom should be discussed, for example, use of the female condom. All women who are at increased risk for STIs should be offered screening and should be counseled to receive the Hepatitis B vaccine. Finally, the Task Force recommends advising, as appropriate, that the use of alcohol or drugs can lead to high-risk sexual behavior (USPSTF, 1996).

In light of the fact that over half of the pregnancies in the United States each year are unintended, the Task Force (1996) recommends counseling all women who are sexually active with male partners about effective contraceptive methods (see Chapter 9). Counseling should be based on information obtained from a detailed sexual history as discussed in Chapters 6 and 18.

Some researchers suggest that preconception counseling should be integrated into the routine women's health visit (Moos, 2003). Certainly, there is strong evidence to support the idea that general wellness counseling serves to improve pregnancy outcomes (Moos). However, women's health care providers should use sensitivity and an understanding and respect for an individual's preferences when initiating preconception counseling. It is important to keep in mind that some women will choose not to conceive, and not all women who conceive will choose to continue the pregnancy.

TOBACCO USE

Tobacco use is the leading preventable cause of death in the United States. Recent morbidity and mortality figures reveal that an average of 178,311 women die from smoking-related illnesses each year (CDC, 2002). The USPSTF strongly recommends that health care providers offer patients who use tobacco counseling on interventions that aid in smoking cessation. Evidence demonstrates that interventions such as screening, brief behavioral counseling, and the use of pharmacotherapeutics increase the number of patients who attempt to quit and who remain abstinent for one year (USPSTF, 2003). A framework provided by the "Five A's" is an effective way in which to engage women who smoke in discussion about cessation (USPSTF). The five A's include:

- *Asking* about tobacco use
- *Advising* to quit through clear personalized messages
- *Assessing* willingness to quit
- *Assisting* to quit
- *Arranging* follow-up and support

The Task Force found insufficient evidence to recommend for or against counseling children and adolescents about tobacco use or efforts to discontinue use by children and adolescents who already use tobacco. There currently is insufficient evidence to suggest that efforts directed at preventing use and assisting in cessation among children and adolescents are effective in the primary care setting. Decisions to initiate such counseling are left to the discretion of the individual provider (USPSTF, 2003).

CONCLUSION

This chapter examines definitions of health and the utilization of those definitions in the provision of primary preventive services, both as a national initiative and for individual health care providers. Secondary prevention is discussed in Chapter 7. Readers are encouraged to use this information in the development of management plans addressing the total health care needs of women across the life span.

REFERENCES

American Association of Poison Control Centers. (2004). *Prevention tips.* Retrieved June 7, 2004, from http://www.aapcc.org/preventi.htm.

American Medical Association. (2003). *H-160.997 AMA Program.* Retrieved April 21, 2004 from http://www.ama-assn.org/apps/pf_new/pf_online.

Centers for Disease Control and Prevention. (1992). Estimated national spending on prevention—United States, 1998. *Morbidity and Mortality Weekly Report 1992, 41,* 529–31.

Centers for Disease Control and Prevention. (2002). Annual smoking-attributable mortality, years of potential life lost, and economic costs—United States, 1995–1999. *Morbidity and Mortality Weekly Report 2002, 51,* 300–303.

Cherry, D., Burt, C., & Woodwell, D. (2003). *National ambulatory medical care survey: 2001 summary* (NCHS Publication No. 337). Washington, DC: Department of Health and Human Services.

Finkelstein, E. A., Fiebelkorn, I. C., & Wang, G. (2004). National medical spending attributable to overweight and obesity: How much, and who's paying?" *Obesity Research 12*(1), 219–226.

Healthy People 2010. (2004). *About healthy people.* Retrieved April 22, 2004 from http://www.healthy people. gov/About/.

Kerns, C., Meehan, N., Carr, R., & Park, L. (2003). Using cross-cultural definitions of health care. *The Nurse Practitioner, 28*(1), 61–62.

Leininger, M. M. (1985). Transcultural care diversity and universality: A theory of nursing. *Nursing and Health Care, 6,* 209–212.

Mokdad, A. H., Marks, J. S., Stroup, D. F., & Gerberding, J. L. (2004). Actual causes of death in the United States, 2000. *Journal of the American Medical Association, 291*(10), 1238–1245.

Moos, M. (2003). Preconceptional wellness as a routine objective for women's health care: An integrative strategy. *Journal of Obstetric, Gynecologic, and Neonatal Nursing, 32*(4), 550–556.

National Center for Health Statistics. (2002a). *Deaths, percent of total deaths, and death rates for the 10 leading causes of death in selected age groups, by race and sex: United States, 2000.* [Data file]. Available from Centers for Disease Control and Prevention Web site, http://www.cdc.gov/.

National Center for Health Statistics. (2002b). *Healthy weight, overweight, and obesity among persons 20 years of age and over, according to sex, age, race, and Hispanic Origin: United States, 1960–62, 1971–74, 1976–80, 1988–94, and 1999–2000* [Data file]. Available from Centers for Disease Control and Prevention Web site, http://www.cdc.gov/.

National Center for Health Statistics. (2003). *Death rates for motor vehicle-related injuries according to sex, race, Hispanic origin, and age: United States, selected years 1950–2001* [Data file]. Available from Centers for Disease Control and Prevention Web site, http://www.cdc.gov/.

National Center for Injury Prevention and Control. (2004). *Community-based interventions to reduce motor vehicle-related injuries: Evidence of effectiveness from systematic reviews.* Retrieved June 7, 2004, from http://www.cdc.gov/ncipc/duip/ mvsafety.htm.

National Information Center on Health Services Research & Health Care Technology [NICHSR]. (2003). *Health Economics Information Resources: A self study course, Module 2.* Retrieved April 20, 2004 from http://www.nlm.nih.gov/nichsr/edu/healthecon/ 02_he_intro.html.

Rogers, M. E. (1970). *An introduction to the theoretical basis of nursing.* Philadelphia: Davis.

Shi, L., & Singh, D. (2004). *Delivering health care in America: A systems approach* (3rd ed.). Boston: Jones & Bartlett.

Sullivan, M. (2003). The new subjective medicine: Taking the patient's point of view on health care and health. *Social Science and Medicine, 56*(7), 1595–1605.

US Preventive Services Task Force. (1996). *Guide to clinical preventive services* (2nd ed.). Baltimore: Williams & Wilkins.

US Preventive Services Task Force. (through 2004). *Guide to clinical preventive service, third edition: Periodic Updates.* Available at http://www.ahcpr.gov/clinic/gcpspu.htm.

Weiss, S. (1999). Economics, ethics, and end-of-life care. *Journal of the American Medical Association, 282*(21), 2076–2081.

World Bank. (2004). *Health, nutrition, and population stats*, [Data file]. Available at http://devdata.worldbank.org/hnpstats/.

World Health Organization. (2003). *WHO definition of health*. Retrieved April 21, 2004, from http://www.who.int/about/definition/en/.

GYNECOLOGIC ANATOMY AND PHYSIOLOGY

NANCY J. HUGHES

NANCY M. STEELE

SUZANNE M. LECLAIRE

The women's health movement encourages women to be knowledgeable about their bodies, to appreciate the unique form and function of the female body, and to take responsibility for caring and making decisions about their bodies that will positively impact their health. The purpose of this chapter is to review female anatomy and physiology that directly impacts gynecologic health and well-being. Female anatomy and physiology is typically referred to as "reproductive" anatomy and physiology, and the term "gynecology" is typically defined as the branch of medicine dealing with the study of diseases and treatment of the female reproductive system. Regardless of whether or not a woman is pregnant or ever intends to reproduce, her gynecologic care has historically focused on reproduction. This example of naming provides insight as to why women often continue to be essentialized to reproductive functions by their care providers.

The authors of this chapter assume that the reader has had basic human anatomy and physiology content. Readers requiring a more in-depth discussion are referred to general anatomy and physiology references.

PELVIC ANATOMY

PELVIC BONES

The primary importance of being able to evaluate the architecture of the pelvis is to assess its accommodation for safe passage of a fetus. The pelvis is composed of four bones: two innominate bones, the sacrum, and the coccyx. Each innominate bone consists of three parts: the pubis, the ischium, and the ilium. The ilium is the posterior and upper portion of the innominate bone. The two ilia form the false pelvis, share with the sacrum the important bony landmark of the sacroiliac notch, and join the sacrum at either side at the sacroiliac synchondroses. The ischium is the medial and lower portion of the innominate

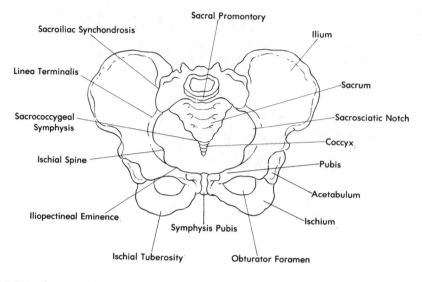

FIGURE 5–1 Bones of the Female Pelvis

bone and provides bony landmarks such as the ischial spine, the ischial tuberosity, and the pelvic sidewall. The pubis is the anterior portion of the innominate bone. The two pubic bones join each other in the front at the symphysis pubis and their inferior angles from the descending rami form the important bony landmark of the pubic arch (Figure 5–1).

The sacrum and the coccyx shape the posterior portion of the pelvis. The sacrum is formed by the fusion of the five sacral vertebrae, includes the important bony landmark of the sacral promontory, and joins the coccyx at the sacrococcygeal symphysis. The coccyx is formed by the fusion of four rudimentary vertebrae, is usually movable, and is itself a key bony landmark. The true pelvis constitutes the bony passageway through which the fetus must maneuver to be born vaginally.

There are four basic pelvic types according to the Caldwell-Moloy classification (1933): gynecoid, android, anthropoid, and platypelloid (Figure 5–2). Each pelvic type is classified in accordance with the characteristics of the posterior segment of the inlet. Most pelves are not pure types but rather a mixture of types.

PELVIC MUSCLES

The pelvic muscles include two muscles that form part of the walls of the pelvic cavity and two muscles that form the floor of the pelvic cavity commonly known as the pelvic diaphragm. In addition to these major muscle groups is the anterior and superficial group that is associated with the genitalia and is called the urogenital diaphragm. The urogenital, or lower pelvic area, is located in the hollow of the pubic arch and consists of the transverse perineal muscles. The strong muscle fibers provide support to the anal canal

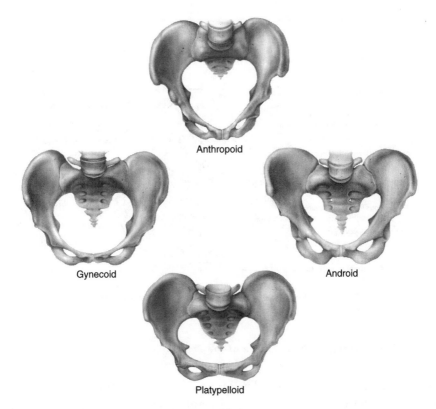

Anthropoid

Gynecoid

Android

Platypelloid

FIGURE 5–2   Caldwell-Moloy Classification of Pelves

during defecation and to the lower vagina during childbirth. These muscles consist of the transverses perinea, the bulbospongiosus, and the ischiocavernosus (Figure 5–3).

Two muscles, the piriformis muscle and the obturator internus muscle, and their fasciae form part of the walls of the pelvic cavity. The origin of the piriformis muscle is the front of the sacrum near the third and fourth sacral foramina. The muscle leaves the pelvis by passing laterally through the greater sciatic foramen and inserts on the upper border of the greater trochanter of the femur. The origin of the obturator internus muscle is the inner surface of the obturator membrane, which closes over most of the obturator foramen, and from the interior surfaces of the pubis and ischium, below the iliopectineal line, and from the pubic ramus. The obturator internus muscle is a fan-shaped muscle, which becomes tendinous as it passes through the lesser sciatic foramen. The tendon inserts on the greater trochanter of the femur (Anderson & Genadry, 2002; Faiz & Moffat, 2002).

The levator ani muscle, a thin sheet of muscle, and the coccygeus muscle form the pelvic floor, and the related fascia form a supportive sling for the pelvic contents. The muscle fibers insert at various points in the bony pelvis and form functional sphincters for

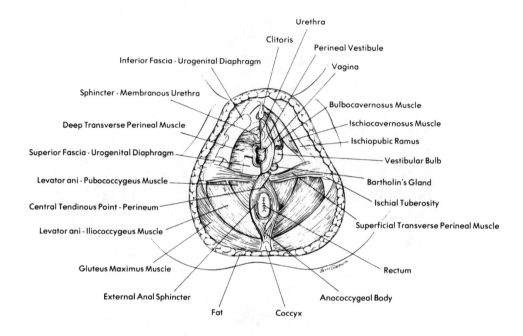

FIGURE 5–3   Superficial Musculature of the Perineum

the vagina, rectum, and urethra. The origin of the levator ani muscle is the pubic bone and the adjacent fascia of the obturator internus muscle. Various portions of this muscular sheet insert on the coccyx (the anococcygeal rapine), and onto a fibrous band lying between the vagina and rectum, known as the perineal body. Although the levator ani muscles are one muscular sheet, they can be subdivided into four different sections depending on the exact origin and insertion of the fibers:

a. The levator prostatae or sphincter vaginae fibers form the sling around the vagina and originate from the posterior surface of the pubis and insert in the perineal body.
b. The puborectalis fibers are considered important in maintaining fecal continence; they originate from the posterior surface of the pubis and form a sling around the rectum.
c. The pubococcygeus fibers originate from the posterior surface of the pubis and insert into the anococcygeal rapine.
d. The iliococcygeus fibers originate from the obturator internus fascia and the ischium and insert into the anococcygeal rapine.

The fan-shaped coccygeus muscle lies anterior to the sacrospinous ligament and originates from the ischial spine and inserts onto the lower part of the sacrum and coccyx and works synergistically to aid the levator ani muscle. The transverse perinei are small straplike muscles that help support the pelvic viscera. They originate from the ischial tuberosity, pass the genitalia, and insert on the central tendon at the midline. The bulbocavernosus muscles aid in strengthening the pelvic diaphragm and in constricting the urinary and vaginal openings. The muscle fibers originate in the perineal body and surround the vaginal openings as the muscle fibers pass forward to insert into the pubis. The ischiocavernous muscle contracts to cause erection of the clitoris during sexual arousal. The muscle fibers originate in the tuberosities of the ischium and continue at an angle to insert next to the bulbocavernosus muscle (Anderson & Genadry, 2002).

FEMALE GENITALIA

Dr. Nelson Soucasaux, a Brazilian gynecologist, has devoted much of her writing to the traditionally typical and symbolic aspects of women's sexual organs and the importance they have toward our understanding of women's nature. She found that historically it was believed that the key to understanding the female psyche was related to a deeper understanding of woman's genital functions (Soucasaux, 1993a; 1993b). By tradition, a woman's uterus was considered "the fundamental organ" and was synonymous with her genital organs. This conception depicted a woman's wholeness to be totally related to her genitals, of which the most important was her uterus. Consequently, there was little appreciation for female genitalia.

The following section describes the multiple organs and anatomical structures that comprise a woman's gynecologic anatomy. Figure 5–4 provides a midsagittal view of a

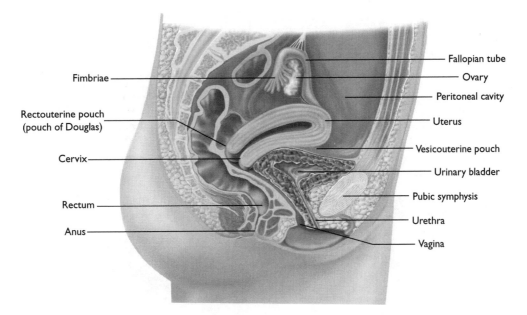

FIGURE 5–4 Midsagittal View of a Woman's Pelvic Organs

woman's gynecologic anatomy. Equally important to the discussion of women's gynecologic anatomy are the multiple nongenital peripheral anatomic structures involved in female sexual responses such as salivary and sweat glands, cutaneous blood vessels, and breasts.

EXTERNAL GENITAL ANATOMY

The Vulva The term "vulva" describes the externally visible outer genitalia (Figure 5–5). The vulva includes the mons pubis, labia minora, labia majora, the clitoris, the urinary meatus, the vaginal opening, and the corpus spongiosum erectile tissue (vestibular bulbs) of the labia minora and the perineum. The vestibule is inside the labia minora and outside of the hymen. On each side of the vestibule is a Bartholin's gland, which secretes lubricating mucus into the introitus during sexual excitement. The mons pubis is the mound-like fatty tissue that covers and protects the symphysis pubis. During puberty, genital hair growth occurs here, covering the pad of tissue.

The labia majora are fused anteriorly with the mons veneris, or anterior prominence of the symphysis pubis, and posteriorly with the perineal body or posterior commissure and assists in keeping the vaginal introitus closed, which in turn assists in the prevention of infection. The labia minora are surrounded by the labia majora and are smaller nonfatty folds covered by nonhair bearing skin laterally and by vaginal mucosa on the medial

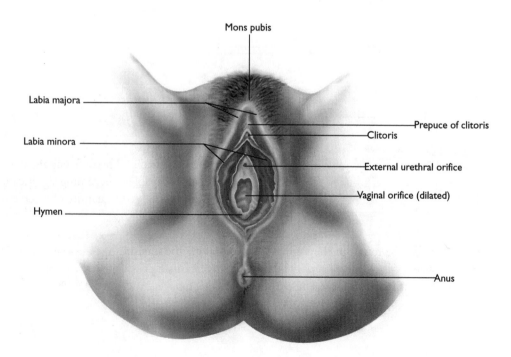

Mons pubis

Labia majora

Labia minora

Hymen

Prepuce of clitoris

Clitoris

External urethral orifice

Vaginal orifice (dilated)

Anus

FIGURE 5–5 The Woman's External Genitalia

aspect. The anterior aspect of the labia minora forms the prepuce of the clitoris and also assists in enclosing the opening of the urethra and the vagina. Women's vulva vary in size, related to the amount of adipose tissue, length, and pigment color of the labia minora or majora, ranging from light pink, dark pink, shades of gray, peach, brown, or black.

Clitoris   This sensitive organ is typically described as analogous to the penis in its erogenous function. During the early 1800s a respected English gynecologist, Isaac Baker Brown, theorized that habitual clitoral stimulation was the cause of the majority of women's diseases because it caused an overexcitement of the woman's nervous system. As a result there was increasing favor for performing clitorectomies, which were believed to rid women of ailments believed to be caused by clitoral stimulation (Duffy, 1963; Hall, 1998). Fortunately this theory and practice has long been refuted and the practice of clitorectomy in the Western world is rare.

Anatomically, the clitoris is formed from the tubercle of undifferentiated common tissue anlagen in the embryo (Boston University School of Medicine [BUSOM], 2004). The clitoris is a small, sensitive organ located at the top of the labia minora and consists of two paired erectile chambers. These chambers are composed of endothelial-lined lacunar spaces, trabecular smooth muscle, and trabecular connective tissue, and are surrounded by a fibrous sheath, the tunica albuginea. The paired corpus spongiosum, or bilateral vestibular bulbs, unite ventrally to the urethral orifice to form a thin strand of spongiosus erectile tissue connection (pars intermedia) that ends in the clitoris as the glans. The clitoris is capped externally by the glans, which is covered by a clitoral hood formed in part by the fusion of the upper part of the two labia minora. The clitoris has numerous nerve endings that contain tissue that fill with blood when sexually aroused. The blood supply to the clitoris includes the dorsal and clitoral cavernosal arteries, which arise from the iliohypogastric pudendal bed. The autonomic efferent motor innervation occurs via the cavernosal nerve of the clitoris arising from the pelvic and hypogastric plexus (BUSOM, n.d.; Moore & Dalley, 1999).

The labia minora together with the clitoris play a critical role in sexual activity. Because of their rich nerve and vascular supply, they are easily sensitized and become engorged with blood during sexual arousal. This vascular erectile tissue is capable of becoming significantly enlarged and tense during sexual excitement. In addition to the great quantity of erectile tissue in the clitoris, erectile tissue is also found inside the labia majora and minora, around the vulvovaginal opening and along the lower third of the vagina. A very small quantity of this tissue can also be found in the vaginal walls and along the urethra. Age-associated female sexual dysfunction from decreased clitoral sensitivity can be associated with histological changes in clitoral cavernosal erectile tissue (BUSOM, n.d.).

Periurethral Glands   There are two Skene's, or paraurethral glands, that open directly into the vulva near the urethral opening. The Skene's glands, which release mucus, form a triangular area of mucous membrane surrounding the urethral meatus from the clitoral glans to the vaginal upper rim or caruncle. The periurethral glands are mobile and can be pushed into and pulled out of the vagina by penile thrusting during coitus (BUSOM, n.d.; Moore & Dalley, 1999).

INTERNAL GENITAL ORGANS

Urethra   The urethra is a short conduit, approximately 3–5-cm long, extending from the base of the bladder and exiting externally in the periurethral glans area. The urethra is composed of three layers of tissue. The muscular layer consists of circular fibers and is continuous, with the bladder extending the whole length of the urethra. A thin layer of spongy erectile tissue, containing a plexus of large veins, is intermixed with bundles of unstriped muscular fibers and lies immediately beneath the mucosal layer. The pale mucosal layer is continuous with the vulva externally and the bladder internally. It is lined by stratified squamous epithelium, which becomes transitional near the bladder. Scattered in the epithelial lining are cells containing 5-HT serotonin (BUSOM, n.d.; Cario, 1999). This submucosal vascular tissue contributes approximately one-third of the normal urethral closing pressure and becomes further vasocongested during sexual arousal.

Halban's Fascia   Halban's fascia is the space between the trigone of the bladder and the anterior part of the vaginal wall. The fascia contains mesenchymal lamina, a fibroelastic sheet made up of collagen, and elastic and muscular fibers. These muscle fibers have an abundantly rich vascular and nerve supply containing pseudo-corpuscular nerve endings or Krause bodies (BUSOM, n.d.; Faiz & Moffat, 2002; Moore & Dalley, 1999).

Ovaries   The ovaries are the women's paired primary sex organs. They produce gametes, or ova, and the sex hormones estrogen and progesterone. Structurally, the ovaries of a sexually mature woman are solid, ovoid structures approximately 2 x 4 cm in size. The color and texture of the ovaries change with a woman's age and reproductive stage. These small, oval-shaped, almond-sized glands are situated on a shallow depression called the ovarian fossa located on either side of the uterus in the upper pelvic cavity. Several ligaments support the ovaries. The broad ligament is the principal supporting membrane of a woman's internal genital organs, including the fallopian tubes and the uterus. The remaining ligaments include the mesovarium, a posterior extension of the broad ligament; the ovarian ligament, which is anchored to the uterus; and a suspensory ligament attached to the pelvic wall. The outermost layer of the ovary is composed of a thin layer of cuboidal epitheal cells called the germinal epithelium. Immediately below this epithelial layer is the tunia albuginea, composed of collagenous tissue (Faiz & Moffat, 2002; Moore & Dalley, 1999; Van De Graff, 1988).

The cortex or the outer region of the ovary contains germinal epithelium with oogonia and ovarian follicles that number about 200,000 at puberty, and the inner and highly vascular medulla. Laced throughout the cortical and medullary layers is the stroma, an ovarian substance in which follicles and blood vessels are imbedded. Nerves, blood vessels, and connective tissue are found in the innermost portion, the hilum, which is the point of entrance for all of the ovarian vessels and nerves.

Circulation is via the ovarian arteries directly from the abdominal aorta, just below the origin of the renal arteries. Ovarian branches of the uterine arteries provide additional circulation. Venous return is through a venous plexus, which collects blood from the adnexal region, draining into the vena cava on the right, and into the renal vein on the left (Faiz & Moffat, 2002; Moore & Dalley, 1999; Van De Graff, 1988).

Innervation of the ovaries is derived from sympathetic and parasympathetic fibers of the ovarian plexus that descend along the ovarian vessels. These nerves supply the ovaries, broad ligaments, and uterine tubes. The parasympathetic fibers in the ovarian plexus are derived from the vagus nerves. The nerve fibers to the ovaries innervate only the vascular networks and not the stroma (Faiz & Moffat, 2002; Moore & Dalley, 1999).

Fallopian Tubes   These paired narrow muscular tubes are positioned between the ovaries and the uterus. Also known as uterine tubes or oviducts, they extend for about 10 cm from each cornu of the body of the uterus, outwards to their openings near the ovaries. The uterine tube has four segments. The pars interstitialis (intramural portion) penetrates the uterine wall. It contains the fewest mucosal folds with the myometrium contributing to its muscularis. The isthmus, the narrow segment adjacent to the uterine wall, contains few mucosal folds. The middle segment known as the ampulla is the widest and longest segment, contains extensive branched mucosal folds, and is the most common site of fertilization. The infundibulum, the funnel-shaped distal segment, opens near the ovary but is not attached (Faiz & Moffat, 2002; Moore & Dalley, 1999). Very fine fingerlike fronds of its mucosal folds, the fimbriae, project from the opening toward the ovary to help direct the oocyte into the lumen of the uterine tube. The inner surface of the tubes has fine hairlike structures called cilia that help to move eggs, released from the ovaries, along the tubes and into the cavity of the uterus. The uterine tube extends medially and inferiorly from the infundibulum into the superior-lateral cavity of the uterine opening (Cario, 1999).

The wall of the uterine tube is composed of three layers: mucosa, muscularis, and serosa. The internal mucosa includes the lamina propria and ciliated columnar epithelium, consisting primarily of two main cell types. On the surface the abundant ciliated columnar cells beat in waves toward the uterus, aiding in egg transport. Shorter, mucus-secreting peg cells are interspersed among the ciliated cells. Cilia propel the film they produce toward the uterus and help to transport the ovum and hinder bacterial access to the peritoneal cavity. The muscularis is the middle layer and has inner circular and outer longitudinal smooth muscle layers. Its wavelike contractions move the ovum toward the uterus. The outer covering of the tubes is the serosa, the lubricative layer, and part of the visceral peritoneum (Coad & Dunstall, 2002).

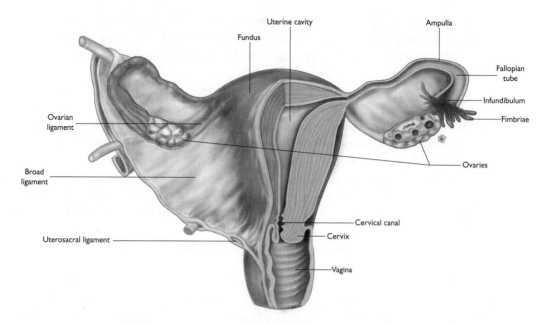

FIGURE 5–6 **Cross-Sectional View of the Woman's Internal Genitalia and Pelvic Contents**

The ovarian and uterine arteries supply blood to the fallopian tubes. The uterine veins, which parallel the arteries, provide the venous drainage. Sympathetic and parasympathetic innervation to the tubes from the hypogastric plexus and pelvic splanchnic nerves regulate the activity of the smooth muscles and blood vessels.

Uterus The uterus is a muscular, inverted pear-shaped, hollow, thick-walled organ that opens to the vagina at the cervix and then widens toward the top where the uterine tubes enter. The anatomic regions include the fundus, body, and cervix (Figure 5–6). The fundus is the uppermost dome-shaped extension of the uterine body above the point of entry of the uterine tubes. The body is the enlarged main portion. The cervix is the downward constricted extension of the uterus that opens into the vagina. The uterus is located anteriorly between the urinary bladder and posteriorly between the sigmoid colon and rectum. When the bladder is empty, the uterus angles forward over the bladder. As the bladder fills, the uterus is lifted dorsally and may become retroflexed, pressing against the rectum. The nulliparous uterus is approximately 7.5-cm long, 5-cm wide, 2-cm thick, and weighs approximately 90 grams (Moore & Dalley, 1999).

The uterine wall of the fundus and body consists of three layers: the endometrium, myometrium, and serosa or adventitia. The uterine mucosa layer consists of simple columnar epithelium supported by a lamina propria. Simple tubular glands extend from the luminal surface into the lamina propria. The stratum functionale is the temporary layer at the luminal surface that responds to ovarian hormones by undergoing cyclic thickening and shedding. The stratum basale is the deeper, thinner, permanent layer that contains the basal portions of the endometrial glands. This layer is retained during menstruation. The epithelial cells lining these glands divide and cover the raw surface of exposed endometrium that occurs during menstruation.

The endometrium receives a double blood supply. In the middle of the myometrium a pair of uterine arteries branch to form the arcuate arteries. The arcuate arteries bifurcate into two sets of arteries: straight arteries to the stratum basale and coiled arteries to the functionalis. The double blood supply to the endometrium is important in the cyclic shedding of the functionalis; the straight arteries are retained as the coiled arteries are lost (Anderson & Genadry, 2002).

The myometrium is composed of four poorly defined layers of smooth muscle that are thickest at the top of the uterus. The middle layers contain the abundant arcuate arteries. The outer layer of the uterus consists of two types of outer coverings. A cap of serosa covers the fundus, and the body is surrounded by an adventitia of loose connective tissue (Anderson & Genadry, 2002).

Structurally, the cervix is made mostly of dense connective tissue, is about 2.5 cm in length, and is covered interiorly by a mucous-secreting ciliated epithelium at the upper regions and by stratified squamous epithelium at the vaginal end. The opening of the cervix into the vagina is almost at a right angle to the long axis of the vagina. Uterine blood supply is via the uterine and ovarian arteries with venous return traveling via the uterine veins. The hypogastric and ovarian nerve plexuses supply sympathetic and parasympathetic fibers as well as carry uterine afferent sensory fibers on their way to the spinal cord at T11 and T12 (Anderson & Genadry, 2002; Faiz & Moffat, 2002).

Vagina The vagina is a canal that extends from the external vulva to the cervix. It is so variable and so capable of distension that it is difficult to accurately determine its dimensions, but on average the vaginal walls are approximately 7.5 cm in length anteriorly and 9 cm long posteriorly (Moore & Dalley, 1999; Van De Graff, 1988). The upper portion of the vagina encircles the vaginal portion of the cervix. The vagina touches the empty bladder on the ventral and superior surface. Inferiorly, the vagina adheres to the posterior wall of the urethra and opens adjacent to the labia minora. The internal mucosal layer has traverse folds, or rugae. This muscular canal extends from the midpoint of the cervix to its opening located between the urethra and rectum. The mucous membrane lining the vagina and musculature is continuous with the uterus. The vaginal walls can be easily separated because their surfaces are normally moist, lubricated by a basal vaginal fluid.

The vaginal wall is composed of three layers: mucosa, muscle, and adventitia. Vaginal epithelium is stratified squamous epithelium supported by a thick lamina propia. The lamina propria has many thin-walled blood vessels that contribute to diffusion of vaginal fluid across the epithelium. The lamina propria of the mucosa contains many elastic fibers as well as a dense network of blood vessels, lymph nodes, and nerve supply. To a much lesser degree than seen in the skin, this epithelium undergoes hormone-related cyclical changes including slight keratinization of the superficial cells during the menstrual cycle (Faiz & Moffat, 2002; Stenchever, Droegemueller, Herbst, & Mishell, 2001).

The epithelium has no glands; therefore it does not secrete mucus. Estrogen causes the epithelium to thicken, differentiate, and accumulate glycogen. Vaginal bacteria metabolize the glycogen to lactic acid, causing the typically low pH of the vaginal environment. Loose connective tissue containing many elastic fibers is found underneath the vaginal epithelium, which has a subdermal layer rich in capillaries. This rich vascular supply is the source for vaginal moisture during sexual stimulation (Coad & Dunstall, 2002). Within the epithelium lie the smooth muscles of the muscularis oriented longitudinally on the outer layer and circular bundles on the inner layer. The outer layer, the adventitia, is made of dense connective tissue with many elastic fibers, which provides structural support for the vagina. It also has an extensive nerve supply and venous capillaries. The adventitia is elastic and rich in collagen, provides structural support to the vagina, and allows for expansion of the vagina during intercourse and childbirth.

The upper two-thirds of the vagina receives efferent innervation through the uterovaginal plexus containing both sympathetic and parasympathetic fibers. The pelvic splanchnic nerves provide the parasympathetic efferent input to the uterovaginal plexus. The proximal two-thirds of the vagina is innervated via the uterovaginal plexus. The lower vagina receives autonomic efferent innervation from the pudendal nerve. The distal one-third of the vagina has primarily somatic sensation; this innervation is from the pudendal nerve and is carried to the sacral spinal cord (Moore & Dalley, 1999; Van De Graff, 1988).

BREAST ANATOMY AND PHYSIOLOGY

It seems common in Western society that a woman's breasts have two functions or roles in her life; one is sexual and the other is maternal. The breasts are visible social sex symbols and they are often a key source of a woman's anxiety about her body. Breasts often define women in the public and private eye.

The breasts are milk-producing glands located over the pectoral muscles. Each consists of a nipple, lobes, ducts, and fibrous and fatty tissue (Figure 5–7). Each breast is composed of 15–20 lobes of glandular tissue. The number of lobes is not related to the size of the breast. The lobes branch to form 20–40 lobules, which are subdivided into many secretory alveoli. These glands are connected together by a series of ducts. The alveoli produce milk and other substances during lactation. Each lobe empties into a single lactiferous duct that travels out through the nipple. As a result, there are 15 to 20 passages through the nipple, resulting in just as many openings in the nipple. Behind the nipple the lactiferous ducts enlarge slightly to form small reservoirs called lactiferous sinuses. Each sinus is 2–4 mm in diameter. Fatty and connective tissues surround the lobes of glandular tissue. The amount of fatty tissue is dependent on many factors including age, percentage of body fat, and heredity. Cooper's ligaments connect the chest

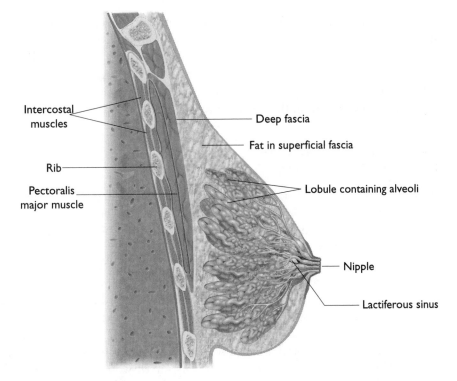

Intercostal muscles

Deep fascia

Fat in superficial fascia

Rib

Pectoralis major muscle

Lobule containing alveoli

Nipple

Lactiferous sinus

FIGURE 5–7   The Structure of a Woman's Breast and Mammary Glands: Sagittal Section

wall to the skin of the breast, giving the breast its shape and elasticity (Moore & Dalley, 1999; Murphy, 1991).

The nipple and areola are located near the center of each breast. They usually have a color and texture that is different from that of the adjacent skin. The color varies and darkens during pregnancy and lactation. The consistency can vary between very smooth to wrinkled and bumpy. The areola is the pigmented area surrounding the nipple. The size of the nipples and areolae varies a great deal from woman to woman, and some size variation is normal from breast to breast on the same woman. The nipple and areola are made of smooth muscle fibers and a thick network of nerve endings. The areola is populated by numerous oil producing Montgomery's glands. These glands may form raised bumps and be responsive to a woman's menstrual cycle. These glands act to protect and lubricate the nipple during lactation. The nipple usually protrudes out from the surface of the breast. Some nipples project inward or are flat with the surface of the breast. Neither flat nor inverted nipples appear to negatively impact a woman's ability to breastfeed.

Reproductive hormones are vital to the development of the breast during puberty and during lactation. Estrogen promotes the growth of the gland and ducts, while progesterone stimulates the development of milk-producing cells. Prolactin, released from the anterior pituitary, stimulates milk production. Oxytocin, released from the posterior pituitary in response to suckling, causes milk ejection from the lactating breast. The lymphatic system is abundant and empties the breast tissue of excess fluid. Lymph nodes along the pathway of drainage monitor for foreign bodies such as bacteria or viruses. The main flow is toward the axilla and anterior axillary nodes, but lymph drainage has been shown to pass in all directions from the breast (Moore & Dalley, 1999; Murphy, 1991).

MENSTRUAL CYCLE PHYSIOLOGY

The initiation of menstruation, called the menarche, usually happens between the ages of 12 and 15 and continues to age 45–50 when menopause occurs. Many women find themselves reluctant to discuss the existence and normality of menstruation. The word "menstruation" has been replaced by such euphemisms as: "the curse," "my period," "my monthly," "my friend," "the red flag," or "on the rag." Most women experience deviations from the average menstrual cycle during their reproductive years. As a result, it is not uncommon for women to display certain preoccupations regarding their menstrual bleeding, not only in relation to the regularity of its occurrence, but also to the characteristics of the flow (volume, duration, associated signs and symptoms, and so on). Unfortunately, society has encouraged the notion that a woman's normalcy is based on her ability to bear children. This misperception has understandably forced women to perseverate over the most miniscule changes in their menstrual cycles. Changes in menstruation are one of the most frequent reasons women visit their practitioners.

There are numerous patterns in the secretion of estrogens and progesterone; thus it is difficult to find two cycles that are exactly the same. Studies that include women of different ethnicities, occupations, nutritional status, and age have demonstrated that the length and duration of different menstrual cycles are as variable as the cycles themselves (Koff, Rierdan, & Stubbs, 1990).

The beginning of menstruation is the most evident external event that indicates the end of a cycle and the beginning of a new one. Widely accepted standards for distinguishing what are regular and irregular or normal versus abnormal are generally based on what is considered average and not necessarily typical for every woman. According to these standards, the normal menstrual cycle is 21–35 days with a menstrual flow lasting 4–6 days, although a flow for as few as 2 days or as many as 8 days is still considered normal (Khan-Sabir & Carr, 2003).

The amount of menstrual flow varies, with the average being 50 ml, but it may be as little as 20 ml or as much as 80 ml. Generally, women are not aware that anovulatory cycles and dysfunctional uterine bleeding are common after menarche and just prior to menopause (Mayo, 1997). Irregular menstrual cycles in adolescent girls are sometimes viewed as an abnormal state, yet approximately 50% of teens do not ovulate during their initial menstrual cycles (Sloane, 2002).

HYPOTHALAMIC-PITUITARY-OVARIAN AXIS

Hypothalamus   The hypothalamus controls anterior pituitary functions via the secretion of releasing and inhibiting factors. The hypothalamus and pituitary regulate hormones that serve as chemical messengers for the regulation of the gynecologic system. The hypothalamus initially releases gonadotropin-releasing hormone (GnRH) in a pulsatile manner. On average, the frequency of GnRH secretion is once per 90 minutes during the early follicular phase, increasing to once per 60–70 minutes, and then decreasing during the luteal phase (Sloane, 2002). The GnRH stimulates the pituitary gland to produce follicle-stimulating hormone (FSH) and luteinizing hormone (LH). Estrogen and progesterone are secreted by the ovaries at the command of FSH and LH and complete the hormonal group necessary for gynecologic health.

The Pituitary Gland   The oval-shaped, pea-sized pituitary gland is located in a small depression in the sphenoid bone of the skull. It is controlled by the hypothalamus, which secretes releasing factors into a special blood vessel network (hypothalamic-hypophyseal portal system) that feeds the pituicytes (Palter & Olive, 2002). These releasing factors cause or inhibit the release of pituitary hormones that travel via the circulatory system to target organs.

   The anterior pituitary synthesizes seven hormones:

- Growth hormone (GH)
- Thyrotropin (TSH)
- Adrenocorticotropin (ACTH)
- Melanocyte-stimulating hormone (MSH)
- Prolactin (Prl)
- Follicle-stimulating hormone (FSH)
- Lutenizing hormone (LH)

The latter two hormones, FSH and LH (gonadotropins), are responsible for regulating gynecologic organ activities. FSH targets the ovaries, where it stimulates the growth and development of the primary follicles and results in the production of estrogen and progesterone. Its release from the pituitary is governed by a negative feedback mechanism involving these steroids. The target for LH is the developing follicle within the ovary. LH is responsible for ovulation, corpus luteum formation, and hormone production in the ovaries. Prolactin is responsible for preparing the mammary gland for lactation and brings about the synthesis of milk (Sherwin, Scoloveno, & Weingarten, 1999).

Ovaries and Uterus   Complex changes occur in the ovaries and the endometrium as a result of the rhythmic fluctuations of gonadotropic hormones. The endometrium emulates the activities of the ovaries; whatever happens in the uterus during the cycle is precisely correlated with whatever is occurring in the ovaries. The object of the ovarian cycle is to produce an ovum, while the object of the endometrial cycle is to prepare a site to nourish and maintain the ovum if it becomes fertilized. The ovarian cycle includes three distinct phases: the follicular phase, ovulation, and the luteal phase. The endometrial cycle can be divided into the proliferative phase, secretory phase, and menstruation.

HORMONAL FEEDBACK SYSTEM

The menstrual cycle is determined by a complex interaction of hormones. The monthly rhythmic functioning of the menstrual cycle is dependent on the changing concentrations of gonadotropic hormones. The release of LH and FSH from the pituitary is dependent on the secretion of GnRH from the hypothalamus, which is modulated by the feedback effects of estrogen and progesterone. The hormones LH and FSH are in turn important for stimulating secretion of estrogen and progesterone. Virtually all hormones are released in short pulses at intervals of 60 to 90 minutes throughout most of the cycle, decreasing in frequency closer to menstruation. Steroid hormones modulate the frequency and amplitude of the pulse, which varies throughout the cycle (Figure 5–8) (Coad & Dunstall, 2002).

Under normal physiological conditions GnRH pulses stimulate the release of FSH and LH. Under the influence of gonadotropic hormone stimulation, the ovarian follicles develop and produce estrogen, which increases in the circulation, reaches the pituitary gland, and affects the amount of FSH and LH secreted without significantly affecting the pulse frequency (negative feedback). When the estrogen level becomes high enough, the negative feedback effect on the pituitary is reversed. Now estrogen causes a midcycle positive feedback effect on the pituitary, which results in a surge of LH and FSH and causes ovulation. Under LH influence, the ruptured follicle becomes the corpus luteum and secretes progesterone. Although the progesterone reduces the frequency of the hypothalamic GnRH pulses, the amount of LH released from the pituitary is proportionally increased to sustain the corpus luteum and the production of progesterone. In the absence of pregnancy, the corpus luteum degenerates, progesterone levels decline, and menstruation occurs. The GnRH pulses return to their frequency at the beginning of the follicular phase and a new cycle begins (Palter & Olive, 2002).

THE OVARIAN CYCLE

The ovarian cycle has three phases: (1) follicular, (2) ovulatory, and (3) luteal.

Follicular Phase   The follicular phase is characterized by the development of ovarian follicles and usually lasts from day 1 to day 14. Folliculogenesis begins during the last few days of the previous menstrual cycle until the release of the mature follicle at ovulation. It is the decrease in estrogen production by the corpus luteum and the dramatic fall of inhibin levels that allow for FSH to rise during the last few days of the menstrual cycle. During days 1 through 4 of the menstrual cycle, a cohort of primary follicles is recruited from a pool of nonproliferating follicles in response to FSH (Coad & Dunstall, 2002). Follicles that have enough granulosa cells will develop receptors for estrogen and FSH on the cells of the granulosa layers and LH receptors on the theca cells. The primary role of

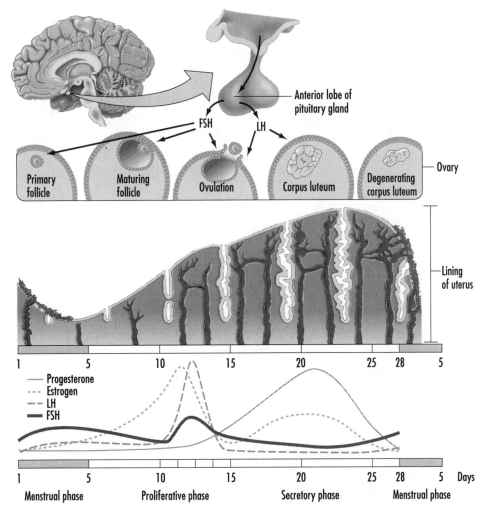

FIGURE 5-8   Influence of Steroid Hormones on the Ovaries and Endometrium.

FSH is to induce the development of increased receptors on the granulose cell to produce estrogen. The preliminary role of LH is to stimulate theca cell production of androgen that will be converted to estrogen by the granulosa layers.

Between cycle days 5 and 7, only one dominant follicle from the cohort of recruited follicles is destined to ovulate during the next menstrual cycle. As menses progresses, FSH levels decline due to the negative feedback of estrogen and the negative effects of the peptide hormone inhibin, which is secreted by the granulosa and theca cells of the developing follicle (Farabee, 2001). The decrease in FSH levels promotes a more androgenic microenvironment within adjacent follicles. By the eighth day of the cycle, the dominant follicle (Graafian follicle) is producing more estrogen than the total amount produced by

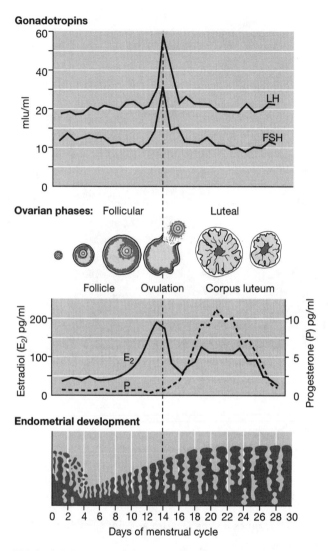

FIGURE 5–9 Ovarian Phases and Endometrial Development

the other developing follicles. In response to the dominant follicle's combination of estrogen and FSH, LH receptors develop on its outermost granulosa layers. The dominant follicle continues to flourish and gradually moves toward the surface of the ovary (Figure 5–9). The Graafian follicle contains the ovum and is surrounded by a layer of granulosa cells, which are further surrounded by the specialized theca interna and theca externa cells. An oocyte maturation inhibitor (OMI) in the follicular fluid suppresses the final maturation of the dominant follicle until the time of ovulation. The OMI's suppressive effects will end hours before the LH surge that causes ovulation (Sloane, 2002).

Ovulatory Phase Ovulation occurs approximately 10 to12 hours after the LH surge. Ovulation and the subsequent conversion of the follicle to the corpus luteum are dependent on the increase of estrogen and the LH surge. During the mid-follicular phase the dominant follicle's FSH levels diminish, but estrogen levels continue to increase. At the end of the follicular phase, estrogen reaches a blood level of approximately 200 picograms/ml that is maintained for up to 50 hours (Sloane, 2002). At this critical time, the high estrogen level initiates a positive feedback of LH, generating the preovulatory LH surge. The LH surge occurs 34 to 36 hours prior to ovulation and provides a relatively accurate predictor for timing ovulation. The LH surge is responsible for many changes in the follicle selected for rupture.

Initially the nuclear membrane around the oocyte breaks down, the chromosomes progress through the rest of the first meiotic division, and the egg moves on to the secondary stage. Meiosis ceases at this time and will only be initiated again if the ovum is fertilized. The LH surge stimulates luteinization of the granulosa cells and stimulates the synthesis of progesterone. Progesterone enhances the positive feedback effect of estrogen on the LH surge and is responsible for promoting enzyme activity in the follicular fluid capable of digesting the follicle wall. High levels of LH and progesterone cause the synthesis of prostaglandins and proteolytic enzymes such as collagenase and plasmin. The exact mechanism is unknown, but the activated proteolytic enzymes and prostaglandins digest collagen in the follicular wall, leading to an explosive release of the ovum (oocyte) with the zona pellucida and corona radiate surrounding it. At ovulation, the ovum is expelled and drawn up by the ciliated fimbriae of the fallopian tube to initiate its migration through the oviduct (Coad & Dunstall, 2002; Khan-Sabir & Carr, 2003).

Luteal Phase Under the influence of LH the follicle's granulosa cells left in the ruptured follicle enlarge, undergo luteinization, and become the corpus luteum. The corpus luteum continues to function for about eight days after ovulation. It secretes increased progesterone and some estrogen that start the negative feedback loop to the hypothalamus and pituitary gland preventing further ovulation within the cycle. In the absence of a fertilized ovum, luteal cells degenerate, causing a decline in estrogen and progesterone levels, and the corpus luteum regresses to become the corpus albicans. As a result of the regression of the corpus luteum, estrogen and progesterone decrease rapidly, removing the negative feedback effect. FSH and LH begin to increase once again to initiate the next menstrual cycle (Coad & Dunstall, 2002; Khan-Sabir & Carr, 2003).

THE ENDOMETRIAL CYCLE

The endometrial cycle has three phases: (1) proliferative, (2) secretory, and (3) menstrual.

Proliferative Phase The proliferative phase is influenced by estrogen and constitutes the regrowth of endometrium after the menstrual bleed. It starts on about the fourth or fifth day of the cycle and usually lasts about 10 days, ending with the release of the ovum. The proliferative phase involves changes in the endometrium, myometrium, and ovaries. The cyclic changes result from fluctuations in gonadotropin and estrogen levels. It is characterized by progressive mitotic growth of the deciduas functionalis in response to increasing levels of estrogen secreted by the ovary. These changes are in preparation for implantation of the fertilized ovum. At the beginning of the proliferative phase, the endometrium is relatively thin and the endometrial glands are straight, narrow, and short. As the phase progresses, the glands become long and tortuous. The endometrium becomes thicker as a result of the glandular hyperplasia and growth of the stroma. The endometrium proliferates from 0.5 to 5 mm in height and increases eight-fold in thickness in preparation for implantation of the fertilized ovum (Sherwin, Scoloveno, & Weingarten, 1999).

Secretory Phase   The secretory phase begins at ovulation. Within a 28-day cycle, it usually lasts from day 15 (after ovulation) to day 28. This phase does not take place if ovulation has not occurred. This phase tends to be the most constant phase, in terms of time. The glands of the endometrium become more tortuous and dilated and fill with secretions primarily as a result of progesterone. The endometrium becomes thick, cushiony, and nutritive in preparation for implantation of the fertilized ovum. In the absence of implantation, the corpus luteum declines and progesterone and estrogen levels subsequently fall. The endometrium begins to regress toward the end of the secretory phase. By days 25 to 26, progesterone and estrogen withdrawal results in increased tortuous coiling and constriction of the spiral arterioles in the thinning layer.

Until the last decade it was believed that decreased blood flow to the superficial endometrial layers resulted in tissue ischemia and resulting menses. Speroff and Fritz (2005) point out that more recent studies do not support the theory of vasoconstriction with resulting hypoxia as causing menstruation. The central theme of the newer model of the initiation of the menstrual cycle is enzymatic autodigestion of the functional layer of the endometrium that is triggered by estrogen–progesterone withdrawal (Speroff & Fritz). As estrogen and progesterone levels fall during the days prior to menses, lysosomal membranes destabilize and the enzymes within are released into the cytoplasm of the epithelial, stromal, and endothelial cells and into the intercellular space. These enzymes are proteolytic, and they digest the cells surrounding them as well as surface membranes. Their actions result in platelet deposition, release of prostaglandins, vascular thrombosis, extravasation of red blood cells, and tissue necrosis in the vascular endothelium (Tabibzadeh, 1996). Enzymatic action progressively degrades the endometrium and eventually disrupts the capillaries and venous system just under the endometrial surface, causing interstitial hemorrhage and dissolution of the surface membrane and allowing blood to escape into the endometrial cavity (Speroff & Fritz). The degeneration continues and extends to the functional layer of the endometrium where rupture of the basal arterioles contributes to the bleeding.

Menstrual Phase   The menstrual phase begins with the initiation of menses and lasts four to six days. Prostaglandins initiate contractions of the uterine smooth muscle and sloughing of the degraded endometrial tissue, leading to menstruation. The composition of menstrual fluid is desquamated endometrial tissue, red blood cells, inflammatory exudates, and proteolytic enzymes. Because some of the clotting factors ordinarily found in blood are lysed by lysosomal enzymes in the uterus, menstrual blood does not clot (Sloane, 2002). For three to five days, there is an average of 20 to 80 ml of blood loss. Approximately two days after the start of menstruation, estrogen stimulates the regeneration of the surface endometrial epithelium, while concurrent simultaneous endometrial shedding is occurring.

CHANGES IN ORGANS DUE TO CYCLIC CHANGES

Cervix   After menstruation, the cervical mucus is scant and viscous. During the late follicular phase, the cervical mucus becomes clear, copious, and elastic. The quantity of cervical mucus increases 30-fold compared to the early follicular phase (Coad & Dunstall, 2002; Khan-Sabir & Carr, 2003). The cervical mucus during this time is clear and stretchable (spinnbarkeit). The cervical mucus displays a characteristic ferning appearance during the ovulatory period if observed under a microscope (Sherwin, Scoloveno, & Weingarten, 1999). After ovulation, when progesterone levels are high, the cervical mucus once again becomes thick, viscous, opaque, and decreased in amount. This thick mucus is hostile and impenetrable to the sperm. Also the increased viscosity reduces the risk of ascending infection at the time of possible implantation. Estrogen increases stromal vascularization and edema and relaxes the myometrial fibers that supply the cervix. Activated collagenase causes the tightly bound collagen bundles to become a loose matrix, triggering the cervix to become softer a few days prior to and at ovulation. The external cervical os everts prior to ovulation. Progesterone causes the cervical muscle to retract, the collagen matrix to tighten, and the cervix to become firmer (Coad & Dunstall, 2002).

Fallopian Tube Mobility   Estrogen stimulates the epithelial cell activity, resulting in increased cilia movement and secretions in the uterine tubes. These special effects assist ovum mobility along the fallopian tube following ovulation. Progesterone reverses these effects, thus inhibiting the peristaltic activity of the fallopian tube smooth muscle.

Vagina   The changes in hormonal levels of estrogen and progesterone have characteristic effects on vaginal epithelium. This information is important when examining cervical cells to relate morphological differences in the stages of the menstrual cycle. During the early follicular phase, exfoliated vaginal epithelial cells have vesicular nuclei and are basophilic. They appear flatter than those in the later phases under the influence of progesterone where they are folded and clumped. The pH of the vagina responds to cyclical changes as estrogen stimulates the growth of lactobacilli. Lactobacilli metabolize glycogen from cervical secretions, producing lactic acid that decreases pH to a level that assists in providing the reproductive tract protection against opportunistic pathogens (Coad & Dunstall, 2002).

REFERENCES

Anderson J. R., & Genadry, R. (2002). Anatomy and embryology. In J. S. Berek (Ed.), *Novak's gynecology* (13th ed., pp. 69–121). Philadelphia: Lippincott Williams & Wilkins.

Boston University School of Medicine: Institute for Sexual Medicine (n.d.). *Female genital anatomy.* Retrieved October 1, 2004, from:http://www.bumc.bu.edu.

Caldwell, W. E., & Moloy, H. C. (1933). Anatomical variations in female pelvic bones and their effect on labor with a suggested classification. *American Journal of Obstetrics and Gynecology, 26,* 479–482.

Cario, H. A. (1999). *Advanced health assessment of women.* Philadelphia: Lippincott & Wilkins.

Coad, J., & Dunstall, M. (2002). *Anatomy and physiology for midwives.* London: Mosby.

Duffy, J. (1963, October 19). Masturbation and clitoridectomy. *The Journal of the American Medical Association, 186,* 246–248.

Farabee, M. J. (2001). *The reproductive system.* Retrieved October 1, 2004, from http://www.emc.maricopa.edu/faculty/farabee/BIOBK/BioBookREPROD.html.

Faiz, O., & Moffat, D. (2002). *Anatomy at a glance.* Oxford, UK: Blackwell.

Hall, L. A. (1998). *The other in the mirror: Sex, Victorians, and historians.* Retrieved October 9, 2004, from http://homepages.primex.co.uk/~lesleyah/sexvict.htm.

Khan-Sabir, N., & Carr, B. R. (2003). *The normal menstrual cycle and the control of ovulation* (Chap. 3). Endotext.com. Retrieved October 9, 2004, from http://www.endocrine-sourcecom/female/female3/female3.htm.

Koff, E., Rierdan, J., & Stubbs, M. I. (1990). Conceptions and misconceptions of the menstrual cycle. *Women and Health, 16*(3–4), 119–136.

Mayo, J. L. (1997). A healthy menstrual cycle. *Clinical Nutrition Insights, 5*(9), 1–8.

Moore, K. L., & Dalley, A. F. (1999). *Clinically oriented anatomy* (4th ed.). Baltimore: Lippincott Williams & Wilkins.

Murphy, P. A. (1991). Anatomy and physiology of the female reproductive system. In R. Lichtman & S. Papera (Eds.), *Gynecology well-woman care* (pp. 3–17). East Norwalk, CT: Appleton & Lange.

Palter, S. F., & Olive, D. L. (2002). Reproductive physiology. In J. S. Berek (Ed.), *Novak's gynecology* (13th ed., pp. 149–168). Philadelphia: Lippincott Williams & Wilkins.

Sherwin, L. N., Scoloveno, M. A., & Weingarten, C. T. (1999). Human reproduction. In *Maternity nursing: Care of the childbearing family* (3rd ed., pp. 103–132). Stamford, CT: Appleton & Lange.

Sloane, E. (2002). *Biology of women* (4th ed.). Albany, NY: Delmar.

Soucasaux, N. (1993a). *Archetypal aspects of the female genitals.* Retrieved September 28, 2004, from: http://www.mum.org/sougenit.htm.

Soucasaux, N. (1993b). *Psychosomatic and symbolic aspects of menstruation.* Retrieved September 24, 2004, from: http://www158.pair.com/hfinley/psychos.

Speroff, L., & Fritz, M. (2005). *Clinical gynecologic endocrinology and infertility* (7th ed.). Philadelphia: Lippincott Williams & Wilkins.

Stenchever, M. A., Droegemueller, W., Herbst, A. L., & Mishell, D. R. (2001). Reproductive anatomy. In *Comprehensive gynecology* (4th ed., pp. 39–68). St. Louis, MO: Mosby.

Tabibzadeh, S. (1996). The signals and molecular pathways involved in human menstruation: A unique process of tissue destruction and remodeling. *Molecular Human Reproduction, 2,* 77–92.

Van De Graff, K. M. (1988). *Human anatomy* (2nd ed., pp. 666–678). Dubuque, IA: Wm. C. Brown.

Chapter 6

GYNECOLOGIC HISTORY AND PHYSICAL EXAMINATION

DEBORAH NARRIGAN

The word gynecology derives from the Greek term gyne meaning "woman—more as queen" and is defined as "a branch of medicine that deals with the diseases and routine physical care of the reproductive system of women" (Merriam-Webster's Collegiate Dictionary, 2001, p. 518). If providers apply this definition of gynecology in practice, then patients will be cared for as royalty. Elevated to a high place, each woman will hold the center of the provider's attention and receive expert, respectful care.

Gynecologic care occurs for two main reasons: to enhance or maintain health and to identify and treat a problem of the reproductive system. This chapter presents the core knowledge and skill base for the gynecologic health history and physical examination. Often the gynecologic examination is embedded in a clinical visit with a wider focus on primary care screening and counseling (see Chapter 7).

HEALTH HISTORY

The purpose of the health history is to establish a relationship with a woman while learning about her health. To a great extent, taking a health history means listening to her story. Both the content and the manner of what she conveys provide important information for a clinician's understanding of what an individual woman wants and needs. To optimize health history taking, several environmental and logistical arrangements should be consistently in place. These include providing a comfortable and private setting, scheduling an appropriate amount of time, and choosing the optimal format and staff member for obtaining the health history.

Privacy is an essential condition for obtaining the health history. Ideally the room or office where the history is taken has a door that can be closed so no noise or traffic interrupts the interview. A closed door ensures confidentiality and conveys the clinician's intent to offer undivided attention to the patient. The woman should remain fully clothed. The provider and patient should be seated a comfortable distance from each other, preferably at a 45° angle, without furniture between them. This seating arrangement promotes a conversational, rather than a confrontational or hierarchical, approach. If an interpreter is present, he or she should be seated so that all three persons can see and hear each other.

Generally the optimal way to gather the health history is to interview the woman alone, because distractions are minimized and privacy is ensured. If however, the patient prefers to have a spouse, friend, or other person with her, she should have this choice. If young children are present, a second adult should be available to attend to them.

If the woman has another person present during the health history, it is essential that at some point the patient is given the opportunity to speak privately with the clinician. This practice is advisable for handling topics that the provider or patient find sensitive, such as the patient's sexual health history. It also allows the clinician to ensure that the choice to have the other adult present was made freely by the woman. For adolescents accompanied by parents or guardians, this policy is particularly important.

Try to listen intently.

> Learn how to listen while being still, achieving 'intellectual repose'. This will help the listener be open to all the messages in the patient's words and body talk. . . . Every one of the interviewer's behaviors should contribute to the communication of empathy and the building of trust essential to a therapeutic partnership. (Seidel, Ball, Dains, & Benedict, 2003, p. 6)

Schedule an appropriate amount of time to allow a woman being seen for an initial visit to tell her story in an unhurried manner. This approach generally yields a rich and pertinent database. Structure the interview around standard questions (Boxes 6–1 and 6–2), but encourage responses to be open ended. The reality of time pressure in ambulatory care settings may make an allocation of 20–30 minutes for obtaining a health history seem like a luxury, but it should be considered a key to excellent care. Many clinicians posit that 90% of the information needed for accurate diagnosis comes directly from the health history.

Choices of format used for obtaining the health history are plentiful, ranging from a self-administered questionnaire to a conversation between the clinician and patient, with information recorded on a prepared form. Trade-offs are obvious in these alternatives. Disadvantages to self-administered health questionnaires include that answers to items may be omitted, questions misunderstood, or terms will be unfamiliar to the respondent. In addition, the entire questionnaire will require visual and verbal review by a nurse or the provider to fill in missing information and clarify answers. Advantages include that some persons may disclose more freely on sensitive topics in writing than if asked verbally, and the total time for this procedure may be less than if all information is obtained in an interview. Regardless which staff person is responsible for obtaining the health history, whoever conducts the interview should be skilled at putting the patient at ease, and in conveying respectful attention through his or her verbal style and behavior.

BOX 6-1   GENERAL HEALTH HISTORY

Reason patient desires care (chief concern)
History of present illness
General medical history
    Current illnesses and diseases
    Past hospitalizations
    Prior surgical procedures
    Immunization status
    Previous serious illnesses
Medications and allergies
    Current medications
    Medication and other allergies
Substance use
    Tobacco
    Alcohol
    Illicit substances
Family health history
    Illnesses and causes of death of first-degree relatives
    Congenital malformations and unexplained mental retardation
Social and occupational history
Safety
Personal habits

GENERAL HEALTH HISTORY

Initially the interviewer briefly introduces herself or himself, states the purposes of the interview, and invites questions from the woman at any point during the visit. The interviewer proceeds next to checking basic demographic data, which is less personal and helps to put the patient at ease.

Reason Patient Desires Care/Chief Concern   Asking, "How may I help you today?" or "What has brought you here today?" are good ways to begin determining what is traditionally referred to as the chief complaint. The woman should be encouraged to describe the problem or reason for the visit in her own words. For example, "I think I want to change from pills to an IUD." She should be interrupted only for specific clarification or to bring her back to the topic if she seems to be digressing too far (Stenchever, Droegmueller, Herbst, & Mishell, 2001).

History of Present Illness   When the woman has finished describing the reason for her visit, the interviewer will need to "give structure to the present problem. . . giving it a chronologic and sequential framework. . . probing for the underlying concerns" (Seidel et al., 2003, p. 17). To maximize understanding of the patient's problem, the health care provider should be sure he or she has answers to the following relevant questions:

1. What were the circumstances at the time the problem started?
2. What has been the sequence of events for symptoms?
3. Has the problem occurred before? If so, what were the circumstances of the previous occurrence and what led to its disappearance?
4. To what extent is the problem interfering with daily life or relationships?
5. What questions does the patient want answered today? What is the patient expecting from today's visit?
6. Have other steps been taken to solve the problem? If so, what were they and how effective have they been?

General Medical History   The woman will need to list any significant health problems she has had in her lifetime, including all hospitalizations and surgical procedures. In addition, the interviewer should ask about specific illnesses that occur frequently, such as diabetes, hypertension, respiratory illnesses, infectious diseases, and mental health problems. A review of adult immunizations is also necessary.

Medications and Allergies   Review all medications the woman is currently taking, including over-the-counter preparations and complementary therapies, and reasons for their use. If she cannot recall the name of a medication she is using, encourage her to bring the package to the next visit. Describe allergic responses to medications, foods, or other substances.

Substance Use   Perhaps the easiest way to proceed with this topic is to inquire about each substance separately, beginning with the legal and most commonly used—tobacco—continuing to alcohol, and ending with illicit substances. When inquiring about tobacco use, find out if she has smoked or is currently smoking, daily number of cigarettes, length of time smoked, number of attempts at quitting, and interest in quitting now. Then ask about alcohol use, again determining amount and type used per day or week, and binge drinking habits. For illicit substances, inquire about types, amount, route, and frequency of use. For interviewers new to the process, positive answers to these questions may elicit surprise or concern, but this is not the time to intervene with counseling. The interviewer needs to stay focused on gathering information. See Chapter 7 for further discussion of screening for substance use.

Family Health History   Gather information about first-degree relatives: parents, grandparents, siblings, and children. A family tree or narrative can be recorded, and information on serious illnesses and causes of death for each of these individuals should be obtained. In addition, occurrences of congenital malformations, unexplained mental retardation, or other disabilities should be covered to offer clues to possible inherited diseases.

Social and Occupational History   Ask the woman about her highest educational level attained, marital status/significant relationships, and employment or vocational history. Information about housing, financial status, family relationships, and potential and actual stressors or social problems should also be elicited.

Safety   Safety issues, primarily the use of seat belts in motor vehicles, and helmets with bicycle or motorcycle use should be checked, as well as presence of firearms in the patient's household. Inquiring about current or past intimate partner violence is often included, but at present it is not clear whether gathering this information from all women should be standard practice (see Chapters 7 and 12).

Personal Habits   Ask the woman about her exercise, sleep, and nutritional patterns.

GYNECOLOGIC HEALTH HISTORY

The gynecologic health history elicits significant details about the woman's reproductive biology that then provide the essential background for the problem-oriented encounter, as well as for a health maintenance visit for a well woman. The standard topics for this health history are listed in Box 6–2. Specific points that should be included about each topic follow.

Menstrual History   The menstrual history is usually the first topic in the gynecologic history, and should cover the following information: age at menarche; length of the cycle, counting from the first day of one menstrual flow until the first day of the next menstrual flow; average number of days of menses; characteristics of the menstrual flow; regularity of cycles; and description of any irregularities and/or accompanying symptoms. In general, cycles range from 21–35 days, and menses last 4–7 days.

BOX 6–2   GYNECOLOGIC HEALTH HISTORY

Menstrual history
Pregnancy history
History of vaginal and pelvic infections
Douching
Gynecologic surgical procedures
Urologic health
Cervical cancer screening
Sexual health
Contraceptive use
Abnormal symptoms

BOX 6–3 GTPAL SYSTEM FOR RECORDING PREGNANCY HISTORY

G—Gravida or pregnancy, the total number of pregnancies the woman has had

T—Term births, those occurring from 37–42 weeks gestation

P—Preterm births, those occurring after the point of viability, which is usually interpreted as gestational age greater than 20 weeks and less than 37 weeks and/or fetal weight greater than 500 grams

A—Abortions, spontaneous and elective terminations prior to 20 weeks gestation

L—Living children

Pregnancy History Begin by asking the patient the total number of times she has been pregnant. Then ask her to describe each pregnancy in chronologic order. As the woman explains her pregnancy history, the interviewer will not only make written notes, but will also complete the GTPAL five-digit numeric summary description of pregnancies (Box 6–3). Specific information to obtain for each pregnancy includes the year it occurred, its duration, type of birth (spontaneous vaginal birth, assisted vaginal birth, or caesarean), gender and weight of the newborn, complications, and whether the child is alive and well now. The category of abortion includes information about elective pregnancy terminations, spontaneous abortions, ectopic pregnancies, and molar pregnancies. For these pregnancies, details of gestational age, procedure, complications, and outcome should be recorded.

History of Vaginal and Pelvic Infections Ask what types of infections, if any, the patient has had; what treatments she has received; how frequently each infection has occurred; and what, if any, complications have occurred. Screening for HIV risk can be done at this point. Ask the woman the number of sexual partners she has at present and has had during her lifetime. Inquire if she is sexually active with persons who present high risk for HIV transmission and whether she uses condoms. Detailed assessment of sexual risk is described in Chapter 18.

Douching Ask the woman about frequency, medication or solutions used, and reasons for douching.

Gynecologic Surgical Procedures Include information on minor procedures such as endometrial biopsies and laparoscopic examinations, as well as major procedures including female circumcision (Box 6–4). The information needed includes year of the procedure, indication, significant complications, and outcome. Obtaining pertinent medical records may also be useful if the patient cannot supply sufficient information.

Urologic Health Topics include the occurrence and frequency of bladder infections, renal infections, incontinence, or other abnormal symptoms.

BOX 6–4   FEMALE CIRCUMCISION

Female circumcision, also known as female genital cutting or mutilation, comprises all procedures involving partial or total removal of the external female genitalia or intentional injury to the female genital organs (World Health Organization, 2000). Circumcisions are classified as follows, from the least to the most extensive excisions:

- *Type I*—Excision of the prepuce, with partial or total excision of the clitoris
- *Type II*—Excision of the clitoris with partial or total excision of the labia minora
- *Type III*—Excision of part or all of the external genitalia and stitching and narrowing of the vaginal opening (infibulation)
- *Type IV*—Other types of genital injuries such as piercing, stretching, and burning

Long-term sequelae of female circumcision include urinary problems, scarring, pain, infertility, and obstetric complications (Nour, 2004; Toubia, 1999; World Health Organization, 2001).

Women may not disclose during the health history that they have been circumcised for a variety of reasons, including fear that the clinician will disapprove or respond negatively to this information. If a woman does disclose that she is circumcised, it may be in describing associated complications noted previously. A woman may also provide this information in response to an open-ended question such as, "Is there anything else you would like me to know about your health background before we begin your examination?" It is important for the clinician to ask when the circumcision occurred, whether the woman has previously had a pelvic examination, and if she is experiencing symptoms of long-term sequelae.

The extent of circumcision will be determined during the inspection of the external genitalia. A pediatric speculum and single digit bimanual examination may be necessary for pelvic examination. A special form for recording health history and physical findings relevant to female circumcision can be helpful (see Campbell, 2004 for a sample form).

Cervical Cancer Screening   Determine whether the patient has had previous cervical cytology screening. If so, find out the approximate date of the last test and whether any have been abnormal. For a woman who has had an abnormal cervical cancer screening result, ask what follow-up occurred, and whether subsequent screening results have been normal.

Sexual Health   Ask if the patient is sexually active and if so, determine whether this is with men, women, or both; whether she is satisfied with her sexual function; and whether she or her partner or partners have any concerns or problems. Further information about assessment of sexual health can be found in Chapter 8.

Contraceptive Use   The contraceptive history is obtained from heterosexual, sexually active women. Determine if she or her partner is currently using a contraceptive method, whether she is satisfied with the method or desires a change, or if she has questions about her current method. Discussing past methods used may be relevant depending on the patient's reason for the visit.

Abnormal Symptoms   Problems such as pelvic pain should be fully described, noting relationship in time with the menstrual cycle, and association with coitus, tampon use, or other factors. Additionally, any vaginal bleeding not related to menstrual flow should be fully described. See Chapters 20 and 25 for detailed information about the assessment of bleeding and pelvic pain.

FINAL STEPS

Closure of the health history should include offering the woman the chance to add comments or ask questions. One approach is simply to say, "I have finished with my questions about your health. Is there anything I have omitted or not covered, or that you would like to add to help me better understand your health or problem today?"

Once the health care provider has completed taking the health history, the next step is to begin to examine, sort, and prioritize the information gathered; and to decide what further assessment measures, such as laboratory tests, are needed. It is often helpful at this time to summarize the findings and offer tentative answers to questions or concerns posed by the patient about her health. An example would be to say, "At this point I think you would be a good candidate for an IUD, but I'd like to wait to discuss this further after I do your physical examination." This type of statement emphasizes the patient and provider's partnership in her care.

PHYSICAL EXAMINATION FOR A GYNECOLOGIC VISIT

Evaluating a new patient usually includes performing a physical examination. The details and description of the techniques, such as auscultation, are beyond the scope of this chapter. Readers are referred to textbooks on physical examination for a review of maneuvers, equipment, and organization of the examination (Bickley, 2004; Seidel et al., 2003). This text assumes that the age range for patients will extend from adolescence through the older adult, or from about 12–70 years of age. Care outside this age range requires specialized pediatric or geriatric skills that go beyond the scope of this chapter.

What constitutes a complete physical examination in the ambulatory gynecology or primary care setting is not standardized. It is customary to evaluate major organ systems briefly and carefully, but not exhaustively. For example, the cardiovascular examination would include complete auscultation of the heart, evaluation of circulation by noting skin color, but would usually omit other maneuvers, such as checking carotid bruits, or palpation of the precordium. When deciding what to include in the physical examination, a principle for novice practitioners to use is: be able to state the rationale for including or excluding any assessment maneuver or particular feature of any organ system. If a rationale for performing any maneuver and obtaining the specific information that maneuver provides can be stated, then including it would be justified.

GENERAL PHYSICAL EXAMINATION

The order of the examination presented below assumes the patient is sitting up to begin the examination. This description proceeds from head to toe, rather than by system.

1. Physical measurements—Obtain and review height, weight, blood pressure, pulse, and temperature (if indicated), before performing the physical examination. Height and weight are most useful when converted to the body mass index (BMI) using Table 6–1. Both BMI and blood pressure should be considered screening tools (see Chapter 7 for further discussion).
2. General appearance—Observe the patient for posture, striking or obvious characteristics or limitations, general emotional state, appropriateness of dress, speech pattern, and social interaction during the visit.
3. Eyes, ears, nose, and throat—Inspect the physical health of eyes, nose, and ears. Examination of the ears with the otoscope, and examination of the eyes with the ophthalmoscope may be performed as indicated. The oropharynx examination includes inspection of the lips, teeth, and gums for dental health, and visualization of the oral cavity for mucosal color, lesions, and tonsillar edema or exudates.
4. Neck—Note range of motion and palpate lymph nodes in the neck and clavicular area.
5. Thyroid—Palpate the gland and isthmus.
6. Chest and lungs—Auscultate the posterior, lateral, and anterior lobes.
7. Spine—Palpate vertebral column, inspect skin.
8. Kidneys—Check costovertebral tenderness.
9. Reflexes—Elicit patellar and additional reflexes as indicated.
10. Peripheral circulation and varicosities—Inspect legs and feet.

Patient then reclines:

11. Heart—Auscultate.
12. Breasts and axillary lymph nodes—See below.
13. Abdomen—Inspect skin, palpate superficially and deeply in all quadrants, and palpate inguinal lymph nodes.

BREAST EXAMINATION

Despite controversy regarding the efficacy of self-breast examination, clinical breast examination performed by health professionals remains a part of the general physical examination (see Chapter 7 for further discussion of breast cancer screening). It is relatively simple and quick, and involves only two types of maneuvers: inspection and palpation. Conditions that promote ease and accuracy in findings are also simple. Adequate lighting helps to reveal subtle variations in skin texture and color. Adequate exposure, or having the

TABLE 6–1   Body Mass Index

Body Mass Index Table

Body Weight (pounds)

Height (inches) / BMI	Normal						Overweight					Obese										Extreme Obesity														
BMI	19	20	21	22	23	24	25	26	27	28	29	30	31	32	33	34	35	36	37	38	39	40	41	42	43	44	45	46	47	48	49	50	51	52	53	54
58	91	96	100	105	110	115	119	124	129	134	138	143	148	153	158	162	167	172	177	181	186	191	196	201	205	210	215	220	224	229	234	239	244	248	253	258
59	94	99	104	109	114	119	124	128	133	138	143	148	153	158	163	168	173	178	183	188	193	198	203	208	212	217	222	227	232	237	242	247	252	257	262	267
60	97	102	107	112	118	123	128	133	138	143	148	153	158	163	168	174	179	184	189	194	199	204	209	215	220	225	230	235	240	245	250	255	261	266	271	276
61	100	106	111	116	122	127	132	137	143	148	153	158	164	169	174	180	185	190	195	201	206	211	217	222	227	232	238	243	248	254	259	264	269	275	280	285
62	104	109	115	120	126	131	136	142	147	153	158	164	169	175	180	186	191	196	202	207	213	218	224	229	235	240	246	251	256	262	267	273	278	284	289	295
63	107	113	118	124	130	135	141	146	152	158	163	169	175	180	186	191	197	203	208	214	220	225	231	237	242	248	254	259	265	270	278	282	287	293	299	304
64	110	116	122	128	134	140	145	151	157	163	169	174	180	186	192	197	204	209	215	221	227	232	238	244	250	256	262	267	273	279	285	291	296	302	308	314
65	114	120	126	132	138	144	150	156	162	168	174	180	186	192	198	204	210	216	222	228	234	240	246	252	258	264	270	276	282	288	294	300	306	312	318	324
66	118	124	130	136	142	148	155	161	167	173	179	186	192	198	204	210	216	223	229	235	241	247	253	260	266	272	278	284	291	297	303	309	315	322	328	334
67	121	127	134	140	146	153	159	166	172	178	185	191	198	204	211	217	223	230	236	242	249	255	261	268	274	280	287	293	299	306	312	319	325	331	338	344
68	125	131	138	144	151	158	164	171	177	184	190	197	203	210	216	223	230	236	243	249	256	262	269	276	282	289	295	302	308	315	322	328	335	341	348	354
69	128	135	142	149	155	162	169	176	182	189	196	203	209	216	223	230	236	243	250	257	263	270	277	284	291	297	304	311	318	324	331	338	345	351	358	365
70	132	139	146	153	160	167	174	181	188	195	202	209	216	222	229	236	243	250	257	264	271	278	285	292	299	306	313	320	327	334	341	348	355	362	369	376
71	136	143	150	157	165	172	179	186	193	200	208	215	222	229	236	243	250	257	265	272	279	286	293	301	308	315	322	329	338	343	351	358	365	372	379	386
72	140	147	154	162	169	177	184	191	199	206	213	221	228	235	242	250	258	265	272	279	287	294	302	309	316	324	331	338	346	353	361	368	375	383	390	397
73	144	151	159	166	174	182	189	197	204	212	219	227	235	242	250	257	265	272	280	288	295	302	310	318	325	333	340	348	355	363	371	378	386	393	401	408
74	148	155	163	171	179	186	194	202	210	218	225	233	241	249	256	264	272	280	287	295	303	311	319	326	334	342	350	358	365	373	381	389	396	404	412	420
75	152	160	168	176	184	192	200	208	216	224	232	240	248	256	264	272	279	287	295	303	311	319	327	335	343	351	359	367	375	383	391	399	407	415	423	431
76	156	164	172	180	189	197	205	213	221	230	238	246	254	263	271	279	287	295	304	312	320	328	336	344	353	361	369	377	385	394	402	410	418	426	435	443

Source: National Heart, Lung, and Blood Institute as a part of the National Institutes of Health and the U.S. Department of Health and Human Services.

woman disrobe to the waist, allows simultaneous observation and comparison of both breasts. Modesty may be a concern for some women. Explaining why this exposure is needed and employing an approach that is gentle but focused on the examination conveys the provider's concern and respect.

Breast Inspection   This maneuver begins with the patient sitting, usually on the examining table, with arms relaxed at her sides, and the examiner standing facing her. Look at each breast and compare them for size, symmetry, contour, skin color, texture, venous patterns, and lesions. Lift the breast with fingertips to inspect the lower and lateral aspects. Breasts vary in shape, and frequently one will be slightly larger than the other. Skin texture should be smooth, contours uninterrupted bilaterally, and venous patterning similar in both breasts. Benign lesions, such as nevi, if longstanding, unchanged, and nontender, are considered normal findings.

Next, inspect the nipples and areolae. The areolae should be round or oval, and bilaterally nearly equal in configuration with a smooth surface. Color ranges from pink to black. Montgomery's tubercles, very small sebaceous glands, may be seen as slightly raised fleshy protuberances, and are a common finding. The nipples also should be equal or nearly equal in size. Most nipples are everted. If one or both are inverted, ask if inversion has been a lifelong characteristic. A newly inverted nipple suggests pathology. A second abnormal finding to note is nipple retraction, or a flattening of the nipple. Look also at the orientation of the nipples. If one points in a different direction from the other, this may be caused by the presence of malignant tissue in the breast. The color of the nipples should be the same as the areolae, while the surface may be smooth or wrinkled and should be without discharge. Supernumerary or extra nipples may also be seen. They are benign, usually small, and are commonly mistaken as moles. They may occur anywhere along a vertical line from the axilla to the inner thigh and are usually unilateral.

The last step in inspection in the sitting position is to have the woman change positions slightly so that the contour and symmetry of the breasts can be assessed completely. The three positions for examination while seated are arms over the head, hands pressed against the hips, and leaning forward at the waist.

Breast Palpation   The patient remains sitting with arms resting freely at her sides. The examiner remains standing facing her. Palpate all four quadrants for nodules and lumps. Use the finger pads because they are more sensitive to touch than fingertips. Press firmly enough to get a good sense of underlying tissue but not so firmly that the tissue is compressed against the rib cage. Rotate the fingers in a clockwise or counter-clockwise direction. Palpating systematically is key to performing a complete examination. Two commonly used patterns for breast palpation are concentric circles starting from the outer edge and spiraling inward to the nipple, and top to bottom in vertical strips. For this latter pattern begin at the top, palpate downward and then upward, working gradually over the entire breast. Either pattern is acceptable as long as the entire breast is palpated.

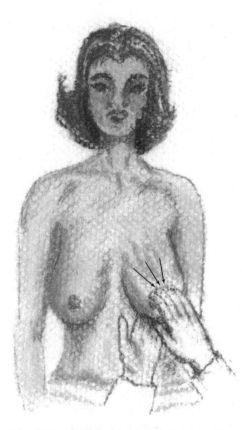

FIGURE 6-1 Palpating Large Breasts *Illustrator:* Marie Hall

Do a complete light palpation followed by a deep palpation. Be aware that a firm transverse ridge of compressed tissue is often found along the lower edge of the breast. This is the inframammary ridge and is a normal finding. For large breasts it may be helpful to place one hand beneath the breast to stabilize it while palpating with the other hand (Figure 6–1).

Breast tissue in adult women feels dense, firm, and elastic. Prior to and during menstruation some women experience cyclical tenderness, swelling, and nodularity. If a mass is felt, note the location, size, shape, consistency, tenderness, mobility, and demarcation of borders.

The Tail of Spence, breast tissue that extends from the upper outer quadrant toward the axilla, must also be palpated because most malignancies develop in the upper outer quadrant (Seidel et al., 2003). This is best done by having the woman raise her arms over her head while the examiner gently compresses the tissue where it enters the axilla between thumb and fingers (Figure 6–2).

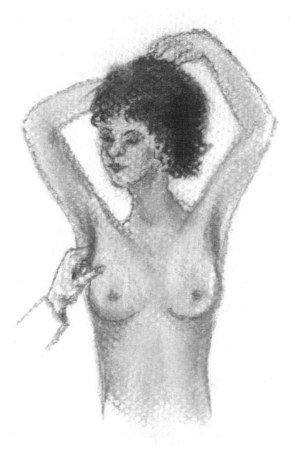

FIGURE 6-2   Palpating the Tail of Spence Illustrator: Marie Hall

Palpation now continues with the woman supine. Place a small pillow or folded towel under the shoulder before beginning the examination of the breast on that side. Use the same palpation technique and pattern for the supine as for the sitting position. Repeat the examination with the woman's arm at her side. This repetition aids in a complete palpation because breast tissue shifts with different positions. After the entire breast is palpated, the nipple should also be gently palpated. Compress the nipple between thumb and index finger to inspect for discharge. This usually causes the nipple to become erect, and may be momentarily painful.

Examination of Lymph Nodes   Have the patient sit with arms flexed at the elbow. The examiner is standing, facing the patient, but is slightly off center. If beginning with the right axilla, use the left hand. Reach deeply into the axillary hollow and press firmly upward with the palmar surfaces of the fingers. Then bring the fingers downward to gently roll the soft tissue against the chest wall. Be sure to examine not only the apex, but also the central and medial aspects along the rib cage, the lateral aspect along the medial surface of the arm, the anterior wall along the pectoral muscles, and the posterior wall along the border of the scapula. Repeat this procedure with the other axilla. Axillary lymph nodes are usually not palpable in adults. The supraclavicular area should also be palpated. Hook the fingers over the clavicle and rotate them over the entire supraclavicular area.

THE PELVIC EXAMINATION

The pelvic examination customarily concludes the physical examination. The description offered here assumes the reader is familiar with the anatomy of the pelvic structures, particularly the reproductive organs, both internal and external (see Chapter 5). A few features of these structures, such as their size and relative locations, are particularly pertinent to performing this examination easily and successfully.

Few experiences that women encounter in the evaluation of their health are as intimate and thus potentially anxiety producing as this examination. All providers who perform the pelvic examination have the professional responsibility to carry it out proficiently, promptly, and respectfully. Each woman brings her own past experiences and her own needs to the present examination. Specific conditions that generally enhance the experience include:

1. Before starting the examination, and at several points during it, explain in general what you are going to do before you do it.
2. Use language that can be understood by the patient. Use common words, not medical terms.
3. Ask the patient if she has any special concerns or questions.
4. Never talk lightly or make jokes about genitalia or the examination. This is entirely inappropriate.
5. Maintain eye contact during the examination as much as is possible, recognizing that women from many cultural groups may not return eye contact. In addition, if the examiner encounters an unexpected finding, conscious attempts should be made to avoid expressing surprise in facial expression or voice, as this will usually raise anxiety. If it is feasible, wait until the examination is completed to discuss the finding. If assistance is needed from another health professional to evaluate an abnormal or unexpected finding, briefly explain the finding and the reason for a second examiner's assessment.
6. Assure the woman that the examination will proceed as gently as possible and ask her to indicate if and when she feels discomfort.
7. Be sure the examination room is a comfortable temperature.
8. Ensure privacy for this examination. Close, or preferably lock, the door to the room.
9. Invite the patient to have someone accompany her for support during the examination if she desires.
10. The health care provider may or may not have an assistant. If the provider is male, it is often policy to have a female assistant present as a legal protection for both patient and provider.

Preparing and Beginning the Pelvic Examination

1. Encourage the patient to empty her bladder for two reasons. First, bimanual examination can be very uncomfortable with a full bladder. Second, a full bladder makes palpation of pelvic organs difficult.
2. Offer the patient the option of a drape. It provides some privacy and warmth and may facilitate her relaxing, but some women may find it intrusive or unnecessary. Its use is optional.
3. Raise the top portion of the examination table to at least 30° and have a pillow at the head of the table. These measures add to patient comfort as well as making it easier for the provider to maintain eye contact with the patient once the examination is in progress.
4. Assist the patient into the lithotomy position, first helping stabilize her feet in the footrests. Place one hand at the edge of the table and instruct her to move down, being sure her buttocks are slightly beyond the edge of the examination table. This detail is important to allow correct positioning of the speculum.
5. After making sure that all examination materials are prepared and within easy reach, wash your hands. Seat yourself on a stool so you are at eye level with the perineum. Don latex or nonlatex gloves (depending on clinician or patient allergy) and start the examination.
6. Ask the patient to separate her legs. Never try to spread her legs, even gently. It is sometimes helpful to touch the *outside* of the woman's knees or thighs and ask her to open her legs toward the examiner's hands. Adjust the light so it illuminates the perineal and vaginal area.
7. The examination is intrusive. Wait a moment until both the examiner and patient are ready, and then tell her the examination will begin. Start with a firm touch of one gloved hand on one of the patient's lower thighs, and then move the examining hand along the thigh toward the external genitalia.
8. If the patient becomes tense or upset during the examination, stop and find out what the problem is. Tell her the examination will not continue until she is at ease. Then make any adjustments that will enable her to cope with the examination before continuing.

Inspection and Palpation of External Genitalia, Vaginal Orifice, and Accessory Glands

1. Inspect, and then palpate the mons pubis, labia majora, and perineum, noting pattern of hair distribution, size and shape of the labia, presence of lesions, scars, rashes, erythema, discharge, or discoloration.
2. Separate the labia majora, inspect and palpate the labia minora, and inspect the urethral orifice and clitoris.
3. Inspect and palpate the vaginal introitus (opening) for presence or absence of the hymen and shape of the opening; note swelling, discharge, or lesions.
4. Insert the index and third fingers to the second joint into the vagina, and press down gently against the posterior vaginal wall. To assess for cystocele, ask the woman to cough or bear down. If she has a cystocele, the anterior vaginal wall will bulge with

this maneuver. Many parous women have a first-degree cystocele. Observe also for rectocele, or bulging of the posterior vaginal wall. This is an abnormal and far less common finding.

5. To assess the tone of the perineal muscles, ask the woman to tighten her muscles around your vaginal examining fingers.

6. Palpate the Bartholin's glands by inserting the index finger of the examining hand about 2 cm into the vagina, turn the hand laterally and gently palpate the tissue behind the vaginal wall between the thumb and index finger on one side, and then rotating the examining hand, palpate in the same manner on the other side of the vagina. Healthy Bartholin's glands are not palpable, but if they are inflamed this maneuver elicits notable pain. If a cyst is present, a fluctuant, nontender mass will be palpable.

7. Palpation of the Skene's glands that lie immediately lateral to the urethral meatus is rapidly performed by turning the examining hand upward and then inserting the index finger into the vagina to the second knuckle and pressing gently upward, then sliding this finger outward. Discharge at the urethral meatus with palpation of the Skene's glands usually indicates infection. This examination lasts only about 10 seconds, but usually causes pain. Some providers think it is necessary to perform this palpation only if gonorrheal infection is suspected (Seidel et al., 2003).

Note that steps 4–7 may be performed with the bimanual examination, according to the provider's preference.

Speculum Examination   It is essential that providers become familiar with how the speculum operates before performing this examination. This ensures women do not experience inadvertent pain caused by its incorrect use. Each provider must also decide which hand to use for holding the speculum. This decision is based entirely on personal preference.

1. Select the appropriate type (Graves or Pederson) and size (pediatric, small, medium or standard, or large) of speculum (Figure 6–3). For most parous women, the standard Graves speculum is used. For very obese women with significant perineal adipose tissue or for grand multiparas, the large Graves speculum will not only allow the best visualization but will also be more comfortable. The wider blade size of the large Graves speculum more effectively holds the lax vaginal walls open, permitting visualization of the cervix. For nulliparous women, the Pederson speculum is the usual choice. Its blades are the same length as the Graves, but are narrower and flat rather than curved. This shape and size minimizes pressure on the anterior and posterior vaginal walls, promoting a more comfortable examination. Use either a plastic or metal speculum (Figure 6–3).

2. Warm the speculum by running it under warm tap water, or equip the examination table drawer with a heating pad where speculums can be stored. Lubricate the end of the speculum blades with water or a small amount (one teaspoon) of water-soluble gel. Wetting the speculum with water instead of lubricating it with water-soluble gel

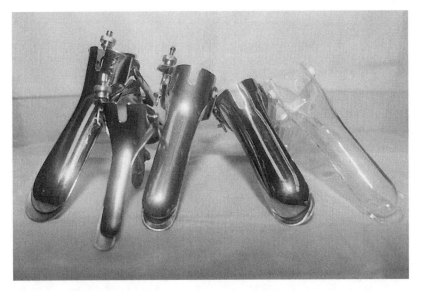

Figure 6–3   Types of Specula From left to right: metal Graves (large size), Pederson, Graves (standard size), and plastic (regular size). *Source:* Reprinted with permission from Varney, H., Kriebs, J. M., & Gegor, C. L. (2004). *Varney's midwifery* (4th ed.). Sudbury, MA: Jones and Bartlett Publishers.

has been thought to be necessary to ensure optimal collection of specimens for cervical cytology. Recently, however, a clinical study examining this practice found that using a small amount of gel on the inferior blade of the speculum does not interfere with cervical cytology specimens or results, and decreases discomfort of the speculum insertion (Amies, Miller, Lee, & Koutsky, 2002).

3. With the index and third fingers of one hand, separate the labia majora and slide these fingers slightly inside the vagina. Tell the woman she is going to feel some pressure, then press these two fingers downward. The very close proximity of the urethra to the anterior vaginal wall can lead to distinct discomfort when the speculum or examining fingers enter and exit the vagina. This maneuver allows good visualization of the opening of the vagina. With the other hand grasp the speculum with index finger over the top of the proximal end of the anterior blade and the other fingers around the handle. This position allows control of the blades as the speculum is inserted.

4. Insert the speculum into the vagina at an oblique angle. Keeping the blades closed, let them slide into the vagina following the direction of the vagina until the blades are all the way in the vagina (Figure 6–4). The length of the blades is six to seven inches, which matches the length of the vagina. Remember that when lying supine, a woman's vagina inclines posteriorly about 45° downward from the vaginal opening toward the sacrum. Keeping the blades at this angle also avoids pressure—and thus discomfort—on the urethra.

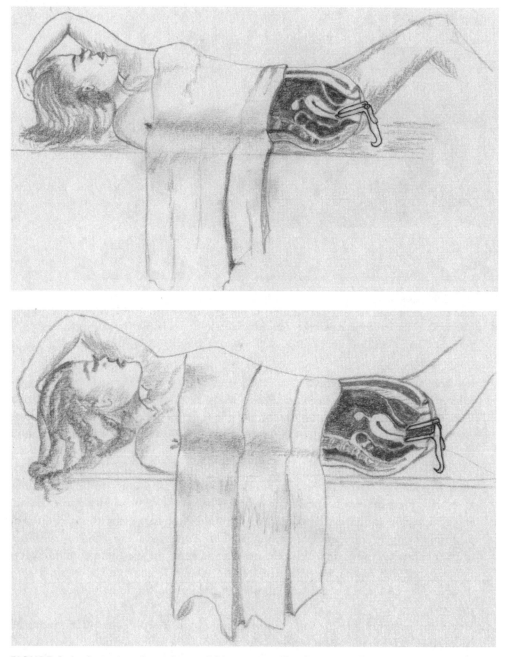

FIGURE 6–4 Speculum Insertion and Placement Top: Insertion; Bottom: Placement
Illustrator: Marie Hall

5. Now rotate the speculum horizontally and open the blades by pressing firmly and steadily on the thumbpiece. The cervix should come into view between the blades at the end of the vagina. If it is not immediately visible with the blades wide open, relax the pressure on the thumbpiece, allowing the blades to close. Then re-position the speculum. Slide the speculum partially out of the vagina, redirect the blades at a slightly different angle, and reinsert it obliquely. Open the blades and the cervix should now come into view. Adequate cervical visualization is essential for obtaining any specimens from the cervix.

6. Once the cervix is visualized, manipulate the speculum a little further into the vagina so that the cervix is well exposed. If using a metal speculum, tighten the screw on the thumbpiece. If using a plastic speculum, click the upper blade onto the notch of the handle. The speculum should remain in place so that both hands can be taken off the speculum, making possible the handling of other equipment.

Inspect the cervix for color, position, size, surface characteristics, shape of the os, and discharge. The cervix is remarkable for the vast variety of shapes, sizes, and appearances that are within the range of health. The color should be pink. Symmetric, circumscribed erythema around the os is a normal finding caused by exposing, or everting, the columnar epithelium lining of the endocervical canal. This eversion results from pressure of the speculum blades against the anterior and posterior fornices.

The position of the cervix correlates to the position of the uterus. The most common position of the cervix is posterior, indicating an anteflexed uterus. The cervix should be located in the midline; deviation may indicate a pelvic mass or adhesions. The diameter of the cervix is about 2–3 cm, and its length is about 3 cm. The os of a nulliparous woman is small and round, while a multiparous os is usually a horizontal slit or may be irregular or stellate. The surface should be smooth. Nabothian cysts may be seen as small white or yellow, raised areas; these are retention cysts of endocervical glands and are a normal variation (see Chapter 22). Note any friable tissue, granular areas, or red or white patchy areas. Note any discharge, and determine if its source is vaginal, which is far more common than from the cervix. Note the color and consistency. Normal vaginal discharge is odorless, creamy or clear, and thick or thin, depending on time in the menstrual cycle.

Three types of specimens are frequently collected at this point in the speculum examination: cervical cells for cytology screening, endocervical sampling for gonorrhea and chlamydia testing, and vaginal secretions for microscopy (see Appendices for procedures). The optimal order for collecting these specimens is unknown because no evidence exists to guide this choice. Opinions also differ among professional organizations. For example, the American College of Obstetricians and Gynecologists (ACOG) recommends collecting specimens for cervical cytology screening before samples for chlamydia and gonorrhea testing (ACOG, 2003). On the other hand, the Centers for Disease Control and Prevention (CDC) note that if a cervical cytology specimen is collected first, bleeding from this sampling could interfere with chlamydia and gonorrhea tests (CDC, 2002).

7. To begin removing a metal speculum, loosen the screw on the thumbpiece, but press on it to keep the blades open as the speculum is withdrawn from around the cervix. If using a plastic speculum, press on the thumbpiece to release it from the notch that has kept the anterior blade open. Once the cervix is no longer within the speculum blades, release most of the pressure on the thumbpiece, and rotate the speculum back to the oblique angle. As the speculum is withdrawn, inspect the vaginal walls. Note color, surface characteristics, and secretions. Vaginal mucosa should be almost the same color as the cervix, and the surface should be moist and smooth or rugated. Normal discharge will appear thin, clear or cloudy, and odorless. After inspection, continue to remove the speculum. Release all pressure on the thumbpiece and the blades will close themselves. Taking care not to pinch the vaginal mucosa, quickly and completely withdraw the speculum in an upward direction, but with downward pressure. This maneuver provides the most comfort for the patient.

8. Deposit the speculum in an appropriate container.

Bimanual Examination   Inform the woman that the next step is examining her reproductive organs internally with your fingers (Figure 6–5). This examination is most easily done with the examiner standing.

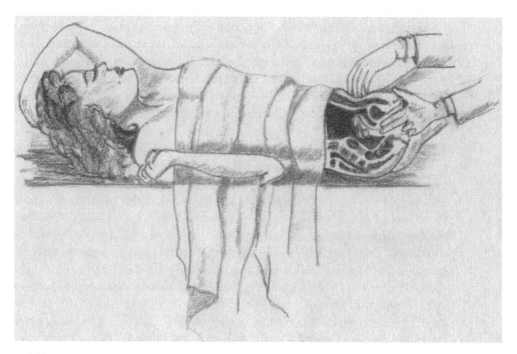

FIGURE 6-5 Bimanual Examination *Illustrator:* Marie Hall

1. Remove the glove from one hand, and lubricate the index and middle fingers of the gloved hand. Generally the dominant hand is gloved and used for the internal examination, but this is a provider preference. Place these two fingers just inside the vaginal orifice, press downward, and gently insert them their full length into the vagina.

2. As the examination continues, be careful of where the thumb of the examining hand is resting. Try to avoid touching the clitoris, which is usually very sensitive.

3. Locate and touch the end of the cervix with the palmar surface of the examining fingers, then run the examining fingers around the circumference of the cervix to feel the size, length, shape, and consistency. A nonpregnant cervix will be firm, like the tip of the nose, while during pregnancy it is softer. Note nodules, surface texture, and position.

4. Assess for cervical motion tenderness by grasping the cervix gently between the examining fingers, moving it from side to side once, and observing the woman for any expression of pain or discomfort. The cervix should move 1–2 cm laterally without discomfort. Painful cervical movement suggests a pelvic inflammatory process.

5. Begin palpation of the uterus by placing the ungloved hand on the abdomen, half way between the umbilicus and the pubis at the midline. Place the intravaginal fingers in front of the cervix in the anterior fornix. Slowly slide the abdominal hand down toward the pubis, pressing downward and forward with the flat surface of all four fingers. At the same time, press upward with the vaginal fingers. This combination of abdominal and vaginal pressure will feel as if the two hands are pressing against each other. The uterus is relatively mobile, usually inclines forward at about 45°, and is essentially flat. It measures about 5–8 cm long, 3.5–5 cm wide, and about 2–3 cm thick. If the uterus is anteflexed or anteverted (Figure 6–6), the fundus will be palpable between the fingers of the two hands at the level of the pubis.

6. If with the previous maneuver the uterus cannot be palpated, place the vaginal fingers together in the posterior fornix with the abdominal hand at the pubis. Press firmly downward with the abdominal fingers. With the vaginal fingers turned upward, press up against the cervix moving it inward. If the uterus is retroverted (Figure 6–6), the fundus should be palpable with this maneuver.

7. If the uterus still is not palpated, move the vaginal fingers to the sides of the cervix pressing the cervix inward as far as is possible. Then move one finger on top and the other beneath the cervix, continuing to press inward, while pressing down with the abdominal fingers. If the uterus is in the midposition (Figure 6–6), it is not possible to palpate the fundus with the abdominal hand. Confirm the location of the uterus as midline, regardless of its anterior, midposition, or posterior position. Also palpate the uterus for size, contour, and consistency. It should feel smooth, firm, round, and flat. It should be mobile in the anterior-posterior plane. This examination should not cause pain, although a sensation of pressure is common.

8. Now continue the bimanual examination by palpating the ovaries and surrounding area, called the adnexae. This term refers to both the areas lateral to the uterus, which are taken up by the broad ligaments, and to the structures located there. Move the abdominal hand to the right lower quadrant. The vaginal fingers remain facing

A

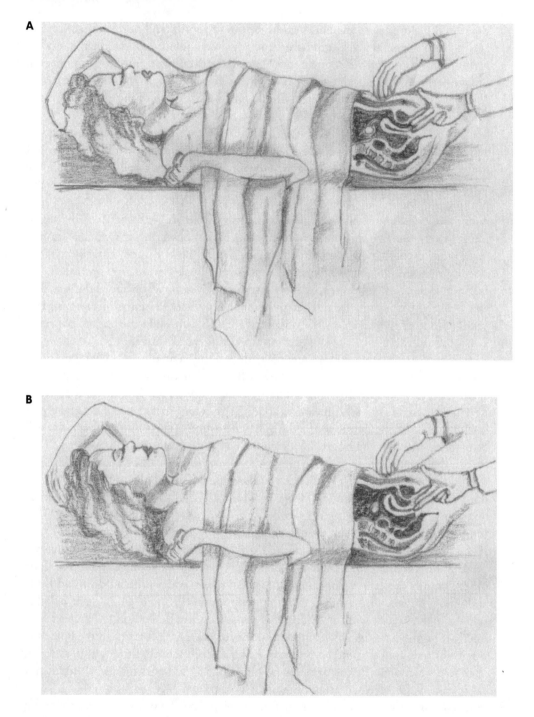

B

Figure 6–6   Variations in Uterine Position A: Anteverted; B: Anteflexed *Illustrator:* Marie Hall
(continues)
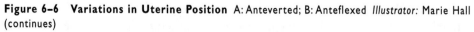

C

D

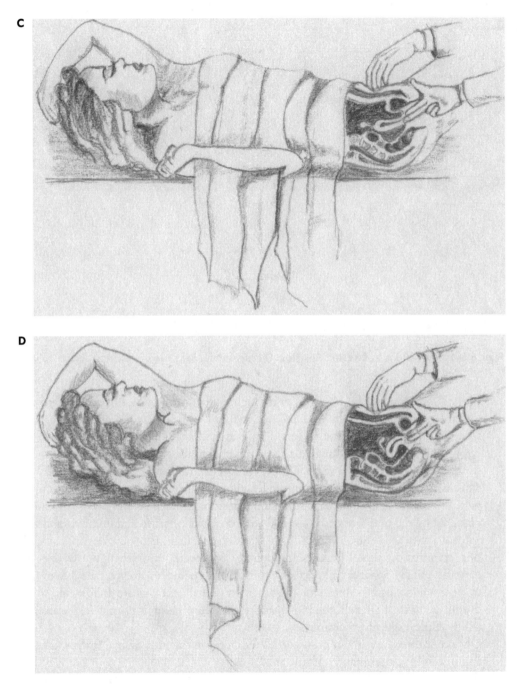

Figure 6–6   Variations in Uterine Position C: Retroverted; D: Retroflexed *Illustrator:* Marie Hall
(continues)

E

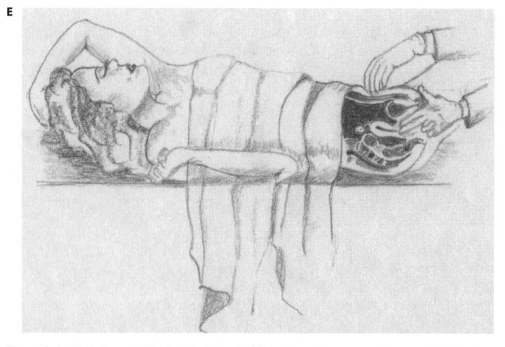

Figure 6–6 Variations in Uterine Position E: Midposition of the uterus *Illustrator:* Marie Hall

upward, but now put both fingers in the right lateral fornix. Press deeply inward and upward toward the abdominal hand. At the same time, with the abdominal hand, sweep the flat surface of the fingers deeply inward and obliquely down toward the pubis. Palpate the entire area in this manner, repeating this sweeping movement, while at the same time the vaginal fingers press upward, inward, and slide downward. This maneuver will be repeated on the left side. Often normal ovaries are difficult to palpate because they are small, sometimes positioned deep in the pelvis, or can be obscured by the presence of abdominal adipose tissue or tense abdominal muscles. If palpable, they are about 3 × 2 × 1 cm, smooth and firm. If the ovaries are palpable, this examination usually causes momentary moderate pain when the ovaries are located. Usually no other adnexal structures are palpable. However, palpable ovaries in post-menopausal women are reason for concern and require follow-up. If the ovaries are not felt after thorough palpation, the examination is normal in the absence of any clinical signs or symptoms.

9. Once the adnexal examination is completed, remove the intravaginal fingers, take off and discard the examination glove.

Rectovaginal Examination This part of the pelvic examination allows palpation to a depth of an additional 2.5 cm, facilitating a more complete evaluation of some pelvic structures.

It is usually an uncomfortable examination, but once mastered, can be very rapidly completed. Many health care providers omit this examination because the vaginal examination has allowed for sufficient palpation of reproductive organs and because digital rectal examination is an inadequate screening strategy for colorectal cancer screening (United States Preventive Services Task Force [USPSTF], 2002). This examination is perhaps most useful if the uterus is retroflexed or retroverted.

1. Before beginning, tell the patient that the rectum and vagina will be briefly examined. Inform her that this may be uncomfortable and may also cause a sensation similar to that of having a bowel movement. Assure her that she will not have one.
2. Put an examination glove on one hand, and lubricate the index and third fingertips with water-soluble gel. Place the third finger against the anus, ask the patient to bear down, and insert this finger into the rectum just past the sphincter. Palpate the anorectal junction and rotate the examining finger to sweep over the anterior and then posterior rectum that can be reached above the sphincter. Note sphincter tone. The mucosal surfaces should feel smooth and uninterrupted.
3. Now also insert the index finger of the examining hand into the vagina as far as it will go. Palpate the septum between the rectum and posterior vaginal wall for thickness. Now ask the woman to bear down, which will bring the uterus about 1 cm closer to your examining finger. Place the vaginal finger in the posterior fornix. With the other hand, press firmly on the abdomen just above the pubis. The posterior surface of the uterus should be palpable, especially if it is retroverted. If the findings of the adnexal examination were questionable, repeat that examination as described above.
4. Gently remove the examining fingers, inspect for secretions, and prepare a specimen for fecal occult blood testing if indicated. Remove and discard gloves, and help the woman to sit up. Give her a moment to regain composure, and then offer her tissues to wipe secretions and lubricant from her perineal area. Leave the examining room to allow her privacy and time to dress. Tell her you will discuss your findings with her after she is clothed.

SUMMING UP AND DOCUMENTING FINDINGS

Having a conversation that summarizes findings from the full physical examination takes little time but is very important. If findings are uniformly normal, describing the examination as "healthy," "fine," or "what is expected" is preferable to characterizing the examination as "normal." If any abnormal findings occurred, these should be explained appropriately. The practitioner should gauge how much detailed explanation, description, and thoughts on a therapeutic plan should be presented based on the individual woman's desire for information and the degree of severity of the finding. If the practitioner is not sure of the implications of the finding, it is reasonable to say so, but also assure the woman that medical consultation will be sought promptly, and that a more complete explanation and therapeutic plan will be forthcoming.

Women also need to be encouraged to voice their concerns, questions, and reactions to the examination. Attention to these issues demonstrates the provider's commitment to understanding and responding to the individual woman.

The final clinical responsibility for this step in management is concise and accurate documentation of findings on the patient's record. Try "to give the patient records a vibrancy that might otherwise be lost" (Seidel et al., 2003, p. 17) by balancing technical documentation with descriptions that highlight the patient's substance and uniqueness.

REFERENCES

American College of Obstetricians and Gynecologists. (2003). *Cervical cytology screening* (ACOG Practice Bulletin No. 45). Washington, DC: Author.

Amies, A. E., Miller, L., Lee, S., & Koutsky, L. (2002). The effect of vaginal speculum lubrication on the rate of unsatisfactory cervical cytology diagnosis. *Obstetrics & Gynecology, 100,* 899–892.

Bickley, L. S. (2004). *Bates' guide to physical examination and history taking* (8th ed.). Baltimore: Lippincott Williams & Wilkins.

Campbell, C. C. (2004). Care of women with female circumcision. *Journal of Midwifery & Women's Health, 49,* 364–365.

Centers for Disease Control and Prevention. (2002). Screening tests to detect *Chlamydia trachomatis* and *Neisseria gonorrhoeae* infection. *Morbidity and Mortality Weekly Review, 51*(RR-15), 1–27. Retrieved October 6, 2004, from http://www.cdc.gov/mmwr/PDF/\RR/RR5115.pdf.

Merriam-Webster's collegiate dictionary (10th ed.). (2001). Springfield, MA: Merriam-Webster.

Nour, N. M. (2004). Female genital cutting: Clinical and cultural guidelines. *Obstetrical and Gynecological Survey, 59,* 272–279.

Seidel, H. M., Ball, J. W., Dains, J. E., & Benedict, W. G. (2003). *Mosby's guide to physical examination* (5th ed.). St Louis, MO: Mosby.

Stenchever, M. A., Droegmueller, W., Herbst, A. L., & Mishell, D. R. (2001). *Comprehensive gynecology* (4th ed.). St. Louis, MO: Mosby.

Toubia, N. (1999). *Caring for women with circumcision: A technical manual for health care providers.* New York: Rainbo.

United States Preventive Services Task Force. (2002). *Screening for colorectal cancer: Recommendations and rationale.* Retrieved January 15, 2005, from http://www.ahcpr.gov/clinic/3rduspstf/colorectal/colorr.pdf.

World Health Organization. (2000, June). *Female genital mutilation* (Fact Sheet No. 241). Retrieved October 5, 2004, from http://www.who.int/mediacentre/factsheets/fs241/en/.

World Health Organization. (2001). *Management of pregnancy, childbirth, and the postpartum period in the presence of female genital mutilation.* Retrieved October 8, 2004, from http://www.who.int/docstore/frh-whd/PDFfiles/Management%20of%20pregnancy%20in%20the%20presence%20of%20FGM.pdf.

CERVICAL CYTOLOGY SCREENING

The goal of this test is to obtain adequate cells from the cervical squamocolumnar junction (SCJ) for cytology screening. The SCJ, or transformation zone, where columnar endocervical epithelium and squamous ectocervical epithelium meet, is where most cervical cancers arise. For many years, specimens were collected using a special wooden spatula (Ayer spatula), sometimes in conjunction with a cotton-tipped swab. The conventional method of preparing the sample for cytology is the Papanicolaou (Pap) smear, which entails applying the specimen to a glass slide. Limitations of this method of specimen collection and preparation are well documented. They include not obtaining sufficient endocervical cells for adequate laboratory cytologic evaluation; unavoidably leaving much of the cellular sample on the collection device when transferring to the glass slide; and obscured detection of abnormal cells due to the presence of blood, mucus, air-drying, or other artifacts on the slide. Newer specimen collection devices and liquid-based preparation methods have been developed to try to overcome these limitations and improve cervical cytology screening.

New specimen collection devices include the endocervical brush (Cytobrush), a broom-like device that can simultaneously sample the ectocervix and endocervix, and extended-tip spatulas (Figure 6A–1). The use of cotton-tipped swabs is no longer recommended. Plastic spatulas are preferable to wooden spatulas, because they retain more cervical cells, and extended-tip spatulas are better than the rounded Ayer spatula. Using an extended-tip spatula and an endocervical brush for specimen collection results in the highest rate of detection of endocervical cells by cytologic examination (Martin-Hirsch, Jarvis, Kitchener, & Lilford, 2000).

Liquid-based methods for cervical cytology screening (ThinPrep, SurePath) allow for more complete removal of cellular material by rinsing the sampling devices in a liquid

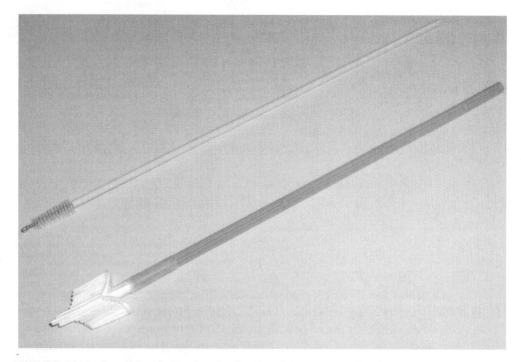

FIGURE 6A-1 Specimen Collection Devices for Cervical Cytology Screening
Endocervical brush (left) and broom (right).

medium. Cells for cytological examination are removed from the medium with a filtering process that minimizes obscuring artifacts. Liquid-based methods appear to increase the sensitivity (fewer false-negative results) of cervical cytology but may decrease the specificity (more false-positive results). Increased sensitivity can improve detection of precancerous lesions, but decreased specificity can result in potentially unnecessary follow-up evaluations and costly treatment of low-grade lesions that can cause psychological distress (ACOG, 2003; USPSTF, 2003). An additional advantage of liquid-based cytology methods is that the sample can also be used to test for human papilloma virus deoxyribonucleic acid (HPV DNA). A disadvantage of liquid-based methods is their higher cost compared to the conventional (Pap) cytology method. These considerations, and the failure of scientific evidence to establish clear superiority of one method over the other, have led to differing recommendations about the use of liquid-based cervical cytology (ACOG, 2003; USPSTF, 2003; Saslow et al., 2002). See Chapter 7 for recommendations. Procedures for both conventional and liquid-based methods for cervical cytology screening using the different specimen collection devices are described in the next section.

CONVENTIONAL METHOD FOR CERVICAL CYTOLOGY SCREENING

1. Assemble materials: a labeled container for one or two standard microscope slides, slides, spatula, endocervical brush, and canister of fixative.
2. Tell the patient that the Pap smear will be performed and that she may feel slight pressure or discomfort, which is caused primarily from the contact of the sampling devices with the endocervix.
3. Visualize the cervix, using the speculum examination procedure described in this chapter.
4. Pick up the spatula, and insert the longer end into the cervical os. Press and rotate the spatula 360°, being sure it stays in direct contact with the inner surface of the cervical os.
5. Pick up the glass slide, press the spatula flat against the surface, and smear the spatula across the slide. Turn the spatula over, and spread the secretions from the second side of the spatula onto the slide. Discard the spatula. Some health care providers prefer to proceed to step 6 and place samples from the spatula and endocervical brush onto the slide after both specimens have been collected.
6. Now insert the endocervical brush so that the bristles are fully in the cervical os and rotate the brush 180° to 360° (one half to one turn).
7. Pick up the glass slide (or second glass slide if using two) and, with firm pressure, roll the bristles of the endocervical brush across the slide surface. If using one slide, recommendations vary as to whether to keep the spatula and endocervical brush samples separate (placing one on each side of the slide), or to place the endocervical brush sample over the spatula sample. Providers should consult their laboratory for the preferred preparation method. Discard the endocervical brush.
8. Spray fixative *promptly* onto the slide, holding the container about 12 inches away from the slide. Allow to air dry for a few minutes before placing the slide in the transport container.
9. Continue the speculum examination or prepare to collect additional specimens.

Note that an assistant, if present, can hold the slides for the provider and apply the fixative.

LIQUID-BASED METHODS FOR CERVICAL CYTOLOGY SCREENING

SPECIMEN COLLECTION WITH THE SPATULA AND ENDOCERVICAL BRUSH

1. Assemble materials: labeled vial of liquid medium, spatula, and endocervical brush. Take the lid off the vial.
2. Prepare the patient as described in step 2 for the conventional method.
3. Visualize the cervix as described in step 3 for the conventional method.

4. Collect specimen with spatula as described in step 4 for the conventional method.
5. Place the spatula into the vial and swirl vigorously 10 times to mix the specimen and the medium. Remove and discard the spatula.
6. Collect specimen with endocervical brush as described in step 6 for the conventional method.
7. Place the endocervical brush into the vial and swirl vigorously 10 times to mix the specimen and the medium. Discard the endocervical brush.
8. Screw the lid tightly and securely onto the vial.
9. Proceed as described in step 9 for the conventional method.

SPECIMEN COLLECTION WITH THE BROOM-LIKE DEVICE

1. Assemble materials: labeled vial of liquid medium and broom-like device. Take the lid off the vial.
2. Prepare the patient as described in step 2 for the conventional method.
3. Visualize the cervix as described in step 3 for the conventional method.
4. Insert the central bristles of the broom into the endocervical canal deep enough to allow the shorter bristles to fully contact the ectocervix. Push gently, and rotate the broom in a clockwise direction five times.
5. Place the broom into the vial and press firmly to the bottom of the vial so that the bristles of the broom are forced apart. Swirl vigorously 10 times to mix the specimen and the medium. Remove and discard the broom.
6. Screw the lid tightly and securely onto the vial.
7. Proceed as described in step 9 for the conventional method.

REFERENCES

American College of Obstetricians and Gynecologists. (2003). *Cervical cytology screening* (ACOG Practice Bulletin No. 45). Washington, DC: Author.

Martin-Hirsch, P., Jarvis, G., Kitchener, J., & Lilford, R. (2000, most recent substantative amendment). Collection devices for obtaining cervical cytology samples (Cochrane Review). In *The Cochrane Library*. Chichester, UK: John Wiley & Sons.

Saslow, D., Runowicz, C. D., Solomon, D., Moscicki, A., Smith, R. A., Eyre, H. J., et al. (2002). American Cancer Society guideline for the early detection of cervical neoplasia and cancer. *CA: Cancer Journal for Clinicians, 52*, 342–362.

United States Preventive Services Task Force. (2003). *Screening for cervical cancer: Recommendations and rationale.* Retrieved October 8, 2004, from http://www.ahcpr.gov/clinic/3rduspstf/cervcan/cervcanrr.pdf.

SCREENING FOR *CHLAMYDIA TRACHOMATIS* AND *NEISSERIA GONORRHOEAE* INFECTIONS

The nucleic acid amplification test (NAAT) is the most sensitive method for detecting *Chlamydia trachomatis* in endocervical samples (CDC, 2002). Several commercial NAAT products are available and use different methods. Providers should follow the manufacturer's instructions. The CDC provides the following general guidelines for the specimen collection procedure:

1. Prepare materials by opening the test kit, labeling the medium container, and placing the swabs provided in the test kit within easy reach.
2. Visualize the cervix using the speculum examination procedure described in this chapter.
3. Remove all secretions and discharge from the cervix with a large swab.
4. Insert the swab supplied by the manufacturer 1–2 cm into the cervical os, rotate it firmly at least twice against the walls of the canal, and allow it to remain in the os for the time recommended by the manufacturer.
5. Withdraw the swab without touching any vaginal surfaces.
6. Place the swab in the appropriate transport medium, or follow the manufacturer's directions provided with the medium collection kit.

Culture is the preferred test method for detecting *Neisseria gonorrhoeae* from the endocervix if "ambient conditions during holding and transport of the specimen are adequate to maintain viability of the organism" (CDC, 2002, p. 10). Collecting an endocervical sample for culture proceeds in the same manner as the *C. trachomatis* NAAT method described previously, but disposition of the swab is different. For a culture, the endocervical specimen is directly inoculated onto a selective nutritive medium such as Martin-Lewis or chocolate agar containing IsoVitaleX. The culture plate should be incubated at

35° to 36.5° Celsius in a carbon dioxide-enriched atmosphere immediately after collection. If these conditions cannot be assured, then a NAAT to detect *N. gonorrhoeae* is recommended. The techniques for endocervical sampling and preparation of the specimen for the *N. gonorrhoeae* NAAT are the same as described previously for *C. trachomatis* screening. Some NAAT products test for both *C. trachomatis* and *N. gonorrhoeae* using the same specimen.

REFERENCES

Centers for Disease Control and Prevention. (2002). Screening tests to detect *Chlamydia trachomatis* and *Neisseria gonorrhoeae* infection. *Morbidity and Mortality Weekly Review, 51*(RR-15), 1–27. Retrieved October 6, 2004, from http://www.cdc.gov/mmwr/PDF/\RR/RR5115.pdf.

PREPARING A SAMPLE OF VAGINAL SECRETIONS FOR MICROSCOPIC EXAMINATION

Vaginal secretions and exudates can be directly examined with a microscope to aid in the diagnosis of vaginal and sexually transmitted infections (see Chapters 17 and 18). Immediately after obtaining the vaginal secretions, mix one sample with normal saline solution, and a second sample with a 10% solution of potassium hydroxide (KOH). *Candida albicans, Trichomonas vaginalis,* clue cells (epithelial cells with indistinct borders due to adherent bacteria) associated with bacterial vaginosis, and white blood cells, can be seen in normal saline solution. Potassium hydroxide lyses trichomonads, white blood cells, and most bacteria, making visualization of *Candida* species easier. The presence of an amine or fishy odor with the addition of KOH to the vaginal secretions should be noted (whiff test), and is associated with but not diagnostic for bacterial vaginosis and trichonomiasis. The CDC (2001) offers the following directions for collecting and preparing these specimens for microscopic examination:

1. Assemble materials: One or two standard glass microscope slides and cover slips, nonsterile cotton tipped swabs, saline solution, and potassium hydroxide solution. Some health care providers also use a small test tube.
2. Using a dropper or single-use blister pack of the solutions, place two to three large drops of saline on one slide and KOH on the second slide. Alternatives include the use of one slide (put drops of both solutions separately on it), or the test tube method (place drops of saline in a test tube and drops of KOH on a slide).
3. Obtain a specimen of vaginal discharge by either swabbing the vaginal walls and posterior fornix with a cotton-tipped swab or by sampling from the concave surfaces of the speculum blade after the speculum has been removed.

4. Mix the sample of discharge with the drops of saline and KOH on the slides. Be sure to put the sample in the saline before the KOH and to keep the saline and KOH solutions separate. If using the test tube method, immerse the swab in the test tube, then use the swab to apply the pre-mixed specimen onto a dry slide.

5. Cover each specimen with a glass cover slip. Avoid trapping air bubbles under the cover slip, which makes the microscopic examination more difficult. Put one edge of the cover slip into the mixed specimen, and then lower the cover slip onto the specimen. Proceed as soon as possible to microscopic examination of the slide.

REFERENCES

Centers for Disease Control and Prevention. (2001). *Program operations guidelines for STD prevention: Appendix ML-B*. Retrieved May 10, 2004, from http://www.cdc.gov/std/program/medlab/ApB-PGmedlab.htm.

7 PERIODIC SCREENING AND HEALTH MAINTENANCE

KATHRYN OSBORNE

Secondary preventive services are those services that enable early identification of risk factors or diagnosis of disease conditions in asymptomatic patients. The initial step in secondary prevention is assessment, which includes obtaining the patient's medical history, performing a physical examination, and evaluating data from laboratory tests. A comprehensive patient history is one of the most valuable screening tools available to the clinician. It affords the clinician an opportunity to receive detailed information about the patient and an opportunity to establish a therapeutic relationship with the patient. A patient's health history forms the basis for determining disease entities for which the patient is at risk, and therefore requires further screening. A management plan is developed once risk factors are identified and should include measures that focus on reducing the short- and long-term consequences of identified risks.

Cost containment is of critical importance today, and therefore it is imperative that clinicians make decisions about testing and treatment that are based on current evidence. Only tests and treatments for which there are proven benefits should be utilized. The yearly performance of routine laboratory tests has not proven to be the most effective tool in the process of delivering preventive health services (US Preventive Services Task Force, [USPSTF] 1996). It is the professional responsibility of every clinician to contain health care costs.

The US Public Health Service gathered together a panel of experts in 1984 to examine the efficacy of preventive health services including screening tests, counseling, immunizations, and chemoprevention. That panel remains active today and presently has 15 experts from various private sector specialty groups. The panel is known as the US Preventive Services Task Force (USPSTF). Their mission is to:

- Evaluate the benefits of individual services.
- Create age-, gender-, and risk-based recommendations about services that should routinely be incorporated into primary medical care.

- Identify a research agenda for clinical preventive care (Agency for Health Research and Quality, 2003).

The initial findings of the Task Force were published in 1989 in the *Guide to Clinical Preventive Services*. These findings were updated in 1996 and include the evaluation of over 200 clinical services. The third edition (2004), consists of online periodic updates that are available on the USPSTF Web site: http://www.ahcpr.gov/clinic/uspstfix.htm. The initial recommendations from the Task Force were not based on cost effectiveness, but the Task Force now recommends that cost effectiveness be considered in all decision making about preventive health services. The intent of the Task Force is to provide clinicians with a framework for decision making about patient management plans that results in improved patient outcomes. The Task Force recognizes the importance of involving the patient in the decision-making process and acknowledges that some patients will prefer to use interventions for which there is no scientific evidence (USPSTF, 1996).

The current recommendation scheme assigns each recommendation to specific categories that serve as a guide for informed and shared decision making (Table 7–1). "A" and "B" designated services are those that the Task Force found sufficient evidence to recommend. The use of services designated as "C" or "I" should be based on the clinical judgment of the clinician, in conjunction with patient education and counseling. Many of the "C" and "I" services are services for which the Task Force found insufficient evidence to either recommend for or against, thus leaving open the opportunity for providers and patients to individualize a management plan. Services with a "D" recommendation are those that the Task Force found to be either of no benefit or potentially harmful.

It is important to remember that these are the screening recommendations for the general population of individuals who do not have risk factors for specific disease entities. Shi and Singh (2004) define risk factors as "attributes that increase the likelihood of developing a particular disease or negative health condition at some time in the future" (p. 42). When no risk factors are found for a particular disease, a woman is considered not at risk for that disease. However, women experience change throughout their lifes. Occasionally, change is accompanied by risk factors. When that happens, there is a subsequent change in the patient's risk status. For example, a 30-year-old woman who is not at

TABLE 7–1   US Preventive Services Task Force Recommendation Scheme, 1998–Present

Quality of Evidence	Net Benefit			
	Substantial	Moderate	Small	Zero/Neg.
Good	A	B	C	D
Fair	B	B	C	D
Poor	Insufficient ("I") evidence to determine the net benefit of the service or to recommend for or against its being routinely provided.			

Source: Reprinted with permission from the US Preventive Services Task Force, 2004.

increased risk for breast cancer experiences a change in risk status when she turns 40. The clinician must be aware of risk factors that may alter the risk status of individual patients so that additional screening is obtained when needed.

This chapter focuses on the recommendations of the USPSTF and provides a brief summary of its evidence-based recommendations. USPSTF recommendations and those from other professional groups are provided so that clinicians may compare and contrast the recommendations from each group (Table 7–2). The USPSTF *Guide to Clinical Preventive Services* provides a more detailed description of the research and implications the recommendations have for clinical practice.

SCREENING RECOMMENDATIONS FOR ALL WOMEN

ALCOHOL MISUSE

The USPSTF assigns a "B" recommendation to screening all adults (including pregnant women) for alcohol misuse (USPSTF, 2004). Historically, research regarding the effects of alcohol on humans and animals has been conducted on males. Only recently has the research focus changed in an attempt to discover the effect of alcohol on females. An initial finding of these studies is that smaller quantities of alcohol can result in more severe damage to women (National Institute on Alcohol Abuse and Alcoholism, 2000). Alcohol consumption is considered hazardous for a woman who has either seven or more drinks in one week or three drinks per occasion. This is considerably less than the threshold allowable for males. Harmful drinking is that which causes physical, social, or emotional harm, but falls short of dependence and addiction (Reid, Fiellin, & O'Connor, 1999). There are a variety of alcohol screening tools that are effective, and many of these can be found at the National Institute on Alcohol Abuse and Alcoholism Web site at: http://www.niaaa.nih.gov.

The USPSTF (2004) suggests using the CAGE questionnaire for alcohol screening. This instrument is short and effective and consists of a series of four questions that can be asked during a health history:

- Do you ever feel the need to **C**ut down your drinking?
- Are you ever **A**nnoyed by people's criticism of your drinking?
- Do you ever feel **G**uilty about drinking?
- Do you ever feel the need for an "**E**ye-opener" in the morning?

Brief questions about the quantity and frequency of alcohol consumption are also helpful. The CAGE questionnaire can be administered to women who are found to consume hazardous amounts of alcohol. Women who answer "yes" to three or four CAGE questions may be alcohol dependent. Those who answer yes to one or two may have alcohol-related problems. Those who answer no to all questions may still be considered at risk for alcohol misuse if they indicated that they consume hazardous amounts of alcohol. The Task Force

TABLE 7-2   A Comparison of Screening Recommendations

	US Preventive Services Task Force (USPSTF)	American College of Obstetricians and Gynecologists (ACOG)	American Cancer Society (ACS)	Other Groups
Cervical Cancer	Pap smear every 1–3 years for all women within 3 years of beginning sexual activity or by age 21. Recommends against screening women over 65 if they have had normal Pap smears and are otherwise not at risk for cervical cancer. Recommends against screening women who have had a total hysterectomy for benign disease Finds that there is insufficient evidence to recommend for or against the use of new technologies to screen for cervical cancer.	Yearly cervical cytology within 3 years of the onset of sexual activity or by age 21. May decrease testing to every 2–3 years after 3 consecutive negative test results if age 30 or older with no history of cervical intraepithelial neoplasia (CIN), HIV or in utero exposure to Diethyl-stilbestrol. Women with a history of hysterectomy for reasons other than carcinoma may discontinue screening. Women with a history of CIN 2 or 3 should be screened yearly until they have 3 consecutive negative vaginal cytology tests.	Yearly Pap smear (using regular Pap tests) for women within three years of beginning vaginal sexual activity. Screening may be done every 2 years if liquid-based tests are used. Testing may be extended to every 2–3 years for women at age 30 who have had 3 normal screens. Screening can be discontinued at age 70 if women have had 3 consecutive normal screens, and is not necessary following total hysterectomy for reasons other than cervical cancer.	
Breast Cancer	Mammogram (with or without clinical breast exam (CBE)) every 1–2 years beginning at age 40. Insufficient evidence to recommend for or against breast self-examination (BSE) or CBE alone at any age.	Mammogram and CBE every 1–2 years for women age 40–49 and yearly for women age 50 and older. Annual CBE for all women. BSE for women of all ages can be recommended.	Mammogram and CBE every year beginning at age 40. CBE every 2–3 years and the performance of monthly BSE for women age 20–39.	

Elevated Cholesterol	Strongly recommends routinely screening women age 45 and older. Also recommends screening women age 20–45 who are at increased risk for coronary artery disease. Makes no recommendation for or against screening women age 20–45 without known risk factors for coronary artery disease.	Nonfasting total cholesterol and HDL every 5 years beginning at age 45.	The National Cholesterol Education Program (sponsored by NIH) recommends screening with total cholesterol and HDL every 5 years.
Osteoporosis	Recommends routine screening for osteoporosis with bone density measurements for all women age 65 and older, and screening for women at increased risk beginning at age 60.	Concurs with the National Osteoporosis Foundation.	The National Osteoporosis Foundation recommends screening all women age 65 and older, and younger postmenopausal women who have had a fracture or who have one or more risk factors for osteoporosis.
Colorectal Cancer	Strongly recommends screening women age 50 and older for colorectal cancer. Found insufficient evidence to determine which strategy is best in terms of the balance of benefits and potential harms or cost-effectiveness.	Concurs with ACS recommendations.	Fecal occult blood testing every year beginning at age 50 and flexible sigmoidoscopy every 5 years. The combination of these is preferable to either one alone. ACS also recommends double contrast barium enema every five years and colonoscopy every 10 years. The American Academy of Family Physicians has recommendations similar to ACS.

(continues)

TABLE 7-2 A Comparison of Screening Recommendations (continued)

	US Preventive Services Task Force (USPSTF)	American College of Obstetricians and Gynecologists (ACOG)	American Cancer Society (ACS)	Other Groups
Ovarian Cancer	Routine screening with tumor markers, ultrasound, or pelvic examination is not recommended. Insufficient evidence to recommend for or against routinely screening asymptomatic women at increased risk of developing ovarian cancer.	No techniques have proven to be effective in the routine screening of asymptomatic low-risk women for ovarian cancer.	During periodic health examinations, a cancer check-up should include health counseling and may include examinations for ovarian cancer.	
IPV	Insufficient evidence to recommend for or against routine screening.	Routinely ask all women direct, specific questions about abuse. Refer to community-based services when identified.		American Academy of Family Physicians advises to remain alert for signs of family violence at every patient encounter.

Sources: American Cancer Society, 2003; American College of Obstetricians and Gynecologists, 2003; US Preventive Services Task Force, 2004.

further recommends that patients who misuse alcohol undergo counseling, either in the primary care setting or with providers specialized in the treatment of alcohol misuse. All pregnant women should be counseled about the harmful effects alcohol has on the developing fetus (USPSTF, 2004).

CERVICAL CANCER

The USPSTF assigns an "A" recommendation to screening for cervical cancer. Screening should begin within three years of the onset of sexual activity or by age 21. The recommended screening test is the Papanicolaou smear, commonly called a Pap smear. There currently is no evidence to support annual Pap smear screening. Annual Pap smears have not demonstrated any improvement in health outcomes. However, the Task Force also recognizes that because of the sensitivity of the Pap smear, many specialty organizations in the United States continue to recommend yearly screening until a minimum number of tests are found to be cytologically normal. Women who are at increased risk for cervical cancer include women infected with human papilloma virus, those who engage in sexual activity at an early age, those who have had multiple sexual partners, and those women who smoke cigarettes (USPSTF, 2004). The Task Force recommends against screening ("D" recommendation) women older than 65 years who are not at increased risk for cervical cancer, and who have a history of cytologically normal screens. The same recommendation against screening is made for women who have had a hysterectomy for reasons other than carcinoma (USPSTF).

DEPRESSION

The USPSTF assigns a "B" recommendation to screening all adults for depression in settings where there is a mechanism in place for follow-up testing and treatment. They assign an "I" recommendation to routinely screening adolescents for depression, although clinicians should be alert for signs of depression in young girls and teens (USPSTF, 2004). Screening for depression is an important aspect of women's health care because the odds are that one in five women will develop clinical depression during their lifetime (National Mental Health Association [NMHA], 2004). Women are two times more likely than men to develop clinical depression (NMHA). There are a variety of depression screening tools available, but perhaps the easiest screening tool is to simply ask a couple of questions about the woman's mood and her ability to find pleasure in activities she usually enjoys. There is no recommended frequency for this type of screening. Patients who elicit a positive screen should be referred to clinicians who are skilled in the diagnosis and treatment of depressive disorders for further testing and management. The Task Force found little benefit in routinely screening patients for whom follow-up is unavailable (USPSTF).

HEIGHT AND WEIGHT

The USPSTF assigns a "B" recommendation to screening all patients for obesity. The body mass index (BMI) is the recommended method of identifying women at increased risk for morbidity and mortality from excessive weight. The BMI is calculated by dividing a woman's weight in kilograms by her height in meters squared (see Chapter 6). Overweight is defined as having a BMI of between 25 and 29.9. Anyone with a BMI of 30 or greater is classified as obese. Patients should be counseled on the importance of maintaining a healthy diet and regular exercise (USPSTF, 2004).

HYPERTENSION

Greater than 50% of all women in the United States will develop hypertension during their lifetimes (National Heart, Lung and Blood Institute, n.d.). The USPSTF assigns an "A" recommendation to screening adults 18 years of age and older for hypertension. The routine screening of children and adolescents is an "I" recommendation. The recommended screening test for hypertension is a blood pressure measurement using a sphygmomanometer. Based on the findings of the Joint National Committee on Prevention, Detection, Evaluation and Treatment of High Blood Pressure (JNC), the recommended frequency of screening is every two years for women with blood pressure readings of less than 130/85, and more frequently for those with higher readings (USPSTF, 2004). The recently released JNC7 recommends a restructuring of traditional blood pressure classifications. The report classifies systolic pressures of 120–139 or diastolic pressures of 80–89 as prehypertensive and recommends that clinicians consider drug therapy for certain individuals that fall within this classification (Joint National Committee on Prevention, Detection, Evaluation and Treatment of High Blood Pressure, 2003). Clinicians are advised to watch for updated recommendations from the USPSTF based on this reclassification.

INTIMATE PARTNER VIOLENCE

The USPSTF assigns an "I" recommendation to screening patients for intimate partner violence (IPV). There are currently no studies that confirm the accuracy of specific screening tools, or that the use of such tools decreases disability or premature death as a result of IPV. Neither are there studies that examine the harmful effects of screening for IPV. Consequently, the Task Force is unable to recommend for or against the use of specific tools to screen for IPV (USPSTF, 2004). According to the National Women's Health Information Center (2003), an estimated four million women per year are victims of IPV. The Task Force recommends that all clinicians remain alert for signs and symptoms of IPV. Women presenting with symptoms or injuries should receive detailed documentation of the injuries, medical treatment, counseling referrals, and a list of community resources that provide shelter and protection (USPSTF). See Chapter 12 for more information on IPV.

OVARIAN CANCER

Routinely screening women for ovarian cancer by measuring serum tumor markers, ultrasound, or pelvic examination receives a "D" recommendation. There is no evidence to demonstrate an improvement in overall health outcomes. The Task Force does not recommend routine screening for ovarian cancer for the general population because of the risks, inconvenience, and cost of follow-up. They have, however, assigned a "C" recommendation to screening women who are at increased risk for ovarian cancer, including women with a family history of ovarian cancer in a first degree relative (USPSTF, 1996). See Chapter 23 for a more in-depth discussion of gynecologic cancers.

RUBELLA IMMUNITY

The USPSTF recommends screening all women of childbearing age for rubella immunity at the time of their first clinical contact. Screening is accomplished by either obtaining a history of vaccination or ordering serologic studies. The USPSTF further recommends that all nonpregnant women of childbearing age receive vaccinations, and those who are pregnant should be vaccinated immediately postpartum. The Task Force recommends against the routine screening of postmenopausal women for rubella (USPSTF, 1996).

TOBACCO USE

The USPSTF assigns an "A" recommendation to screening all adults for tobacco use. The recommended screening tool is careful questioning by the clinician about the patient's tobacco use during the routine health history. The most recent data suggest that over 20% of American women smoke cigarettes (National Center for Health Statistics, 2003). While the average number of cancer deaths attributed to smoking fell for men between the years 1995 and 1999, the average number of cancer deaths attributed to smoking rose for women during the same time (Centers for Disease Control and Prevention [CDC], 2002). As discussed in Chapter 4, the Task Force recommends implementation of interventions to promote smoking cessation in all patients who use tobacco. Scientific evidence demonstrates that patients who quit using tobacco are likely to have substantial overall health benefits, regardless of the number of years of tobacco use (USPSTF, 2004).

SPECIAL POPULATIONS

SCREENING RECOMMENDATIONS FOR ADOLESCENTS

Chlamydia   The USPSTF assigns an "A" recommendation to screening all women, age 25 years and younger, and all women who are at an increased risk for a sexually transmitted infection, for chlamydia. The most significant risk factor for infection is age. Adolescents and women through 20 years of age are at highest risk, although an increased prevalence is also seen in women aged 20 to 25 years. Additionally, women at increased risk of infection include unmarried women, African-American women, women with a history of sexually transmitted infections, those with multiple partners, women with cervical ectopy, and those who inconsistently use barrier methods of contraception. In addition to individual risk factors, chlamydia infection is seen more frequently in particular communities. Health care providers should be aware of prevalence rates of infection in the communities in which they practice (USPSTF, 2004).

There are a number of screening tests available (see Chapter 6). The choice of screening test is based on cost, convenience, and feasibility. The Centers for Disease Control and Prevention (CDC) has summarized the advantages and disadvantages of each test. This summary can be found at http://www.cdc.gov/STD/LabGuidelines.

SCREENING RECOMMENDATIONS FOR OLDER WOMEN

Breast Cancer   Screening mammography, with or without a clinical breast examination (CBE), for women age 40 years and older receives a "B" recommendation from the USP-STF. There is a lack of evidence that a CBE without mammography and breast self-examination (BSE) has any affect on breast cancer mortality. Some evidence suggests that CBE and BSE may actually increase the likelihood of further testing and biopsy while doing little to improve outcomes, and therefore CBE and BSE are an "I" recommendation. The recommended frequency for mammography screening is every 12 to 33 months. Women at an increased risk for developing breast cancer should begin having mammograms at an earlier age and benefit from the increased frequency of screening. The following factors place women at an increased risk for breast cancer: (1) history of breast cancer in a mother or sister, (2) women who had their first child after age 30, and (3) women with a previous breast biopsy that revealed atypical hyperplasia (USPSTF, 2004). Please refer to Chapter 13 for a more in-depth discussion of breast cancer.

Colorectal Cancer   The USPSTF recommends screening all adults age 50 years and older for colorectal cancer ("A" classification). Individuals with existing risk factors for colon cancer have about a 20% occurrence rate of disease. In light of the fact that colon cancer occurs frequently in individuals who are considered at average risk, the Task Force suggests that earlier initiation of screening for women at higher risk of colorectal cancer is reasonable. Risk factors for colorectal cancer are: (1) history of colorectal cancer in a first degree relative, (2) rare genetic disorders such as familial adenomatous polyposis or hereditary nonpolyposis colorectal cancer, (3) chronic ulcerative colitis, (4) history of polyps or colorectal cancer, and (5) those with a family history of adenomatous polyps that were diagnosed before the age of 60 years. Screening tests include home fecal occult blood testing (FOBT), flexible sigmoidoscopy, FOBT combined with flexible sigmoidoscopy, colonoscopy, and double-contrast barium enema. Each of these options has advantages and disadvantages for the patient and the practice setting. Clinicians should discuss the risks and benefits of each screening test, and include patient preference in choosing a screening method. The optimal interval for screening depends upon the screening test used and can vary from yearly FOBT to colonoscopy every 10 years (USPSTF, 2004). Clinicians who provide health care for women who require screening should familiarize themselves with the risks, costs, and benefits of the various screening options.

Elevated Cholesterol Levels   The USPSTF assigns an "A" recommendation to screening all women 45 years of age and older for lipid disorders. Screening cholesterol levels in women aged between the years 20 and 44 with pre-existing risk factors for coronary artery disease receives a "B" recommendation. The recommended screening tool is a serum measurement of total cholesterol and high-density lipoprotein cholesterol with the patient fasting or nonfasting. The optimal frequency of screening is unknown; however, the Task Force recommends screening every five years for the general population, and more frequently for individuals with high normal lipid levels, and less frequently for women with repeatedly low levels. All women should receive counseling about the benefits of a healthy diet (low in saturated fats and high in fruits and vegetables), regular exercise, and maintaining a healthy weight (USPSTF, 2004).

Hearing Impairment   The USPSTF assigns a "B" recommendation to screening all older adults for hearing impairment. The recommended screening method is to ask the patient about her perception of changes in hearing. Patients should be informed that although changes in hearing often occur with aging, they are not considered a normal aging process, and utilization of hearing devices often can improve hearing. Women in whom hearing loss is suspected should be referred to specialists for further testing. Traditional hearing screens involve the use of audiometry, a series of auditory tones that, upon recognition, elicit an affirmative response from the patient. There is insufficient evidence to recommend for or against the use of audiometry, and therefore audiometry is a "C" recommendation. There is no recommended frequency of testing, and therefore it is left to the discretion of the clinician (USPSTF, 1996).

Osteoporosis   Screening women over age 65 for osteoporosis receives a "B" recommendation. The USPSTF recommends routine screening beginning at age 60 for women who are at increased risk of osteoporosis. There is evidence that earlier screening may prevent some fractures; however, there is not enough evidence to demonstrate that early screening outweighs the risk associated with screening and treatment.

The USPSTF assigns a "C" recommendation to routinely screening women younger than 60 years of age for osteoporosis. Factors associated with increased risk for the development of osteoporosis include low body weight (less than 70 kg), cigarette smoking, sedentary lifestyle, family history, decreased lifetime calcium intake, increased alcohol and caffeine intake, and white or Asian ethnicity. Low body weight appears to be the best predictor of risk for developing osteoporosis. The best predictor of hip fracture is bone density testing using dual-energy x-ray absorptiometry of the head of the femur. The USPSTF recognizes that bone density testing of peripheral sites using other modalities can also be effective in predicting increased risk of fracture. Optimal frequency of screening has not been studied, but evidence suggests it may take up to two years to identify changes in bone density. More frequent screening may be appropriate in women with low baseline bone density measurements. Women in whom osteoporosis is identified should be counseled on the risks and benefits of various treatment options (USPSTF, 2004). See Chapter 11 for further information about osteoporosis.

Visual Changes   The USPSTF assigns a "B" recommendation to screening older adults for visual impairment. Visual changes leading to accidental injury are more prevalent after the age of 65 years (USPSTF, 1996). The Task Force also concluded that while the effect of routine screening for visual changes in the elderly has not been assessed, there is fair evidence that routine screening can result in overall improvements in acuity and offers little likelihood of serious harm as a result of the screening. The recommended screening tool is the Snellen Acuity Chart. The Task Force leaves the determination of frequency to the discretion of the clinician because there is no recommended frequency for visual screening.

ADDITIONAL OBSERVATIONS

It is important to remember that the screening recommendations discussed in this chapter are for healthy, asymptomatic women. In addition to these screening recommendations, the USPSTF recommends that clinicians remain alert for findings that are suggestive of conditions found in Table 7–3. As noted in Chapter 6, the gynecologic history and physical examination provide excellent opportunities to gather important screening informa-

TABLE 7-3 Additional Observations

Condition	Population
Symptoms of peripheral arterial disease	Older women, smokers, women with diabetes
Skin lesions with malignant features	All women, especially those with increased risk factors (white race; presence of atypical moles; increased number of common moles or freckles; family or personal history of skin cancer; history of severe sunburns in childhood; light skin, hair, and eye color)
Signs and symptoms of oral cancer or premalignancy	Women who use tobacco and older women who drink alcohol regularly
Subtle or nonspecific signs and symptoms of thyroid dysfunction	Older women, postpartum women, and women with Downs syndrome
Signs and symptoms of hearing impairment	All women
Spinal curvatures	Adolescents
Change in functional performance	Older women
Suicidal ideation	Women with established risk factors for suicide (history of previous attempts or threats, previous psychiatric diagnosis or treatment, substance abuse, recent loss)
Family violence	All women
Drug abuse	All women
Untreated tooth and gum disease	All women

Source: Adapted from the US Preventive Services Task Force, 2004.

tion about the patient. Answers to a few direct questions, and close attention during the physical examination can give the clinician important information and should always be part of a routine patient encounter.

REFERENCES

Agency for Healthcare Research and Quality. (2003, January). *About the USPSTF* (Publication No. 00-P046). Retrieved September 27, 2004, from http://www.ahrq.gov/clinic/uspstfab.htm.

American Cancer Society. (2003). *Cancer facts and figures.* Retrieved September 27, 2004, from http://www.cancer.org/downloads/STT/CAFF2003PWSecured.pdf.

American College of Obstetricians and Gynecologists. (2003, November). *Primary and preventive care: Periodic assessments* (Committee Opinion No. 292) Washington, D.C.: Author.

Centers for Disease Control. (2002). Annual smoking-attributable mortality, years of potential life lost, and economic costs—United States, 1995–1999. *Morbidity and Mortality Weekly Report*, 51, 300–303.

Joint National Committee on Prevention, Detection, Evaluation and Treatment of High Blood Pressure. (2003). *JNC7 Express.* Retrieved June 8, 2004, from http://www.nhlbi.nih.gov/guidelines/hypertension/jncintro.htm.

National Center for Health Statistics. (2003). *Current cigarette smoking by persons 18 years of age and over according to sex, race, and age: United States, selected years 1965–2001* [Data file]. Retrieved June 8, 2004, from http://www.cdc.gov/.

National Heart, Lung and Blood Institute. (n.d.). *Facts about heart disease in women: Preventing and controlling high blood pressure.* Retrieved June, 8, 2004, from http://www.nhlbi.nih.gov/health/public/heart/hbp/hdw_hbp.htm.

National Institute on Alcohol Abuse and Alcoholism. (2000). *Gender differences in alcohol intake.* Retrieved June, 8, 2004, from http://www.niaaa.nih.gov/extramural/gendiff.htm.

National Mental Health Association. (2004). *Clinical depression in women.* Retrieved June 8, 2004 from http://www.nmha.org/ccd/support/women.cfm.

National Women's Health Information Center (2003). *Intimate partner violence fact sheet.* Retrieved January 5, 2005 from http://www.4woman.gov/.

Reid, M.C., Fiellin, D.A., & O'Connor, P.G. (1999). Hazardous and harmful alcohol consumption in primary care. *Archives of Internal Medicine, 159*(15), 1681–1689.

Shi, L., & Singh, D. (2004). *Delivering health care in America: A systems approach* (3rd ed.). Sudbury, MA: Jones & Bartlett.

United States Preventive Services Task Force. (1996). *Guide to clinical preventive services* (2nd ed.). Baltimore: Williams & Wilkins.

United States Preventive Services Task Force. (2004). *Guide to clinical preventive service* (3rd ed.) [update through 2004]. Retrieved June 8, 2004, from http://www. ahcpr.gov/clinic/gcpspu.htm.

Chapter 8

SEXUALITY

CATHERINE INGRAM FOGEL

Despite the unalterable fact that women are sexual beings, it is difficult for many women and their clinicians to view sexual health as an essential component of health care or to discuss sexual concerns. Yet sexuality is an organic, normal, physical, and emotional function that is inextricably woven into the fabric of human life (Northrup, 1998). All women have a right to intimate and sexual lives and relationships that are voluntary, wanted, pleasurable, and noncoercive (Alexander, 1997). Women often ask questions and express concerns regarding sexuality and sexual activity to their clinicians and expect nonjudgmental, open and direct communication regarding sexual matters, sexual information, counseling, or therapy from them. Clinicians providing sexual health care need to understand the adverse impact that illnesses and their treatments can have on sexuality and sexual functioning. Additionally, an awareness of the detrimental impact of violence and coercive sexual experiences on sexual enjoyment is essential. All women are entitled to education regarding their health, including the provision of sexual information and resources, and to counseling to improve or sustain current sexual relationships or to solve a particular problem.

The goal of this chapter is to develop a solid knowledge base about sexuality for use in clinical practice from which sexual concerns may be addressed. This chapter will focus on sexual desire, women's views of themselves and presentations to society, sexual response, and factors that influence sexual response, function, and dysfunction. Additionally, strategies for assessment will be discussed as a foundation for management of female sexual dysfunction, which is addressed in Chapter 14.

FEMALE SEXUALITY

Female sexuality is defined as the integrated, unique expression of self that includes the physiologic and psychologic processes inherent in sexual development. Included in sexual development are a view and presentation of one's self as a female, sexual desire, sexual response, and sexual orientation (Fogel, 2003). The complex process known as sexuality is coordinated by the neurologic, vascular, and endocrine systems (Phillips, 2000). It encompasses a woman's values, attitudes, behaviors, physical appearance, beliefs, emotions, personality, and social and cultural orientations. Further, sexuality is a fundamental component of every woman's life and an important aspect of her health throughout her life. A woman's ability to express herself sexually lasts from birth to death, and there are few women for whom sex has not been important at some time in their lives. Sexual expression is influenced by ethical, cultural, moral, and spiritual factors and is expressed differently at different times—alone, with one partner, or with many. In addition, no two women will express their sexuality exactly the same way. Women express their identities and their need for emotional and physical closeness with others, in part, through their sexual relationships. Expressed positively, sexuality can bring much pleasure; however, sexuality also has the potential to cause great pain. A woman's sexuality is not limited by age, attractiveness, partner availability or participation, or sexual orientation.

COMPONENT OF SEXUALITY

The unique human quality that is sexuality has several dimensions including sexual desire, presentation of self as a sexual being, sexual orientation, and sexual lifestyles and relationships. Sexuality combines both sex or one's anatomical characteristics as male or female, with gender, or one's view and presentation of self as a man or a woman. Sexuality is more than just sexual intercourse, and involves a wide range of behaviors including fantasy, self-stimulation, noncoital pleasuring, erotic stimuli other than touch, communication about needs and desires, and the ability to define what is wanted and pleasurable in a relationship (Alexander, 1997). While acknowledging the influence of biology on sexuality, sexuality is also a social construct based on prescribed arrangements and sexual scripts that provide guidelines for appropriate sexual behaviors (Amaro, Navarro, Conron, & Raj, 2002).

Sexual desire or libido is manifested by an interest in sexual experience (Charlton & Quatman, 1997). Kaplan (1979) considered sexual desire as the innate urge for sexual activity, which is produced by the activation of a specific system in the brain and experienced as a specific sensation that motivates an individual to seek or respond to sexual experience. The amount of sexual desire experienced varies from woman to woman, differs across a woman's life, and can be suppressed or repressed by many different factors. Although Kaplan considers sexual desire to be a physical need, similar to hunger, a more accurate representation would also include a recognition of women's needs for intimacy as a strong influence on sexual desire (Basson, 2000). Additional factors in the development of sexual desire include experiencing feelings of pleasure, enjoyment, dissatisfaction, or pain during sexual activity. Sexual desire can also develop from an interest in sexual activity, a preferred frequency of activity, and a gender preference for a sexual partner (Fogel, 2003). These scripts vary by gender, from culture to culture, and by cultural subgroups. In addition, an individual's expression of these scripts can vary due to cultural prescriptions and their personal situations (Amaro et al., 2002).

A view of self as a female and presentation of self as a sexual being begins to form in early childhood and evolves throughout a woman's life as life circumstances shape her identity. A woman's view of herself as female includes her gender identity, or the personal, private conviction that each person has about being feminine (sense of self as a woman); her sense of having characteristics customarily defined as feminine, masculine or both (gender role); and body image (mental picture of one's body and its relationship to the environment) (Fogel, 2003). While gender identity can be influenced by one's biologic or anatomic sex, it is not necessarily consistent with biologic sex (Alexander & LaRosa, 1994).

Presentation of self as a woman (gender role behaviors) includes all those behaviors that women use to indicate to society that they are women including dress, hairstyle, speech patterns, and walk. Gender role behaviors are a reflection of a woman's internalization of societal and cultural stereotypes and expectations of what a woman's behavior should be (Alexander & LaRosa, 1994). Gender role prescriptions and expectations shape sexual expression. Beliefs about women and men and assumptions regarding appropriate behaviors for both affect sexual behavior, communication patterns, and expectations of sexual relationships.

Sexual orientation is the erotic or romantic attraction or preference for sharing sexual expression with persons of a specific gender. It also refers to the preference an individual develops for a partner, or the preference for the gender of the person with whom one has an emotional and physical attraction, and with whom one wishes to share sexual intimacy. Sexual preferences exist on a continuum ranging from total orientation to the same sex, through bisexuality, to total orientation to the other sex. Sexual orientation may be determined before birth, although orientation can also be influenced by social factors and personal experiences. It is important to note that one's sexual practices may not necessarily indicate sexual orientation.

Sexual lifestyles and relationships provide the pattern and context for one's sexuality. While many options exist for women today, not all are equally accepted by society (Bernhard, 1995). The most frequently acknowledged pattern for women is heterosexual, marital monogamy, which is assumed to be the most desirable status by the majority of societies. In contrast, women who engage in serial heterosexual monogamy have an established pattern of conducting one monogamous relationship followed by another. Women who choose a pattern of nonmonogamous heterosexual marriage participate in sexual activity with other individuals or couples while married. Other women have elected to have sexual relations with one or more concurrent male partners without marriage (heterosexual coupling without marriage). A woman is considered to be bisexual when her sexual and affectional preferences are directed toward individuals of either sex. Bisexual women may be married, have partners of both sexes simultaneously or serially, or have lesbian relationships as well as previous sexual relationships with men. Women who partner with a woman (lesbians) direct their sexual and affectional preferences toward women. Lesbians may be coupled or single with one or many partners; however, the most common pattern is serial monogamy. The celibate lifestyle involves the conscious choice to abstain from sexual activity. Women may view this choice positively as a means of giving one's time and energy and total attention to other activities, or celibacy may be involuntary, as when women are between relationships.

SEXUAL HEALTH

Defining sexual health is difficult and for many it is not something that is considered until its absence is noticed. While experts do not agree on a definition of sexual health, the World Health Organization (1975) provides a beginning point: Sexual health is the integration of somatic, emotional, intellectual, and social aspects of sexual beings in ways that are positively enriching and that enhance personality, communication, and love. Essential elements of this definition include the capacity to enjoy and control sexual and reproductive behavior in accordance with a social and personal ethic; freedom from shame, fear, guilt, and misconceptions that inhibit sexual response and harm sexual relationships; and freedom from disease, illness, organic disorders, and deficiencies that interfere with sexual functioning. Essential to sexual health is an acceptance of one's gender identity, body image, sexual identity, and sexual orientation. Also important is the ability to comfortably communicate one's sexual feelings, needs, and desires. Thus sexual health may be considered the factors that enable women to enjoy and control their sexual and reproductive lives, including a physical and emotional state of well-being, and the quality of sexual and other close relationships.

Definitions of sexual health and sexual practices may contain value-laden terms that are susceptible to different interpretations. Cultural norms often dictate what is acceptable or normal behavior. Before clinicians can provide sexual health care, they must be aware of how they define normal and abnormal sexual practices. Because it is not always easy to distinguish between aberrant and merely unconventional practices, clinicians should consider the questions found in Box 8–1 in order to identify the attitudes and beliefs they hold regarding sexual practices.

SEXUAL RESPONSE IN WOMEN

Sexual response involves capacity, or what a woman is capable of experiencing, and activity, or what she actually experiences. Emotion and physiology are interwoven in a woman's sexual response cycle. Traditionally the Masters and Johnson (1966) model of

BOX 8-1   ASSESSING A SEXUAL BEHAVIOR

The following questions can be used when considering whether or not a particular behavior or practice is abnormal:

- What does the behavior mean to the woman?
- Does the behavior enrich or impoverish the sexual life of the woman and those with whom she shares sexual relations?
- Is the behavior tolerable to society?
- Is the behavior between two consenting adults?
- Does the behavior cause physical or psychological harm to the woman or her partner?
- Does the behavior involve coercion?

Source: MacLauren, 1995.

sexual response, adapted by Kaplan (1979), has been used to explain sexual response in both men and women. Although Masters and Johnson began the modern movement toward an understanding of the sexual response cycle, their description focused solely on physiologic responses to stimuli. The two principal physiologic responses to sexual stimulation are vasocongestion and muscle tension, and are represented differently throughout the phases of the woman's sexual response cycle. Later authorities incorporated both biologic and psychological components (Kaplan; American Psychiatric Association, 1994). However, the focus on genital responses and customary indicators of desire, such as sexual fantasies and the need for self-stimulation, ignores important components of women's sexual satisfaction, including intimacy, trust, and comfort with vulnerability, communication, respect, affection, and pleasure associated with sensual touching (Basson, 2000; Leiblum, 1998; Tiefer, 1991). Basson suggests that women's sexual response more commonly arises from needs for intimacy rather that a desire for physical sexual arousal, and that women's sense of sexual arousal arises only minimally from an awareness of genital congestion and other physiological changes.

The traditional female sexual response cycle as described by Masters and Johnson and Kaplan, modified to include the element of consent (Chalker, 1994), consists of four sequential phases: desire, excitement, orgasm, and resolution. The desire phase consists of sexual fantasy, thoughts, and awareness that sexual stimulation is wanted without physiologic changes. Vasocongestion, muscle tension, and other physiologic changes build, peak and release, then resolve during the excitement, orgasm, and resolution phases respectively. During the cycle, there is progression from a subjective sense of anticipation and pleasure to release and finally to relaxation.

While this model is useful for understanding male sexual response and dysfunction, it does not account for four fundamental aspects of women's healthy sexual functioning (Basson, 2000). First, women have a lower biologic urge to be sexual for the release of sexual tension than men. Second, women's motivations for sexual experiences are related to rewards that are not sexual in nature, and that are in addition to and may be more relevant than their biologic urges. Although these rewards are not irrelevant to men, they may often be less of a motivating force. Men may experience their desire independent of context, and thus desire may be more accurately labeled "drive." Third, women's sexual arousal is a subjective mental excitement that may or may not be associated with an awareness of genital vasocongestion and other physical nongenital arousal symptoms. In fact, genital awareness may or may not be an erotic stimulus for women. Finally, women may or may not experience orgasmic release of sexual tension. When orgasmic release does occur, it can happen in a variety of ways, even in the same woman (Basson).

Basson (2000) suggests that while the Masters and Johnson model as modified by Kaplan may represent the beginning of a new understanding of sexual relationships for women, it is not truly representative of women's long-term sexual relationships, and that a different model would be more appropriate (Figure 8–1). Women move from a sexually neutral state to seeking sexual stimuli when they sense either an opportunity to be sexual or a partner's need, or when they have an awareness of one or more of the potential benefits of sexual activity. Sexual desire may be experienced as a craving for sexual sensations for their own sake, a desire to experience physical and subjective arousal, or possibly a release of sexual tension. In this model, sexual desire is a response rather than a spontaneous event. Although a woman may experience spontaneous desire in the form of sexual dreams, thoughts, or fantasies, she is more likely to be at a baseline neutral state at the onset of a partner experience (Basson).

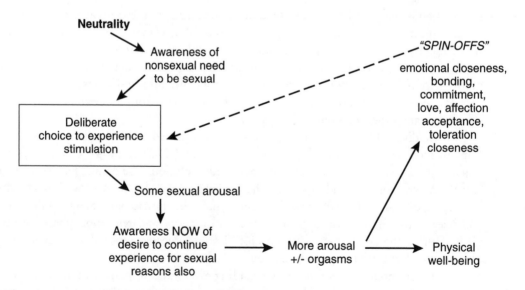

FIGURE 8–1   A Woman's Sex Response Cycle
Source: Copyright 2000 from The female sexual response: A different model by Rosemary Basson. Reproduced by permission of Taylor & Francis, Inc., http://www.taylorandfrancis.com.

According to Cawood and Bancroft (1996), many sexually functional and satisfied women do not have conventional markers of spontaneous sexual desire. For many women sexual arousal and responsive sexual desire occur simultaneously after the decision to experience sexual stimulation. Choice is initially based on needs other than a desire for physical sexual response and release. Women may experience physical well-being without orgasms and subsequent release. Emotional closeness with its attendant commitment, bonding, tolerance of imperfections in a relationship, and the appreciation of a partner's satisfaction, are valued emotional rewards for women and will act as motivators to activate the next sexual cycle. Further, these rewards may be sufficient by themselves, or they may be accompanied by physical sexual hunger. Although a woman may be motivated to be sexual by experiencing increased intimacy, she also needs a pleasant physical experience in order for the motivation to continue over time.

FACTORS INFLUENCING SEXUALITY

DEVELOPMENTAL FACTORS

Adolescence   Adolescence, the ages from 12 to 19 years, is a period of rapid physical change. It is also a time of potentially stressful psychosocial demands, including a time of awareness and change in sexual feelings. The development of adolescent sexuality focuses on five aspects:

- Physical changes of puberty and their relationship to self-esteem and body image
- Learning about normal bodily functions and sensual and sexual responses and needs
- Developing one's sense of self as a woman (gender identity) and comfort with one's sexual orientation
- Learning about sexual and romantic relationships
- Developing a personal sexual value system (Masters, Johnson, & Kolodney, 1995; Zwelling, 1997)

Sexuality is often defined through activities such as dating. During this time, adolescent females select companions, test ideas regarding themselves, and eventually experience sexual pleasure.

As adolescents develop a capacity for sexual intimacy, sexual curiosity and experimentation are common. Few very young teenage girls have had intercourse, with 8 in 10 girls being sexually inexperienced at age 15. In contrast, about 40% of all adolescents between 15 and 19 years old have had sexual intercourse (Singh & Darroch, 1999). In addition, 45.5% of adolescent females and 50.8% of adolescent males report having had two or more sexual partners in the past year (Hall, Holmqvist, & Sherry, 2004). In the United States, the likelihood of adolescents having sexual intercourse increases steadily with age (Alan Guttmacher Institute, 1999). Unwanted sexual experiences are common for adolescent girls with 25% to 40% of them reporting unwanted sexual experiences (Moore, Driscoll, & Lindberg, 1998; Wilson & Klein, 2002). The younger a woman is when she first has sexual intercourse, the more likely she is to have had unwanted or nonvoluntary coitus. Further, young women who begin sexual activity early have greater numbers of lifetime sexual partners (Seidman & Reider, 1994). Adolescents often face peer pressure to be sexually active. An additional motivation for sexual activity for girls may be a desire for sexual intimacy rather than a wish for the physical act of intercourse.

Early Adulthood and Midlife   In early adulthood (ages 20 to 40 years), women achieve maturity in a sexual role and in the relationship tasks started in adolescence, including developing intimacy with another individual and development of long-term commitment to a sexual relationship. Important career and personal decisions are made and increasing responsibilities assumed; balancing relationships, career, and children is often a concern. Women face choices regarding sexual lifestyles and often experience several before settling into one. During these years a woman continues to develop her personal sexual value system and must learn to be tolerant of others' sexual values. At some point during a woman's twenties and thirties, she faces decisions about childbearing. Throughout these years, frequency of sexual activity typically decreases (Fogel, 2003).

In midlife, 40 to 60 years of age, women's sexuality is as varied as are women (Doress-Worters & Ditzion, 1998; Sang, Warshow, & Smith, 1991; Taylor & Sumral, 1993). Some women report that sex is very good, possibly the best ever. Others report that sex is not the driving force it once was, or that sex is less exciting and gratifying. Although decreased libido can impact a woman at any age, up to one-third of postmenopausal women report a loss of sexual interest during menopause (Murray, 2000). The physiologic changes associated with menopause can affect sexual desire, expression, and functioning. Fluctuating levels of estrogen and related vasomotor instability can result in sleep disturbances associated with hot flashes. The resulting fatigue can adversely affect sexual desire. In the years immediately before and after menopause, women may report a loss of sexual desire associated with decreased vaginal lubrication, vaginal dryness, dyspareunia, painful spasms of the vaginal muscles, loss of clitoral sensations, fewer orgasms, or decreased depth of orgasm (Bachmann & Leiblum, 2004; Northrup). In contrast, other women may report increased sexual desire, increased clitoral sensitivity, increased responsiveness, and an increase in orgasms (Northrup). For some women, a decreased concern of becoming pregnant may increase sexual desire and lessen inhibitions.

Older Adulthood   During older adulthood (after age 65), women continue to be sexual and enjoy sexual activity. Although sexual frequency may decline, sexual enjoyment sometimes increases with age, and patterns of sexual behavior remain similar to those in midlife (Alexander & LaRosa, 1994; Steinke, 1988, 1994). The need for excitement, pleasure, and intimacy does not fade with aging. A critical issue for older women's sexual expression and activity is availability of a partner. Another important factor is health, as good health is positively associated with sexual interest and activity (B. K. Johnson, 1996).

Postmenopausal women are not immune to the universal psychosocial stressors that have been shown to decrease libido in younger women (Butcher, 1999; Klock, 1999). The increased responsibilities of different roles that accrue with age can increase marital strain and depression, and have a negative impact on libido (Murray, 2000). Satisfaction with one's sexual function is also influenced by self-evaluation within the context of personal desires and expectations. Personal expectations are often based on cultural and social factors as well as past sexual experiences. The prevailing cultural view of older women as asexual beings can negatively affect sexual expression and activity, and often becomes a self-fulfilling prophecy. Further, the current cultural emphasis on youth, beauty, and thinness also contributes to the societal expectation of asexuality in older women.

The physiologic changes associated with aging (decreased estrogen supply, decreased tissue elasticity, thinning of vaginal tissues) can cause irritation or discomfort with penetration and contribute to lessened desire and activity. The vascular changes that occur in arousal and the intensity of muscular contractions with orgasm may diminish moderately after the ages 55 to 60 (Alexander, 1997). Loss of fatty tissue of labia and mons pubis may result in tenderness and easily damaged tissue or abrasions, and may also decrease sexual libido and functioning. Orgasms may decrease in intensity and, in some women, become painful. Breast size also decreases and the breasts may sag. While these changes may alter a woman's sexual view of herself, they do not alter her ability to respond sexually. Body changes may require that a woman and her partners alter how they engage in sexual activity. With aging, sexual practices may include the use of a water-soluble lubricant, increased foreplay for arousal, different sexual positions, and planning intercourse for times when energy levels are highest.

Childbearing   Sexuality is often a concern for many women and their partners during pregnancy and postpartum as they experience the changes associated with childbearing. At the same time, these changes offer an opportunity to obtain a sexuality assessment and provide education for a couple's changing needs (Alteneder & Hartzell, 1997). Women may experience changes in sexuality, including levels of libido and frequency of sexual activity, with each trimester of pregnancy. During the first trimester, desire and functioning may be inhibited by nausea and vomiting, breast tenderness, fatigue, and anxiety about the pregnancy. In the second trimester, women often express heightened desire as they feel better, although some may be inhibited by increasing weight and bodily changes. Women may experience diminished sexual desire and activity during the third trimester associated with physical discomfort related to increasing size, especially near term. Fears about the effect of intercourse on pregnancy maintenance and harming the fetus may decrease sexual interest or pleasure at any time during pregnancy. A woman's partner may also experience decreased interest in sexual activity as his view of a woman shifts from partner to mother. Both may experience reticence associated with the presence of a third person (the fetus) in their relationship (Fogel, 2003).

During the postpartum period, women report lessened sexual desire and decreased sexual activity for up to six months (Byrd, Hyde, DeLamater, & Plant, 1998). Reasons for decreased desire and activity are physical discomfort, lessened physical strength, dissatisfaction with appearance, and fatigue (Ellis & Hewat, 1985; Fischman, Rankin, Socken, & Lenz, 1986). Early postpartum physical symptoms, such as lochia and increased vaginal discharge, are often not conducive to sexual desire or activity. Once the initial vaginal discharge has subsided, women may notice marked vaginal dryness associated with decreased estrogen and progesterone. Although vaginal dryness is more common among women who are breastfeeding, it can occur in any postpartum woman and may require some form of lubrication to prevent dyspareunia. Finally, motherhood allows little privacy and little rest, both of which are necessary for sexual pleasure.

Infertility   Struggles with infertility and repeated attempts to conceive can negatively impact sexual self-esteem, sexual expression, activity, and desire. Women may find the concepts of "woman" and "infertile" to be mutually exclusive (C. L. Johnson, 1996). Fertility and virility seem to be inextricably linked in our society. A diagnosis of infertility may negatively affect a woman's sense of sexuality, her self-image, and even her marriage. For women who desire pregnancy, stress and the need to time intercourse may interfere with pleasure and communication, as couples no longer have sex for pleasure, but rather only for procreation. Years of attempting to conceive and bear a child make spontaneous sex difficult to maintain. Sexuality is an important source of communication and growth in the development of a couple's relationship. When the desired end result of sexual activity is reproduction, sex can become mechanical or demanding. Women may initiate sexual activity around the time of ovulation even if they are experiencing low or decreased desire. Reacting to a feeling of threat or resentful of "sex on demand," men may experience reactive impotence, or the inability to perform sexually, especially around the time of ovulation.

SOCIOCULTURAL INFLUENCES

Women's sexuality exists within the context of cultural expectations, individual experiences, and biologic potential. Social influences on sexuality first begin within the family. Through socialization of the individual, a family conveys its own, as well as societal, sexual attitudes and behaviors, and may contribute to later sexual dysfunction. Restrictive family upbringing or a belief that expressions of intimacy or sexuality are shameful or taboo may contribute to a woman's inability to express herself sexually. Poor parent–child interactions can contribute indirectly to sexual problems through decreased self-esteem or through an inability to cope with intimacy (Sheaham, 1989) Unsatisfactory relationships with fathers may contribute to orgasmic difficulties (Bernhard, 1995). Messages such as "sex is something to endure," or "women who enjoy sex are no good," may inhibit sexual expression or enjoyment.

Religion also influences sexual attitudes, beliefs, and values, and can exert a strong influence throughout a person's life. Religious proscriptions can contribute to sexual concerns or problems. For example, a view that sexual intercourse is acceptable only for procreation may raise concerns when pleasurable sensations are felt. Accepting or rejecting premarital sex, allowing or limiting contraception to prevent pregnancy, beliefs about monogamy for men and women, and condoning or rejecting homosexuality are examples of religious influences in a woman's life.

Society and culture are inextricably interwoven with sexuality and influence it as much as physiology and psychology. Society defines what sexual behavior is, defines the norms for that behavior, and guides the behavior of the individuals in a given culture. In part, women form their ideas of what is sexually appropriate and desirable from years of cultural scripting. These scripts are frequently different for men and women and can be the basis for many of the issues women experience in sexual relationships. The notions that men who are sexually aggressive are "macho" or "studs" and that sexually aggressive women are "whores" and "easy" are examples of such cultural beliefs. Current sex role stereotypes prescribe that men initiate sexual activity and that women exercise control.

Sexual myths are common in every culture and society, are a source of sexual misinformation, and can be related to many sexual problems. Often they interfere with women reaching full sexual potential and establishing fulfilling sexual relationships. Many sexual myths exist today (Fogel, 2003; Smith, 1997). Examples of such myths include: that women's needs are secondary to men's, that large amounts of sexual stimulation are needed to arouse a woman, and that when a woman says "no" she doesn't mean it. There are also sexual myths that are specific to elderly women, such as older women are not interested in or capable of sexual expression, or that older women are physically unattractive and sexually undesirable.

A specific behavior may be defined as desirable by one cultural group and evil by another. Different views often exist regarding premarital, extramarital, and marital sex; appropriate sexual positions; accepted foreplay activities; and duration of coitus. Certainly cultural practices that physically alter sexual response, such as female circumcision (see Chapter 6), will affect sexuality.

HEALTH-RELATED INFLUENCES

A number of health-related factors, including illness, surgery, disability, medications, and substance abuse, can influence sexuality and sexual performance. Illness can affect sexuality in a number of ways, and a variety of medical conditions can cause sexual dysfunction in women (Box 8–2). Chronic illness with its associated fatigue, pain, and stress affects sexual desire and arousal more often than it affects orgasm. Many medications can alter sexual functioning and cause sexual dysfunction including anorgasmia and inadequate lubrication (Box 8-3). The degree of impairment is often dose related. Depending on the dosage and an individual's mental and physical states, some medications known to inhibit sexual function may instead enhance it. Examples of such drugs include the benzodiazepine tranquilizers and chlorpheniramine (Roberts, Fromm, & Bartlik, 1998).

All cancers can impact sexuality and intimacy. Treatment that affects the vascular system or causes nerve damage may alter sexual function. Changes in body image and self-concept may have a profound influence on sexuality (Rogers & Kristjanson, 2002). For example, in our society where breasts are sexual, a woman with breast cancer may have

BOX 8-2 MEDICAL CONDITIONS ASSOCIATED WITH ALTERED SEXUAL FUNCTIONING IN WOMEN

Arthritis
Cancers
Cerebrovascular accident
Chronic obstructive pulmonary disease
Coronary artery disease
Diabetes mellitus
Hypertension
Malnutrition
Neurologic disorders
Renal failure
Thyroid disorders

Source: EngenderHealth, 2004.

BOX 8-3 MEDICATIONS ADVERSELY AFFECTING SEXUAL FUNCTIONING

Anorectics
Anticancer drugs
Anticonvulsants
Antihistamines
Antihypertensives
    Alpha blockers
    Angiotensin converting enzyme inhibitors
    Beta blockers
    Calcium channel blockers
Histamine H_2-receptor blockers
Psychotropics
    Antipsychotics/neuroleptics
    Anxiolytics
    Monoamine oxidase inhibitors
    Mood stabilizers
    Phenothiazines
    Selective serotonin reuptake inhibitors
    Tranquilizers
    Tricyclic antidepressants

Source: Roberts, Fromm, & Bartlik, 1998.

sexuality concerns. Greater sexuality problems may be experienced by women who dislike their breasts, have a negative self-image, have been sexually abused, lack a support system, or are uncomfortable discussing personal or sexual concerns (Bernhard, 1995). Treatment of gynecologic cancer is also associated with less frequent intercourse, sexual excitement, and arousal (Andersen, Anderson, & DeProsse, 1989; Schover, Fife, & Gershenson, 1989). Women with endometrial cancer have stressed the negative effect of symptoms such as vaginal bleeding on sexual expression. Further, the fatigue and lethargy associated with cancer treatment adversely influence sexual functioning (Lamb & Sheldon, 1994). Results of studies on the effect of a hysterectomy on sexuality vary considerably and no longer document negative effects only (Bernhard, 1992; Katz, 2002).

Disability can affect a woman's sexuality in various ways. Disabled women are often viewed as asexual by health providers and the public alike (Cesario, 2002), and as such are not encouraged to express their sexual feelings or to be sexually active. The attitude that a disability somehow neuters a woman interferes with her right to sexual feelings and sexual expression (Nosek et al., 1994; Blackwell-Stratton, Breslin, Mayerson, & Bailey, 1988; Sawin, 2003). A critical issue for some women who are disabled is body image as they may view their bodies as a problem and a source of anxiety rather than pleasure. The reactions of others may also suggest that a woman's body is unacceptable or unattractive (Nelson, 1995). The specific physical effects of a given disability on sexual activity differ according to the condition. For example, women with spinal cord injuries commonly report autonomic dysreflexia and bladder incontinence (Jackson & Wadley, 1999). These women may also experience alterations in desire, establishing adequate vaginal lubrication, the ability to reach or feel orgasm, and difficulty finding a comfortable position for intercourse (Cesario, 2002).

Sexually transmitted infections (STIs), including the human immunodeficiency virus (HIV), are transmitted within the context of an interpersonal relationship and have the potential to affect a woman's sexuality and sexual functioning. Women who have been diagnosed with an STI often experience depression, low self-esteem, guilt, lack of trust, and anger (Fogel, 2003). The adoption of safer sex practices necessitates altered sexual practices. Sexual risk-reduction practices require individuals to give up behavior that has been enjoyable, gratifying, highly reinforced, and often of long duration, and replace it with alternatives that are almost always less gratifying, more awkward, or inconvenient, and more difficult than current behaviors (Kelly & Kalichman, 1995). Women may decide to avoid risk by being celibate, by decreasing the number of their partners, or avoid certain partners, and by changing or avoiding specific sexual activities that increase risk. The risk of sexual coercion may be great for women in power-imbalanced relationships with men who resist using condoms. Sex roles and sexual double standards may hinder a woman's ability to ask for safer sex practices and contribute to a man's resistance to implement these practices.

Chemical dependency can have an adverse effect on sexual functioning and sexuality. Sexual dysfunction, especially sexual desire disorders, can occur with the use of substances such as alcohol, amphetamines, cocaine, opioids, sedatives, and tranquilizers (Klein,

1997; Zerbe, 1999). Women who use illicit substances may also trade sex for drugs and money.

RELATIONSHIP AND PARTNER FACTORS

Women are more likely than men to associate sex with love and commitment, and a woman's subjective perception of sexual pleasure is influenced by her perception of her relationship with her partner. Women have reported that their most pleasurable sexual feelings were in response to intercourse with a partner, though their most profound physical responses occurred through masturbation (Darling, Davidson, & Jennings, 1991). Relationship discord may precipitate sexual dysfunction; so much so that many sex therapists believe that sexual dysfunction is a symptom of underlying relationship dysfunction. Open communication of one's sexual preferences, feelings, and desires is essential for sexual satisfaction. One or both partners may experience difficulty after disclosure of sexual activity outside the relationship. Sexual communication difficulties can be exacerbated by distrust, feelings of betrayal, and fear of disease. Sexual dysfunction in one partner may precipitate dysfunction in the other partner. For example, erectile difficulty in the male is often accompanied by lack of vaginal lubrication, orgasmic difficulties, and impaired desire disorders in the female.

Loss of one's partner can adversely affect sexuality. Many women define their identity through their relationships, and thus loss of a partner can create a loss of sense of self. Further, the typical image of a widow is that of a grieving woman whose sexual life has ended. Factors that may be related to a woman's sexuality after loss of a partner are her extramarital sexual experiences, age, and sexual satisfaction in the marriage (Bernhard, 1995). Remarriage is correlated with age; the older a woman is when she loses a partner, the less likely she is to remarry.

SEXUAL ASSESSMENT

In order to provide satisfactory sexual health care, clinicians must be comfortable with their own sexuality, aware of their own biases, and have a sincere desire to assist their patient. When sexual health care is provided, it is essential that clinicians not make assumptions regarding a woman's sexual attitudes, values, feelings, or behavior. Additionally, clinicians need to know how various health problems, diseases, and their treatment affect sexual functioning and sexuality. Sexual health assessment includes a physiological, psychological, and sociocultural evaluation through obtaining a history, conducting a physical examination, and laboratory tests.

HISTORY

The sexual history is the most important aspect of the assessment process in relation to sexuality. Yet clinicians are often reluctant to ask about their patient's sexual histories or lifestyles (Warner, Rowe, & Whipple, 1999). Factors contributing to clinicians not obtaining adequate information about a woman's sexuality include not seeing the woman's sexual history as relevant to her health problem, inadequate training, embarrassment, and fear of offending.

Clinicians should take responsibility for introducing topics of sexual health problems. As with any interview, it is important to establish a positive tone before beginning. Rapport needs to be developed and sufficient time for trust to build needs to be allowed before soliciting information the woman may consider highly personal or intimate. Choose a quiet, private place where the woman can be comfortable and where interruptions can be minimized. Have the woman remain dressed and sit at eye level with her. Such measures foster a sense of acceptance and respect for the patient and reduce her possible feelings of intimidation. Do not allow anyone other than the patient to be present during this portion of the history in order to obtain candid, open discussion. Women should be assured that information obtained during an oral history is confidential although chart documentation is not. Further, any information that is obtained from a form completed by the patient also may not be confidential. It is not necessary to collect all the information at the same time, and a sexual history can be collected over several patient visits, especially when the woman is very anxious. It is essential for clinicians to continually monitor their own responses for negative or uncomfortable feelings because these are easily conveyed to patients. Usually more information is obtained if you begin with open-ended questions and allow the woman to tell her story in the way she is most comfortable. Women should be told why questions are being asked. Limits can be set if women offer excessive or irrelevant information. Patients should be redirected if information becomes tangential, and encouragement should be provided if progress is slow.

It is best to begin with less threatening material, such as her obstetrical history or childhood sexual education, and move to more sensitive topics such as her current sexual practices. A general guide is to begin with questions about an individual's sexual education history (e.g., How did you learn about sex?), proceed to personal attitudes and beliefs about sexuality, and finally to assess actual sexual behaviors.

Avoid using excessive medical terminology during an interview; both the clinician and the woman need to know the meaning of terms used. Euphemisms such as "slept with" should not be used. Only one question should be asked at a time and the woman given enough time to answer. Statistical questions such as "How many times a week do you have sexual intercourse?" are not helpful because normal practices vary extensively among individuals. Rather than asking about a particular sexual experience, which people tend to deny, it is better to ask how many times the experience has occurred. This technique suggests that the experience is normal. Techniques such as "universalizing" or prefacing questions by comments such as "Many people..." or "Other women I have talked with have said" may make a woman feel more comfortable when answering sensitive questions.

A sexual history can be incorporated into a total health history, or it can be more formal and inclusive. A number of formats are available for use, and the reader is referred to references (Fogel, 2003; Heiman, 1995; MacLauren, 1995; Zwelling, 1997). In most cases, sexual concerns or problems can be uncovered by asking a few questions (Box 8–4). While the

> ## BOX 8-4 QUESTIONS INCLUDED IN A SEXUAL HISTORY
>
> - Are you sexually active? Alternate questions are "Are you sexually involved?" and "Are you having sexual relations?"
> - Are you having any sexual difficulties or problems at this time? Do you have any pain?
> - Has (illness, pregnancy, surgery) interfered with your being a partner? Has any (illness, surgery, medication, treatment) changed how you feel about yourself as a woman? Has any (disease, surgery, medication, treatment) altered your ability to function sexually?
> - Is sex pleasurable for you (desire)? Are you having difficulty with lubrication during sex (arousal)? Are you able to have an orgasm/climax (orgasm)? Do you have any pain or discomfort during sexual activity (pain)?
> - Are you satisfied with your sexual activity? Is it satisfactory? Are you happy with it?
> - Do you have any sexual problems or questions?
> - Do you limit physical contact with your partner because you are afraid it will lead to sex?
> - Do you become irritated when your sexual partner initiates sex?
> - Do you feel that having sex is an imposition?

specific form of sexual history to be used will vary depending on the woman, it is essential to include questions about her body image, concerns relating to sexual functioning, changes that have occurred in sexual function in the past six months or since the last visit, degree of satisfaction with sex life, and health conditions, medications, or treatments that affect sexual function. Women can also be asked to describe their present relationship and to rate this relationship with respect to communication, affection, sexual needs met, and sexual communication. If the woman is in more than one relationship, inquire about each relationship. A complete gynecologic history (see Chapter 6) is relevant and should also be obtained. Detailed assessment of risk for STIs can be found in Chapter 18.

PHYSICAL EXAMINATION AND DIAGNOSTIC STUDIES

When it is indicated by history, reason for seeking care, treatment goals, or need for referral, a physical examination may be performed. While there are no studies specific to sexual assessment, often the history and physical examination may suggest a specific laboratory test. Physical examination and diagnostic studies to be considered in the evaluation of sexual concerns can be found in Chapter 14.

CONCLUSION

Sexuality begins with conception and develops throughout a woman's life. Sexual problems are among the most common of human concerns and will be experienced by most people, if only briefly, at some point in their lives. It is essential for clinicians caring for women to have a working knowledge of sexual functioning and to provide a nonjudgmental, supportive approach so that women are comfortable in discussing sexuality. Providers can promote healthy sexual functioning by fostering communication, providing accurate information and counseling, and when needed, making appropriate referrals to other health professionals.

REFERENCES

Alan Guttmacher Institute. (1999). *Facts in brief: Teen sex and pregnancy.* Retrieved October 8, 2004, from http://www.agi-usa.org/pubs/fb_teen_sex.html.

Alexander, B. A. (1997). Women's sexuality: A paradigm shift. In J. A. Rosenfeld (Ed.), *Women's health in primary care.* Baltimore: Williams & Wilkins.

Alexander, L. L., & LaRosa, J. H. (1994). *New dimensions in women's health.* Sudbury, MA: Jones & Bartlett.

Alteneder, R. R., & Hartzell, D. (1997). Addressing couples' sexuality concerns during the childbearing period. *Journal of Obstetric, Gynecologic, and Neonatal Nursing, 26*(4), 651–658.

Amaro, H., Navarro, A. M., Conron, K. J., & Raj, A. (2002). Cultural influences on women's sexual health. In G. M. Wingood & R. J. DiClemente (Eds.), *Handbook of women's sexual and reproductive health.* New York: Kluwer Academic/Plenum.

American Psychiatric Association. (1994). *Diagnostic and statistical manual of mental disorders* (4th ed.). Washington, DC: Author.

Andersen, B. L., Anderson, B., & DeProsse, C. (1989). Controlled prospective longitudinal study of women with cancer: I. Sexual functioning outcomes. *Journal of Consulting and Clinical Psychology, 57,* 683–691.

Bachmann, G. A., & Leiblum, S. R. (2004). The impact of hormones on menopausal sexuality: A literature review. *Menopause: The Journal of the North American Menopause Society, 11*(1), 120–130.

Basson, R. (2000). The female sexual response: A different model. *Journal of Sex & Marital Therapy, 26,* 51–65.

Bernhard, L. A. (1992). Consequences of hysterectomy in the lives of women. *Health Care for Women International, 13,* 281–291.

Bernhard, L. (1995). Sexuality in women's lives. In C. I. Fogel & N. F. Woods (Eds.), *Women's health care.* Thousand Oaks, CA: Sage.

Blackwell-Stratton, M., Breslin, M. L., Mayerson, A. B., & Bailey, S. (1988). Smashing icons: Disabled women and the disability women's movements. In M. Eine & A. Asch (Eds.), *Women with disabilities: Essays in psychology, culture and politics.* Philadelphia: Temple University Press.

Butcher, J. (1999). ABC of sexual health: Female sexual problems I: Loss of desire: what about the fun? *British Medical Journal, 318,* 41–43.

Byrd, J. E., Hyde, J. S., DeLamater, J. D., & Plant, A. (1998). Sexuality during pregnancy and the year postpartum. *Journal of Family Practice, 47*(4), 305–308.

Cawood, H. H., & Bancroft, J. (1966). Steroid hormones, the menopause, sexuality, and well-being of women. *Psychological Medicine, 26,* 925–936.

Cesario, S. K. (2002). Spinal cord injuries: Nurses can help affected women & their families achieve pregnancy, birth. *Association of Women's Health, Obstetric, and Neonatal Nurses Lifelines, 6,* 224–232.

Chalker, R. (1994). Updating the model of female sexuality. *Sexuality Information and Education Council of the United States, 22,* 1–6.

Charlton, R. S., & Quatman, T. (1997). A therapist's guide to the physiology of sexual response. In R. S. Charlton (Ed.), *Treating sexual desire.* San Francisco: Jossey-Bass.

Darling, C. A., Davidson, J. K., & Jennings, D. A. (1991). The female sexual response revisited: Understanding the multiorgasmic experiences in women. *Archives of Sexual Behavior, 20,* 535.

Doress-Worters, P., & Ditzion, J. (1998). Women growing older. In Boston Women's Health Collective,

Our bodies, ourselves for the new century. New York: Simon & Schuster.

Ellis, D. J., & Hewat, R. J. (1985). Mother's postpartum perceptions of spousal relationships. *Journal of Obstetric, Gynecologic, and Neonatal Nursing, 14*(2), 140–146.

EngenderHealth (2004). *Sexuality and sexual health: Online minicourse.* Retrieved November 9, 2004 from http://www.engenderhealth.org/res/onc/sexuality/index.html.

Fischman, S. H., Rankin, E. A., Socken, K. L., & Lenz, E. R. (1986). Changes in sexual relationships in postpartum couples. *Journal of Obstetric, Gynecologic, and Neonatal Nursing, 15*(1), 58–63.

Fogel, C. I. (2003). Women and sexuality. In E. Q. Youngkin & M. S. Davis (Eds.), *Women's health: A primary care clinical guide* (3rd ed.). Upper Saddle River, NJ: Pearson Prentice Hall.

Hall, P. A., Holmqvist, M., & Sherry, S. B. (2004). Risky adolescent sexual behavior: A psychological perspective for primary care clinicians. *Topics in Advanced Practice Nursing Journal, 4*(1), 1–10.

Heiman, J. R. (1995). Evaluating sexual dysfunction. In D. P. Lemke, J. Pattison, L. A. Marshall, & D. S. Cowley (Eds.), *Primary care of women.* Norwalk, CT: Appleton & Lange.

Jackson, A., & Wadley, V. (1999). Multicenter study of women's self-reported reproductive health after spinal cord injury. *Archives of Physical Medicine and Rehabilitation, 80*(11), 1420–1428.

Johnson, B. K. (1996). Older adults and sexuality: A multidimensional perspective. *Journal of Gerontological Nursing, 22*(2), 6–15.

Johnson, C. L. (1996). Regaining self-esteem: Strategies and interventions for the infertile woman. *Journal of Obstetric, Gynecologic, and Neonatal Nursing, 25*(4), 291–295.

Kaplan, H. (1979). *Disorders of sexual desire and other new concepts and techniques in sex therapy.* New York: Brunner/Mazel.

Katz, A. (2002). Sexuality after hysterectomy. *Journal of Obstetric and Gynecologic and Neonatal Nursing, 31*(3), 256–262.

Kelly, J. A., & Kalichman, S. C. (1995). Increased attention to human sexuality can improve HIV-AIDS prevention efforts: Key research issues and directions. *Journal of Consulting and Clinical Psychology, 63*(6), 907–918.

Klein, M. (1997). Disorders of desire. In R. S. Charlton (Ed.), *Treating sexual desire.* San Francisco: Jossey-Bass.

Klock, S. (1999). Psychological aspects of women's reproductive health. In K. J. Ryan (Ed.), *Kistner's gynecology and women's health* (7th ed.). St. Louis, MO: Mosby.

Lamb, M. A., & Sheldon, T. A. (1994). The sexual adaptation of women treated for endometrial cancer. *Cancer Practice, 2*(2), 103–113.

Leiblum, S. R. (1998). Definition and classification of female sexual disorders. *International Journal of Impotence Research, 10,* S102–S106.

MacLauren, A. (1995). Comprehensive sexual assessment. *Journal of Nurse-Midwifery, 40*(2), 104–119.

Masters, W., & Johnson, V. (1966). *The human sexual response cycle.* Boston: Little, Brown.

Masters, W. H., Johnson, V. E., & Kolodney, R. C. (1995). *Human sexuality* (5th ed.). New York: Harper-Collins.

Moore, K. A., Driscoll, A. K., & Lindberg, L D. (1998). *A statistical portrait of adolescent sex, contraception, and childbearing.* Washington, DC: National Campaign to Prevent Teen Pregnancy.

Murray, W. (2000). Decreased libido in postmenopausal women. *Nurse Practitioner Forum, 11*(4), 219–224.

Nelson, M. R. (1995). Sexuality in childhood disability. *Physical Medicine and Rehabilitation: State of the Art Reviews, 9*(2), 451–462.

Northrup, C. (1998). *Women's bodies, women's wisdom.* New York: Bantam Books.

Northrup, C. (2001). *The wisdom of menopause.* New York: Bantam Books.

Nosek, M. A., Howland, C. A., Young, M. E., Georgiou, D., Rintala, D. H., Foley, C. C., Bennett, J. L., & Smith, Q. (1994). Wellness models and sexuality among women with physical disabilities. *Journal of Applied Rehabilitation Counseling, 25*(1), 50–58.

Phillips, N. A. (2000). Female sexual dysfunction: Evaluation and treatment. *American Family Physician, 62,* 127–136, 141–142.

Roberts, L. W., Fromm, L. M., & Bartlik, B. D. (1998). Sexuality of women through the life phases. In L. A.

Wallis (Ed.), *Textbook of women's health.* Philadelphia: Lippincott-Raven.

Rogers, M., & Kristjanson, L. J. (2002). The impact on sexual functioning of chemotherapy-induced menopause in women with breast cancer. *Cancer Nursing, 25*(1), 57–65.

Sang, B., Warshow, J., & Smith, A. J. (1991). *Lesbians at midlife: The creative transition.* Minneapolis, MN: Spinster's Ink.

Sawin, K. J. (2003). Health care concerns for women with physical disability and chronic illness. In E. Q. Youngkin & M. S. Davis (Eds.), *Women's health: A primary care clinical guide* (3rd ed.). Upper Saddle River, NJ: Pearson Prentice Hall.

Schover, L. R., Fife, M., & Gershenson, D. M. (1989). Sexual dysfunction and treatment for early stage cervical cancer. *Cancer, 63*, 204–212.

Seidman, S. N., & Reider, R. O. (1994). A review of sexual behavior in the United States. *American Journal of Psychiatry, 151*(3), 330–341.

Sheaham, S. L. (1989). Identifying female sexual dysfunction. *Nurse Practitioner, 14*, 25–26, 28, 30, 32, 34.

Singh, S., & Darroch, J. E. (1999). Trends in sexual activity among adolescent American women: 1982–1995. *Family Planning Perspective, 31*(5), 212–219.

Smith, R. P. (1997). *Gynecology in primary care.* Baltimore: Williams & Wilkins.

Steinke, E. E. (1988). Older adults' knowledge and attitudes about sexuality and aging. *Image: Journal of Nursing Scholarship, 20*(2), 93–95.

Steinke, E. E. (1994). Knowledge and attitudes of older adults about sexuality in aging: A comparison of two studies. *Journal of Advanced Nursing, 19*, 477–485.

Taylor, D., & Sumral, A. C. (1993). *The time of our lives. Women write on sex after 40.* Freedom, CA: The Crossing Press.

Tiefer, L. (1991). Historical, scientific, clinical, and feminist criticisms of "the human sexual response cycle." *Annual Review of Sex Research, 2*, 1–23.

Warner, P. H., Rowe, T., & Whipple, B. (1999). Shedding light on the sexual history. *American Journal of Nursing, 99*(6), 34–40.

Wilson, K. M., & Klein, J. D. (2002). Health care and contraceptive use among adolescents reporting unwanted sexual intercourse. *Archives of Pediatrics and Adolescent Medicine, 156*, 341–344.

World Health Organization. (1975). *Education and treatment in human sexuality: The training of health professionals.* (WHO Technical Report Series, No. 572). Geneva, Switzerland: Author.

Zerbe, K. J. (1999). *Women's mental health in primary care.* Philadephia: Saunders.

Zwelling, E. (1997). Sexuality during pregnancy. In F. H. Nichols & E. Zwelling (Eds.), *Maternal-newborn nursing theory and practice.* Philadelphia: Saunders.

CONTRACEPTION

PATRICIA AIKINS MURPHY
KATHERINE MORGAN
FRANCES E. LIKIS

Contraceptive management is often a challenging undertaking, but providing family planning services offers clinicians the opportunity to empower people by helping them to make choices that can truly alter their life courses. There are more than 60 million women of reproductive age in the United States. Seven in ten of these women, or about 42 million women, are sexually active and do not want to become pregnant. The average woman in the United States desires two children and thus must use contraception for approximately three decades of her life. Sixty-one percent of US women of reproductive age in the United States who practice contraception use reversible methods of contraception. Three million unintended pregnancies occur each year in the United States. Women who use no contraception account for 47% of these pregnancies. Women who use some contraceptive method account for the remaining 53% of unintended pregnancies; the majority of these result from inconsistent or incorrect use (Alan Guttmacher Institute, 2004).

Thus the challenge lies in helping each woman choose the method that best meets her needs and providing education so that the chosen method can be used correctly and consistently. Unfortunately, there is no perfect contraceptive method—one that requires no effort, never fails, has no side effects, is easily affordable, and reverses immediately. The good news is that there are more contraceptive options available now than ever before.

Contraceptive users today want more than efficacy from a method. They desire a method that is safe, convenient, cost-effective, and has few side effects. How a method affects a woman's life, from side effects such as daily spotting to the need to remember to do something every day, may be a major determinant in consistency of use. In addition, knowledge about the noncontraceptive health benefits of methods is increasing; thus women can make contraceptive choices that can have positive implications for their health. Most therapeutic uses of contraception (for example, treatment of menorrhagia with the levonorgestrel intrauterine system [LNG-IUS]) are not approved by the Food and Drug Administration (FDA), although many are supported by evidence. Clinicians frequently prescribe medications for conditions other than those for which they have FDA approval, and this off-label use is within the scope of the prescriptive privilege when sound rationale and evidence are used (Cranston, Williams, Nielsen, & Bezman, 1998).

Contraceptive counseling should never be guided by a provider's biases about what is best for a particular person. The best method for any woman is the one that she wants and is motivated to use. Providers should present all of the choices that are reasonable (i.e., those that are acceptable in light of the individual history) and assist the woman to find her own best option. Clinicians should use evidence-based contraindications to avoid unnecessarily restricting contraceptive options when determining whether the patient's history makes a particular method acceptable. The Medical Eligibility Criteria for Contraceptive Use developed by the World Health Organization (WHO) (2004) are helpful in determining whether or not a woman is a candidate for a particular method (Appendix 9–A). A thorough knowledge of the contraceptive methods available is imperative for providing contraceptive counseling that leads to informed choice. Women usually use contraception in the context of a relationship, and thus partners may need education as well. A woman may at times need supportive counseling to negotiate contraceptive issues within her relationship.

This chapter provides an overview of the various methods of contraception. Data on efficacy and effectiveness, safety and side effects, noncontraceptive benefits, and the advantages and disadvantages of each method are presented. Full discussion of contraceptive counseling and management is beyond the scope of this chapter. Interested readers are referred to the bibliography at the end of the chapter.

CONTRACEPTIVE EFFICACY AND EFFECTIVENESS

The effectiveness of contraceptive methods is described in several ways. "Efficacy," sometimes referred to as "method failure" or "perfect use" failure rates, describes the likelihood that an unintended pregnancy will occur even when the method is used consistently and exactly as prescribed. In most research studies, pregnancies that result from inconsistent use or incorrect use are not included in "method failure" rates. "Effectiveness," also termed "user failure" or "typical use" failure rates, describes all unintended pregnancies that occur if a method is not used properly (Trussell, 2004). Not all contraceptive failures are "user failures": all contraceptive methods have inherent failure rates. Unintended pregnancies occur even with highly effective methods such as sterilization (Table 9–1). Methods that are highly dependent on user consistency may have higher failure rates, but not all unintended pregnancies occur as a result of user errors. Providers should try to avoid implying that unintended pregnancies are the user's fault.

Several factors affect contraceptive failure rates. Most failures are concentrated in early usage: more fertile women will have earlier failures, and women who use contracep-

TABLE 9–1   Percentage of Women Experiencing an Unintended Pregnancy during the First Year of Typical Use and the First Year of Perfect Use of Contraception and the Percentage Continuing Use at the End of the First Year, United States

Method	% of Women Experiencing an Unintended Pregnancy within the First Year of Use		% of Women Continuing Use at One Year[3]
	Typical Use[1]	Perfect Use[2]	
(1)	(2)	(3)	(4)
No method[4]	85	85	
Spermicides[5]	29	18	42
Withdrawal	27	4	43
Periodic abstinence	25		51
Calendar		9	
Ovulation method		3	
Sympto-thermal[6]		2	
Post-ovulation		1	
Cap[7]			
Parous women	32	26	46
Nulliparous women	16	9	57
Sponge			
Parous women	32	20	46
Nulliparous women	16	9	57
Diaphragm[7]	16	6	57
Condom[8]			
Female (Reality)	21	5	49
Male	15	2	53
Combined pill and minipill	8	0.3	68
Evra patch	8	0.3	68
NuvaRing	8	0.3	68
Depo-Provera	3	0.3	56
Lunelle	3	0.05	56
IUD			
ParaGard (copper T)	0.8	0.6	78
Mirena (LNG-IUS)	0.1	0.1	81

(continues)

TABLE 9–1 continued

Method	% of Women Experiencing an Unintended Pregnancy within the First Year of Use		% of Women Continuing Use at One Year[3]
	Typical Use[1]	Perfect Use[2]	
(1)	(2)	(3)	(4)
Norplant and Norplant-2	0.05	0.05	84
Female sterilization	0.5	0.5	100
Male sterilization	0.15	0.10	100

Emergency Contraceptive Pills: Treatment initiated within 72 hours after unprotected intercourse reduces the risk of pregnancy by at least 75%.[9]

Lactational Amenorrhea Method: LAM is a highly effective, temporary method of contraception.[10]

1   Among typical couples who initiate use of a method (not necessarily for the first time), the percentage who experience an accidental pregnancy during the first year if they do not stop use for any other reason. Estimates of the probability of pregnancy during the first year of typical use for spermicides, withdrawal, periodic abstinence, the diaphragm, the male condom, the pill, and Depo-Provera are taken from the 1995 National Survey of Family Growth corrected for underreporting of abortion; see the text for the derivation of estimates for the other methods.

2   Among couples who initiate use of a method (not necessarily for the first time) and who use it perfectly (both consistently and correctly), the percentage who experience an accidental pregnancy during the first year if they do not stop use for any other reason. See the text for the derivation of the estimate for each method.

3   Among couples attempting to avoid pregnancy, the percentage who continue to use a method for 1 year.

4   The percentages becoming pregnant in columns (2) and (3) are based on data from populations where contraception is not used and from women who cease using contraception in order to become pregnant. Among such populations, about 89% become pregnant within 1 year. This estimate was lowered slightly (to 85%) to represent the percentage who would become pregnant within 1 year among women now relying on reversible methods of contraception if they abandoned contraception altogether.

5   Foams, creams, gels, vaginal suppositories, and vaginal film.

6   Cervical mucus (ovulation) method supplemented by calendar in the pre-ovulatory and basal body temperature in the post-ovulatory phases.

7   With spermicidal cream or jelly.

8   Without spermicides.

9   The treatment schedule is one dose within 120 hours after unprotected intercourse, and a second dose 12 hours after the first dose. Both doses of Plan B can be taken at the same time. Plan B (1 dose is 1 white pill) is the only dedicated product specifically marketed for emergency contraception. The Food and Drug Administration has in addition declared the following 18 brands of oral contraceptives to be safe and effective for emergency contraception: Ogestrel or Ovral (1 dose is 2 white pills), Alesse, Lessina, or Levlite (1 dose is 5 pink pills), Levlen or Nordette (1 dose is 4 light-orange pills), Cryselle, Levora, Low-Ogestrel, or Lo/Ovral (1 dose is 4 white pills), Tri-Levlen or Triphasil (1 dose is 4 yellow pills), Portia, Seasonale, or Trivora (1 dose is 4 pink pills), Aviane (one dose is 5 orange pills), and Empresse (one dose is 4 orange pills).

10 However, to maintain effective protection against pregnancy, another method of contraception must be used as soon as menstruation resumes, the frequency or duration of breastfeeds is reduced, bottle feeds are introduced, or the baby reaches 6 months of age.

Source: Reprinted with permission from Trussell, J. (2004). Contraceptive efficacy. In R. A. Hatcher, J. Trussell, F. Stewart, A. Nelson, W. Cates, F. Guest, et al. (Eds.), *Contraceptive technology* (18th ed.). New York: Ardent Media.

tion incorrectly or inconsistently will get pregnant sooner. In addition, older women are less fecund (able to get pregnant) than younger woman; thus, any method used by younger women will have a higher failure rate than the same method used by older women. Other factors contributing to contraceptive success are the fertility of the male partner, motivation to avoid pregnancy (as opposed to simply wanting to space pregnancies), relationship status, and frequency of sexual intercourse (Trussell, 2004).

NONHORMONAL METHODS

The nonhormonal contraceptive methods can be grouped into three general categories:

- *Physiologic Methods*—Abstinence, coitus interruptus, lactational amenorrhea method (breastfeeding), and fertility awareness-based (FAB) methods
- *Barrier Methods*—Male condoms, vaginal barrier methods, and spermicides
- *Sterilization*—Male and female

One additional contraceptive method that does not contain hormones—the copper intrauterine device—is covered in the section on intrauterine contraception. The reversible nonhormonal contraceptive options (physiologic and barrier methods) generally require motivated users, and most of these methods necessitate taking action with every act of sexual intercourse. In general, their efficacy is less than that of hormonal methods, but systemic side effects are avoided. In addition, many barrier methods do not require involvement of a health care provider. Nonhormonal methods may also be chosen because they fit within the woman's cultural beliefs. The irreversible contraceptive options, male and female sterilization, are the only permanent forms of contraception and require certainty that future childbearing is not desired.

PHYSIOLOGIC METHODS

Abstinence   Abstaining from penile-vaginal intercourse is the only certain way to avoid pregnancy. Abstinence is most often practiced in conjunction with FAB methods or prior to becoming sexually active. Although abstinence is generally promoted as the method of choice for adolescents, counseling should include all contraceptive options.

Efficacy and Effectiveness   Abstinence is 100% effective at preventing pregnancy.

Safety and Side Effects   There are no contraindications to or side effects from using abstinence.

Noncontraceptive Benefits   There are no noncontraceptive benefits of abstinence.

Advantages and Disadvantages Abstinence is readily available and completely effective. Abstinence prevents sexually transmitted infections (STIs), including human immunodeficiency virus (HIV) via penile-vaginal transmission, but users must be cautioned to avoid other sexual practices (e.g., oral sex and anal sex) that put them at risk for STIs (see Chapter 18). The major disadvantage of abstinence is that it is unrealistic for most couples in long-term relationships to use abstinence exclusively for an extended period of time.

Coitus Interruptus Coitus interruptus, also known as withdrawal, is the removal of the penis from the vagina prior to ejaculation. Coitus interruptus prevents pregnancy by keeping sperm from entering the vagina. While only 3% of contracepting women in the United States use coitus interruptus as their current method, 35–46% of women (percentages vary with age) report having used withdrawal at some time in their lives (Abma, Chandra, Mosher, Peterson, & Piccinino, 1997; Piccinino & Mosher, 1998).

Efficacy and Effectiveness The theoretical efficacy of coitus interruptus is high, but typical use failure rates demonstrate the difficulty of using this contraceptive method consistently and correctly (Table 9–1). Even when the method is used correctly, pregnancy may result from sperm in preejaculatory fluid.

Safety and Side Effects There are no contraindications to or side effects from using coitus interruptus.

Noncontraceptive Benefits There are no noncontraceptive benefits of coitus interruptus.

Advantages and Disadvantages Coitus interruptus is readily available, requires no supplies or cost, and is user controlled. Couples can use coitus interruptus intermittently when other methods are unavailable. Disadvantages include the need to use this method with every act of intercourse, and the need to exert the self-discipline and control necessary to stop intercourse. Coitus interruptus does not prevent STI transmission because penile-vaginal contact occurs, and HIV and other STIs can be present in preejaculatory fluid. Women who use coitus interruptus should be educated about emergency contraception as a back-up method.

Lactational Amenorrhea Method Infant suckling during breastfeeding increases maternal prolactin levels, which in turn inhibit ovulation; this is the physiological basis of lactational awareness method (LAM). Three conditions must be met for LAM to be effective: (1) exclusive or near exclusive (>90%) breastfeeding, (2) amenorrhea, and (3) infant is less than 6 months old (Kennedy, Labbok, & Van Look, 1996). Breastfeeding education and support are beneficial for women using LAM.

Efficacy and Effectiveness Breastfeeding is an extremely effective method of contraception if the conditions for use are met (Table 9–1). Failures typically occur when breastfeeding is nonexclusive or after the infant is 6 months old. In these instances, the likelihood of ovulation increases and the woman may be unaware of her return to fertility.

Safety and Side Effects   There are no contraindications to LAM, but breastfeeding is not recommended for women who are HIV positive in countries such as the United States where infant formula is accessible, or for women who are taking medications that could be harmful to the infant. The only side effects of LAM are those associated with breastfeeding, such as sore nipples and mastitis.

Noncontraceptive Benefits   Women who breastfeed their infants have decreased risk of ovarian, endometrial, and breast cancers (Collaborative Group on Hormonal Factors in Breast Cancer, 2002; Newcomb & Trentham-Dietz, 2000; Whittemore, 1994). Breastfeeding also has numerous benefits for infant health.

Advantages and Disadvantages   LAM is readily available, free, and can be used immediately postpartum. The disadvantages of LAM are that it is only available to women who are breastfeeding, duration of use is limited, and women may have difficulty sustaining the patterns of breastfeeding required for effectiveness. In addition, LAM does not provide protection from STI/HIV.

Fertility Awareness-Based Methods   FAB methods involve determining when a woman is most fertile during each month and using either abstinence or barrier contraception during that time to prevent pregnancy. The "fertile window" or time when intercourse is most likely to result in pregnancy comprises the five days before plus the day of ovulation (Wilcox, Weinberg, & Baird, 1995). FAB methods are also referred to as natural family planning and the rhythm method. Among women in the United States who use contraception, 2–3% use FAB methods (Piccinino & Mosher, 1998).

The fertile window can be identified with calendar methods or by using signs and symptoms of ovulation. Calendar methods require counting the days in the menstrual cycle. The calendar rhythm method entails the woman recording the length of 6–12 menstrual cycles and determining the longest and shortest cycles. She uses that information to identify the first (days in shortest cycle minus 18) and last (days in longest cycle minus 11) fertile day each month. Calculations must be updated with each cycle (Jennings, Arevalo, & Kowal, 2004). This method requires careful calculations that can be confusing; thus the Standard Days Method (SDM) was developed as a simpler calendar method. Women using the SDM are advised to use abstinence or a barrier contraceptive on days 8–19 of the menstrual cycle. A color-coded set of beads called CycleBeads can be used in conjunction with the SDM to help women keep track of their fertile window (http://www. cyclebeads.com). The SDM is recommended for women whose cycles are 26–32 days in length (Arévalo, Jennings, & Sinai, 2002). The postovulation method is another variation on the calendar method. The woman subtracts 14 days from her average cycle length to predict the day of ovulation. Abstinence or a barrier method is used during the first half of the cycle until the fourth morning after the predicted day of ovulation. This method requires the longest period of abstinence or use of additional contraception.

Signs and symptoms of ovulation include a rise of the basal body temperature (BBT) and changes in cervical mucus. The BBT rises at the time of ovulation and remains elevated for the rest of the cycle. Using BBT charting in conjunction with postovulation is beneficial, but predicting the fertile period with BBT is difficult because ovulation has already occurred once the rise in temperature is observed. The Billings Ovulation Method uses assessment of cervical mucus to determine the fertile window. Women check daily for the increased, clear, stretchy, slippery cervical secretions associated with ovulation. The fertile time lasts from the day ovulatory cervical secretions are first observed until four days after they are last observed (Billings, 2001). The Two-Day Method is a simplified version of the ovulation method. The woman checks daily for cervical secretions and is considered fertile any day that she has cervical secretions present or had them present the day before (Arévalo, Jennings, Nikula, & Sinai, 2004). The symptothermal method involves observing multiple indicators of the fertile window. The most common combination is assessment of cervical mucus and daily BBT charting. The cervical secretions can be used to identify the beginning of the fertile window, and the BBT can be used to detect the end. Some women using the symptothermal method also assess cervical position and signs of ovulation (e.g., mittelschmerz). Home ovulation tests originally used for women with infertility (e.g., Clearblue Easy Fertility Monitor) can be used in conjunction with the calendar, ovulation, or symptothermal methods to improve effectiveness (Fehring, 2005). The detailed information required for patient education about FAB methods is beyond the scope of this chapter. Readers are referred to the Web sites in Box 9–1 for further information, including training courses for providers.

Efficacy and Effectiveness   Theoretical efficacy for FAB methods varies according to the specific technique used (Table 9–1). The typical use failure rate reflects the difficulty of using these methods correctly and consistently.

Safety and Side Effects   There are no health concerns with the use of FAB methods, but certain circumstances or conditions complicate their use. These include the postpartum period, breastfeeding, immediately after an abortion, recent menarche or perimenopause

---

BOX 9–1 WEB SITES FOR FERTILITY AWARENESS-BASED METHODS INFORMATION

Billings Ovulation Method: http://www.billingsmethod.com
Institute for Natural Family Planning: http://www.marquette.edu/nursing/nfp/index.html
Institute for Reproductive Health: http://irh.org
Taking Charge of Your Fertility: http://www.tcoyf.com

when cycles may be irregular, medications that alter the regularity of cycles or fertility signs, vaginal discharge, irregular vaginal bleeding, and conditions associated with elevated body temperature (WHO, 2004). There are no side effects of FAB methods.

Noncontraceptive Benefits   The principles of FAB methods can be used to conceive when couples decide they want children.

Advantages and Disadvantages   Patients may have to pay for FAB methods training or supplies (e.g., basal body thermometer, CycleBeads), but there is no ongoing cost unless a barrier contraceptive is used during the fertile window. These methods are user controlled and may be the only acceptable form of contraception for some religions and cultures. Disadvantages include the need for detailed education, ongoing attention to identifying the fertile window, and abstaining from intercourse or using an additional contraceptive method several days a month. FAB methods do not protect from STI, and users should be educated about emergency contraception.

BARRIER METHODS

The use of physical and chemical barriers for contraception is as old as history. In ancient times, women used vaginal suppositories of crocodile dung, wool, seaweed, or crushed root, often mixed with honey and herbs. Other methods included sea sponges moistened with lemon or vinegar. Condoms made of linen or animal intestines were also commonly used (Tone, 2001). With the development of technology for vulcanized rubber in the mid-1800s, manufacture of condoms and "womb veils" (term used for devices such as diaphragms and caps) increased dramatically. By the 1870s, women in the United States could purchase these devices from mail order companies, pharmacies, dry-goods stores, and rubber vendors. Until the development of hormonal and intrauterine contraception in the latter half of the 1900s, these were the only methods other than FAB methods that were available to couples desiring to control their fertility (Tone).

All barrier methods are coitus-dependent. They must be applied at the time of intercourse, before any penile penetration (as sperm are present in preejaculatory fluid) and ideally before any genital contact (thus avoiding disruption in sex play). This may be a problem for some couples due to the need to "plan ahead," or for others who find application disruptive. Couples can be taught to make application or insertion of the barrier method part of their sex play. The coitus-dependent nature of barrier methods may be an advantage for couples who have infrequent intercourse.

Although less effective in preventing pregnancy than contemporary hormonal or intrauterine methods, interest in barrier contraception is on the rise again. This is due in part to its hormone-free aspects and in large part to its potential role as dual protection against pregnancy and STIs, including HIV. The cervix is the point of entry for many sexually transmitted pathogens. Protecting the cervix via chemical or physical barriers is an expanding area of research in the prevention of STIs. Finally, barrier contraceptives can be used by most people because contraindications to the use of these methods are rare (WHO, 2004).

Male Condoms   The condom is a thin sheath that is placed over the erect penis. It serves as a barrier to pregnancy by trapping seminal fluid and sperm and offers protection against STIs. In fact, early descriptions of condom use in the 1500s emphasized the condom's role in protection from syphilis and other diseases (Tone, 2001). Latex condoms were first introduced in the mid-1800s. With few exceptions, the design has changed little since then. They are manufactured and packaged with a rolled rim, designed to be applied to the tip of the penis and then rolled down over the erect penis. It is important to note that there is a right side and a wrong side when the condom is rolled up; applying the condom with the wrong side out will prevent it from being placed properly, and potentially contaminate the outside of the condom with seminal fluid. Minor design changes over the years to this rolled rim construction have included enlarged tips to contain ejaculated fluid (Figure 9–1), as well as variety of colors, sizes, flavors, and textured surfaces that are purported to enhance sexual pleasure. Some condoms add lubricants as well, including spermicidal lubricants.

Nonlatex condoms were developed in response to several concerns about latex condoms. These condoms are made of polyurethane or a latexlike material called styrene ethylene butylene styrene (SEBS). Nonlatex condoms are odorless, colorless, and non-allergenic. They transmit body heat better, and have a looser fit, theoretically allowing

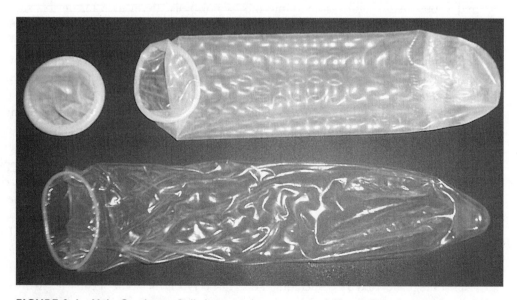

FIGURE 9–1   Male Condoms. Rolled rim condom as packaged. Unrolled condoms with rounded and extended tips.

more sensitivity. They can be used with any lubricant, and do not usually deteriorate with the use of oil-based lubricants or under adverse storage conditions. Most consumers prefer the polyurethane condom over latex with regard to appearance, lack of odor, comfort, sensitivity, and "natural feel" (Rosenberg, Waugh, Solomon, & Lyszkowski, 1996). Users of the SEBS nonlatex condom also preferred this condom to its latex comparison for many of the same reasons. These preferences may translate into more consistent use of condoms. Consistent use and consumer familiarity with and education about the product may reduce the higher rates of breakage and slippage that have been reported in studies.

Efficacy and Effectiveness   When used correctly and consistently, latex condoms are an effective form of contraception (Gallo, Grimes, & Schulz, 2003) (Table 9–1). Condom failures are commonly related to breakage of the condom, or slippage during intercourse or while removing the condom. In general, pregnancy rates for nonlatex condoms are slightly higher than latex condoms, but within the range considered acceptable for barrier methods. However, nonlatex condoms have higher reported rates of breakage and slippage than latex condoms (Frezieres, Walsh, Nelson, Clark, & Coulson, 1999; Gallo et al., 2003). It is unclear whether this is related to the product, or to a lack of familiarity with the product.

Safety and Side Effects   Latex condoms should not be used by persons with known latex allergies. Some women report genital irritation and discomfort from the use of condoms. This may be related to the condom or to concomitant lubricant use. Some condoms are lubricated with a spermicide (nonoxynol-9), which may produce genital irritation in some women (see the section on spermicides). One study of a polyurethane condom evaluated genital irritation in both men and women. Although there were no differences between the men in each group, the female partners in the polyurethane group had significantly less genital pain, pruritis, and vaginal pain than the latex condom group (Steiner, Dominik, Rountree, & Dorflinger, 2003).

Noncontraceptive Benefits   Condoms are routinely recommended for their noncontraceptive benefit of protection from STIs. Consistent use of latex condoms in at-risk populations can result in an 80% reduction in the incidence of HIV infection (Weller & Davis, 2001). The evidence is less strong regarding the condom's effectiveness in preventing other STIs, but in general, experts feel that condoms likely offer protection for infections transmitted by cervical and vaginal secretions (such as gonorrhea, chlamydia, and trichomoniasis). It is less clear whether condoms offer significant protection against viral infections such as human papillomavirus (HPV), or genital ulcer infections such as herpes, syphilis, and chancroid. However, studies do suggest that latex condom use may reduce the risk of HPV-associated diseases such as cervical neoplasia in women (National Institute of Allergy and Infectious Diseases, 2001).

BOX 9–2   ADVANTAGES AND DISADVANTAGES OF BARRIER METHODS

Advantages:

- Nonhormonal
- Do not require daily action
- Some are available without prescription.
- Some offer protection against STIs.

Disadvantages:

- Require planning
- Require application at the time of intercourse and may be interruptive
- Breakage or slippage of barrier methods at time of intercourse may increase risk of unintended pregnancy.

Note: All women relying on barrier or coitus-dependent methods should be aware of emergency contraception and be offered an advance prescription.

Advantages and Disadvantages   Condoms have the advantage of being widely available over-the-counter, without the need for provider visit or prescription. The nonlatex condoms tend to be more expensive than their latex counterparts. Condoms are coitus-dependent (Box 9–2). Correct use is critical to prevent breakage, slippage, and resulting unintended pregnancy. A potential disadvantage of using condoms as a contraceptive method is that they are male controlled. Women who are in relationships where they cannot negotiate condom use with their partners need a method they can control.

Spermicides   Spermicides are chemical barriers that are used alone or in conjunction with a physical barrier (such as a condom, diaphragm, or sponge) to prevent pregnancy. In earlier centuries, douching with chemical substances, insertion of cocoa butter or gelatin suppositories, and foaming tablets made of sodium bicarbonate with boric acid or quinine were popular, albeit not very effective, methods of contraception (Tone, 2001).

All spermicides currently marketed in the United States contain nonoxynol-9 (N-9). The product may be formulated as a gel, cream, foam, suppository, foaming tablet, or film, and is generally provided in 50–150 milligram (mg) dosages. There are other spermicidal compounds available in other countries, such as octoxynol-9, benzalkonium chloride, or menfegol. According to the 1995 National Survey of Family Growth, less than 5% of women use spermicides alone or with a barrier method for contraception (Abma et al., 1997). In Title X family planning clinics, an estimated 2% of women report using N-9 formulations as their sole method of contraception (Centers for Disease Control and Prevention, 2002).

Efficacy and Effectiveness   Studies comparing N-9 in various formulations (vaginal contraceptive film, foaming tablets, suppositories, and gels), each used without condoms or other physical barriers, showed typical use pregnancy rates over six months that ranged from 10–15% up to 28% (Raymond, Chen, & Luoto, 2004; Raymond & Dominik, 1999) (Table 9–1). These rates are higher than those for other barrier contraceptives. Formulations containing at least 100 mg of N-9 had lower rates. Although the effectiveness of spermicides used as a sole agent is less than that of other contraceptive methods, spermicide use is more effective than using no method.

Safety and Side Effects   N-9 is a surfactant, and surfactants can disrupt cell membranes. By extension, many believed that the surfactant would also act against pathogenic organisms and protect against gonorrhea, chlamydia, herpes, and syphilis. Studies from the late 1980s suggested that N-9 could inactivate HIV and other STIs (Louv, Austin, Alexander, Stagno, & Cheeks, 1988; Malkovsky, Newell, & Dalgleish, 1988; Polsky et al., 1988).

Other studies have shown that N-9 is an irritant to both animal and human tissue. Frequent use is associated with increased complaints of vaginal irritation. As an irritant, N-9 has the potential to disrupt or damage epithelial tissue in both the vagina and rectum. Studies have shown that the risk of disruption increases with frequency of use and dose (Wilkinson, Tholandi, Ramjee, & Rutherford, 2002). Because intact tissue is the first defense against infection, N-9 could thus potentially increase the risk of transmission of infection by causing microabrasions in the epithelium. Recent reviews of the literature provide good evidence that N-9 does *not* reduce STIs among sex workers or women attending STI clinics (Wilkinson et al., 2002), and in fact may even *increase* the risk of HIV acquisition in high-risk women (Van Damme et al., 2002).

Current recommendations for the use of N-9 based spermicides are:

- N-9 should not be used for purpose of STI protection.
- N-9 should not be used by women with multiple daily acts of intercourse.
- N-9 should not be used by women at high risk for HIV acquisition.
- N-9 should not be used rectally.

However, for women at low risk of HIV acquisition, N-9 products can remain a contraceptive option (WHO, 2001). In fact, N-9 is intended to be used with other female cervicovaginal barriers.

The likelihood of women using N-9 for contraception developing specific genitourinary symptoms after 6 to 7 months of use is 13–17% for a yeast infection, 8–12% for bacterial vaginosis, 19–27% for vulvovaginal irritation, and 11–15% for urinary tract symptoms (but only 3–6% for culture-proven urinary tract infection). The likelihood of irritation and other genitourinary symptoms in the male partner is 6–14% after 6 to 7 months of use. There was no comparison group in these studies to indicate if these rates are higher, lower, or the same as symptoms in the general population of sexually active contracepting women (Raymond et al., 2004). However, the reported rates are high enough to warrant counseling women to report symptoms so that they can be evaluated, diagnosed, and properly treated.

Noncontraceptive Benefits   Despite concerns about the potential for cervicovaginal epithelial disruption with N-9-based spermicides, the appeal of vaginally applied chemical barriers remains high. This is due to their potential as dual protection: both spermicidal and microbicidal. Woman-controlled, vaginally applied, lubricating microbicides offer great potential for protection against STIs, including HIV. At the time this chapter was written, there were more than 60 potential microbicides in development and 18 were already being studied in clinical trials.

Advantages and Disadvantages   Spermicides containing N-9 are widely available over-the-counter and do not require a prescription or provider visit. Thus they are readily accessible to women who need personally controlled, discreet, low-cost contraception. Spermicides are coitus-dependent (Box 9–2). Disadvantages include the low contraceptive effectiveness and the potential for symptoms of cervicovaginal irritation. As noted above, women with multiple daily acts of intercourse or who are at high risk for STI/HIV should avoid use of spermicides containing N-9.

Diaphragms   The traditional diaphragm has a long history as a contraceptive device (Tone, 2001). Currently only about 2% of contracepting women in the United States use the diaphragm (Piccinino & Mosher, 1998). However, the device is reemerging as a candidate for a woman-controlled method that provides not only contraceptive protection, but also potential protection against some STIs.

Efficacy and Effectiveness   The contraceptive efficacy of the diaphragm is similar to that of the male condom (Table 9–1). Traditional diaphragms are designed to be used in conjunction with a spermicide. There have been no studies of differences in the contraceptive effectiveness of a diaphragm depending on whether or not spermicide is used. During sexual excitement the upper part of the vagina expands; thus diaphragms and other devices that might be in contact with the vaginal walls during fitting may no longer provide a complete physical barrier to sperm migration during intercourse. Theoretically, an additional and important function of the diaphragm would be to maintain spermicide in contact with the cervical os, thus ensuring that sperm are trapped by the chemical barrier.

Safety and Side Effects   Spermicide side effects discussed above may also be experienced by diaphragm users. Diaphragms in the United States are generally made of latex and should not be used by women with latex allergies. Silicone diaphragms are an option for these women. Irritation or even abrasions of the vaginal mucosa have been noted in women with improperly sized diaphragms or prolonged retention in the vagina. Although no clear association with toxic shock syndrome has been demonstrated, diaphragms and other devices should not be left in the vagina for more than 24 hours, and their use during menses is discouraged.

Urinary tract infections are more common in diaphragm users than among women using hormonal contraceptives. There are two possible reasons for this. The first is mechanical; the rim of the diaphragm may cause pressure against the urethra, which might be perceived as frequency or dysuria, or incomplete bladder emptying, and may lead to infection. The second reason is that the spermicides used with the diaphragm can alter normal vaginal flora and may increase the likelihood of *E. Coli* bacteriuria.

Noncontraceptive Benefits   Researchers are interested in the diaphragm's possible value in protecting the cervix from infection, but data regarding any possible protective effect are not currently available.

Advantages and Disadvantages   Diaphragms are user controlled, nonhormonal methods that are only needed at the time of intercourse (Box 9–2). The devices come in multiple sizes, from 50 to 105 mm in diameter; sizes increase in 5 mm increments (Figure 9–2). They must be fit by a clinician and require a prescription to purchase. Thus, they have a higher initiation cost than condoms, but can be used for years with proper care. The only additional cost is the spermicide that must be used with the diaphragm. Diaphragms are washable and reusable. Proper use is important. Users should be counseled on the timing of insertion and removal, use of spermicide, appropriate care of the device, and need for periodic reevaluation of the size.

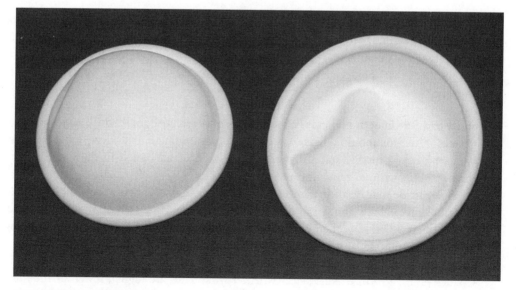

FIGURE 9–2   Diaphragms

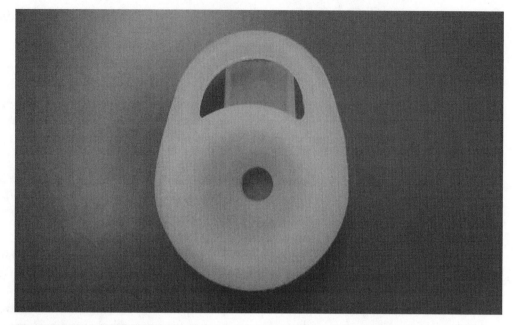

FIGURE 9–3 Lea's Shield. *Source:* Reprinted with permission from Yama, Inc.

Lea's Shield   Lea's Shield (Figure 9–3) is a new vaginal barrier contraceptive device. It is made of silicone, not latex. Thus it is not allergenic, has less odor problems, and does not deteriorate with petroleum-based lubricants. It is about the same size as a diaphragm, but comes in only one size, and is washable and reusable.

Efficacy and Effectiveness   An early study of Lea's Shield found an annual failure rate of about 15%, within the range of pregnancy rates for other barrier methods (Mauck et al., 1996). Like the diaphragm, it is intended to be used with a spermicide. The manufacturer recommends that the device be coated with spermicide, to maximize contraceptive effectiveness.

Safety and Side Effects   There is no known association with toxic shock syndrome, but in general, clinicians should advise women not to use vaginal barrier devices during menses. Package labeling further states that the device should not be left in the vagina for more than 48 hours without removing and washing it.

Spermicide may be an irritant to the cervical or vaginal mucosa for some women, and the same precautions about spermicide use previously discussed apply to this method. Approximately 6% of women in a clinical trial of Lea's Shield noted abnormal bleeding or spotting, and 6% were found to have vaginitis, cervicitis, or abnormal Pap test. Seventeen percent of the women reported pelvic pain or dyspareunia at some point during the study (Mauck et al., 1996). It is not clear whether these rates are higher, lower, or the same as would be found in the general population.

Noncontraceptive Benefits   There are no data on whether Lea's Shield offers protection against STI, but the theoretical potential of female physical barrier methods for protecting the cervix might apply to this device.

Advantages and Disadvantages   Lea's Shield shares the advantages and disadvantages of all nonhormonal, coitus-dependent barrier contraceptives (Box 9–2). Lea's Shield is a prescription product in the United States, although it is available over-the-counter in other countries. It can be purchased through US Planned Parenthood affiliates or directly from Yama, the manufacturer/distributor (http://www.leasshield.com). It does not require clinician fitting, as it is available in only one size. There would be an initial cost for the device; recurrent costs would be for spermicide.

Cervical Caps   Cervical caps are cuplike devices that cover the cervix. Smaller than diaphragms or vaginal barriers, they maintain their position over the cervix by suction, adhering to the cervix, or via a design that uses vaginal walls for support. Caps have long been popular in Europe, where several types of latex caps and a disposable silicone cap are available. The Prentif cap and the FemCap are the only cervical cap devices approved in the United States.

The Prentif cervical cap is a thimble-shaped device with a firm rim that fits snugly over the cervix (Figure 9–4). Made of latex, it is held in place by suction and support of the vaginal wall. Although women in research studies were permitted to use the cap for up

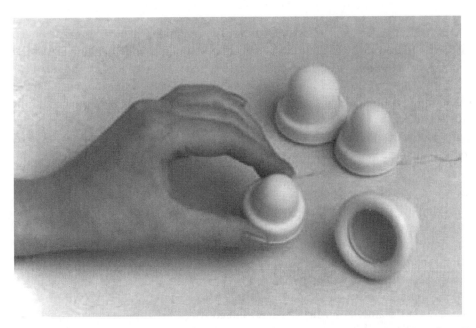

FIGURE 9–4   Prentif Cavity-Rim Cervical Cap. *Source:* Reprinted with permission from Cervical Cap Ltd.

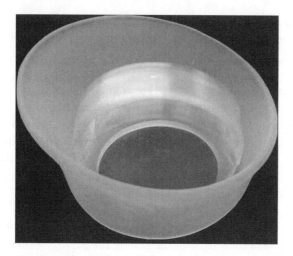

FIGURE 9–5 **FemCap.** *Source:* Reprinted with permission from FemCap Inc.

to 72 hours, most did not. The FDA guidelines set a maximum time of wear after insertion at 48 hours. The FemCap is made of silicone and has a design like an inverted sailor's cap (Figure 9–5). Its fit is less snug than the Prentif cap. The FemCap can also be worn for up to 48 hours, and as with all vaginal devices, should not be used during menses. Both devices are designed to be used with spermicide.

Efficacy and Effectiveness   The Prentif cap is comparable to a diaphragm in efficacy (Gallo, Grimes, & Schulz, 2002). The FemCap was not as effective in preventing pregnancy as the traditional diaphragm in clinical studies; the extrapolated annual failure rates would be a bit over 20%. However, there were some design issues that were felt to contribute to the failure rates in the research studies (Mauck, Callahan, Weiner, & Dominik, 1999). These were corrected in a subsequent design of the cap, and the device that was approved by the FDA is the modified design. Cervical caps may be less effective in women who have had children than in those who have not (Table 9–1).

Safety and Side Effects   In research studies, Prentif cap users had a slight increase in cervical cytology changes after 3-months use as compared to diaphragm users. US package labeling suggests a Pap smear be repeated after three months of use. Prentif cap users also had a lower risk of vaginal ulcerations or lacerations in studies. There is no evidence of an increase in episodes of vaginitis, bacterial vaginosis, candidiasis, or urinary tract infection among users of this cap (Gallo et al., 2002).

In a randomized trial comparing FemCap to the traditional diaphragm, FemCap users had significantly fewer urinary tract infections (7.5%) than those in the diaphragm group (12.4%). In this same study, there were no differences in vaginitis, irritation, dysmenorrhea, or Pap test changes between the groups (Mauck et al., 1999).

Noncontraceptive Benefits   As with all barrier methods, protection of the cervix by the cervical cap offer some noncontraceptive benefit in the prevention of STIs, especially those that are acquired via the cervix.

Advantages and Disadvantages   Cervical caps are coitus-dependent (Box 9–2), and may be appropriate for women who do not want or cannot use hormonal contraception. The latex-free FemCap is also appropriate for women who have, or whose partners have, latex allergies. Insertion and removal of cervical caps may be complex for some women. These women will need additional teaching and counseling. In a comparative study, there were more insertion and removal problems with FemCap than with the traditional diaphragm. About 10–15% of potential research subjects could not be fit with the FemCap, or were unable to insert or remove it (Mauck et al., 1999).

Caps require an initial cost for fitting and purchase, but should last for about two years with proper care. Ongoing costs would only be for spermicides. Both the Prentif cap and the FemCap are available only with a prescription. These cervical caps are available through Planned Parenthood affiliates, local distributors or dispensing pharmacies, or may be ordered directly from the companies. The Prentif cap (http://www.cervcap.com) and FemCap (http://www.femcap.com) Web sites provide detailed information about obtaining these devices.

Vaginal Sponge   The vaginal sponge is a soft, synthetic, absorbent sponge saturated with a spermicide. There are several types of sponges, although at the time of this writing, none are available in the United States. The Today sponge is a single-use polyurethane device that contains approximately 1000 mg of nonoxynol-9 spermicide; when moistened, the sponge gradually releases 125–150 mg of spermicide over 24 hours of use (Figure 9–6). Its primary contraceptive effectiveness is from the gradual release of spermicide; it also provides a physical barrier of the cervix and absorbs semen. It can be used for multiple episodes of coitus over 24 hours without inserting more spermicide.

The Today sponge was available in the United States until 1995, when the sole manufacturer ceased production after the FDA imposed new manufacturing standards. Another company purchased the rights to the sponge in 1998 and has been working with the FDA for marketing approval in the United States. At the time of this writing, the Today sponge is being marketed in Canada.

Efficacy and Effectiveness   Pregnancy rates are somewhat higher among women who use contraceptive sponges than among women who use diaphragms (Kuyoh, Toroitich-Ruto, Grimes, Schulz, & Gallo, 2003). As with the cap, these higher rates appear to be among women who have had children, as opposed to women who have never given birth (McIntyre & Higgins, 1986) (Table 9–1).

Safety and Side Effects   Women who use the sponge tend to discontinue use of their method at higher rates than women who use the diaphragm; over 40% of the women

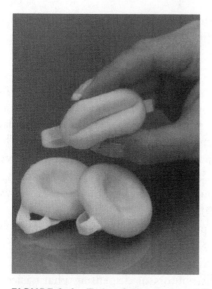

FIGURE 9–6 Today Sponge. *Source:* Reprinted with permission from Allendale Pharmaceuticals

who use both methods stopped using them in research studies. Allergic-type reactions, such as dermatitis, erythema, irritation, and vaginal itching were more common with the sponge, although they occurred in only about 4% of users (Kuyoh et al., 2003). During the time the sponge was available in the United States, 13 cases of toxic shock syndrome related to use of the sponge were reported. Some of these were associated with menstruation, recent childbirth, or other risk factors for the syndrome, and may not have been attributable to sponge use. Even so, given the number of sponges sold during that time, experts estimated that the risk of toxic shock syndrome was extremely low: approximately 1 case per 2 million sponges used ("Leads from the *MMWR*", 1984).

Noncontraceptive Benefits   The sponge may offer some noncontraceptive benefit in the prevention of STIs by physical protection of the cervix. However, this is a theoretical advantage and actual protection has not been demonstrated.

Advantages and Disadvantages   The sponge shares the advantages and disadvantages of other nonhormonal barrier, coitus-dependent methods (Box 9–2). It does not require a clinician visit or fitting and will be available over-the-counter. Its single use application may be more expensive over time than methods that can be reused.

Female Condom   The female condom was developed as an alternative to male condoms, to give women a nonprescription barrier contraceptive method that they could control, and also use to reduce their exposure to STIs. It has been available in the United States since 1993 (Hoffman, Mantell, Exner, & Stein, 2004). The female condom is a polyurethane sheath about 6.5 inches long that has a flexible ring at both ends (Figure

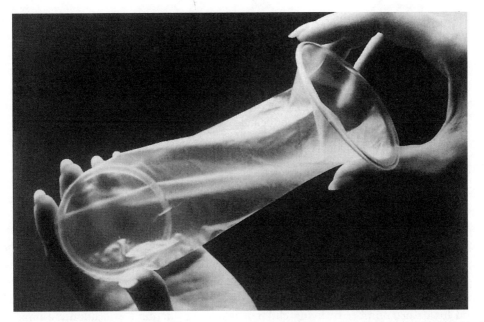

Figure 9-7   Female Condom. *Source:* Reprinted with permission from Varney, H., Kriebs, J. M., & Gegor, C. L. (2004). *Varney's midwifery* (4th ed.). Sudbury, MA: Jones and Bartlett.

9–7). The smaller ring, at the closed end of the sheath, is inserted high in the vagina. The larger ring rests outside the vagina against the vulva and acts as a guide during penetration. This ring also maintains the sheath covering the full length of the vagina, and prevents it from "bunching up" inside the vagina. The sheath is coated with a silicone-based, nonspermicidal lubricant, and women can use additional lubricant as well. The female condom should not, however, be used simultaneously with a male condom, as the risk of breakage increases.

Efficacy and Effectiveness   Studies of the effectiveness of the female condom in preventing pregnancy demonstrate that its efficacy is in the same range as that of other barrier methods (Farr, Gabelnick, Sturgen, & Dorflinger, 1994) (Table 9–1).

Safety and Side Effects   Female condoms are made of polyurethane and so do not present problems for people with latex allergies.

Noncontraceptive Benefits   Laboratory studies demonstrate that polyurethane can block smaller viruses such as herpes virus and HIV. Studies suggest that the female condom is at least as effective as male condoms in preventing STIs (Hoffman et al., 2004).

Advantages and Disadvantages   The female condom is a nonhormonal, female-controlled method that is available over-the-counter. A randomized crossover trial suggests that most users prefer the male condom to the female condom (Kulczycki, Kim, Duerr, Jamieson, & Macaluso, 2004). The population in this study may not be representative of women who desire female-controlled barrier methods and protection from STIs.

Some women find the female condom difficult to insert, although this problem decreases with proper education. Although it is a female-controlled method, male partner cooperation may still be necessary for consistent use; partner's lack of acceptance is often cited as a reason for discontinuation. Female condoms can be used only once and thus can be costly over time.

STERILIZATION

Sterilization is one of the most prevalent contraceptive methods in the United States. Approximately 11 million women rely on sterilization, and there are about 700,000 tubal sterilizations and 500,000 vasectomies performed annually in the United States (American College of Obstetricians and Gynecologists [ACOG], 2003). In 1995, nearly one quarter (24.2%) of US women aged 15–44 were surgically sterile for contraceptive reasons (Abma et al., 1997). Sterilization is considered a permanent procedure. People choose sterilization when they are sure they want no more children. Thus, the person's age and his or her number of living children when considering sterilization are important determining factors.

Female Sterilization   Female sterilization involves permanently blocking the fallopian tubes, which prevents sperm ascending the reproductive tract from meeting and fertilizing an egg released from the ovary. Female sterilization can be performed postpartum, postabortion, or as an "interval" procedure unrelated to pregnancy. Few sterilization procedures in the United States are performed in conjunction with abortion; about half are done postpartum, and half are interval procedures. The most common surgical approaches include laparoscopy, minilaparotomy, and procedures concurrent with a cesarean section. Newer approaches include microlaparoscopy and transcervical methods (Pati & Cullins, 2000).

A variety of methods exist for occluding the fallopian tubes. These include unipolar or bipolar electrothermal coagulation; mechanical occlusion using clips, rings, bands, or plugs; and ligation or salpingectomy, using one of several techniques. All of these methods are generally effective immediately. A newly approved transcervical method involves placing micro-inserts of metal and fibers into the fallopian tubes via a hysteroscopic procedure. During the three to four months following this procedure, tissue grows into the insert, effectively blocking the tubes. Other transcervical methods currently under investigation include the deposition of chemical substances into the tubes via hysteroscopy (ACOG, 2003; Pati & Cullins, 2000).

Efficacy and Effectiveness   Tubal sterilization is a highly effective contraceptive method (Table 9–1). The overall failure rate is low, but failures do occur and are more frequent in women who are younger at the time of sterilization. Failure rates are similar to those of other highly effective, long-term methods such as implants and intrauterine contraception. The most effective sterilization methods are postpartum partial salpingectomy and unipolar coagulation. The method with the highest failure is laparoscopic spring clip application (Peterson et al., 1996). Many experts recommend timing an interval procedure during the follicular phase of the menstrual cycle and using a highly sensitive pregnancy test prior to surgery to reduce the risk of luteal phase pregnancies that are conceived but not recognized before the procedure is performed.

Safety and Side Effects   Sterilization is a very effective method of contraception, but when pregnancy does occur after tubal sterilization, the risk of ectopic pregnancy is high. In the largest study done of sterilization, one-third of all poststerilization pregnancies were ectopic (Peterson et al., 1997). Other risks are related to the surgical procedures and include infection, hemorrhage, anesthesia complications, and surgical trauma or injury. The likelihood of these is very low, occurring in less than 1% of all procedures.

A "post-tubal syndrome" has been described; this usually refers to increased dysmenorrhea and abnormalities in the menstrual cycle. Most authorities believe such symptoms are more likely related to discontinuing hormonal contraceptives, or simply getting older and entering the perimenopause. There is no consistent evidence of a true post-tubal syndrome within the first two years after the procedure (Peterson et al., 2000).

Noncontraceptive Benefits   Studies in the United States and other countries suggest there is a decreased risk of ovarian cancer following tubal sterilization. In addition, some studies have shown a lower risk of pelvic inflammatory disease (PID) among women who have been sterilized when compared to women who have not (Westhoff & Davis, 2000). Reasons for this are not entirely clear but could be related to mechanical blockage of an ascending spread of pathologic organisms.

Advantages and Disadvantages   Tubal sterilization is a highly effective permanent method of birth control, suited for women who have completed their families. The surgical procedures are expensive and insurance coverage is variable. Additional barriers to access include requirements for a waiting period after signing consent and minimum age requirements. Studies in the United States suggest that women who have been sterilized are less likely to return for annual checkups or to use other preventive health services such as Pap tests. They are also less likely to use condoms for prevention of STIs. Counseling for women contemplating or undergoing sterilization should focus on the continued need for preventive health services (Winkler et al., 1999).

The younger the woman is at the time of her sterilization, the more likely she is during subsequent years to express regret about having the procedure. Younger women are also more likely to inquire about or seek a reversal of the procedure than older women (Hillis, Marchbanks, Tylor, & Peterson, 1999).

Male Sterilization   Male sterilization, or vasectomy, cuts or blocks both the right and the left vas deferens, which are the small tubes that carry sperm from the testes to become part of the seminal fluid. Sperm compose only about 5% of the semen that is produced by the prostate and other glands; thus, there is only a minimal decrease in the amount of seminal fluid. Vasectomies have no effect on sex drive, male hormone production, or sexual function. Approximately 1 in 6 US men over the age of 35 has had a vasectomy (Abma et al., 1997).

Two types of vasectomy procedures are currently in use and both can be performed in an outpatient setting (Sokal, McMullen, Gates, & Dominik, 1999). The traditional vasectomy requires small incisions in the scrotum. The vas is lifted out through the incision and tied off, cauterized, or blocked using surgical clips. The opening is then sutured. With the "no scalpel" method, the skin of the scrotum is pierced and the vas exposed and blocked through an opening so small it does not require stitches.

Vasectomy is not immediately effective birth control. Sperm are continually produced and transported through the male reproductive tract and therefore some sperm will remain distal to the site of the vasectomy. Generally it takes between 15 and 20 ejaculations to clear all sperm from the reproductive tract and be assured of contraception (Jamieson et al., 2004). Men are usually advised to have a follow-up visit and examination of ejaculate to ensure the absence of sperm before stopping other contraceptive methods.

Efficacy and Effectiveness   The first-year failure rate for vasectomy is estimated to be very low, but good research is lacking. Recent attempts to systematically review and summarize studies of vasectomy have led to the conclusion that most studies are of poor quality and better research is needed. Vasectomy failure rates appear to be lower than those for female sterilization (Jamieson et al., 2004) (Table 9–1).

Safety and Side Effects   Most men will experience some degree of postoperative discomfort; infection and scrotal hematoma occur infrequently. Some men will develop epididymitis or orchitis (defined as painful, swollen, and tender epididymis or testis), which are easily treated (Alderman, 1991). After a vasectomy, the testes continue to make sperm, which are absorbed by the body. Some men develop antisperm antibodies after the procedure; however, this does not increase the risk of autoimmune disease (Mullooly, Wiest, Alexander, Greenlick, & Fulgham, 1993).

Noncontraceptive Benefits   No benefits other than contraceptive have been demonstrated to date for vasectomy.

Advantages and Disadvantages   Vasectomy is a simple procedure that is less complicated and less costly than female sterilization for couples wishing permanent birth control. As is true with tubal sterilization, regret may occur with certain unanticipated life changes.

Reversal may have a better chance of success in men who have not developed antisperm antibodies (Hendry, 1994). Men need to be counseled that they might still be at risk for STIs.

HORMONAL METHODS

The FDA approval of combined oral contraceptives (COCs) in 1960 marked a revolutionary change in reproductive rights and responsibilities for women around the world. For the first time, women had access to a nearly 100% effective form of contraception that did not require the participation of the male partner and was independent of the act of coitus. COCs (or "The Pill") are some of the best studied and widely used medications available today and remain the most popular form of reversible contraception in the United States (Alan Guttmacher Institute, 2004).

There are two types of hormonal contraceptives: those that contain progestin (progestin-only), and those that contain progestin and estrogen (combined). Progestin, the synthetic version of the endogenous hormone progesterone, is highly effective alone as a contraceptive, but may cause irregular bleeding. The addition of estrogen to progestin in combined methods results in more predictable bleeding patterns due to stabilization of the endometrium. Estrogen as a single agent for contraception would require doses that would cause unacceptable risks of serious side effects, such as thromboembolic events and endometrial hyperplasia. The synergistic activity of estrogen and progestin makes it possible to combine these hormones in lower doses for successful contraception than would be possible using either hormone alone (Wallach & Grimes, 2000).

The combined contraceptive methods are COCs, the patch, and the vaginal ring. The progestin methods are progestin-only pills, the depot medroxyprogesterone acetate (DMPA) injection, and the subdermal implant. Each method is described in this section. An additional method that contains progestin, the LNG-IUS, is discussed later in the chapter in the section on intrauterine contraception.

Both progestin and estrogen inhibit the hypothalamic-pituitary-ovarian axis and subsequent steroidogenesis. Progestins have several contraceptive effects, including preventing the luteinizing hormone (LH) surge and thus inhibiting ovulation; thickening the cervical mucus, which inhibits sperm penetration and transport; changing the motility of the fallopian tubes so that transport of sperm or ova is impaired; and causing the endometrium to become atrophic, although it is unknown if these changes are sufficient to prevent implantation in the rare event that fertilization occurs. Estrogen suppresses follicle-stimulating hormone (FSH), thus preventing the selection and emergence of a dominant follicle. The primary mechanism of action of all hormonal contraceptive methods, with the exception of progestin-only pills (POPs), is preventing ovulation. Other contraceptive effects of progestin provide secondary mechanisms to prevent pregnancy should ovulation occur. POPs do not consistently inhibit ovulation, and their primary mechanism of action is thickening the cervical mucus. None of the hormonal methods provide

STI/HIV protection, so it is important to stress the concomitant use of barrier methods in women who are at risk of exposure to STIs.

COMBINED HORMONAL METHODS

Early formulations of COCs contained unnecessarily high doses of hormones, with 80–100 micrograms (mcg) of either ethinyl estradiol or mestranol and 1–5 mg of progestins. The trend, since the 1970s, has been to develop lower dose formulations that are equally effective, safer, and have a better side effect profile. In addition to improving COC formulations, alternative delivery systems for combined contraception have been developed that allow women to avoid a daily dosing schedule. These newer methods include the combined contraceptive injection, patch, and vaginal ring. They allow the circulating doses of estrogen and progestin to be lowered even further. This section begins with information about COCs that is followed by a discussion of the patch and ring. The combined injectable contraceptive (Lunelle) is not included in this chapter because it is no longer available in the United States, and there are no plans for the product to return to the US market as of this writing.

Combined Oral Contraceptives   Since the milestone introduction of COCs in the United States in 1960, many formulations of "The Pill" have been developed. Each is unique while on patent, but today there are more generic formulations than there are patented, and thus the same formulation can have several names. COCs are classified as monophasic or multiphasic (biphasic or triphasic), depending on whether the dosage of hormones is constant or varies. There is no evidence that monophasic or multiphasic formulations are superior.

Most of the COCs available today contain 20–35 mcg of ethinyl estradiol, although there are a few COCs available with 50 mcg of ethinyl estradiol or mestranol, the methyl ether of ethinyl estradiol. Approximately 30% of mestranol is lost as it is converted to ethinyl estradiol thus a 50 mcg mestranol pill is bioequivalent to a 35 mcg ethinyl estradiol pill.

COCs also contain one of several different progestins. The progestins are often referred to as first, second, or third generation, but this is an inappropriate categorization. With the exception of drospirenone, all progestins available in the United States are derived from 19-nortestosterone. These derivatives can be divided into two categories: the estranes or chemical derivatives of norethindrone (norethindrone, norethindrone acetate, and ethynodiol diacetate), and the gonanes or chemical derivatives of norgestrel (norgestrel, its active isomer levonorgestrel, desogestrel, and norgestimate). These categories differ in terms of both bioavailability and half-life. Caution should be exercised when comparing the potency or purported androgenicity of the various type of progestin by category. Rather, formulations should be judged on the clinical response of the patient. Drospirenone, the only non-testosterone derived progestin, is an analogue of the diuretic spironolactone. Drospirenone has a mild potassium-sparing diuretic effect, necessitating potassium levels to be checked during the first cycle in women using angiotensin converting enzyme inhibitors (ACE), chronic daily nonsteroidal anti-inflammatory drugs (NSAIDS), angiotensin-II-receptor antagonists, potassium-sparing diuretics, heparin, and aldosterone antagonists (Berlex Laboratories, 2003). Women with conditions that predispose them to hyperkalemia should not use COCs containing drospirenone.

The initial choice of a particular COC should be made with the goal of providing the woman with safe, effective contraception. All low-dose (less than 50 mcg) COCs meet this requirement, so it is reasonable to provide a woman with whatever formulation is most cost-effective, or whatever pill she requests by name.

Instructions contained in the pill package insert include options for a Sunday start, a first day start, and a day five start. These are all based on the principle that as long as COCs are begun within the first five days of the menses, there is contraceptive protection in the first cycle. The Sunday start has been the traditional approach in the United States, because the appearance of COC packages often reflects that regimen, and the withdrawal bleed does not usually occur on the weekend, which couples may find preferable. The advantage of the first day start is that no backup contraceptive method is required in the first cycle. Women are advised to use additional contraception, such as condoms, with the other start regimens for the first seven days. A new approach is to utilize a "quick start" by beginning the pill regardless of where the woman is in her menstrual cycle, if pregnancy is excluded and with additional contraception for the first seven days. Instructions are given to take a pregnancy test in two to three weeks if there was unprotected sex during the cycle. This has been shown to increase continuation and is not associated with an increased incidence of adverse bleeding patterns (Westhoff et al., 2002; Westhoff, Morroni, Kerns, & Murphy, 2003).

According to the traditional schedule, women take 21 days of active COCs followed by 7 days of inactive pills or no pills. During the hormone-free week, bleeding from the withdrawal of estrogen and progestin occurs. This is technically a withdrawal bleed, rather than a menses, and is based primarily on convention rather than science. Extended (omitting the hormone-free week for 2 or more cycles) and continuous (omitting the hormone-free week indefinitely) COC regimens are becoming increasingly popular, both for medical indications and convenience. Monophasic pills are generally preferred for this use.

Efficacy and Effectiveness   COCs require the woman's daily adherence to the dosing schedule, which can be compromised by many factors resulting in a gap between efficacy and effectiveness (Table 9–1). Based on worldwide levels of pill use in the year 2000, over 2 million women become pregnant unintentionally each year due to incorrect pill use (Zlidar, 2000). Common reasons for COC failure include not starting a new pack on time, missing pills, "taking a break" from the pill, and discontinuing the pill in response to normal side effects. The counseling and education provided by the clinician is critical to the ultimate success of the woman in avoiding unwanted pregnancy.

The most important pills to take in each cycle are the first and last active COCs, keeping the hormone-free interval to no longer than seven days. During the hormone-free week, pituitary stimulation of the ovary by FSH is likely to resume and follicular development may begin in many women (Elomaa et al., 1998; Killick, Bancroft, Oelbaum, Morris, & Elstein, 1990). Immature follicles stimulated during the hormone-free phase generally regress once the hormonal pills are resumed, and seven consecutive days of pill use have been shown to be sufficient in suppressing any follicular function (Letterie & Chow, 1992). Hormone-free intervals of less than seven days may become the standard recommendation in the future. Patient instructions must stress the importance of starting a new pack on time and not taking longer than seven days off of the active pills. If a woman does extend the hormone-free interval beyond seven days, she should be instructed to abstain from intercourse or use additional contraception until seven consecutive pills have been taken.

Missing pills is almost universal among women who choose the pill for contraception. Missing a random pill now and then, however, is unlikely to lead to a method failure. This fact may actually lead to complacency regarding the importance of daily adherence to the schedule as women come to feel that inconsistent pill use is adequate. The probability of pill failure increases with repeated missed pills. This is complicated by the fact that instructions for women who miss a pill can be confusing. Simplified instructions include a "seven-day rule." This states that if the first pill in the pack is missed, or if two or more pills in a row are missed in the cycle, the woman should abstain or use barrier methods for seven days. If only one pill is missed, the next pill should be taken as soon as possible, but no backup is required. In the case where a woman has missed three or more consecutive pills, and if a withdrawal bleed has begun, she may discard the old pill pack and begin a new cycle. Again, she should not have more than seven days of inactive pills or pill-free days.

Many women incorrectly believe that temporarily discontinuing or "taking a break from" COCs is beneficial. It is important to convey to patients that there is no accumulation of hormones in the body, and the fact that a withdrawal bleed occurs is evidence that the endometrium is responding to the absence of hormones. There are no differences in the long-term fertility of women who use the pill intermittently and those who use the pill for many years. Among women who take a break, however, the rate of unintended pregnancy increases 25% (Guillebaud, 2000).

As many as 32% of women in the United States who begin taking oral contraceptives, discontinue use before the end of one year (Table 9–1). A misunderstanding about the management of side effects may compound this dissatisfaction. Clear information about the common side effects during the first three cycles of pill use should be given. Whenever a woman begins a new COC, she should be advised to contact the provider prior to discontinuing the pills if she experiences unwanted side effects. This way a different pill may be substituted without interrupting effective contraception. There are many references to assist the clinician in fine-tuning COC formulations to each woman's needs (see bibliography at end of chapter).

A number of medications can impact the effectiveness of COCs. Pharmacologic mechanisms that alter medication metabolism include induction of liver enzymes, alterations in sex hormone binding globulin (SHBG), and medications that impact the first-pass effect in the gut. Medications that can reduce the effectiveness of COCs include rifampin, griseofulvin, and some anticonvulsants (e.g., carbamazepine and phenytoin). Emerging research indicates the over-the-counter herbal supplement St. John's wort may also interfere with oral contraceptives (Hall et al., 2003). Broad-spectrum oral antibiotics have been blamed for COC failures; however, pharmacologic evidence is lacking to support this (Dickinson, Altman, Nielsen, & Sterling, 2001). Given the prevalence of antibiotic use, any pill failures are more likely to be coincidence or to be associated with missed pills. Women who are concerned about reduced COC efficacy while on antibiotics can shorten or eliminate the placebo pills used, or use an additional contraceptive, but it is not necessary to routinely recommend these precautions.

Safety and Side Effects   COCs are one of the most extensively studied medications available and are known to be extremely safe for healthy women. Many of the side effects are bothersome but not dangerous; however, serious complications are possible and are the basis of contraindications to COC use. Contraindications may be related to the direct effects of either the hormonal ingredient, as in breast cancer, or as the result of hormonal effects on other systems, as in thromboembolism. The WHO Medical Eligibility Criteria for Contraceptive Use (2004; see Appendix 9–A) provide an evidence-based guide to the contraindications to COC use. One must always weigh the risks of pregnancy in relation to the risks associated with contraceptive use.

All COCs increase the risk of venous thromboembolism (VTE). The risk appears to be related to the dose of estrogen and is greatest for women with known clotting disorders, such as Factor V Leiden, or a family history of thrombosis. There is a difference between the various progestin components that may contribute to the risk of VTE; however, the difference between pills is small, and the studies showing the risk are subject to methodological errors (Speroff & Fritz, 2005). COCs containing less than 50 mcg of estrogen do not appear to increase the risk of arterial thrombosis (myocardial infarction or stroke) in healthy, nonsmoking women, including women over 40 years old. COCs may increase blood pressure in some women through an increase in plasma angiotensin. Because hypertension is a cofactor in the development of cardiovascular disease, blood pressure should be monitored in oral contraceptive users.

Metabolic effects of COCs include development of benign hepatocellular adenomas, although this is very rare with the low-dose pills. There does not appear to be an association with these benign tumors and the development of liver cancer. Low-dose COCs appear to create negligible changes in insulin levels or glucose levels and have no effect on the development of diabetes. There is no difference in weight gain in pill users versus nonusers in large studies; however, there are a few women who experience an anabolic response to oral contraceptives and are able to lose weight once the oral contraceptive is discontinued (Speroff & Fritz, 2005).

Numerous studies have shown that a history of COC use, regardless of duration, does not have an effect on the number of breast cancer cases diagnosed in the population when viewed over a lifetime. Current COC users experience an increase in the number of breast cancer cases; however, the risk is small, and it most likely represents a detection bias, as pill users are more likely to receive regular screening (Marchbanks et al., 2002; Speroff & Fritz, 2005). Recent studies have noted an increase in the incidence of cervical cancer in COC users (Moodley, 2004; Smith et al., 2003). Further study is needed to exclude the effects of early intercourse, HPV infection, smoking, and detection bias.

Mood changes and changes in libido have been noted among pill users and may respond to a change in the pill formulation. Depression, although rare, may justify the use of alternate methods of contraception. Other effects specific to estrogen include: nausea, cervical ectopy and leukorrhea, telangiectasis, chloasma (darkening of sun-exposed skin), growth of breast tissue (ductal tissue or fat deposition), increase in the cholesterol content within the bile (which can lead to gallstones), benign hepatocelluar adenomas, and changes in the clotting cascade. Effects specific to the androgenic impact of progestins include increased appetite and subsequent weight gain, mood changes and depression, fatigue, complexion changes, changes in carbohydrate metabolism, increased low-density lipoprotein (LDL) and decreased high-density lipoprotein (HDL) cholesterol, decreased libido, and pruritis. Effects that can be either estrogen or progestin related include headaches, hypertension, and breast tenderness. Studies have shown that many side effects women associate with COCs occur either during the seven hormone-free days or appear to be associated with the demise of follicles recruited during the hormone-free interval (Sulak, Scow, Preece, Riggs, & Kuehl, 2000). Therefore, a trial of extended use as described previously may improve symptoms women experience at predictable times in their pill cycles.

Noncontraceptive Benefits　The noncontraceptive benefits of COCs are numerous and underappreciated. There is evidence that women who use the pill for a total of four years reduce their risk of ovarian cancer by 60%. Pill use does not need to be consecutive, and the reduction in risk persists at least 20 years after pills are discontinued (Gross & Schlesselman, 1994; Ness et al., 2001; Rosenberg et al., 1994). Likewise, COC use reduces the risk of endometrial cancer by 50%. Risk lessens with increasing duration of use and persists for many years after the COCs are stopped (Schlesselman, 1997). Women on COCs experience lower rates of PID requiring hospitalization, fewer ectopic pregnancies, and a lower incidence of endometriosis. These are the most common causes of infertility; thus, it can be said that the pill helps preserve fertility, not by conservation of ovulation but through prevention of causes of subfertility. Other well-documented noncontraceptive benefits of the pill include improvement in acne and hirsutism, and reduced incidence of benign breast disease (Hatcher et al., 2004). Older studies demonstrated reduced risk of developing functional ovarian cysts while on COCs, but this effect is less profound with the lower doses of hormones in currently used COCs. There is limited evidence that COCs may also preserve bone density, reduce the risk of uterine fibroids, and improve rheumatoid arthritis (Borgelt-Hansen, 2001; Burkman, Collins, Shulman, & Williams, 2001).

In addition to being effective contraception, COCs have many other therapeutic uses. COCs regulate cycles and are useful in the management of abnormal bleeding patterns. While taking COCs, women experience lighter "periods" (withdrawal bleeds) that may treat or improve anemia. COCs can also be an effective treatment for mittelschmerz, dysmenorrhea, endometriosis, premenstrual symptoms, and the vasomotor symptoms of perimenopause. Women who experience catamenial conditions, those that rise and fall in synchronicity with the menstrual cycle such as menstrual migraines, may also find improvement with COCs. Decreasing the number of withdrawal bleeding episodes per year may further diminish these problems.

Advantages and Disadvantages   COC use is unrelated to coitus. Most women in the United States are familiar with the instructions for COC use, and this method is widely available in pharmacies and clinics. There is confidence in the product due to the fact it has been on the market for over for over 40 years and has been continually researched. Additionally, there are over 45 different formulations of the pill, allowing individualization based on response to the products. The obvious disadvantage to COCs is the need for daily pill taking. Ongoing cost of the method can also be problematic. Particularly for young women, lack of privacy may also be an issue. Finally, some women experience side effects with COCs that they are unable to tolerate.

Combined Contraceptive Patch and Ring   The contraceptive patch (Ortho Evra) and vaginal ring (NuvaRing) share many similarities with COCs, yet they have some distinct differences. The patch and ring utilize delivery systems that allow for simpler dosing than daily pill taking. Both methods avoid the first-pass metabolism of oral contraceptives, allowing for lower dose administration and potentially avoiding interactions with other medications.

The patch releases 20 mcg/day of ethinyl estradiol and 150 mcg/day of the progestin norelgestromin, the active metabolite of norgestimate. These active ingredients are rapidly absorbed and reach therapeutic serum concentrations within 48 hours, with a half-life of approximately 28 hours (Association of Reproductive Health Professionals, 2002.). The thin, beige patch is approximately the size of a matchbook (Figure 9–8). It is applied by the woman and worn for one week at a time. The patch is changed weekly on the same day of the week for three weeks and then no patch is worn for one week to allow for a withdrawal bleed. As with oral contraceptives, no more than seven days should pass between removal of the last patch and the beginning of the next patch cycle. The patch can be worn on the buttocks, upper arm, abdomen, and anywhere on the upper torso except the breasts.

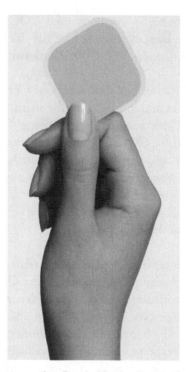

FIGURE 9–8 Combined Contraceptive Patch (Ortho Evra). *Source:* Reprinted with permission from Ortho McNeil Pharmaceutical.

The ring is colorless and flexible with an outer diameter of about 2 inches (Figure 9–9). The ring releases 15 mcg/day of ethinyl estradiol and 120 mcg/day of the progestin etonogestrel, the active metabolite of desogestrel. The active ingredients of the ring rapidly diffuse across the mucus membrane of the vagina and reach a steady state in the serum. The ring is left in place in the vagina for 21 days and then removed for one week allowing for a withdrawal bleed. The ring provides a steady delivery of hormones allowing for a very low serum concentration, approximately half of the serum concentration found with a 30 mcg oral contraceptive (Timmer & Mulders, 2000).

Efficacy and Effectiveness   The patch and ring have the same theoretical efficacy and typical use failure rates as COCs (Table 9–1). There is less opportunity for user error with the patch and ring as these methods need not be remembered daily. Each patch remains at therapeutic levels for at least nine days (Abrams, Skee, Natarajan, Wong, & Anderson, 2002). The ring also remains at therapeutic levels after three weeks; therefore, there is also some margin of error if women forget to change the products on time (Mulders & Dieben, 2001). Neither product is currently recommended for extended use, although

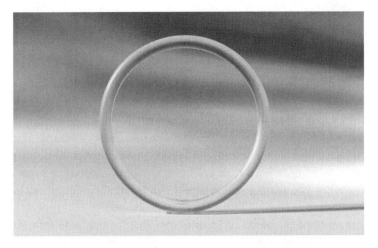

FIGURE 9-9   Combined Contraceptive Ring (NuvaRing). *Source:* Reprinted with permission from Organon USA Inc. NuvaRing is a registered trademark of N.V. Organon.

studies are underway. Higher failure rates have been documented in women weighing more than 198 lbs. (90 kg) with the patch as well as with lower dose COCs. These were very limited studies, and the contraceptive methods were still very effective. Thus women of greater weights should be cautioned about the possibility of increased failure rates but not denied the methods. The patch is only effective if it is completely attached to the skin; even partial detachment necessitates replacement. The exact placement of the ring in the vagina is not critical to its efficacy.

Safety and Side Effects   The WHO Medical Eligibility Criteria for Contraceptive Use (2004; see Appendix 9–A) are currently the same for COCs, the patch, and the ring. It is theoretically possible that the nonoral delivery systems may result in different safety and side effect profiles, but there is no evidence of this to date. Providers are cautioned to not presume the patch and ring are "safer" than COCs. A woman who is not a candidate for COCs should not be given the patch or ring either.

In general, the side effects of the patch and ring are very similar to those of COCs, such as breakthrough bleeding and nausea. In clinical trials, women using patches reported more breast tenderness than women using COCs, but this resolved over the first three months of use (Audet et al., 2001). The patch and ring also have unique side effects related to their delivery systems. About 20% of women in studies of the patch experienced some skin irritation at the site of application, but less than 3% discontinued use for this reason (Audet et al.). The ring may be felt during intercourse; however, this is not commonly cited as a reason for discontinuation. There is no increase in vaginitis or cervical cytological changes with the vaginal ring (Veres, Miller, & Burington, 2004).

Noncontraceptive Benefits It is theoretically plausible that the noncontraceptive benefits of COCs apply to the patch and ring because these methods affect the hypothalamic-pituitary-ovarian axis in the same way as COCs; however, epidemiologic studies to support this do not yet exist. Caution must be exercised in attributing the same long-term benefits of COCs to the patch and ring in the absence of evidence.

Advantages and Disadvantages The intrinsic advantage of the patch and ring is the absence of daily dosing, which may lead to greater effectiveness. A specific advantage of the vaginal ring is there is no visible evidence of use, which may appeal to some women, particularly adolescents, who want to keep their contraceptive use private. The patch may appeal to women who are not comfortable with vaginal placement, but desire a nondaily method.

One current disadvantage of the patch and ring is that there is only one formulation of each method. A variety of products may allow for individual variations in response to hormones, and patch color choices may appeal to some women as well. These methods also require ongoing costs. A final disadvantage of the patch and the ring is that both methods still contain large amounts of active ingredients at disposal. This has prompted environmental concerns about the effect of high doses of estrogen and progestin seeping into the water supply. There may be a recommendation in the future to place the used devices into a biohazard waste container instead of landfills.

PROGESTIN HORMONAL METHODS

Progestin contraceptives are used continuously; there is no hormone-free week as with combined methods. Progestin contraceptive methods are generally considered safer for women who are unable to take estrogen. In spite of this, the product labeling for some progestin-only products mimics the labeling for products containing estrogen. The WHO Medical Eligibility Criteria for Contraceptive Use (2004; see Appendix 9–A) are useful for determining appropriate candidates for progestin-only contraception. Progestin contraceptives do not provide the same cycle control as methods with estrogen.

Progestin-Only Pills The POPs or "minipills" in the United States contain either 0.35 mg of norethindrone (brand names are Camila, Errin, Micronor, and Nor-QD) or 0.075 mg of norgestrel (Ovrette). Each pill contains active ingredients; there is no hormone-free week as with COCs. POPs must be taken not only daily, but also at the same time each day.

Efficacy and Effectiveness POPs do not suppress ovulation as reliably as COCs and thus rely primarily on the contraceptive effect of thickened cervical mucus. In a woman who ovulates while taking the progestin-only pill, taking the pill as few as three hours late may allow the cervical mucus to return to its fertile spinnbarkeit state and render the contraceptive effect temporarily void. When POPs are used in combination with lactation, the two are nearly 100% effective.

Safety and Side Effects   Contraindications to POP use can be found in Appendix 9–A. Irregular bleeding and spotting are the most common side effects associated with POPs (Hatcher et al., 2004). Other side effects include breast tenderness, mood changes and depression, benign ovarian cysts, and decreased effectiveness when used in combination with medications that induce liver enzymes, such as anticonvulsants, rifampin, and perhaps St. John's wort.

Noncontraceptive Benefits   Similar to other hormonal methods, there is a reduction in menorrhagia and dysmenorrhea with the POP (Hatcher et al., 2004). Other possible noncontraceptive benefits include a decrease in premenstrual symptoms and a decrease in upper reproductive tract infections due to the thickened cervical mucus. The reductions in ovarian and endometrial cancer seen with COCs have not been reported with POPs.

Advantages and Disadvantages   Each package of POPs contains one type of pill (versus two or more in a package of COCs), and there may be less confusion about which pill is to be taken. The POP is a safe method for many women who cannot take estrogen for medical reasons. Similarly, women who are sensitive to even low-estrogen pills, as manifested by nausea, breast tenderness, or hypertension, but who still want an oral contraceptive may do well on the POP. POPs are preferable to COCs for lactating women because they do not cause adverse effects on the volume or quality of breast milk. Weight gain is rarely a problem for women taking POPs (Hatcher et al., 2004). The contraceptive effect ends immediately upon discontinuation of the POP. Disadvantages, other than the side effects previously mentioned, include the need for careful adherence to the dosing schedule. Utilizing an alarm or watch that beeps daily at the same time may enhance compliance.

Progestin Injection   DMPA (Depo-Provera) has been approved for contraception since 1995, although the clinical trials were conducted in the 1960s and 1970s and the medication was used for the treatment of endometriosis and as an off-label contraceptive prior to FDA approval. Currently, 150 mg of DMPA is given by intramuscular injection every 11 to 13 weeks. A 104 mg subcutaneous injection to be given monthly is pending FDA approval at this writing. DMPA is a synthetic progestogen in the pregnane family, different than the estrane and gonane progestins found in oral contraceptives. When given at 12-week intervals, DMPA is a powerful inhibitor of the hypothalamic-pituitary axis at the level of the hypothalamus (Schwallie & Assenzo, 1973). Ovulatory suppression often lasts longer than 13 weeks, but because in a minority of women the contraceptive effect expires, all women are instructed to return for repeat doses at 12-week intervals.

Ideally, the first DMPA injection should be given during the first five days of the menses or at six weeks postpartum prior to the resumption of intercourse, and it can be provided immediately postabortion. If these circumstances are not practical, it is reasonable to provide the injection once pregnancy has been ruled out. In this case, the woman should be advised to take a highly sensitive pregnancy test two to three weeks after the first injection, as amenorrhea may be interpreted as a normal effect of the method. If DMPA is given in early pregnancy, there is no evidence of fetal anomalies or miscarriage (it was previously used to prevent miscarriage), but it is important to detect pregnancy as soon as possible to facilitate entry to prenatal care or abortion care. Women given DMPA "off cycle" (outside the previously mentioned ideal parameters for initiation of the method) should be instructed to use a barrier method for the first seven days while the serum levels are reaching adequate concentrations. The same instructions apply to women who are late for their injections. If there has been unprotected intercourse in the previous five days, a woman should be offered emergency contraception as well.

Efficacy and Effectiveness   The failure rates for DMPA are listed in Table 9–1. The difference between theoretical efficacy and typical use probably reflect the impact of patients not returning on time for subsequent injections.

Safety and Side Effects   Like POPs, DMPA is safer than combination products overall and can be used by women who are not candidates for estrogen. Refer to Appendix 9–A for a complete list of contraindications and precautions regarding DMPA use. As with all progestin-only methods, side effects associated with DMPA include changes in bleeding patterns, with breakthrough bleeding and spotting occurring in the majority of women in the first six months of use. By 12 months of use, approximately 73% of women will have become amenorrheic (Mainwaring et al., 1995). With appropriate counseling, many women see amenorrhea as a benefit of DMPA.

Weight gain with DMPA has been widely reported. The package insert lists an average weight gain in the first year of 5.4 pounds rising to a total of 13.8 pounds after 4 years of use (Pharmacia & Upjohn Company, 1999). Further studies show that weight gain is more likely to be concentrated in those who have a high body mass index (BMI) at initiation of use (Risser, Gefter, Barratt, & Risser, 1999). With obesity and its attendant health risks at epidemic proportions, counseling about healthy weight management is essential for all women, with close attention paid to women using DMPA. Other side effects reported in a small minority of women on DMPA include abdominal pain, dizziness, headache, weakness or fatigue, and nervousness.

Noncontraceptive Benefits   Noncontraceptive benefits of DMPA include a reduction in the number of seizures in women with epilepsy and seizure disorders. DMPA is not affected by the anticonvulsant medications, making it ideal for the patient with seizure disorders who does not want to become pregnant (Guberman, 1999). DMPA is also associated with a reduction in sickle cell crisis in patients with sickle cell disease (Kaunitz, 1998). DMPA is also not affected by any medications except aminoglutethimide, which is used to treat Cushing's disease.

Like all hormonal contraception, women have less menorrhagia and less dysmenorrhea with DMPA. Ectopic pregnancy, PID, and endometriosis are all common causes of infertility. Because of the high degree of ovulatory suppression, ectopic pregnancies are decreased when compared to women using no contraception. PID may also be decreased, as with other hormonal methods, and DMPA is also a successful treatment for endometriosis. Altogether, DMPA may have the effect of preserving fertility by avoiding these conditions. Another unique benefit of DMPA is that it is private, which has contributed to the appeal of this method among the adolescent population. The widespread acceptance of DMPA among adolescents is one reason cited for the drop in adolescent pregnancy seen in the past decade (Alan Guttmacher Institute, 2002).

Advantages and Disadvantages   Advantages of DMPA include its high degree of efficacy and long-term nature that does not interfere with coitus. There is no evidence of use for women who want to keep their contraceptive choice private. DMPA can be used during lactation without compromise of the breast milk quality or quantity. Women 35 years of age and older who smoke are able to use DMPA even during the later reproductive years, a time when prevention of pregnancy can be as critical as for the younger woman. DMPA has long been used among women with mental disabilities in order to achieve amenorrhea in women who cannot manage their menses.

The long-term nature of DMPA may also be considered a disadvantage, as the contraceptive effect may not cease immediately upon discontinuation. In fact, the average return to fertility is 10 months, with a range of 4 to 33 months (Pharmacia & Upjohn Company, 1999). Another major disadvantage of DMPA is its effect on bone mineral density. DMPA is associated with very low estradiol levels, due to its thorough ovulatory suppression, that may lead to osteopenia in some women (Scholes, LaCroix, Ichikawa, Barlow, & Ott, 2004). This bone loss appears to recover within a few years of DMPA discontinuation but raises concerns about the long-term impact of use in adolescents who have not achieved peak bone mass as well as in women near menopause (Taneepanich-skul, Intaraprasert, Theppisai, & Chaturachinda, 1997). Pregnancy and lactation can increase the risk of osteopenia; therefore as with all contraceptives, the risk of pregnancy must be compared to the risks associated with contraception. All teens require education about adequate calcium intake, regardless of contraceptive method. DMPA has also been noted to cause changes in the lipid profile, reducing HDL cholesterol.

DMPA requires intramuscular injections be provided by a trained health care provider. The new subcutaneous formulation may be able to be self-administered, which might improve continuation for women who find it hard to get to a provider's office. However, there remains the possibility of allergic reaction to either the progestin or the vehicle used for injection, or vagal reactions to the injection itself. As with all hormonal methods, there is no protection for STIs.

Progestin Implant   Subdermal progestin implants are the most effective reversible methods of hormonal contraception and are even more effective than sterilization. At the time this chapter was written, it was anticipated that the single-rod implant (Implanon) would be available on the US market in 2005. The single implant is 40 mm long and 2 mm in diameter and contains 68 mg of etonogestrel released slowly over three years. As with its predecessors (Norplant and Norplant-2), training of providers will be needed to ensure appropriate placement and skilled removal. Removal of the new implant is reported to be easier than previous multiple-rod systems because it is a single rod, is slightly larger in size, and is made of ethylene vinyl acetate, which is less flexible than the silastic used to make older rods. The implant should be inserted during the first seven days of the menses, post-partum, or postabortion, to avoid pregnancy in the first cycle. Fertility returns rapidly after removal, with one-year pregnancy rates similar to those of women discontinuing barrier methods (Glasier, 2002).

Efficacy and Effectiveness   Among a research study of 53,530 cycles, there were no preg-nancies, the lowest rate of any contraceptive method (Croxatto & Makarainen, 1998). This high rate of efficacy is related to the intrinsic efficacy of the product and the fact that once inserted, there is no room for user error.

Safety and Side Effects   Based on worldwide data, subdermal implants are as safe as other progestin-only methods with similar side effects, such as irregular bleeding and amenor-rhea (Booranabunyat & Taneepanichskul, 2004). Irregular bleeding is the most common reason for discontinuation (Glasier, 2002). Low-dose subdermal contraception has a his-tory of association with the development of benign follicular cysts that rarely require intervention, but can be a cause for anxiety among women when encountered. Other side effects of the method include injury and irritation at the insertion site, acne, breast ten-derness, weight increase, breast pain, and mood changes.

Noncontraceptive Benefits   As with other progestin-only methods, subdermal implants may provide decreased menorrhagia and dysmenorrhea, suppression of cyclic symptoms associated with menses, and decreased risk for PID.

Advantages and Disadvantages   Advantages of the subdermal implant include the pres-ence of highly effective contraception following a single insertion procedure. The contra-ceptive effect is immediately reversible upon removal of the device. The implant is discreet but palpable, providing reassurance to the woman that it is in place and has not migrated. Disadvantages of subdermal contraception include the recency of market intro-duction and limited provider experience with the method, as well as a corresponding shortage of research on its use in the United States. However, if the Norplant experience proves educational, it is likely that the method will be well received among appropriately counseled women who are cared for by trained providers who are skilled in insertion and removal techniques. High initial cost and a second fee for insertion may be barriers to use of the implant for some women.

INTRAUTERINE CONTRACEPTION

The use of medical devices placed in the uterus to prevent pregnancy dates back to the early 1900s. Infection risk was high with early devices, but design improvements led to a variety of available intrauterine devices (IUDs) in the 1960s and 1970s (Tone, 2001). Popular devices were generally of inert plastic, with single filament threads that protruded through the cervix into the vagina. The one memorable exception to this was the Dalkon Shield, introduced in 1970. This device quickly became associated with a high risk of pelvic infection. It had a multifilament tail enclosed in a sheath. When the strings were cut, the protective sheath was compromised and bacteria could ascend into the uterus inside the sheath (Nelson, 2000). Although other IUDs did not have the same design flaw, the adverse publicity and lawsuits associated with the Dalkon Shield tainted all IUDs and use of the device fell out of favor by the late 1970s. Recent developments in design and scientific review of the risks and benefits associated with intrauterine contraception have led to a revival of interest in this method of birth control.

There are two intrauterine contraceptives available in the United States (others are used in other countries). The copper IUD (T380A, Paragard) is a T-shaped device of polyethylene with copper wire wound around the stem and arms (Figure 9–10). A monofilament polyethylene thread is attached to a ball on the end of the stem. The copper adds additional spermicidal and other effects that allow the device to be smaller than a

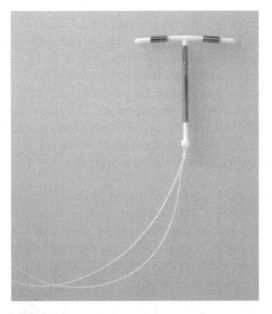

FIGURE 9–10   Copper T380A Intrauterine Device (ParaGard). *Source:* Reprinted with permission from FEI Women's Health.

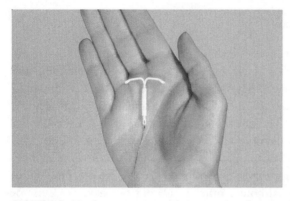

FIGURE 9–11 Levonorgestrel Intrauterine System (Mirena). *Source:* Reprinted with permission from Berlex.

plain plastic device. The primary contraceptive effect is provided by the reaction to having a foreign body in the reproductive tract: a sterile inflammatory response that is spermicidal (Alvarez et al., 1988). The LNG-IUS (Mirena) is also T-shaped, but contains no copper. Instead it has a reservoir that releases levonorgestrel at a rate of 20 mcg per day (Figure 9–11). The local delivery of progestin produces thickening of the cervical mucus and an endometrial reaction, in addition to the foreign body (Jonsson, Landgren, & Eneroth, 1991). It also has a monofilament thread. The copper IUD is effective and may stay in place for at least 10 years, and the LNG-IUS is effective and may stay in place for at least five years.

The copper IUD may be inserted at any time during the menstrual cycle when pregnancy can be ruled out. The LNG-IUS is inserted within seven days of the onset of menses. Many providers perform insertion of either device during menses to be certain the woman is not pregnant. Postabortion, postplacental (within 10 minutes after expulsion of the placenta), and immediate postpartum (within the first week after childbirth and preferably the first 48 hours) insertion may also be performed. The procedures for copper IUD and LNG-IUS insertion differ and are beyond the scope of this chapter. The manufacturers provide insertion training for clinicians and can be contacted via their websites (http://www.paragard.com and http://www.mirena-us.com).

Effectiveness and Efficacy Intrauterine contraception is extremely effective (Table 9–1). The copper IUD and LNG-IUS can be spontaneously expelled from the uterus. While expulsion may be associated with cramping or bleeding, it may be unnoticed. Women should be taught to check periodically for the strings to ensure the device is still placed properly. There is little room for user error with intrauterine contraception, other than not checking the strings and thus not recognizing an expulsion.

Safety and Side Effects Despite the negative experience associated with the Dalkon Shield, contemporary intrauterine contraceptives with monofilament threads are very safe for appropriate candidates (see Appendix 9–A). There is no evidence that they increase the risk of PID or infertility. There is a temporary increase in infection rates during the first weeks after insertion, and this is probably related to improper insertion techniques or preexisting infection prior to insertion (Farley, Rosenberg, Rowe, Chen, & Meirik, 1992; Grimes, 2000). Use of an IUD does not increase the rate of ectopic pregnancy. When an IUD user becomes pregnant, the pregnancy is more likely to be ectopic, but because the chance of pregnancy itself is so rare, the actual rate of ectopic pregnancy is very low. Perforation of the uterus during insertion is a rare but possible risk. Perforations are more likely to occur in lactating women in the early postpartum period. Perforation risk can be reduced by waiting until involution is complete.

The most common side effects associated with the copper IUD are bleeding and dysmenorrhea; five to 15% of women discontinue using the device within one year due to these side effects (Sivin et al., 1991). Menstrual blood loss increases with copper IUDs, as does the length of the menses (by about 1–2 days).

Irregular bleeding is common with the LNG-IUS. Initially intermenstrual bleeding may occur. As the duration of use increases, there is a reduction in menstrual flow and often amenorrhea develops. Counseling prior to insertion of the device may help reduce anxiety about the irregular bleeding. Women should be counseled that the bleeding does not represent hormonal fluctuations, but rather the shedding of the endometrial lining as an atrophic state is achieved. Other side effects with the LNG-IUS include lower abdominal pain, complexion changes, back pain, breast tenderness, headaches, mood changes, and nausea, although these all decline with time, and are present in a minority of patients. In general, the hormonal side effects are few with this low dose of progestin. As with other progestin-only methods, benign follicular cysts are common occurring in 8% to 12% of users. Most cysts resolve spontaneously (Pakarinen, Suvisaari, Luukkainen, & Lahteenmaki, 1997).

Noncontraceptive Benefits   There is some evidence to suggest that copper-containing IUDs are associated with a reduced risk of endometrial and invasive cervical cancer (Hill, Weiss, Voigt, & Beresford, 1997).

Menstrual flow is reduced up to 90% with the LNG-IUS (Milsom, Andersson, Andersch, & Rybo, 1991), and the device can be useful in treating the menorrhagia associated with perimenopause and uterine leiomyomas if there is no distortion of the uterine cavity. The LNG-IUS provides therapy for menorrhagia that is equivalent to endometrial ablation, while preserving fertility (Majorbanks, Lethaby, & Fahrquhar, 2003). The LNG-IUS may also be useful in the treatment of endometrial hyperplasia, endometriosis, and adenomyosis (McGavigan & Cameron, 2003). The progestin in the device is sufficient to protect the endometrium as a component of hormone therapy. The LNG-IUS can be inserted in the late reproductive years and then left in place through the transition to menopause. Another emerging noncontraceptive benefit is that the cervical mucus barrier and atrophic endometrium created by the LNG-IUS may actually protect the user from PID (Li, Lee, & Pun, 2004). Studies show the risk of PID to be equal in IUD users and nonusers and related to the risk of STIs rather than IUD use (Otero-Flores, Guerrero-Carreno, & Vasquez-Estrada, 2003).

Advantages and Disadvantages   Intrauterine contraception has the advantage of providing long-term contraception that is not coitus-dependent and does not require adjustments to daily activities (such as remembering to take a pill every day). Contemporary intrauterine contraception has effectiveness rates that are nearly comparable to those of sterilization. Unlike permanent sterilization, intrauterine contraception has the added advantage of being rapidly reversible, making this method ideal for young women who desire long-term birth control. They are discreet and private methods. Copper devices are hormone-free. The reduced bleeding with the LNG-IUS can lead to substantial savings in the cost of sanitary products.

There is a high upfront cost for intrauterine contraception. The copper IUD and LNG-IUS cost several hundred dollars, and a visit to a skilled clinician is needed for insertion. Many providers also require a pre-insertion visit to test for infections, and a post-insertion visit after the first menses to ensure the device has not been expelled. However, these are long-term contraceptives with no additional costs, and thus are among the least expensive methods over time.

EMERGENCY CONTRACEPTION

Emergency contraception is the use of regular contraceptive methods *after* intercourse to prevent pregnancy. There are three emergency contraceptive methods: POPs, COCs, and the copper IUD. Emergency contraception works by preventing or delaying ovulation, preventing fertilization, and/or preventing implantation. Emergency contraception does not cause an abortion, has no effect on an established pregnancy, and does not offer any protection for STI/HIV. Access to emergency contraception has the potential to reduce the incidence of unintended pregnancy by as much as 50% (Trussell, Stewart, Guest, & Hatcher, 1992), which would have a tremendous positive impact on the lives of women, men, and their families, by reducing the need for abortion and the social costs associated with unplanned pregnancy and childbearing (see Chapter 15).

Progestin-only emergency contraceptive pills (ECPs) must contain 0.75 mg of levonorgestrel per dose. The dedicated progestin ECP product in the United States is Plan B; POPs (Ovrette, 20 pills per dose) can also be used. Combined ECPs must contain at least 100 mcg of ethinyl estradiol and 0.50 mg of levonorgestrel per dose. Numerous COCs can be used as combined ECPs (see Table 9–1, Footnote 9). The first dedicated combined ECP product in the United States, Preven, was withdrawn from the market in 2004. The traditional ECP regimen is to take the first dose within 72 hours of unprotected intercourse, and a second dose 12 hours after the first. Newer research has demonstrated that ECPs are effective if taken up to 120 hours after unprotected intercourse (Ellertson et al.,

2003; Rodrigues, Grou, & Joly, 2001; von Hertzen et al., 2002). In addition, both doses of progestin-only ECPs can be given together in a single dose (Arowojolu, Okewole, & Adekunle, 2002; von Hertzen et al., 2002).

As of this writing, the over-the-counter availability of progestin-only ECPs (Plan B) is still pending. Until ECPs are available over-the-counter, clinicians should do everything they can to increase access to emergency contraception, including providing advance prescriptions for ECPs to all patients of reproductive age. Studies have shown that having the product at home increases the likelihood that it will be used when needed and does not promote sexual risk taking (Glasier & Baird, 1998; Raine, Harper, Leon, & Darney, 2000). Providing the prescription to new patients over the phone as needed is another way to increase access.

The copper IUD can be inserted up to five days after unprotected intercourse. This method is rarely utilized as emergency contraception in the United States because it is restricted to women who are appropriate IUD candidates. In addition, use of the copper IUD is not cost-effective if utilized only for the single cycle in which it is inserted for emergency contraception.

Efficacy and Effectiveness   The effectiveness of emergency contraception is measured by its reduction of expected pregnancies after unprotected intercourse. If 1,000 women have a single act of unprotected intercourse mid-cycle, 80 will become pregnant without emergency contraception. If combined ECPs are used, 20 women will become pregnant (74% reduction). If progestin-only ECPs are used, 12 women will become pregnant (89% reduction). If a copper IUD is inserted, 1 woman will become pregnant (99% reduction).

Safety and Side Effects   ECPs should not be given to women with a known or suspected pregnancy, not because they would be harmful but rather because they would be ineffective. There are no medical conditions with which ECPs should not be used or have risks that outweigh their benefits. The usual contraindications and precautions for ongoing COC and POP use do not apply to ECPs (WHO, 2004). The usual contraindications and precautions to copper IUD use apply when using this method for emergency contraception (see Appendix 9–A).

Combined ECPs cause nausea in about 50% of women and vomiting in about 25%. Progestin ECPs are associated with less nausea (23%) and vomiting (6%) (Task Force on Postovulatory Methods of Fertility Regulation, 1998). The copper IUD can cause the side effects discussed in the section on intrauterine contraception.

Advantages and Disadvantages   Emergency contraception is the only birth control method that can be used after intercourse. Progestin ECPs are preferable to combined because they are more effective and cause less side effects. Emergency contraception cannot be used as an ongoing method and provides no STI/HIV protection.

REFERENCES

Abma, J. C., Chandra, A., Mosher, W. D., Peterson, L. S., & Piccinino, L. J. (1997). Fertility, family planning, and women's health: New data from the 1995 National Survey of Family Growth. *Vital and Health Statistics, 23*(19), 1–114.

Abrams, L. S., Skee, D. M., Natarajan, J., Wong, F. A., & Anderson, G. D. (2002). Pharmacokinetics of a contraceptive patch (Evra/Ortho Evra) containing norelgestromin and ethinyloestradiol at four application sites. *British Journal of Clinical Pharmacology, 53*, 141–146.

Alan Guttmacher Institute. (2002*). Teen pregnancy: Trends and lessons learned.* Retrieved November 2, 2004, from http://www.guttmacher.org/pubs/ib_1-02.html.

Alan Guttmacher Institute. (2004). *Facts in brief: Contraceptive use.* Retrieved October 8, 2004, from http://www.guttmacher.org/pubs/fb_contr_use.html.

Alderman, P. M. (1991). Complications in a series of 1224 vasectomies. *The Journal of Family Practice, 33*, 579–584.

Alvarez, F., Brache, V., Fernandez, E., Guerrero, B., Guiloff, E., Hess, R., et al. (1988). New insights on the mode of action of intrauterine contraceptive devices in women. *Fertility and Sterility, 49*(5), 768–773.

American College of Obstetricians and Gynecologists. (2003). Benefits and risks of sterilization. (ACOG Practice Bulletin No. 46). *Obstetrics and Gynecology, 102*, 647–658.

Arévalo, M., Jennings, V., Nikula, M., & Sinai, I. (2004). Efficacy of the new TwoDay Method of family planning. *Fertility and Sterility, 82*, 885–892.

Arévalo, M., Jennings, V., & Sinai, I. (2002). Efficacy of a new method of family planning: The Standard Days Method. *Contraception, 65*, 333–338.

Arowojolu, A. O., Okewole, I. A., & Adekunle, A. (2002). Comparative evaluation of the effectiveness and safety of two regimens of levonorgestrel for emergency contraception in Nigerians. *Contraception, 66*, 269–273.

Association of Reproductive Health Professionals. (2002). *A clinical update on transdermal contraception* (Clinical Proceedings). Retrieved November 2, 2004, from http://www.arhp.org/healthcareproviders/cme/onlinecme/transdermalcp/index.cfm?ID=311.

Audet, M. C., Moreau, M., Koltun, W. D., Waldbaum, A. S., Shangold, G., Fisher, A. C., et al. (2001). Evaluation of contraceptive efficacy and cycle control of a transdermal contraceptive patch versus an oral contraceptive: A randomized controlled trial. *Journal of the American Medical Association, 285*, 2347–2354.

Berlex Laboratories. (2003). *Yasmin* [Package insert]. Wayne, NJ: Author.

Billings, E. L. (2001). *Teaching the Billlings Ovulation Method* (3rd ed.). Retrieved September 30, 2004, from http://www.woomb.org/bom/lit/teach/teach.pdf.

Booranabunyat, S., & Taneepanichskul, S. (2004). Implanon use in Thai women above the age of 35 years. *Contraception, 69*, 489–491.

Borgelt-Hansen, L. (2001). Oral contraceptives: An update on health benefits and risks. *Journal of the American Pharmaceutical Association, 41*, 875–886.

Burkman, R. T., Collins, J. A., Shulman, L. P., & Williams, J. K. (2001). Current perspectives on oral contraceptive use. *American Journal of Obstetrics and Gynecology, 185*(Suppl. 2), S4–S12.

Centers for Disease Control and Prevention. (2002). Nonoxynol-9 spermicide contraception use: United States, 1999. *Morbidity and Mortality Weekly Report, 51*, 389–392.

Collaborative Group on Hormonal Factors in Breast Cancer. (2002). Breast cancer and breastfeeding: Collaborative reanalysis of individual data from 47 epidemiological studies in 30 countries, including 50302 women with breast cancer and 96973 women without the disease. *Lancet, 360*, 187–195.

Cranston, J. W., Williams, M. A., Nielsen, N. H., & Bezman, R. J. (1998). Report of the Council on Scientific Affairs: Unlabeled indications of Food and Drug Administration-approved drugs. *Drug Information Journal, 32*, 1049–1061.

Croxatto, H. B., & Makarainen, L. (1998). The pharmacodynamics and efficacy of Implanon: An overview of the data. *Contraception, 58*(Suppl. 6), 91S–97S.

Dickinson, B. D., Altman, R. D., Nielsen, N. H., & Sterling, M. L. for the Council on Scientific Affairs, American Medical Association. (2001). Drug interactions between oral contraceptives and antibiotics. *Obstetrics and Gynecology, 98*, 853–860.

Ellertson, C., Evans, M., Ferden, S., Leadbetter, C., Spears, A., Johnstone, K., et al. (2003). Extending the time limit for starting the Yuzpe regimen of emergency contraception to 120 hours. *Obstetrics and Gynecology, 101*, 1168–1171.

Elomaa, K., Rolland, R., Brosens, I., Moorrees, M., Deprest, J., Tuominen, J., et al. (1998). Omitting the first oral contraceptive pills of the cycle does not automatically lead to ovulation. *American Journal of Obstetrics and Gynecology, 179*, 41–46.

Farley, T. M., Rosenberg, M. J., Rowe, P. J., Chen, J. H., & Meirik, O. (1992). Intrauterine devices and pelvic inflammatory disease: An international perspective. *Lancet, 339*, 785–788.

Farr, G., Gabelnick, H., Sturgen, K., & Dorflinger, L. (1994). Contraceptive efficacy and acceptability of the female condom. *American Journal of Public Health, 84*, 1960–1964.

Fehring, R. J. (2005). New low and high tech calendar methods of family planning. *Journal of Midwifery and Women's Health, 50*, 31–38.

Frezieres, R. G., Walsh, T. L., Nelson, A. L., Clark, V. A., & Coulson, A. H. (1999). Evaluation of the efficacy of a polyurethane condom: Results from a randomized, controlled clinical trial. *Family Planning Perspectives, 31*, 81–87.

Gallo, M. F., Grimes, D. A., & Schulz, K. F. (2002). Cervical cap versus diaphragm for contraception (Cochrane Review). In *The Cochrane Library.* Chichester, UK: John Wiley & Sons.

Gallo, M. F., Grimes, D. A., & Schulz, K. F. (2003). Nonlatex versus latex male condoms for contraception (Cochrane Review). In *The Cochrane Library.* Chichester, UK: John Wiley & Sons.

Glasier, A. (2002). Implantable contraceptives for women: Effectiveness, discontinuation rates, return of fertility, and outcome of pregnancies. *Contraception, 65*, 29–37.

Glasier, A., & Baird, D. (1998). The effects of self-administering emergency contraception. *New England Journal of Medicine, 339*, 1–4.

Grimes, D. A. (2000). Intrauterine device and upper-genital-tract infection. *Lancet, 356*, 1013–1019.

Gross, T. P., & Schlesselman, J. J. (1994). The estimated effect of oral contraceptive use on the cumulative risk of epithelial ovarian cancer. *Obstetrics and Gynecology, 83*, 419–424.

Guberman, A. (1999). Hormonal contraception and epilepsy. *Neurology, 53*(4, Suppl. 1), S38–S40.

Guillebaud, J. (2000). *Contraception today: A pocketbook for general practitioners* (4th ed.). London: Martin Dunitz.

Hall, S. D., Wang, Z., Huang, S. M., Hamman, M. A., Vasavada, N., Adigun, A. Q., et al. (2003). The interaction between St John's wort and an oral contraceptive. *Clinical Pharmacology and Therapeutics, 74*, 525–535.

Hatcher, R. A., Zieman, M., Cwiak, C., Darney, P. D., Creinen, M. D., & Stosur, H. R. (2004). *Managing contraception: 2004-2005.* Tiger, GA: Bridging the Gap Foundation.

Hendry, W. F. (1994). Vasectomy and vasectomy reversal. *British Journal of Urology, 73*, 337–344.

Hill, D. A., Weiss, N. S., Voigt, L. F., & Beresford, S. A. (1997). Endometrial cancer in relation to intra-uterine device use. *International Journal of Cancer, 70*, 278–287.

Hillis, S. D., Marchbanks, P. A., Tylor, L. R., & Peterson, H. B. (1999). Poststerilization regret: Findings from the United States Collaborative Review of Sterilization. *Obstetrics and Gynecology, 93*, 889–895.

Hoffman, S., Mantell, J., Exner, T., & Stein, Z. (2004). The future of the female condom. *Perspectives on Sexual and Reproductive Health, 36*, 120–126.

Jamieson, D. J., Costello, C., Trussell, J., Hillis, S. D., Marchbanks, P. A., Peterson, L. S., et al. (2004). The risk of pregnancy after vasectomy. *Obstetrics and Gynecology, 103*, 848–850.

Jennings, V. H., Arévalo, M., & Kowal, D. (2004). Fertility awareness-based methods. In R. A. Hatcher, J. Trussell, F. Stewart, A. L. Nelson, W. Cates, et al. (Eds.), *Contraceptive technology* (18th ed., pp. 317–329). New York: Ardent Media.

Jonsson, B., Landgren, B. M., & Eneroth, P. (1991). Effects of various IUDs on the composition of cervical mucus. *Contraception, 43*, 447–458.

Kaunitz, A. M. (1998). Injectable depot medroxyprogesterone acetate contraception: An update for U.S. clinicians. *International Journal of Fertility and Women's Medicine, 43*, 73–83.

Kennedy, K. I., Labbok, M. H., & Van Look, P. F. A. (1996). Consensus statement: Lactational amenorrhea method for family planning. *International Journal of Gynecology and Obstetrics, 54*, 55–57.

Killick, S. R., Bancroft, K., Oelbaum, S., Morris, J., & Elstein, M. (1990). Extending the duration of the pill-free interval during combined oral contraception. *Advances in Contraception, 6,* 33–40.

Kulczycki, A., Kim, D. J., Duerr, A., Jamieson, D. J., & Macaluso, M. (2004). The acceptability of the female and male condom: A randomized crossover trial. *Perspectives on Sexual and Reproductive Health, 36,* 114–119.

Kuyoh, M. A., Toroitich-Ruto, C., Grimes, D. A., Schulz, K. F., & Gallo, M. F. (2003). Sponge versus diaphragm for contraception: A Cochrane review. *Contraception, 67,* 15–18.

Leads from the *MMWR.* Toxic-shock syndrome and the vaginal contraceptive sponge. (1984). *Journal of the American Medical Association, 251,* 1015–1016.

Letterie, G. S., & Chow, G. E. (1992). Effect of "missed" pills on oral contraceptive effectiveness. *Obstetrics and Gynecology, 79,* 979–982.

Li, C. F., Lee, S. S., & Pun, T. C. (2004). A pilot study on the acceptability of levonorgestrel-releasing intrauterine device by young, single, nulliparous Chinese females following surgical abortion. *Contraception, 69,* 247–250.

Louv, W. C., Austin, H., Alexander, W. J., Stagno, S., & Cheeks, J. (1988). A clinical trial of nonoxynol-9 for preventing gonococcal and chlamydial infections. *The Journal of Infectious Disease, 158,* 518–523.

Mainwaring, R., Hales, H. A., Stevenson, K., Hataska, H. H., Poulson, A. M., Jones, K. P., et al. (1995). Metabolic parameter, bleeding, and weight changes in U.S. women using progestin only contraceptives. *Contraception, 51,* 149–153.

Majorbanks, J., Lethaby, A., & Fahrquhar, C. (2003). Surgery versus medical therapy for heavy menstrual bleeding (Cochrane Review). In *The Cochrane Library.* Chichester, UK: John Wiley & Sons.

Malkovsky, M., Newell, A., & Dalgleish, A. G. (1988). Inactivation of HIV by nonoxynol-9. *Lancet, 1*(8586), 645.

Marchbanks, P. A., McDonald, J. A., Wilson, H. G., Folger, S. G., Mandel, M. G., Daling, J. R., et al. (2002). Oral contraceptives and the risk of breast cancer. *New England Journal of Medicine, 346,* 2025–2032.

Mauck, C., Callahan, M., Weiner, D. H., & Dominik, R. (1999). A comparative study of the safety and efficacy of FemCap, a new vaginal barrier contraceptive, and the Ortho All-Flex diaphragm. The Fem-Cap Investigators' Group. *Contraception, 60,* 71–80.

Mauck, C., Glover, L. H., Miller, E., Allen, S., Archer, D. F., Blumenthal, P., et al. (1996). Lea's Shield: A study of the safety and efficacy of a new vaginal barrier contraceptive used with and without spermicide. *Contraception, 53,* 329–335.

McGavigan, C. J., & Cameron, I. T. (2003). The Mirena levonorgestrel system. *Drugs Today, 39,* 973–984.

McIntyre, S. L., & Higgins, J. E. (1986). Parity and use-effectiveness with the contraceptive sponge. *American Journal of Obstetrics and Gynecology, 155,* 796–801.

Milsom, I., Andersson, K., Andersch, B., & Rybo, G. (1991). A comparison of flurbiprofen, tranexamic acid, and a levonorgestrel-releasing intrauterine contraceptive device in the treatment of idiopathic menorrhagia. *American Journal of Obstetrics and Gynecology, 164,* 879–883.

Moodley, J. (2004). Combined oral contraceptives and cervical cancer. *Current Opinions in Obstetrics and Gynecology, 16,* 27–29.

Mulders, T. M., & Dieben, T. O. (2001). Use of the novel combined contraceptive vaginal ring NuvaRing for ovulation inhibition. *Fertility and Sterility, 75,* 865–870.

Mullooly, J. P., Wiest, W. M., Alexander, N. J., Greenlick, M. R., & Fulgham, D. L. (1993). Vasectomy, serum assays, and coronary heart disease symptoms and risk factors. *Journal of Clinical Epidemiology, 46*(1), 101–109.

National Institute of Allergy and Infectious Diseases, National Institutes of Health, Department of Health and Human Services. (2001). *Workshop summary: Scientific evidence on condom effectiveness for sexually transmitted disease (STD) protection.* Retrieved October 8, 2004, from *http://www.niaid. nih.gov/dmid/stds/condomreport.pdf.*

Nelson, A. L. (2000). The intrauterine contraceptive device. *Obstetrics and Gynecology Clinics of North America, 27,* 723–740.

Ness, R. B., Grisso, J. A., Vergona, R., Klapper, J., Morgan, M., & Wheeler, J. E. (2001). Oral contraceptives, other methods of contraception, and risk reduction for ovarian cancer. *Epidemiology, 12,* 307–312.

Newcomb, P. A., & Trentham-Dietz, A. (2000). Breast feeding practices in relation to endometrial cancer risk, USA. *Cancer Causes & Control, 11,* 663–667.

Otero-Flores, J. B., Guerrero-Carreno, F. J., & Vazquez-Estrada, L. A. (2003). A comparative randomized study of three different IUDs in nulliparous Mexican women. *Contraception, 67,* 273–276.

Pakarinen, P. I., Suvisaari, J., Luukkainen, T., & Lahteenmaki, P. (1997). Intracervical and fundal administration of levonorgestrel for contraception: Endometrial thickness, patterns of bleeding, and persisting ovarian follicles. *Fertility and Sterility, 68,* 59–64.

Pati, S., & Cullins, V. (2000). Female sterilization. Evidence. *Obstetric and Gynecology Clinics of North America, 27,* 859–899.

Peterson, H. B., Jeng, G., Folger, S. G., Hillis, S. A., Marchbanks, P. A., Wilcox, L. S., et al. (2000). The risk of menstrual abnormalities after tubal sterilization. U.S. Collaborative Review of Sterilization Working Group. *New England Journal of Medicine, 343,* 1681–1687.

Peterson, H. B., Xia, Z., Hughes, J. M., Wilcox, L. S., Tylor, L. R., & Trussell, J. (1996). The risk of pregnancy after tubal sterilization: Findings from the U.S. Collaborative Review of Sterilization. *American Journal of Obstetrics and Gynecology, 174,* 1161–1168.

Peterson, H. B., Xia, Z., Hughes, J. M., Wilcox, L. S., Tylor, L. R., & Trussell, J. (1997). The risk of ectopic pregnancy after tubal sterilization. U.S. Collaborative Review of Sterilization Working Group. *New England Journal of Medicine, 336,* 762–767.

Pharmacia & Upjohn Company. (1999). *Depo-Provera contraception injection* [Package labeling]. Kalamazoo, MI: Author.

Piccinino, L. J., & Mosher, W. D. (1998). Trends in contraceptive use in the United States: 1982–1995. *Family Planning Perspectives, 30,* 4–10, 46.

Polsky, B., Baron, P. A., Gold, J. W., Smith, J. L., Jensen, R. H., & Armstrong, D. (1988). In vitro inactivation of HIV-1 by contraceptive sponge containing nonoxynol-9. *Lancet, 1*(8600), 1456.

Raine, T., Harper, C., Leon, K., & Darney, P. (2000). Emergency contraception: Advance provision in a young, high-risk clinic population. *Obstetrics and Gynecology, 96,* 1–7.

Raymond, E. G., Chen, P. L., & Luoto, J. (2004). Contraceptive effectiveness and safety of five nonoxynol-9 spermicides: A randomized trial. *Obstetrics and Gynecology, 103,* 430–439.

Raymond, E., & Dominik, R. (1999). Contraceptive effectiveness of two spermicides: A randomized trial. *Obstetrics and Gynecology, 93,* 896–903.

Risser, W. L., Gefter, L. R., Barratt, M. S., & Risser, J. M. (1999). Weight change in adolescents who used hormonal contraception. *Journal of Adolescent Health, 24,* 433–436.

Rodrigues, I., Grou, F., & Joly, J. (2001). Effectiveness of emergency contraceptive pills between 72 and 120 hours after unprotected sexual intercourse. *American Journal of Obstetrics and Gynecology, 184,* 531–537.

Rosenberg, L., Palmer, J. R., Zauber, A. G., Warshauer, M. E., Lewis, J. L., Jr., Strom, B. L., et al. (1994). A case-control study of oral contraceptive use and invasive epithelial ovarian cancer. *American Journal of Epidemiology, 139,* 654–661.

Rosenberg, M. J., Waugh, M. S., Solomon, H. M., & Lyszkowski, A. D. (1996). The male polyurethane condom: A review of current knowledge. *Contraception, 53,* 141–146.

Schlesselman, J. J. (1997). Risk of endometrial cancer in relation to use of combined oral contraceptives. A practitioner's guide to meta-analysis. *Human Reproduction, 12,* 1851–1863.

Scholes, D., LaCroix, A. Z., Ichikawa, L. E., Barlow, W. E., & Ott, S. M. (2004). The association between depot medroxyprogesterone acetate contraception and bone mineral density in adolescent women. *Contraception, 69,* 99–104.

Schwallie, P. C., & Assenzo, J. R. (1973). Contraceptive use: Efficacy study utilizing medroxyprogesterone acetate administered as an intramuscular injection once every 90 days. *Fertility and Sterility, 24,* 331–339.

Sivin, I., Stern, J., Coutinho, E., el Mahgoub, S., Diaz, S., Pavez, M., et al. (1991). Prolonged intrauterine contraception: A seven-year randomized study of the levonorgestrel 20 mcg/day (LNg 20) and the Copper T380 Ag IUDS. *Contraception, 44,* 473–480.

Smith, J. S., Green, J., Berrington de Gonzalez, A., Appleby, P., Peto, J., Plummer, M., et al. (2003). Cervical cancer and use of hormonal contraceptives: A systematic review. *Lancet, 361,* 1159–1167.

Sokal, D., McMullen, S., Gates, D., & Dominik, R. (1999). A comparative study of the no scalpel and standard incision approaches to vasectomy in 5 countries. The Male Sterilization Investigator Team. *Journal of Urology, 162,* 1621–1625.

Speroff, L., & Fritz, M. (2005). *Clinical gynecologic endocrinology and infertility* (7th ed.). Baltimore: Lippincott Williams & Wilkins.

Steiner, M. J., Dominik, R., Rountree, R. W., & Dorflinger, L. (2003). Contraceptive effectiveness of a polyurethane condom and a latex condom: A randomized controlled trial. *Obstetrics and Gynecology, 101*, 539–547.

Sulak, P. J., Scow, R. D., Preece, C., Riggs, M. W., & Kuehl, T. J. (2000). Hormone withdrawal symptoms in oral contraceptive users. *Obstetrics and Gynecology, 95*, 261–266.

Taneepanichskul, S., Intaraprasert, S., Theppisai, U., & Chaturachinda, K. (1997). Bone mineral density in long-term depot medroxyprogesterone acetate acceptors. *Contraception, 56*, 1–3.

Task Force on Postovulatory Methods of Fertility Regulation. (1998). Randomized controlled trial of levonorgestrel versus the Yuzpe regimen of combined oral contraceptives for emergency contraception. *Lancet, 352*, 4284–4233.

Timmer, C. J., & Mulders, T. M. (2000). Pharmacokinetics of etonogestrel and ethinylestradiol released from a combined contraceptive vaginal ring. *Clinical Pharmacokinetics, 39*, 233–242.

Tone, A. (2001). *Devices and desires: A history of contraceptives in America.* New York: Hill & Wong.

Trussell, J. (2004). Contraceptive failure in the United States. *Contraception, 70*, 89–96.

Trussell, J., Stewart, F., Guest, F., & Hatcher, R. A. (1992). Emergency contraceptive pills: A simple proposal to reduce unintended pregnancies. *Family Planning Perspectives, 24*, 269–273.

Van Damme, L., Ramjee, G., Alary, M., Vuylsteke, B., Chandeying, V., Rees, H., et al. (2002). Effectiveness of COL-1492, a nonoxynol-9 vaginal gel, on HIV-1 transmission in female sex workers: A randomised controlled trial. *Lancet, 360*, 971–977.

Veres, S., Miller, L., & Burington, B. (2004). A comparison between the vaginal ring and oral contraceptives. *Obstetrics and Gynecology, 104*, 555–563.

von Hertzen, H., Piaggio, G., Ding, J., Chen, J., Song, S., Bártfaim, G., et al. (2002). Low dose mifepristone and two regimens of levonorgestrel for emergency contraception: A WHO multicentre randomised trial. *Lancet, 360*, 1803–1810.

Wallach, M., & Grimes, D. A. (Eds.). (2000). *Modern oral contraception.* Totowa, NJ: Emron.

Weller, S., & Davis, K. (2001). Condom effectiveness in reducing heterosexual HIV transmission (Cochrane Review). In *The Cochrane Library.* Chichester, UK: John Wiley & Sons.

Westhoff, C., & Davis, A. (2000). Tubal sterilization: Focus on the U.S. experience. *Fertility and Sterility, 73*, 913–922.

Westhoff, C., Kerns, J., Morroni, C., Cushman, L. F., Tiezzi, T., & Murphy, P.A. (2002). Quick Start: A novel oral contraceptive initiation method. *Contraception, 66*, 141–145.

Westhoff, C., Morroni, C., Kerns, J., & Murphy, P.A. (2003). Bleeding patterns after immediate versus conventional oral contraceptive initiation: A randomized controlled trial. *Fertility and Sterility, 79*, 322–329.

Whittemore, A. S. (1994). Characteristics relating to ovarian cancer risk: Implications for prevention and detection. *Gynecologic Oncology, 55*(Pt. 2), S15–S19.

Wilcox, A. J., Weinberg, C. R., & Baird, D. D. (1995). Timing of sexual intercourse in relation to ovulation. *New England Journal of Medicine, 333*, 1517–1521.

Wilkinson, D., Tholandi, M., Ramjee, G., & Rutherford, G. W. (2002). Nonoxynol-9 spermicide for prevention of vaginally acquired HIV and other sexually transmitted infections: Systematic review and meta-analysis of randomised controlled trials including more than 5000 women. *Lancet Infectious Diseases, 2*, 613–617.

Winkler, H. A., Anderson, P. S., Fields, A. L., Runowicz, C. D., De Victoria, C., & Goldberg, G. L. (1999). Compliance with Papanicolaou smear screening following tubal ligation in women with cervical cancer. *Journal of Women's Health, 8*, 103–107.

World Health Organization. (2001). *WHO/CONRAD technical consultation on nonoxynol-9: Summary report.* Retrieved October 8, 2004, from http://www.who.int/reproductive-health/rtis/nonoxynol9.html.

World Health Organization. (2004). *Medical eligibility criteria for contraceptive use* (3rd ed.). Retrieved October 8, 2004, from http://www.who.int/reproductive-health/publications/RHR_00_2_medical_eligibility_criteria_3rd/index.htm.

Zlidar, V. M. (2000). Helping women use the pill. (Series A, No. 10). *Population Reports, 28*(2).

WEB SITES

Association of Reproductive Health Professionals: http://www.arhp.org

Contraception Online: http://www.contraceptiononline.org

BIBLIOGRAPHY

Dickey, R. P. (2004). *Managing contraceptive pill patients* (12th ed.). Dallas, TX: EMIS Medical.

Hatcher, R. A., Trussell, J., Stewart, F., Nelson, A., Cates, W., Guest, F., et al. (Eds.). (2004). *Contraceptive technology* (18th ed.). New York: Ardent Media.

Hatcher, R. A., Zieman, M., Cwiak, C., Darney, P. D., Creinen, M. D., & Stosur, H. R. (2004). *Managing contraception: 2004-2005.* Tiger, GA: Bridging the Gap Foundation.

Speroff, L., & Fritz, M. (2005). *Clinical gynecologic endocrinology and infertility* (7th ed.). Baltimore: Lippincott Williams & Wilkins.

Speroff, L., & Darney, P. D. (2001). *A clinical guide for contraception* (3rd ed.). Baltimore: Lippincott Williams & Wilkins.

Appendix
9–A

SELECTED MEDICAL ELIGIBILITY CRITERIA FOR CONTRACEPTIVE USE

The World Health Organization (WHO) Medical Eligibility Criteria for Contraceptive Use is a comprehensive, evidence-based guide for determining whether women have relative or absolute contraindications to contraceptive methods. WHO uses the following four classification categories of whether a person can use or should not use a method:

- *Category 1*—A condition for which there is no restriction for the use of the contraceptive method
- *Category 2*—A condition where the advantages of using the method generally outweigh the theoretical or proven risks
- *Category 3*—A condition where the theoretical or proven risks usually outweigh the advantages of using the method
- *Category 4*—A condition that represents an unacceptable health risk if the contraceptive method is used

The following table is a summary of selected criteria for contraceptive use. The table is a quick reference and not inclusive of the full guidelines. Readers are referred to the complete Medical Eligibility Criteria (available online, see citation at the end of the appendix) for clarifications of category classification, complete references, and conditions and contraceptive methods that are not included in this table. Abbreviations for the methods in the table are as follows:

- *COC/P/R*—Low-dose (≤ 35 mcg ethinyl estradiol) combined oral contraceptives, patch, and vaginal ring
- *POP*—Progestin-only pills
- *DMPA*—Depot medroxyprogesterone acetate injection
- *Implants*—Levonorgestrel/etonogestrel implants
- *Cu-IUD*—Copper intrauterine device
- *LNG-IUD*—Levonorgestrel intrauterine device

When there is a differentiation between criteria for initiation and continuation of a method, these are noted with the abbreviations "I" and "C" next to the category number.

Personal Characteristics and Reproductive History

Condition	COC/P/R	POP	DMPA	Implants	Cu-IUD	LNG-IUD
Age	Menarche to < 40 = 1	Menarche to < 18 = 1 18–45 = 1 > 45 = 1	Menarche to < 18 = 2 18–45 = 1 > 45 = 2	Menarche to < 18 = 1 18–4 = 1	Menarche to < 20 = 2 ≥ 20 = 1	Menarche to < 20 = 2 ≥ 20 = 1
Parity						
a) Nulliparous	1	1	1	1	2	2
b) Parous	1	1	1	1	1	1
Breastfeeding						
a) < 6 weeks postpartum	4	3	3	3		
b) 6 weeks to < 6 months primarily breastfeeding	3	1	1	1		
c) ≥ 6 months	2	1	1	1		
Postpartum (not breastfeeding)						
a) < 21 days	3	1	1	1		
b) ≥ 21 days	1	1	1	1		
Postpartum (breastfeeding or non-breastfeeding women, including post-cesarean section)						
a) < 48 hours					2	3
b) ≥ 48 hours to < 4 weeks					3	3
c) ≥ 4 weeks					1	1
d) Puerperal sepsis					4	4
Post-abortion						
a) First trimester	1	1	1	1	1	1
b) Second trimester	1	1	1	1	2	2
c) Immediate post-septic abortion	1	1	1	1	4	4

Condition	COC/P/R	POP	DMPA	Implants	Cu-IUD	LNG-IUD
Past Ectopic Pregnancy	1	2	1	1	1	1
History of Pelvic Surgery (including cesarean section, see also postpartum section)	1	1	1	1	1	1
Smoking						
a) Age < 35	2	1	1	1	1	1
b) Age ≥ 35						
i) < 15 cigarettes/day	3	1	1	1	1	1
ii) ≥ 15 cigarettes/day	4	1	1	1	1	1
Obesity ≥ 30 kg/m² body mass index (BMI)	2	1	1	1	1	1
Cardiovascular Disease						
Multiple Risk Factors for Arterial Cardiovascular Disease (such as older age, smoking, diabetes, and hypertension)	3/4	2	3	2	1	2
Hypertension						
a) History of hypertension, where blood pressure *cannot* be evaluated (including hypertension during pregnancy)	3	2	2	2	1	2
b) Adequately controlled hypertension, where blood pressure *can* be evaluated	3	1	2	1	1	1

(continues)

Condition	COC/P/R	POP	DMPA	Implants	Cu-IUD	LNG-IUD
Hypertension (continued)						
c) Elevated blood pressure levels (properly taken measurements)						
i) systolic 140–159 or diastolic 90–99	3	1	2	1	1	1
ii) systolic > 160 or diastolic > 100	4	2	3	2	1	2
d) Vascular disease	4	2	3	2	1	2
History of High Blood Pressure During Pregnancy (where current blood pressure is measurable and normal)	2	1	1	1	1	1
Deep Venous Thrombosis (DVT)/Pulmonary Embolism (PE)						
a) History of DVT/PE	4	2	2	2	1	2
b) Current DVT/PE	4	3	3	3	1	3
c) Family history (first-degree relatives)	2	1	1	1	1	1
d) Major surgery						
i) with prolonged immobilization	4	2	2	2	1	2
ii) without prolonged immobilization	2	1	1	1	1	1
e) Minor surgery without immobilization	1	1	1	1	1	1
Known Thrombogenic Mutations (e.g., Factor V Leiden; Prothrombin mutation; Protein S, Protein C, and antithrombin deficiencies)	4	2	2	2	1	2

Condition	COC/P/R	POP	DMPA	Implants	Cu-IUD	LNG-IUD
Superficial Venous Thrombosis						
a) Varicose veins	1	1	1	1	1	1
b) Superficial thrombophlebitis	2	1	1	1	1	1
Current and History of Ischemic Heart Disease	4	I2/C3	3	I2/C3	1	I2/C3
Stroke (history of cerebrovascular accident)	4	I2/C3	3	I2/C3	1	2
Known Hyperlipidemias (screening is *not* necessary for safe use of contraceptive methods)	2/3	2	2	2	1	2
Valvular Heart Disease						
a) Uncomplicated	2	1	1	1	1	1
b) Complicated (pulmonary hypertension, atrial fibrillation, history of subacute bacterial endocarditis)	4	1	1	1	2	2
Neurologic Conditions						
Headaches						
a) Non-migrainous (mild or severe)	I1/C2	I1/C1	I1/C1	I1/C1	1	I1/C1
b) Migraine						
i) Without aura						
Age < 35	I2/C3	I1/C2	I2/C2	I2/C2	1	I2/C2
Age = 35	I3/C4	I1/C2	I2/C2	I2/C2	1	I2/C2
ii) With aura (at any age)	I4/C4	I2/C3	I2/C3	I2/C3	1	I2/C3
Epilepsy	1	1	1	1		1
Depressive Disorders	1	1	1	1		1
Depressive Disorders						

(continues)

Condition	COC/P/R	POP	DMPA	Implants	Cu-IUD	LNG-IUD
Reproductive Tract Infections and Disorders						
Vaginal Bleeding Patterns						
a) Irregular pattern *without* heavy bleeding	1	2	2	2	1	I1/C1
b) Heavy or prolonged bleeding (includes regular and irregular patterns)	1	2	2	2	2	I1/C2
Unexplained Vaginal Bleeding (suspicious for serious conditions) Before evaluation	2	2	3	3	I4/C2	I4/C2
Endometriosis	1	1	1	1	2	1
Benign Ovarian Tumors (including cysts)	1	1	1	1	1	1
Severe Dysmenorrhea	1	1	1	1	2	1
Trophoblast Disease						
a) Benign gestational trophoblastic disease	1	1	1	1	3	3
b) Malignant gestational trophoblastic disease	1	1	1	1	4	4
Cervical Ectropion	1	1	1	1	1	1
Cervical Intraepithelial Neoplasia (CIN)	2	1	2	2	1	2
Cervical Cancer (awaiting treatment)	2	1	2	2	I4/C2	I4/C2
Breast Disease						
a) Undiagnosed mass	2	2	2	2	1	2
b) Benign breast disease	1	1	1	1	1	1
c) Family history of cancer	1	1	1	1	1	1
d) Cancer						
i) Current	4	4	4	4	1	4
ii) Past and no evidence of current disease for 5 years	3	3	3	3	1	3

Condition	COC/P/R	POP	DMPA	Implants	Cu-IUD	LNG-IUD
Endometrial Cancer	1	1	1	1	I4/C2	I4/C2
Ovarian Cancer	1	1	1	1	I3/C2	I3/C2
Uterine Fibroids						
a) Without distortion of the uterine cavity	1	1	1	1	1	1
b) With distortion of the uterine cavity	1	1	1	1	4	4
Anatomical Abnormalities						
a) That distort the uterine cavity					4	4
b) That do not distort the uterine cavity					2	2
Pelvic Inflammatory Disease (PID)						
a) Past PID (assuming no current risk factors of STIs)						
i) with subsequent pregnancy	1	1	1	1	I1/C1	I1/C1
ii) without subsequent pregnancy	1	1	1	1	I2/C2	I2/C2
b) ID-current	1	1	1	1	I4/C2	I4/C2
STIs						
a) Current purulent cervicitis or chlamydial infection or gonorrhea	1	1	1	1	I4/C2	I4/C2
b) Other STIs (excluding HIV and hepatitis)	1	1	1	1	I2/C2	I2/C2
c) Vaginitis (including trichomonas vaginalis and bacterial vaginosis)	1	1	1	1	I2/C2	I2/C2
d) Increased risk of STIs	1	1	1	1	I2-3/C2	I2-3/C2

(continues)

Condition	COC/P/R	POP	DMPA	Implants	Cu-IUD	LNG-IUD
HIV/AIDS						
High Risk of HIV	1	1	1	1	I2/C2	I2/C2
HIV-infected	1	1	1	1	I2/C2	I2/C2
AIDS	1	1	1	1	I3/C2	I3/C2
Clinically well on ARV therapy (see Antiretroviral Therapy below)						
Other Infections						
Schistosomiasis						
a) Uncomplicated	1	1	1	1	1	1
b) Fibrosis of the liver	1	1	1	1	1	1
Tuberculosis						
a) Non-pelvic	1	1	1	1	I1/C1	I1/C1
b) Known pelvic	1	1	1	1	I4/C3	I4/C3
Malaria	1	2	2	2	1	1
Endocrine Conditions						
Diabetes						
a) History of gestational disease	1	1	1	1	1	1
b) Non-vascular disease						
i) non-insulin dependent	2	2	2	2	1	2
ii) insulin dependent	2	2	2	2	1	2
c) Nephropathy/retino-pathy/neuropathy	3/4	2	3	2	1	2
d) Other vascular disease or diabetes of > 20 years' duration	3/4	2	3	2	1	2
Thyroid Disorders						
a) Simple goiter	1	1	1	1	1	1
b) Hyperthyroid	1	1	1	1	1	1
c) Hypothyroid	1	1	1	1	1	1

Condition	COC/P/R	POP	DMPA	Implants	Cu-IUD	LNG-IUD
Gastrointestinal Conditions						
Gallbladder Disease						
a) Symptomatic						
i) treated by cholecystectomy	2	2	2	2	1	2
ii) medically treated	3	2	2	2	1	2
iii) current	3	2	2	2	1	2
b) Asymptomatic	2	2	2	2	1	2
History of Cholestasis						
a) Pregnancy-related	2	1	1	1	1	1
b) Past COC–related	3	2	2	2	1	2
Viral Hepatitis						
a) Active	4	3	3	3	1	3
b) Carrier	1	1	1	1	1	1
Cirrhosis						
a) Mild (compensated)	3	2	2	2	1	2
b) Severe (decompensated)	4	3	3	3	1	3
Liver Tumors						
a) Benign (adenoma)	4	3	3	3	1	3
b) Malignant (hepatoma)	4	3	3	3	1	3
Anemias						
Thalassemia	1	1	1	1	1	1
Sickle Cell Disease	2	1	1	1	2	1
Iron-Deficiency Anemia	1	1	1	1	2	1

(continues)

Condition	COC/P/R	POP	DMPA	Implants	Cu-IUD	LNG-IUD
Drug Interactions						
Drugs That Affect Liver Enzymes						
a) Rifampicin	3	3	2	3	1	1
b) Certain anticonvulsants (phenytoin, carbamazapine, barbiturates, primidone, topiramate, oxcarbazepine)	3	3	2	3	1	1
Antibiotics (excluding rifampicin)						
a) Griseofulvin	2	2	1	2	1	1
b) Other antibiotics	1	1	1	1	1	1
Antiretroviral Therapy	2	2	2	2	I2-3/C2	I2-3/C2

Source: Adapted from World Health Organization. (2004). *Medical eligibility criteria for contraceptive use* (3rd ed.). Retrieved October 8, 2004, from http://www.who.int/reproductive-health/publications/RHR_00_2_medical_eligibility_criteria_3rd/index.htm.

GYNECOLOGIC HEALTH CARE FOR LESBIANS

LINDA A. BERNHARD

Health is experienced in the context of each individual's life. "A feminist understanding of women's health conceptualizes the experience of health not as the experiences of a woman's body but rather as inseparable from the everyday experiences of an embodied life" (McDonald, McIntyre, & Anderson, 2003, p. 705). Health, and specifically gynecologic health, is experienced biologically, psychosocially, sexually, and spiritually. This is as true for lesbians as it is for all other women. Lesbians have the same health care needs as other women, but they also have unique experiences of health because they are lesbian. Too often, "women's health" has not explicitly included lesbian health, but a feminist approach to women's health must. This chapter will provide an overview about who lesbians are, examples of how health care is affected for lesbians, and some current research for lesbian health. Suggestions for providing culturally competent care to lesbians are included throughout the chapter.

WHO ARE LESBIANS?

Lesbians are women who love women; that is their only commonality. Lesbians differ from one other in every other way: race, ethnicity, class, age, religion, geographic location, citizenship, and ability status. Indeed, lesbians are found in every subgroup of women. Lesbians are also diverse in what they call themselves (e.g., lesbian, gay, dyke, queer, etc.), with whom they partner, and with whom they have sexual relationships. Although many lesbians only have sexual relationships with women, others have had sexual relationships with men in the past or may currently be having sexual relationships with men. The term "lesbian" is used in this chapter, but clinicians can ask their patients how they want to be identified.

DEFINING SEXUAL ORIENTATION AND GENDER IDENTITY

There is no standard definition for lesbian or sexual orientation; however, three components—sexual identity, behavior, and attraction or desire—are increasingly being used to define sexual orientation for research and educational purposes (Solarz, 1999). Sexual identity refers to one's self-definition of being heterosexual, homosexual, or bisexual. Sexual behavior refers to one's sexual partners: women, men, both, or neither. Attraction or desire refers to whether one sexually desires or fantasizes about women, men, or both. Sexual attraction is sometimes described as sexual preference.

Traditionally, lesbians have been defined by their sexual behavior. That is, having sex with women meant one was a lesbian. However, this is a label given to women, not necessarily self-claimed. When women claim their own labels and identities, women who have sex with women identify themselves as heterosexual or bisexual, as well as lesbian (McGonigle, 2003; Powers, Bowen, & White, 2001). Furthermore, women who have sex only with men may identify themselves as lesbian. Sexual identity and sexual behavior are not always consistent. Lesbians may also be celibate.

"Sex" typically refers to biology, and "gender" refers to the social expression of oneself as female or male (Colebrook, 2004). Some individuals may claim a gender identity as transgender. Transgender includes a wide variety of persons, including transsexuals and others. Transgender individuals claim both female and male characteristics. Transsexual persons are those born biologically one sex, who believe themselves rightfully to be the other sex. These persons may or may not undergo surgical procedures or take hormones so that their physical bodies are consistent with their mental self-perceptions. Transgender individuals may also have a sexual identity as heterosexual, homosexual, or bisexual.

Sexual orientation and gender identity are flexible and changing. Women may vary in their sexual identity, behavior, and attraction at different times in their life, and in different places, or with different people (LeMoncheck, 1997).

HOW MANY LESBIANS ARE THERE?

It is impossible to know the actual number of lesbians in the United States. This is partially because of the difficulty in defining them, but also because many lesbians are afraid to disclose their lesbian identity for fear of discrimination or other personal harm. Thus, lesbians are an invisible minority. Nonetheless, estimates of the number of lesbians ranges from 2–10% of the population (Solarz, 1999). In addition, it is even more difficult to know the diversity among lesbians because of racial, ethnic, and religious proscriptions against homosexuality in some cultures.

HOMOPHOBIA AND HETEROSEXISM

Homophobia is an individual's irrational fear or hate of homosexual people. In health care, lesbians experience homophobia when providers and others think they are sick or immoral (Fone, 2000). Lesbians may feel hassled, unwanted, or unsafe. Providers who are homophobic may avoid lesbian patients.

Heterosexism is the societal institutionalization of a dichotomy where one group of people—heterosexuals—are valued, and another group of people—homosexuals—are devalued and oppressed (Herek, 1995). In that way it is similar to other dichotomies, such as racism or classism. Heterosexism is the belief that heterosexuality is the best sexual orientation and that all people are, or should be, heterosexual.

The experience of homophobia and heterosexism is also affected by other personal characteristics of a lesbian, such as race, age, class, religion, and ability status. These characteristics cannot be divided; a lesbian may experience all of them simultaneously. That is, an African-American lesbian who is 80 years old and in a wheelchair can experience racism, heterosexism, sexism, agism, and ableism all at the same time. She is an integrated human being, not only lesbian or African-American or any of the other qualities that she possesses.

HEALTH CARE FOR LESBIANS IN A SOCIETAL CONTEXT

Social intolerance of homosexuality is still largely acceptable in US society. Violence against lesbians (and other sexual and gender minority persons) is common. Consequently, lesbians live with a great deal of stress in a society that does not accept them. Stress comes either from *hiding* her sexual orientation (i.e., being "in the closet"), so that she can avoid discrimination and loss, or from being "out" (of the closet) and thus risking discrimination and hate crimes because others know that she *is* a lesbian. In many places it is legal to discriminate against homosexuals, so the threat is real. Lesbians lack the legal rights of marriage and can experience discrimination in child custody situations, as well as in employment and housing.

"Coming out" is a developmental process that includes identifying and accepting oneself as lesbian, and then identifying oneself as lesbian to others. It is usually a gradual process, often accompanied by significant stress, because the girl or woman is afraid of what will happen to her and what kinds of changes she will experience if and when she does come out. Thus, lesbians may be out in some aspects of their life and not in others. For example, she may be out to family and close friends, but not out at work. Coming out can occur at any time in a woman's life. In addition, coming out is a never-ending process because whenever a lesbian meets someone she does not know, like a health care provider, she has a choice to be out or not.

An important part of the coming out process is becoming involved in lesbian and/or gay culture and community. Similar to other cultural groups, there is a sense of security in being with persons like oneself. With regard to health care, lesbians have found security by developing health clinics and support groups for themselves outside the mainstream health care system. Lesbians are also known to be high users of complementary and alternative medicine (CAM) or integrative health and wellness systems, often because CAM providers are thought to be more holistic in their care (Bowen, Anderson, White, Powers, & Greenlee, 2002; Mathieson, Bailey, & Gurevich, 2002). Nonetheless, Matthews (1998) found in her study of lesbians using an alternative health care system (the Lesbian

Community Cancer Project in Chicago), that none of them had abandoned completely traditional allopathic health care.

HEALTH CARE FOR LESBIANS IN AN INSTITUTIONAL CONTEXT

Institutions of health care include outpatient facilities as well as hospitals. Health care for lesbians is often limited by institutional policies that define family in traditional ways, such as nuclear family or blood relatives. Another limitation is staff who enforce outdated policies that prevent lesbians from being recognized as partners or family members. When such policies are implemented, lesbians may be denied access to information, participation in treatment decisions, or visitation.

One way that some lesbians protect themselves from such situations is by obtaining a Durable Power of Attorney for Health Care. This document allows a person to appoint another person, such as a lesbian partner, to make health care decisions for her when she is unable to do so for herself. This document serves as the proof of her intentions for future health care and can provide access to institutions and providers for the designee.

Lesbians may also seek legal guardianship for their children or for partners who become disabled. In some states lesbians may legally adopt another person, regardless of age, as a way to maintain a legal relationship for health care and other purposes, such as inheritance.

DEVELOPMENT OF A RESEARCH BASE FOR LESBIAN HEALTH

Lesbian health care has only become a topic of significant discussion and research since the 1980s. The first major study to identify lesbian physical and mental health care needs and concerns was the National Lesbian Health Survey (Bradford & Ryan, 1987). This national survey of 1900 self-identified lesbians is now classic. It was the first attempt to ask lesbians throughout the United States to describe their own health care needs, and it became a model that other researchers have used to describe lesbian health needs—locally, regionally, and nationally.

Lesbian health activism began to grow in the early 1990s with breast cancer activism, after the national media brought attention to the possible increased risk for breast cancer among lesbians (Gessen, 1993). Where previously lesbians were often working in isolation, they began to work together and found strength in numbers. Activism surrounding breast cancer has evolved into a larger and more general social movement for lesbian health.

In 1993 a group of lesbian activists met with then US Secretary of Health and Human Services (HHS), Donna Shalala, and other governmental officials, resulting in the initiation of a variety of activities for lesbian health within HHS. The most important result was that in 199, for the first time ever, the Institute of Medicine (IOM) constituted a committee to study lesbian health. The landmark publication of *Lesbian Health: Current Assessment and Directions for the Future* (Solarz, 1999) represents full recognition of the importance of lesbians and their health as worthy of attention and study. The eight recommendations were broad, including multiple topics for research, funding for research, conferences, and other mechanisms for dissemination of information about lesbian health.

In an attempt to maintain the momentum for lesbian health brought about by the release of the IOM report, the Gay and Lesbian Medical Association invited the HHS Office on Women's Health (OWH) and the National Institutes of Health (NIH) Office of Research on Women's Health (ORWH) to cosponsor a workshop to discuss implementation of the recommendations from the IOM report. On March 23 and 24, 2000, the Scientific Workshop on Lesbian Health (2000) was held in Washington, DC. In addition to ORWH and OWH, several other government agencies and lesbian, gay, bisexual, and transgender (LGBT) health organizations sponsored the workshop. More than 100 lesbian health experts, government, and foundation representatives were in attendance.

The majority of the workshop consisted of discussions in 10 working groups:

- Cancer
- Cardiovascular disease and obesity
- Health promotion and intervention
- Human immunodeficiency/acquired immune deficiency syndrome (HIV/AIDS) and sexually transmitted diseases
- Life span development
- Mental health and substance abuse
- Research career development
- Research methodology
- Resiliency and health effects of homophobia
- Service delivery and access to services

Reports of new and ongoing efforts in lesbian health, such as the inclusion of questions on sexual identity and behavior in the National Health and Nutrition Examination Survey (NHANES) were also presented. Participants concluded their discussions by identifying a total of 70 specific steps for implementing the recommendations in the IOM report, and thus creating an action plan with a set of priorities for lesbian health research (*Scientific Workshop on Lesbian Health*, 2000).

Since the Scientific Workshop, NIH has funded lesbian health research, HHS created a Committee on Disparities Related to Sexual Orientation, and Healthy People 2010 announced that it will include sexual orientation as a population group. In addition, lesbian health activists joined with other sexual minority activists, and they created the National Coalition for Lesbian, Gay, Bisexual and Transgender Health in October 2000.

The coalition's purpose is to improve the health of LGBT persons by focusing on research, policy, education, and training. In 2002 the coalition held the first Lesbian, Gay, Bisexual, Transgender, and Intersex Health Summit, now a biennial event. In 2003 they sponsored the first National LGBT Health Awareness Week, now an annual event. Lesbian health activists recognize that lesbians share health concerns with other sexual minorities and also have unique health concerns as lesbians, so both movements will continue to work for better health for lesbians.

BARRIERS TO HEALTH CARE FOR LESBIANS

Barriers to quality health care for lesbians result from the homophobia and heterosexism in society and prevent equal access to health care for all persons. Lesbians experience many internal and external barriers to obtaining quality health care. Internal barriers are those that lesbians themselves hold, and include reluctance to disclose their lesbian identity and their distrust of medical institutions. External barriers are those within the health care system and among health care providers. In addition to the barriers that exist, many lesbians avoid seeking health care because of bad experiences they have had at some time in the past, or because they have heard about other lesbians' bad experiences.

Many lesbians are also reluctant to disclose their sexual identity to providers because they are afraid of homophobic responses, mistreatment, and judgments being made about them if they disclose. However, providers cannot give complete care if they do not have complete information about their patients. Three types of disclosure are possible: planned, passive, and unplanned (Bernhard, 2001).

Planned disclosure is when a lesbian decides consciously that she will come out to the provider. This is the safest form of disclosure for the lesbian because she is in control, and can also plan her actions, based on possible reactions to her coming out. Results of research suggest that higher education is associated with more disclosure to health care providers, and disclosure to providers is associated with greater utilization of health care (Bergeron & Senn, 2003). Passive disclosure occurs when the lesbian does not specifically tell the provider that she is lesbian, but assumes that the provider knows that she is lesbian, perhaps because of her appearance. She does nothing to affirm or deny what she thinks the provider knows. Unplanned disclosure occurs when a lesbian had explicitly planned *not* to come out to a provider, but something occurs during the interaction that causes her to think that she must disclose. It could be an unnecessary procedure, such as a pregnancy test that she does not need, or feeling challenged by a provider for not using contraception when she says that she is sexually active. This is a very unsafe situation for the lesbian because she did not consider options for how to deal with an unpleasant situation that developed.

The most significant external barrier to lesbian health care is the assumption by health care providers that all of their patients are heterosexual. In gynecologic offices this is obvious when providers assume that all women who come to them are seeking contraception. Although some lesbians may need contraception, most do not. The heterosexual assumption is also made when there are no representations of lesbians in the office. This could include pictures or posters of lesbian couples, with or without children, as well as health information materials directed toward lesbians. It is also seen in intake materials that include a space for "husband," rather than partner or significant other.

A barrier related to the heterosexual assumption is when providers lack knowledge about lesbians and their health. Although research on lesbian health has been limited, evidence is increasing and providers must be as aware of the growing body of knowledge about lesbian health, as they are aware of other health advances.

Another barrier to health care for lesbians can be financial. Lesbians may not have health insurance because they work in jobs that do not provide insurance. Some heterosexual women also are unable to receive health insurance through their work. The difference is that many of those heterosexual women have health insurance from their husbands' employment. Although employers are increasingly providing domestic partner benefits, they are not available to many lesbians who could use them. Domestic partner benefits also reflect coverage for children, and lesbian parents may have difficulty obtaining coverage for their children who are not "related" to them through birth or adoption.

EATING DISORDERS AND LESBIANS

Societal norms for beauty and attractiveness require women to be extremely thin and fit to be happy and valued in society. Women may develop eating disorders, such as binging and purging or highly restrictive diets, in an effort to attain or maintain thinness. However, lesbians are often presumed to have less body dissatisfaction, dieting, and disordered eating behaviors than heterosexual women because lesbians are more able to resist societal norms. Studies consistently demonstrate that lesbians have higher body weight (Cochran et al., 2001; Valanis et al., 2000) and body mass index (BMI) than heterosexual women (Mays, Yancey, Cochran, Weber, & Fielding, 2002; Moore & Keel, 2003), including their own heterosexual sisters (Roberts, Dibble, Nussey, & Casey, 2003). Increased weight puts lesbians at increased risk for cardiovascular disease and other health problems (Roberts et al., 2003).

Weight often increases as women age, and both older heterosexual and lesbian women have reported more body dissatisfaction than younger women (Moore & Keel, 2003; Yancey, Cochran, Corliss, & Mays, 2003). Race was shown to be an independent predictor of higher BMI in lesbians and bisexual women, with African-American women having a higher BMI (Yancey et al., 2003).

The most current research suggests that there may be more similarities than differences between heterosexual and lesbian women with regard to body image. Body image in women may be more related to gender than to sexual orientation (Moore & Keel, 2003;

Share & Mintz, 2002). Although heterosexual women may have a preferred lower body weight, lesbians who did not have partners had a lower BMI than lesbians living with partners (Yancey et al., 2003), suggesting that single lesbians may be similar to single heterosexual women who are dating.

Buffers that may help lesbians avoid viewing themselves negatively, having a poor body image, or developing eating disorders include having a more positive lesbian identity (Joshua, 2003) and more participation in lesbian social activities (Heffernan, 1999). However, feminist identity and activities do not appear to buffer (Guille & Chrisler, 1999; Heffernan, 1999).

SEXUALLY TRANSMITTED INFECTIONS, BACTERIAL VAGINOSIS, AND LESBIANS

When caring for women with STIs, sexual *behavior* is more important than sexual *identity* because sexual identity and sexual behavior are not always congruent. For example, in one study, fewer women who had only female sexual partners reported a history of STIs than did women who identified as lesbian (Bauer & Welles, 2001). Some of those who identified as lesbian reported only male sexual partners. Sexual partners and specific sexual behaviors are what place women at risk for contracting and transmitting STIs.

Although both lesbians and health care providers have thought that lesbians are at extremely low risk for development of STIs, that perception is inaccurate. The myth that lesbians are at low (or no) risk for STIs has been perpetuated based on the belief that lesbians do not have sex with men. That belief has been challenged through research that demonstrates that most lesbians have had sex with men at some time in their lives, and many continue to have sex with men (Bauer & Wells, 2001; Diamant, Schuster, McGuigan, & Lever, 1999). Thus, some lesbians may acquire STIs from male sexual partners and then transmit those infections to female sexual partners.

STIs are also transmitted between lesbian partners. Research has demonstrated that human papillomavirus (HPV) (Marrazzo, 2000; Marrazzo, Koutsky, Kiviat, Kuypers, & Stine, 2001) and herpes simplex virus (HSV) types 1 and 2 (Marrazzo, Stine, & Wald, 2003) can be sexually transmitted from woman to woman. In addition, case reports suggest that trichomoniasis (Kellock & O'Mahony, 1996) and syphilis (Campos-Outcalt & Hurwitz, 2002) are also sexually transmissible between women.

The prevalence of STIs in lesbians and women who have sex with women (WSW) is not well known, but reports clearly demonstrate that STIs in this population should be acknowledged, screened, and treated. In a study of WSW, conducted in Minneapolis and St. Paul, Minnesota, the self-reported incidence of STIs among lesbians and WSW was highest for genital warts (8%). Trichomoniasis and chlamydia were reported by 6%, genital herpes by 5%, and gonorrhea by 2% (Bauer & Welles, 2001). These rates are higher than another study of lesbians in the Seattle area in which the rates of *diagnosed* STIs for WSW were: trichomoniasis found in 2% of women, chlamydia in 1.1%, and syphilis in 0.7% (Marrazzo, Koutsky, & Handsfield, 2001). The prevalence of HPV when tested by polymerase chain reaction in another study was 13% (Marrazzo, Koutsky, Kiviat, et al., 2001). In the first study of HSV among lesbians, the seroprevalence of HSV-1 was 46% and of HSV-2 was 8%; however, only 6.1% of the lesbians in the study self-reported genital herpes (Marrazzo et al., 2003).

HIV has been identified in lesbians and women who report sex only with women (Kwakwa & Ghobrial, 2003). However, lesbians themselves and health care providers often assume that lesbians are immune to HIV. Recent studies show that many lesbians think they are at low risk (Fishman & Anderson, 2003) or no risk (Montcalm & Myer, 2000) for contracting HIV.

The number of AIDS cases in WSW, and how they contracted the disease, is unclear for several reasons. First, in half of the cases of AIDS in women reported to the Centers for Disease Control and Prevention (CDC), it is unknown whether they had ever had sex with women (CDC, 2003). This is because either the provider did not ask or the woman did not give that information. Nonetheless, the CDC says that 2% of women with AIDS have had sex with women, and 16% of those have had sex only with women. But that is clearly an underestimate. Second, the CDC uses a transmission-reporting system that is arranged hierarchically, and the first category in which an individual fits is defined as the (only) transmission source for that individual. The categories are: men who have sex with men, injecting drug use, men who have sex with men and inject drugs, hemophilia/coagulation disorder, heterosexual contact, receipt of blood transfusion, blood components, or tissue, and other/risk nor reported or identified. The majority of women with AIDS who reported sex only with women had another exposure category, usually injection drug use, and consequently, nearly all lesbians who have HIV have been classified as having acquired the infection through injection drug use. It is impossible to know whether their mode of infection was via sex with women. Multiple factors may account for transmission, and female to female transmission may have occurred prior to, or consequent with, injection drug use or heterosexual transmission. Some states and cities have added sexual orientation to their surveillance form (*Scientific Workshop on Lesbian Health*, 2000) as a way of identifying potential multiple modes of transmission in anyone diagnosed with HIV or AIDS. Although HIV can be transmitted between women, it appears to be rare.

Bacterial vaginosis (BV) is caused by a bacterial imbalance in the vagina that apparently does not affect men; thus, it is not currently considered an STI. Nonetheless, research has demonstrated that BV can be sexually transmitted between women (Berger et al., 1995; Marazzo et al., 2002). Because BV is not a reportable communicable disease, its prevalence is unclear. The CDC (2000), however, estimates that up to 16% of pregnant women in the United States have BV, with higher incidence in African-Americans, and lower incidence in Asian-Americans and Caucasians.

Bacterial vaginosis appears to be quite prevalent in lesbians and WSW and may be more common in WSW than among heterosexual women (Fethers, Marks, Mindel, & Estcourt, 2000; Skinner, Stokes, Kirlew, Kavanagh, & Forster, 1996). The reported prevalence of BV in lesbians and WSW ranges from 8% (Fethers et al., 2000) to 33% (Skinner et al., 1996). Concordance was demonstrated between partners in 81% (Berger et al., 1995) to 95% of female couples (Marrazzo et al., 2002) for both the presence and absence of BV. Interestingly, couples with concordant BV did not participate in different sexual activities than those who did not have BV.

Because of the perception of lesbian immunity to STIs, lesbians may engage in risky sexual behaviors without an awareness of the risk. Risky sexual behaviors that lesbians may use include unprotected oral, anal, or vaginal sex with female or male partners whose HIV status is positive or unknown; sex during menses; sharing sex toys; and sado-masochistic activities that result in a break in the skin. Low-income lesbians, especially if they are women of color or addicted to drugs, may also perform sex work for money or drugs, which additionally increases their risk for STIs (Arend, 2003). Other risky behaviors that lesbians may engage in that could result in HIV transmission through transfer of blood are sharing razors, and brushing or flossing teeth prior to having sex (Fishman & Anderson, 2003).

Providers should counsel their patients about ways to prevent the spread of STIs and encourage them to be tested, especially for HIV. Women should know their own and their partners' HIV status, and use barriers consistently and correctly. Lesbians can use dental dams as a barrier during oral sex with female partners, but many women find them too small or difficult to use. Providers can suggest using clear plastic wrap instead. Providers can also encourage lesbians to use gloves during penetrative sex and not to share sex toys.

GYNECOLOGIC CANCERS AND LESBIANS

Like most other women, lesbians are afraid of cancer. When lesbians were asked to rank the health issues of greatest concern to them, breast cancer was rated number one, with cervical and ovarian cancers in the top ten (White & Dull, 1998). Like other women, including women who have a family history of breast cancer, lesbians also overestimate their risk for breast cancer (McTiernan et al., 2001). This section will include information about cancer risk, screening, diagnosis, and interventions—showing similarities and differences between lesbians and heterosexual women.

CANCER RISK

In 1992 work by Suzanne Haynes at the National Cancer Institute, in which she concluded that lesbians were at increased risk for breast cancer, was presented in the media that lesbians had a one in three risk of developing breast cancer (Gessen, 1993). This resulted in a major concern among lesbians that remains today. Haynes' analysis—not empirical research—was based on evidence suggesting that lesbians are less likely to have children, more likely to delay childbirth until after age 30, more likely to drink alcohol, and more likely to be overweight than heterosexual women. These risk factors have been associated with breast cancer; however, they are each risk factors that are not unique to lesbians or common to all lesbians.

There are still no prospective empirical studies to determine whether lesbians are at higher risk for breast cancer. Lesbians in the Women's Health Initiative did have higher self-reports of breast cancer (7%), compared to heterosexuals (4.9%), but bisexuals had the highest prevalence in that study (8.4%) (Valanis et al., 2000). The authors did not suggest any explanation for that finding. In another case-control study of 21- to 45-year-old women with and without breast cancer, the relative risk was higher for lesbians than for nonlesbians (Kavanaugh-Lynch, White, Daling, & Bowen, 2002). Risk factors that explained the difference were parity, breast feeding, BMI, and use of alcohol.

In contrast, results of two retrospective studies challenge the assumption of increased risk, and suggest that there is no increased risk of breast cancer for lesbians when compared to other women (Cochran et al., 2001; Roberts, Dibble, Scanlon, Paul, & Davids, 1998). Roberts et al. reviewed medical records of 1019 women attending the Lyon-Martin Women's Health Services in San Francisco between 1995 and 1997, and found differences in risk factors, but no significant differences in the prevalence of breast cancer between lesbians and heterosexual women. Cochran et al. compiled results of seven previous surveys of lesbian health that included a total of about 12,000 women. Approximately 0.9% of lesbians 18–75 years of age reported a positive history of breast cancer. Although this under-represents the prevalence of breast cancer, because these were survivors of breast cancer, the authors compared the result to some 109,000 women 18–75 years of age in the NHANES III study and found the estimated prevalence of breast cancer in that sample also to be 0.9%. This would suggest that lesbians do not have a higher risk for developing breast cancer than the general population of women.

Lesbians may not have greater risks for cancers than heterosexual women, but they may have different risk factors. This is true not only for breast cancer, as previously noted, but also for ovarian cancer. Results of a retrospective study of risk factors for ovarian cancer revealed differences in risk factors between lesbian and heterosexual women (Dibble, Roberts, Robertson, & Paul, 2002). Not surprisingly, lesbians had lower parity and less use of oral contraceptives than did heterosexual women. Both higher numbers of pregnancies and longer use of oral contraceptives are believed to protect against ovarian cancer. Lesbians also had a higher BMI, but heterosexual women had higher rates of smoking, both additional risk factors for ovarian cancer (Dibble et al.).

CANCER SCREENING

Regardless of whether or not lesbians are at higher risk for various cancers than other women, all women should have access to cancer screening. Clark, Bonacore, Wright, Armstong, and Rakowski (2003) conducted focus groups with legally unmarried women to discuss barriers to screening for breast, cervical, and colon cancer. Barriers included the cost of screening and lack of insurance, and pain—mostly associated with colon cancer. The most important barrier was lack of acknowledgment and validation of women in the context of their lives. These women were distressed with intake forms that did not allow them to identify emotional support persons. They also reported feeling devalued in offices that focused on reproductive health. Women who partner with women specifically reported being discriminated against if they disclosed their sexual orientation and delayed or avoided screening because of feeling blamed or guilty about the size and shape of their bodies. Although these feelings were somewhat more frequent in women who were overweight or had large breasts, they were not unique to those women (Clark et al., 2003). Older lesbians may avoid cancer screening specifically because they fear being identified as lesbian or because of the hostility that they expect to receive from health care providers based on their experiences with health care in the past (Dibble & Roberts, 2003). Inadequate screening may increase the likelihood of later diagnosis of cancer, and greater morbidity and mortality.

There is no clear evidence that lesbians participate in mammography screening more or less frequently than other women. Some studies show that lesbians are equally as likely as heterosexual women to have mammograms (Diamant, Schuster, & Lever, 2000; Valanis et al., 2000). Others show that lesbians are significantly more likely than heterosexual women (Aaron et al., 2001) or less likely to have mammograms (Powers et al., 2001).

However, research clearly demonstrates that lesbians are less likely than heterosexual women to have regular Pap tests (Aaron et al., 2001; Mays et al., 2002; Powers et al., 2001). Mays et al. found that African-American and Hispanic, but not Asian-American, lesbians were significantly less likely to have had Pap tests within two years than African-American and Hispanic heterosexual women. Using the transtheoretical model in a large Internet-based survey of women, McGonigle (2003) found that lesbians were less likely to be in the maintenance stage of change than either bisexual or heterosexual women. Maintenance was defined as cervical screening on a regular basis. Younger lesbians (under 35) and less educated lesbians were also less likely than other women to have regular Pap smears (Diamant et al., 2000).

One important reason why some lesbians have not had Pap tests is that health care providers have told them they did not need one because they were not having sex with men (Marrazzo, Koutsky, Kiviat, et al., 2001). Not surprisingly then, women who have not had sex with men are less likely to have regular Pap screening (Marrazzo, Koutsky, Kiviat, et al.). Unfortunately, older lesbians in the Women's Health Initiative who reported never having had sex with men had higher self-reports of cervical cancer than lesbians who reported having had sex with men (Valanis et al., 2000).

CANCER DIAGNOSIS AND TREATMENT

Lesbians have many similarities to heterosexual women concerning their responses to newly diagnosed breast cancer (Fobair et al., 2001). They also do not receive different treatments for breast cancer than heterosexual women (Dibble & Roberts, 2002). Fobair et al. compared responses of lesbian and heterosexual women with breast cancer who had completed surgical treatment. Because of the difficulty in obtaining lesbians to participate in the research, there was a significant difference in the time since diagnosis between the groups: 7 months for heterosexual women and 15 months for lesbians. Nonetheless, there were no differences between the groups in emotional distress, expression of feelings, and sexual satisfaction; however, lesbians were significantly less fatalistic, more likely to express anger, and to use active coping than were heterosexuals. Lesbians had fewer body image problems and were more able to show their bodies to others. Lesbians received significantly more social support from their partners and friends, while heterosexual women received significantly more support from relatives. Lesbians were also significantly less satisfied with their physicians' care and inclusion of their partners in treatment discussions than were heterosexual women (Fobair et al., 2001). The only difference between lesbians and heterosexual women concerning treatment for breast cancer identified by Dibble and Roberts (2002) was that lesbians had more side effects from chemotherapy than heterosexual women did.

INTERVENTIONS FOR LESBIANS AND CANCER

The legally unmarried women in Clark et al. (2003) study also made suggestions to health care providers for increasing the likelihood of their participation in cancer screening. Most importantly, they wanted a trusting relationship with a provider whom they felt knew them and cared about them as whole persons. They wanted to make their own, informed decisions about health care and have those decisions respected by the provider. And as a practical matter, they wanted to be able to schedule appointments for screening several months in advance and have multiple exams scheduled on the same day.

Dibble and Roberts (2003) provided an intervention to women in senior centers for gay, lesbian, bisexual, and transgender (GLBT) persons to enhance cancer screening for older lesbians. The intervention (a one-hour didactic presentation by a lesbian health care provider, followed by a 15-minute question and answer period) had a positive impact, based on a six-month follow-up, with lesbians seeking mammography and pelvic exams. However, there was a very high (20%) refusal rate because these older lesbians were afraid of exposure and perceived lack of anonymity, even with a lesbian presenter and in a place known to them.

A 12-week Supportive-Expressive group therapy intervention for lesbians with breast cancer resulted in a significant increase in mood and family relations and a decrease in stress for the lesbians who participated (Fobair et al., 2002). There were no changes in body image or sexuality. These lesbians did report significantly less instrumental (helpful assistance) and informational (provision of knowledge) social support following the intervention, but that could have been because they no longer needed assistance or information.

PROVIDING CULTURALLY COMPETENT CARE

Lesbians will feel most comfortable and safe in health care environments when they think that their sexual orientation is *not* an issue, and it will not be the primary part of themselves being treated. To make that happen, health care providers must educate themselves about lesbians and lesbian health, and create environments that are welcoming, non-threatening, and normalized to lesbians. Being educated includes knowledge about the provision of care to lesbians, as well as knowledge about the content of health care for lesbians.

Regarding the provision of care, providers must use good communication skills. Specifically, providers should use gender-neutral language, avoiding the heterosexual assumption. Ask how a woman chooses to be identified, what she prefers to be called, and who her family, partners, and important relationships are. Providers should use a non-threatening, nonjudgmental approach, and work specifically to make lesbians feel at ease, comfortable, and safe. If the provider is relaxed, it will help the patient to relax.

Providers should encourage disclosure of sexual orientation when it is relevant to the presenting need, and may also disclose their own sexual orientation, especially if they are a sexual minority themselves and are able to come out. However, providers should also ask the lesbian whether and how she wants that information documented in her medical record. To avoid lesbians believing that their sexuality is what is being treated, providers should always consider the full range of physical and psychosocial health problems for which a lesbian may be seeking care, and explain why they are asking the questions they ask.

To educate themselves, providers can read or attend conferences. They can also talk with individual lesbians in their communities who are out and willing to assist with educating health care providers who want to learn. Providers can also work with local community lesbian or gay agencies. Two examples are Stonewall Columbus, in Columbus, Ohio, which has a Rural Lesbian Health Project to provide culturally sensitive health care to lesbians in rural Ohio (http://www.stonewallcolumbus.org), and the GLBT Health Access Project in Massachusetts, which provides training to health providers and GLBT populations to promote the health of GLBT persons in Massachusetts (http://www.glbthealth.org).

In addition, there is a national training project for health care providers called Removing the Barriers. This program was developed by the Mautner Project, a national lesbian health organization based in Washington, DC, in collaboration with the CDC. Removing the Barriers is designed to improve providers' skills in working with lesbians and women who partner with women and to enhance health care environments so that health care for lesbians will be improved (Scout, Bradford, & Fields, 2001). The Mautner Project partners with sites in any community across the United States. They have recently expanded the project to include training of trainers, so that more people can be educated. Providers can contact The Mautner Project (http://www.mautnerproject.org) to determine whether there is an opportunity available in their local communities to participate in the training, and if there is not, to initiate such a project.

Lesbians also want providers who are competent (Saulnier, 2002). To educate themselves about the content of health care for lesbians, providers should read current research and other literature about lesbian health. They should also be willing to search for information, rather than simply dismiss questions that lesbians might ask.

To make the health care environment acceptable to lesbians, providers should first consider the physical environment. Having images of lesbians, health information designed for lesbians, or lesbian magazines in the waiting area makes lesbians feel like they are welcome. Lesbians will also feel accepted when intake forms ask for significant or important relationships, rather than husband or spouse. Reception staff must also be fully trained to be sensitive to the special needs of lesbian patients, and to protect their privacy. Finally, providers should be aware of community resources and referrals, such as support groups for lesbians with cancer, that are specific to lesbians or sexual minorities, as well as mainstream referrals that are culturally sensitive to lesbians.

HEALTH CARE FOR SPECIAL GROUPS OF LESBIANS

YOUTH AND ADOLESCENT LESBIANS

Youth and adolescents are less likely to identify themselves as lesbian or gay, regardless of their sexual behaviors (D'Augelli, 2004). Adolescents want to be like their friends, and coming out as lesbian sets them apart in many ways. Self-identification as lesbian or gay is typically the last step in the process of coming out (D'Augelli). Thus, health care providers should not presume that girls for whom they provide care—even if they report being heterosexual—are not having sex with girls. Although providers should not make the assumption of heterosexuality with women of any age, it may be even more true with youth.

Lesbian youth and adolescents engage in activities that put them at high risk for STIs (including HIV), pregnancy, and cervical cancer. Although lesbian girls are no more likely than heterosexual girls to report ever having had sex with men, they currently have sex more frequently than heterosexual girls, and they are more likely to become pregnant (Saewyc, Bearinger, Blum, & Resnick, 1999). About one-third of lesbian girls in one study did not use contraception, and among those who did use contraception, they used less effective methods, such as withdrawal or rhythm. Some lesbian girls reportedly think that they will not become pregnant if they have sex with gay boys.

In addition to unprotected sex, lesbian youth are likely to have body piercings or tattoos. Piercings of the tongue, abdomen, or genitalia, most commonly the clitoral hood or labia, can place youth at risk for bacterial infections and other STIs, especially during the initial healing period, with transfer of body fluids (Peterkin & Risdon, 2003). Full healing may take six to eight weeks.

Smoking cigarettes is now recognized as an important risk factor for the development of cervical cancer. Although research on adult lesbians shows conflicting evidence about smoking prevalence, a recent study shows that lesbian and bisexual girls are significantly more likely than heterosexual girls to use tobacco (Austin et al., 2004). Lesbian and bisexual girls, ages 12–17, were far more likely to report having smoked cigarettes in the past week, month, and year, and to report that most or all of their friends smoked also (Austin et al.). Health care providers should encourage all adolescents not to begin smoking and assist those who have started smoking to stop.

When asked about the characteristics of health care providers and health care sites that would help them to trust a provider or site, 14- to 23-year-old sexual minority youth in Philadelphia indicated that they wanted providers who maintain confidentiality, demonstrate respect and honesty, and are well educated (Ginsburg et al., 2002). Providers should be good listeners, nonjudgmental, and sensitive to GLBT issues. That is, they should not assume that GLBT youth have HIV or that they engage in risky sexual behaviors, and they should be understanding of same sex partners' needs.

Concerning health care sites, the most important thing these youth said was that the place should be clean (Ginsburg et al., 2002). They also wanted a diverse staff, including race, gender, and sexual orientation. They wanted GLBT posters or magazines, making the place inviting, although those who were less out wanted GLBT health information available in private places, which could be individual examining rooms or restrooms.

OLDER LESBIANS

Older women experience age and sex discrimination, and older lesbians can also experience heterosexism. Many lesbians who are 55 years and older today lived their lives deeply in the closet, trying hard not to be identified as lesbian, or specifically trying to "blend in" with other people in their communities (Jones & Nystrom, 2002). These women are still afraid of being identified as lesbian. In the Women's Health Initiative, only 0.6% of women were identified as lesbian; however, 2.8% did not answer the question, and those women may very well be lesbians who were afraid of being "outed."

Some older lesbians were previously married to men and have children and grandchildren. Others do not have biological children, but have children that they consider "theirs" (Claes & Moore, 2000). These older women have created networks of significant others who are their "chosen family." Health care providers need to be aware of the possibility of lesbian intergenerational relationships that are important to these women.

Older lesbians have similar concerns as other older women, such as housing, finances, illness, and wanting to maintain control over their own lives. In addition, their concerns for aging may include the impact of death of a partner, family, and friends that may or may not be recognized by society (Jones & Nystrom, 2002). Some lesbians will experience widowhood, although widowhood is rarely acknowledged for lesbians, except by their most immediate friends or family. The lack of social acceptance or acknowledgment of their loss can make the experience even more painful, and may increase lesbians' risk for depression or other mental health problems.

LESBIANS WITH DISABILITIES

All women with disabilities face barriers to health care. For lesbians with disabilities, their disability is one more factor that makes health care difficult. Disabilities range from blindness or deafness to mobility problems to mental health problems, and vary by whether the disability is visible or invisible and whether it is lifelong or acquired. Consequently, lesbians with disabilities are an extremely heterogeneous group. Moreover, they share issues of disability with heterosexual women (e.g., the myth that women who are disabled are not sexually active) at the same time that they share issues of lesbian health with other lesbians (e.g., fear of disclosure to providers). Consequently, lesbians with disabilities may feel even more unsafe in gynecologic offices than other lesbians (O'Toole, 1996). It is incumbent upon health care providers to provide the same quality of care for lesbians with disabilities as it is for all lesbians and for all women.

CONCLUSION

Lesbians are a diverse group of women who have health and gynecologic health care needs similar to all women, but who also have unique needs because they are lesbians. Barriers to quality health care exist in society generally and in specific health care settings. The most obvious barrier is providers who assume that all their patients are heterosexual. Providers who individualize care, create a safe and affirming health care environment, and who try to provide culturally competent care to all their patients—whether they have STIs, gynecologic cancers, or eating disorders—will earn the trust of lesbians and, in so doing, improve the health care that lesbians receive.

REFERENCES

Aaron, D. J., Markovic, N., Danielson, M. E., Honnold, J. A. Janosky, J. E., & Schmidt, N. J. (2001). Behavioral risk factors for disease and preventive health practices among lesbians. *American Journal of Public Health, 91*, 972–875.

Arend, E. D. (2003). The politics of invisibility: HIV-positive women who have sex with women and their struggle for support. *Journal of the Association of Nurses in AIDS Care, 14*(6), 37–47.

Austin, S. B., Ziyadeh, N., Fisher, L. B., Kahn, J. A., Colditz, G. A., & Frazier, A. L. (2004). Sexual orientation and tobacco use in a cohort study of U.S. adolescent girls and boys. *Archives of Pediatrics & Adolescent Medicine, 158*, 317–322.

Bauer, G. R., & Welles, S. L. (2001). Beyond assumptions of negligible risk: Sexually transmitted diseases and women who have sex with women. *American Journal of Public Health, 91*, 1282–1286.

Berger, B. J., Kolton, S., Zenilman, J. M., Cummings, M. C., Feldman, J., & McCormack, W. M. (1995). Bacterial vaginosis in lesbians: A sexually transmitted disease. *Clinical Infectious Diseases, 21*, 1402–1405.

Bergeron, S., & Senn, C. Y. (2003). Health care utilization in a sample of Canadian lesbian women: Predictors of risk and resilience. *Women & Health, 37*(3), 19–35.

Bernhard, L. A. (2001). Lesbian health and health care. *Annual Review of Nursing Research, 19*, 145–177.

Bowen, D. J., Anderson, J., White, J., Powers, D., & Greenlee, H. (2002). Preferences for alternative and traditional health care: Relationship to health behaviors, health information sources, and trust of providers. *Journal of the Gay and Lesbian Medical Association, 6*, 3–7.

Bradford, J., & Ryan, C. (1987). *The National Lesbian Health Care Survey.* Washington, DC: National Lesbian and Gay Health Foundation.

Campos-Outcalt, D., & Hurwitz, S. (2002). Female-to-female transmission of syphilis: A case report. *Sexually Transmitted Diseases, 29*, 119.

Centers for Disease Control and Prevention (2000). *Tracking the Hidden Epidemics 2000: Trends in STDs in the United States.* Retrieved September 26, 2004, from http://www.cdc.gov/nchstp/od/news/RevBrochure1pdf.htm.

Centers for Disease Control and Prevention. (2003, July). *HIV/AIDS and U.S. Women Who Have Sex with Women (WSW).* Retrieved September 26, 2004, from http:/www.cdc.gov/hiv/pubs/facts/wsw.htm.

Claes, J. A., & Moore, W. (2000). Issues confronting lesbian and gay elders: The challenge for health and human services providers. *Journal of Health and Human Services Administration, 23*(2), 181–202.

Clark, M. A., Bonacore, L., Wright, S. J., Armstrong, G., & Rakowski, W. (2003). The cancer screening project for women: Experiences of women who partner with women and women who partner with men. *Women & Health, 38*(2), 19–33.

Cochran, S. D., Mays, V. M., Bowen, D., Gage, S., Bybee, D., Roberts, S. J., et al. (2001). Cancer-related risk indicators and preventive screening behaviors among lesbians and bisexual women. *American Journal of Public Health, 91*, 591–597.

Colebrook, C. (2004). *Gender.* New York: Palgrave Macmillan.

D'Augelli, A. R. (2004). High tobacco use among lesbian, gay, and bisexual youth. *Archives of Pediatrics & Adolescent Medicine, 158*, 309–310.

Diamant, A. L., Schuster, M. A., & Lever, J. (2000). Receipt of preventive health care services by lesbians. *American Journal of Preventive Medicine, 19*, 141–148.

Diamant, A. L., Schuster, M. A., McGuigan, K., & Lever, J. (1999). Lesbians' sexual history with men: Implications for taking a sexual history. *Archives of Internal Medicine, 159*, 2739–2736.

Dibble, S. L., & Roberts, S. A. (2002). A comparison of breast cancer diagnosis and treatment between lesbian and heterosexual women. *Journal of the Gay and Lesbian Medical Association, 6*, 9–17.

Dibble, S. L., & Roberts, S. A. (2003). Improving cancer screening among lesbians over 50: Results of a pilot study. *Oncology Nursing Forum, 30*, E71–E79.

Dibble, S. L., Roberts, S. A., Robertson, P. A., & Paul, S. M. (2002). Risk factors for ovarian cancer: Lesbian and heterosexual women. *Oncology Nursing Forum, 29*, 29.

Fethers, K., Marks, C., Mindel, A., & Estcourt, C. S. (2000). Sexually transmitted infections and risk behaviours in women who have sex with women. *Sexually Transmitted Infections, 76*, 345–349.

Fishman, S. J., & Anderson, E. H. (2003). Perception of HIV and safer sexual behaviors among lesbians. *Journal of the Association of Nurses in AIDS Care, 14*(6), 48–55.

Fobair, P., Koopman, C., Dimiceli, S., O'Hanlan, K., Butler, L. D., Classen, C., et al. (2002). Psychosocial intervention for lesbians with primary breast cancer. *Psycho-Oncology, 11*, 427–438.

Fobair P., O'Hanlan, K., Koopman, C., Classen, C., Dimiceli, S., Drooker, N., et al. (2001). Comparison of lesbian and heterosexual women's response to newly diagnosed breast cancer. *Psycho-Oncology, 10*, 40–51.

Fone, B. (2000). *Homophobia.* New York: Picador USA.

Gessen, M. (1993, February 9). Lesbians and breast cancer. *The Advocate*, 45–48.

Ginsburg, K. R., Winn, R. J., Rudy, B. J., Crawford, J., Zhao, H., & Schwarz, D. F. (2002). How to reach sexual minority youth in the health care setting: The teens offer guidance. *Journal of Adolescent Health, 31*, 407–416.

Guille, C., & Chrisler, J. C. (1999). Does feminism serve a protective function against eating disorders? *Journal of Lesbian Studies, 3*(4), 141–148.

Heffernan, K. (1999). Lesbians and the internalization of societal standards of weight and appearance. *Journal of Lesbian Studies, 3*(4), 121–127.

Herek, G. M. (1995). Psychological heterosexism in the United States. In A. R. D'Augelli & C. J. Patterson (Eds.), *Lesbian, gay, and bisexual identities over the lifespan* (pp. 321–346). New York: Oxford University Press.

Jones, T. C., & Nystrom, N. M. (2002). Looking back. . . Looking forward: Addressing the lives of lesbians 55 and older. *Journal of Women & Aging, 14*(3/4), 59–76.

Joshua, M. D. (2003). A model of the development of disordered eating among lesbians. *Dissertation Abstracts International, 63*(9), 4375.

Kavanaugh-Lynch, M. H. E., White, E., Daling, J. R., & Bowen, D. J. (2002). Correlates of lesbian sexual orientation and the risk of breast cancer. *Journal of the Gay and Lesbian Medical Association, 6,* 91–95.

Kellock, D. J., & O'Mahoney, C. P. (1996). Sexually acquired metronidazole-resistant trichomoniasis in a lesbian couple. *Genitourinary Medicine, 72,* 60–61.

Kwakwa, H. A., & Ghobrial, M. W. (2003). Female-to-female transmission of human immunodeficiency virus. *Clinical Infectious Diseases, 36,* e40–e41.

LeMoncheck, L. (1997). *Loose women, lecherous men: A feminist philosophy of sex.* New York: Oxford University Press.

Marrazzo, J. M. (2000). Genital human papillomavirus infection in women who have sex with women: A concern for patients and providers. *AIDS Patient Care and STDs, 14,* 447–451.

Marrazzo, J. M., Koutsky, L. A., Eschenbach, D. A., Agnew, K., Stine, K., & Hillier, S. L. (2002). Characterization of vaginal flora and bacterial vaginosis in women who have sex with women. *Journal of Infectious Diseases, 185,* 1307–1313.

Marrazzo, J. M., Koutsky, L. A., & Handsfield, H. H. (2001). Characteristics of female sexually transmitted disease clinic clients who report same-sex behavior. *International Journal of STD & AIDS, 12,* 41–46.

Marrazzo, J. M., Koutsky, L. A., Kiviat, N. B., Kuypers, J. M., & Stine, K. (2001). Papanicolaou test screening and prevalence of genital human papillomavirus among women who have sex with women. *American Journal of Public Health, 91,* 947–952.

Marrazzo, J. M., Stine, K., & Wald, A. (2003). Prevalence and risk factors for infection with herpes simplex virus type-1 and −2 among lesbians. *Sexually Transmitted Diseases, 30,* 890–895.

Mathieson, C. M., Bailey, N., & Gurevich, M. (2002). Health care services for lesbian and bisexual women: Some Canadian data. *Health Care for Women International, 23,* 185–196.

Matthews, A. K. (1998). Lesbians and cancer support: Clinical issues for cancer patients. *Health Care for Women International, 19,* 193–203.

Mays, V. M., Yancey, A. K., Cochran, S. D., Weber, M., & Fielding, J. E. (2002). Heterogeneity of health disparities among African American, Hispanic, and Asian American women: Unrecognized influences of sexual orientation. *American Journal of Public Health, 92,* 632–639.

McDonald, C., McIntyre, M., & Anderson, B. (2003). The view from somewhere: Locating lesbian experience in women's health. *Health Care for Women International, 24,* 697–711.

McGonigle, T. H. (2003). Surveying for sexuality in cyberspace: Sexual orientation and stage of change for cervical cancer screening. Unpublished doctoral dissertation, Ohio State University.

McTiernan, A., Kuniyuki, A., Yasui, Y., Bowen, D., Burke, W., Culver, J. B., et al. (2001). Comparisons of two breast cancer risk estimates in women with a family history of breast cancer. *Cancer Epidemiology, Biomarkers & Prevention, 10,* 333–338.

Montcalm, D. M., & Myer, L. L. (2000). Lesbian immunity from HIV/AIDS: Fact or fiction? *Journal of Lesbian Studies, 4,* 131–147.

Moore, F., & Keel, P. K. (2003). Influence of sexual orientation and age on disordered eating attitudes and behaviors in women. *International Journal of Eating Disorders, 34,* 370–374.

O'Toole, C. J. (1996). Disabled lesbians: Challenging monocultural constructs. In D. M. Krotoski, M. A. Nosek, & M. A. Turk (Eds.), *Women with physical disabilities: Achieving and maintaining health and well-being* (pp. 135–151). Baltimore: Paul H. Brooks.

Peterkin, A., & Risdon, C. (2003). *Caring for lesbian and gay people: A clinical guide.* Buffalo, NY: University of Toronto Press.

Powers, D., Bowen, D. J., & White, J. (2001). The influence of sexual orientation on health behaviors in women. *Journal of Prevention & Intervention in the Community, 22*(2), 43–60.

Roberts, S. A., Dibble, S. L., Nussey, B., & Casey, K. (2003). Cardiovascular disease risk in lesbian women. *Women's Health Issues, 13,* 167–174.

Roberts, S. A., Dibble, S. L., Scanlon, J. L., Paul, S. M., & Davids, H. (1998). Differences in risk factors for breast cancer: Lesbian and heterosexual women. *Journal of the Gay and Lesbian Medical Association, 2,* 93–101.

Saewyc, E. M., Bearinger, L. H., Blum, R. W., & Resnick, M. D. (1999). Sexual intercourse, abuse and pregnancy among adolescent women: Does sexual orientation make a difference? *Family Planning Perspectives, 31*(3), 127–131.

Saulnier, C. F. (2002). Deciding who to see: Lesbians discuss their preferences in health and mental health care providers. *Social Work, 47,* 355–365.

Scientific workshop on lesbian health: Steps for implementing the IOM report. (2000). Washington, DC: United States Department of Health and Human Services, Office on Women's Health.

Scout, Bradford, J., & Fields, C. (2001). Removing the barriers: Improving practitioners' skills in providing health care to lesbians and women who partner with

women. *American Journal of Public Health, 91,* 989–990.

Share, T. L., & Mintz, L. B. (2002). Differences between lesbians and heterosexual women in disordered eating and related attitudes. *Journal of Homosexuality, 42*(4), 89–106.

Skinner, C. J., Stokes, J., Kirlew, Y., Kavanagh, J., & Forster, G. E. (1996). A case-controlled study of the sexual health needs of lesbians. *Genitourinary Medicine, 72,* 277–280.

Solarz, A. L. (Ed.). (1999). *Lesbian health: Current assessment and directions for the future.* Washington, DC: National Academy Press.

Valanis, B. G., Bowen, D. J., Bassford, T., Whitlock, E., Charney, P., & Carter, R. A. (2000). Sexual orientation and health: Comparisons in the Women's Health Initiative sample. *Archives of Family Medicine, 9,* 843–853.

White, J. C., & Dull, V. T. (1998). Room for improvement: Communication between lesbians and primary care providers. *Journal of Lesbian Studies, 2*(1), 95–110.

Yancey, A. K., Cochran, S. D., Corliss, H. L., & Mays, V. M. (2003). Correlates of overweight and obesity among lesbian and bisexual women. *Preventive Medicine, 36,* 676–683.

Chapter 11

MENOPAUSE

IVY M. ALEXANDER
LINDA C. ANDRIST

Menopause, often thought of as the closure of reproductive capability, has emerged as one of the predominant health issues for midlife women. A major reason that menopause is receiving so much attention is the increasing numbers of women reaching middlescence. The baby boom generation, people born between 1945 and 1960, is the largest middle-aged cohort ever recorded. Population experts project that by 2030, 20% of Americans will be 65 years of age and older (Administration on Aging, 2004). Because the life span continues to increase, women will live one-third of their lives after menopause.

The emphasis on the end of reproduction ignores the myriad issues facing women at midlife. Midlife brings with it changes, such as children leaving home, illness or death of parents, and career changes. Transitions that accompany midlife include adjusting to the idea of mortality, adapting to changes in family relationships, becoming more authentic, and assessing and appreciating one's life experiences (Sampselle, Harris, Harlow, & Sowers, 2002).

During middlescence, described as ages 35–65 by many resources, women continue to grow and develop psychologically. Increasingly, menopause is being understood as another life stage with potential for growth and development. The challenges experienced during this transition may serve as the basis for personal reflection and growth (Busch, Barth-Olofsson, Rosenhagen, & Collins, 2003).

Researchers have elucidated women's unique growth and development, such as Gilligan (1982), who found that relationship was a priority for women. Jordan and colleagues (1991) found that women develop in relationship with others, and development means increasing complexity, connection, and mutuality. Collins (1990) recognized the uniqueness of African-American women's experience. The major premise in much of the published works is the importance of recognizing the variation in women's development based on culture, race, and socioeconomic variables.

To that end, Sampselle et al. (2002) conducted focus groups with 32 Caucasian and African-American women to identify factors that enhanced midlife women's well-being, and whether these factors differed between the two groups. They found that Caucasian participants were concerned about menopause as a sign of aging and the loss of youthful appearance, while the African-American women were welcoming of menopause as a normal event. All of the women identified child bearing and child launching as major stages in women's lives. The potential for further personal development was enhanced by fewer childcare demands, and women felt few feelings of loss.

Quinn (1991) developed a theoretical model, "Integrating a New Me," through a qualitative study with 12 women. She found four processes that women experienced:

- *Tuning into me*—The beginning of the awareness of entering the perimenopause
- *Facing a paradox of feelings*—Includes both positive and negative feelings about situations such as getting older, reproduction, physical vulnerability, and uncertainty about the future
- *Contrasting impressions*—Encompasses the processing of conflicting information, women developing their own symbolic meaning through integrating interactions with others, and their own self-appraisal
- *Making adjustments*—Refers to the changes and alterations that women make in response to their emotional, physical, and life changes in daily living

Building on Sheehy's (1976, 1995) work, Wilmoth (1996) proposed a conceptual framework that includes *disassembling, evaluating,* and *reassembling,* to find one's own truth. *Disassembling* is the taking apart of our psychological lives and examining them from a new perspective. Part of this includes a natural mourning process for lost youth, loss of procreative abilities, and lost opportunities, and is similar to Quinn's first process. The *evaluation* process that accompanies disassembling requires that women look into themselves to see who they are and whether they like themselves. Wilmoth argues that the context of each woman's experience is dependent on her lived experience and life situation; thus the variation in women's experiences. *Reassembling* incorporates a coming of age and a movement toward mastery.

Ballard, Kuh, and Wadsworth (2001) described the menopause transition as a status passage based on a longitudinal study, which includes five stages: (1) expectations of symptoms, (2) experience of symptoms and loss of control, (3) confirmation of the menopause, (4) regaining control, and (5) freedom from menstruation.

All of the models discussed previously include three major phases: assessment, adjusting to change, and acceptance. It is noteworthy that many researchers have found that menopause itself, the cessation of menstruation, is just one event in the overall context of midlife women's lives.

TABLE 11–1   Recommended Hormone Therapy Terminology*

Term	Abbreviation/Explanation
Estrogen therapy alone	ET
Estrogen/progestogen therapy	EPT
Hormone therapy	HT, Encompassing term for ET/EPT
Continuous-combined daily estrogen/ progestogen therapy	CC-EPT
Continuous-sequential estrogen/ progestogen therapy (estrogen daily, progestogen added on a set sequence)	CS-EPT
Preparations of ET or EPT that have a systemic, not solely vaginal, effect	Systemic ET/EPT
Preparations of ET that have a predominantly vaginal, not systemic, effect	Local ET
Progestogen	Encompassing term for progesterone and progestin

*The North American Menopause Society (NAMS) has urged clinicians, researchers, and the media to standardize terminology, which they consider essential for accurate communication. Note that the word "replacement" has been deleted from the terms "hormone replacement therapy" and "estrogen replacement therapy."
Source: Adapted from NAMS, 2003.

THE MEDICALIZATION OF MENOPAUSE: A HISTORICAL PERSPECTIVE

Menopause is a remarkable example of the medicalization of women's bodies throughout the 20th century. The biomedical model perpetuated menopause as a deficiency disease (MacPherson, 1981) or endocrinopathy (Utian, 1987). Science attempted to establish hormone therapy (HT, Table 11–1) as the panacea for prevention of diseases in old age, and pharmaceutical corporations aggressively marketed their products as "the fountain of youth."

In 1938, researchers in England produced the first synthetic estrogen, diethylstibesterol, which was heralded as the cure for postmenopausal symptoms. Premarin was the first nonsynthetic estrogen produced from the urine of pregnant mares and was introduced by Wyeth-Ayerst in 1942. Although it was prescribed for many women, the prevalence of HT did not increase significantly until the 1960s, particularly after the publication of *Feminine Forever* by gynecologist Robert Wilson (1966). The major message in this highly popular book, 100,000 copies of which were sold in the first seven months, was that after menopause women would become eunuchs with withered breasts and begin a "living decay" (Wilson, p. 43). Estrogen use, referred to then as hormone replacement therapy (HRT), promised women the fountain of youth and was praised by Wilson as "one of the greatest biological revolutions in the history of civilization" (Wilson, 1966, p. 16). Interestingly, Wilson's work was funded by Ayerst, Searle, and Upjohn.

Between the years 1967 and 1975, sales of Premarin (conjugated equine estrogens or CEE) tripled. By the time it was linked with endometrial cancer, Premarin was the fifth most popular drug in the United States. In 1975 researchers began to link estrogen use with an increased incidence of endometrial cancer, and the sales of Premarin dropped dramatically. By 1979 the National Institute on Aging convened a consensus conference and agreed that because HRT increases the risk for endometrial cancer, "women using estrogens should take them only for the shortest possible time, in the lowest possible dose" (US Department of Health, Education, and Welfare, 1979, p. 1). Additionally, the committee concluded that HT was effective only for hot flashes and vaginal dryness (National Women's Health Network, 2000). It is noteworthy that this is the same recommendation put forward by the North American Menopause Society (NAMS) in 2003.

During the 1980s epidemiological data demonstrated that the addition of a progestogen to estrogen therapy (ET) lowered the risk of endometrial cancer. Once again, HT increased in popularity. When researchers demonstrated that HT could decrease the risk of osteoporosis in the early 1980s (Weiss, Ure, Ballard, William, & Daling, 1980), the promotion of HT changed from relieving symptoms to prevention of disease in old age. By the late 1980s several observational studies showed that HT was protective against heart disease and until the release of the findings of the Women's Health Initiative (WHI) data in 2002, health care providers were recommending HT to nearly all postmenopausal women for long-term prevention of heart disease. The US Preventive Services Task Force (USPSTF) made the recommendation in the 1990s that all women should be counseled about and *consider* preventative HT (USPSTF, 1996). The USPSTF did not, however, offer a recommendation about whether women should actually *take* HT. Studies linking estrogen use and breast cancer were glossed over, and women were told that the risk of heart disease outweighed the risk of breast cancer. Studies were published linking the use of HT and reduced risk of Alzheimer's, memory loss, skin integrity, and colon cancer.

The WHI is the largest clinical trial ever to be conducted on health risks of postmenopausal women. Nearly 17,000 women were randomized into HT or placebo groups between 1993 and 1998. The estrogen with progestogen arm of the study was halted in 2002, after a mean of 5.2 years of follow-up, because the health risks outweighed the benefits. These included increased risk of breast cancer, coronary events, stroke, and pulmonary embolism (Rossouw et al., 2002). In March 2004, the estrogen arm of the study was also stopped because researchers found an increased risk of stroke. The study group also reported that estrogen did not appear to increase or decrease heart disease or breast cancer (National Institutes of Health [NIH], 2004; Anderson et al., 2004). Results from the WHI established that ET prevents osteoporosis-related hip fractures as well as protecting the spine and small bones. While CEE are still indicated for the prevention of postmenopausal osteoporosis, most experts recommend the use of nonestrogen medications (Liu, 2004).

Some experts have pointed out the limitations of the WHI results, such as the age of participants. The mean age was 63 years, which is significantly older than newly menopausal women. The study also used only one HT product, Prempro, which contains CEE and medroxyprogesterone acetate (MPA). Although findings from the WHI may apply to all HT products, additional clinical trials are needed to clarify the risks and benefits of other products. Finally, the WHI did not address quality of life issues for women with moderate to severe vasomotor symptoms. In fact, these women were excluded from the study. It is therefore difficult to evaluate differences in HT response between women who initiate HT before the cessation of menses and those who begin later (Wysocki, Alexander, Schnare, Moore, & Freeman, 2003).

Additional study of HT use in women is planned. A multicenter, randomized, controlled longitudinal trial evaluating effects of HT in women as they enter menopause is in development (Grady, 2004). This research likely will offer some answers to questions raised by the WHI and add further questions for clinicians to consider regarding HT use for menopausal women.

The NAMS released a position statement on the treatment of vasomotor menopausal symptoms in 2004. Key points in the statement include:

- The primary indication for systemic ET and estrogen-progestin therapy (EPT) is the treatment of moderate to severe menopausal symptoms, including hot flashes.
- All women with an intact uterus should receive systemic progestogen with estrogen to decrease the risk of endometrial hyperplasia and adenocarcinoma.
- Current data from the WHI and Heart and Estrogen/Progestin Replacement Study (HERS) support a link between EPT and risks for coronary heart disease, breast cancer, stroke, thromboembolism, and dementia.
- ET and EPT should be prescribed for the shortest possible amount of time and are not to be used for prevention of coronary heart disease.

We are now witnessing the dismantling of menopause as a disease, particularly in nursing. Over 20 years ago, MacPherson (1981) challenged nurses to begin deconstructing the biomedical paradigm. Since then, nurse researchers have been at the forefront of published studies of women's experiences of menopause and midlife. Feminist scholars have reclaimed menopause as another developmental stage in women's lives (Andrist & McPherson, 2001).

NATURAL MENOPAUSE

Menopause is defined as the point in time following 12 consecutive months of amenorrhea and occurs in response to normal physiologic changes in the hypothalamic-pituitary-ovarian axis (see Chapter 5 for a detailed description of the menstrual cycle). During the perimenopausal period, occurring two to eight years prior to the last menstrual period, and for the 12 months of amenorrhea preceding menopause, fewer ovarian follicles develop in each menstrual cycle. The follicles that do develop are less responsive to follicle-stimulating hormone (FSH), and the ovaries produce less estradiol, progesterone, and androgens. Thus, the usual negative feedback effect from elevated estrogen and progesterone levels on hypothalamic production of gonadotropin-releasing hormone (GnRH) is lost, and anterior pituitary production of FSH and leutenizing hormone (LH) continues. Irregular menstrual cycles, characterized by longer or shorter cycles, heavier or lighter flow, periods of amenorrhea, and worsening or newly developing premenstrual symptoms, are common during this time. Eventually, ovarian follicle production stops, estrogen and progesterone levels remain low, FSH and LH levels remain high, and menstruation ceases. The postmenopausal period refers to the first five years or so following menopause when hormonal fluctuations are often still present (NAMS, 2002; Soules et al., 2001; Utian, 1999a, 1999b, 2001).

A woman is born with approximately 1.2 million ovarian follicles. Throughout her life some follicles are used during ovulation, but most are lost through atresia until menopause when about 1000 follicles remain although it is currently believed that the number of ovarian follicles in women is finite; a recent study identified new ovarian follicle development in adult female mice (Johnson, Canning, Kaneko, Pru, & Tilly, 2004). It remains to be seen whether or not this phenomenon is true in humans.

Although it sounds like a smooth process, the perimenopausal transition is anything but smooth for most women. Hormone levels can fluctuate wildly from day to day, causing many of the symptoms associated with the perimenopause and menopause transition (Table 11–2). Hormone fluctuation is related to many factors including the reduced number of responsive ovarian follicles.

TABLE 11–2   Symptoms Associated with Perimenopause and Menopause

Acne	Arthralgia	Asthenia
Decreased libido	Decreased vaginal lubrication	Depression
Dizziness	Dry eyes	Dry/thinning hair
Dyspareunia	Dysuria	Fatigue
Forgetfulness	Formication	Headache
Hirsutism/virilization	Hot flashes/flushes	Irregular menses/bleeding
Irritability/mood disturbances	Mastalgia	Myalgia
Nervousness/anxiety	Night sweats	Nocturia
Odor	Palpitations	Paresthesia
Poor concentration	Recurrent cystitis	Recurrent vaginitis
Sleep disturbances/insomnia	Skin dryness/atrophy	Stress urinary incontinence*
Urinary frequency	Urinary urgency	Vaginal atrophy
Vaginal/vulvar burning	Vaginal/vulvar irritation	Vaginal/vulvar pruritis

*Data are inconclusive.

Sources: Alexander et al., 2003; Avis et al., 2001; Greendale, Lee, & Arriola, 1999; Jacobs Institute on Women's Health, 2003; McKinlay, 1996.

Contrary to popular belief, women do continue to produce estrogen and androgens after menopause. There are three different types of estrogen. Estradiol (E_2), the most potent estrogen, is the main estrogen produced during the reproductive years, and is present in low amounts in the postmenopausal years following peripheral conversion of androstenedione. Estriol (E_3) is secreted by the placenta and synthesized from androgens produced by the fetus during pregnancy, and is present in nonpregnant women in small amounts as a byproduct of estradiol and estrone. Estrone (E_1), the weakest estrogen, is the primary estrogen present in postmenopausal women, children, and men. In the postmenopausal period, estrone is produced by adipose conversion of androstenedione secreted by the adrenals (95%), and to a lesser extent the ovaries (5%), and metabolism of estradiol.

Although the ovaries no longer produce functional follicles, the corticostromal and hilar cells of the stromal tissue are steroidogenic and produce significant levels of both androstenedione and testosterone for many years. Circulating levels of androstenedione in postmenopausal women are approximately half those of premenopausal women. Conversely, circulating levels of testosterone remain relatively constant in women who are either pre- or postmenopausal, partly due to the effect of high FSH and LH levels that stimulate the ovarian stromal tissue to increase testosterone production.

Natural menopause occurs for most women between the ages of 48 and 55 years. Fifty-one is the average age for women in the Western world (Soules et al., 2001; Utian, 1999b). The age at menopause is difficult to predict for an individual woman, but does correlate with the age when her mother or older sisters had menopause (Cramer, Xu, & Harlow, 1995; de Bruin et al., 2001). A number of factors that may affect the age at menopause have been studied, such as parity, age at menarche, obesity, height, and oral contraceptive use. However, only smoking has consistently been found to have a relationship, and is associated with menopause occurring one and one half years earlier among smokers versus nonsmokers (Bromberger et al., 1997; Cooper, Sandler, & Bohlig, 1999; Gold et al., 2001; van Noord, Dubas, Dorland, Boersma, & te Velde, 1997). Ethnicity also may have an effect on age at menopause. A few studies have found that African-American women experience menopause slightly earlier, with an average age at menopause of 49.6 years and a median age of 49.3 or 50 years (Bromberger et al., 1997; Palmer, Rosenberg, Wise, Horton, & Adams-Campbell, 2003). However, no significant difference in age at menopause was identified in black versus white women (average age 51.4 years for both groups) in the Study of Women's Health across the Nation (SWAN) (Gold et al., 2001). Interestingly, the SWAN study did identify statistically significant differences in average age at menopause among Hispanics (51.0 years) and Japanese-Americans (51.8 years), as compared with Caucasians (51.4 years).

MENOPAUSE FROM OTHER CAUSES

Menopause can also occur due to several other causes (NAMS, 2002; Utian, 1999a). *Induced menopause* occurs either following surgical excision of both ovaries (bilateral oopherectomy) or ovarian function ablation from medication, chemotherapy, or radiation. Menstruation and fertility cease immediately following surgical menopause, but menstruation and fertility may remain for several months after ablative treatments. *Premature menopause* is menopause that occurs before the age of 40. Premature menopause often follows the pattern of natural menopause with the permanent loss of menstruation and fertility. *Idiopathic ovarian insufficiency or premature ovarian failure* (POF) also occurs in women under 40 years old; however, it is not the same as premature menopause because POF is not always permanent and is often associated with other health problems, such as autoimmune and genetic disorders. *Temporary menopause* can occur at any age when normal ovarian function is lost and then resumes. Temporary menopause can be idiopathic, related to a disease entity, or induced by medications. Women who experience induced or premature menopause have early loss of fertility and often experience more severe symptoms. They are at greater risk for developing cardiovascular disease (CVD) and osteoporosis, and may also face significant health problems related to underlying disease processes.

DIAGNOSING MENOPAUSE

Menopause is most accurately diagnosed based on the clinical absence of menses for 12 consecutive months. Serial FSH testing that revealed levels sustained at under 40m IU/L was used in the past to determine menopause status. However, because FSH levels can return to normal and estrogen levels can unexpectedly rise high enough to trigger the LH surge needed for ovulation, serum FSH testing is no longer recommended for determining perimenopausal or menopausal status (Bastian, Smith, & Nanda, 2003; NAMS, 2002). Similarly, perimenopause is most accurately identified based on a variety of factors including age and symptoms such as hot flashes, irregular menses, and vaginal dryness. Due to the potential for unexpected ovulation, women who are perimenopausal need to continue to use a reliable form of birth control (see Chapter 9 for information about contraception). Exceeded only by adolescents, perimenopausal women experience the second highest rate of unintended pregnancies. In fact, 95% of pregnancies are unintended for adolescents aged 15–19 years, 42% for women aged 30–34 years, 56% for women aged 35–39 years, and 77% for women aged 40–44 years (US Department of Health and Human Services, 1998; USPSTF, 2003).

DIFFERENTIAL DIAGNOSES TO CONSIDER

Other health problems can mimic the symptoms of menopause and must also be considered when a woman presents with perimenopausal and menopausal symptoms (NAMS, 2002). These diagnoses may include diabetes, hypertension, arrhythmias, thyroid disorders (hypothyroid or hyperthyroid), anemia, depression, tumors, or carcinoma. A sample list of differential diagnoses is provided in Table 11–3. Medications, alcohol, or drug use can also cause many symptoms similar to perimenopause and menopause. Each woman presenting

TABLE 11–3 Sample of Differential Diagnoses That Have Symptoms Similar to Perimenopause and Menopause

Diagnosis	Symptoms Similar to Perimenopause/Menopause
Anemia	Fatigue Cognitive changes
Anovulation Pregnancy	Amenorrhea Irregular bleeding
Arrhythmias	Fatigue Palpitations
Arthritis	Joint aches/pain
Depression	Fatigue Moodiness Anxiety Sleep disturbances, insomnia
Diabetes	Fatigue Hot flashes/heat intolerance
Hypertension	Headaches
Hyperthyroid	Sleep disturbance, insomnia Nervousness, irritability Heat intolerance
Hypothyroid	Fatigue Dry skin Cognitive problems
Infections (viral illnesses, HIV, influenza, fever, tuberculosis, sexually transmitted infections)	Vasomotor symptoms Dyspareunia Cystitis symptoms Vaginitis
Pregnancy Spontaneous abortion Uterine fibroids Uterine polyps Endometriosis Adenomyosis Ovarian cysts Ovarian tumors	Menstrual changes Menorrhagia
Vulvar dystrophy	Vaginal atrophy Dyspareunia

with menopausal symptoms must be carefully evaluated through history and a physical examination, and selective laboratory testing (such as complete blood count, fasting glucose, and serum thyroid stimulating hormone level) to accurately identify the cause of her symptoms. Often a woman has several diagnoses to contend with at once, such as hypertension, diabetes, and menopause. Controlling her diabetes and hypertension may also reduce her menopausal symptoms enough so that they no longer are bothersome for her.

PRESENTATION AND VARIATION OF THE MENOPAUSE EXPERIENCE

The menopause experience is unique and personal. Some women have severe symptoms that disrupt all aspects of their lives, while others find it almost a "nonevent" and report no bothersome symptoms. Most symptoms are related to reduced levels of estrogen and progesterone. Two types of estrogen receptors have been identified (alpha and beta) and are located in the cognitive and vasomotor centers of the brain, eyes, skin, heart, vascular system, gastrointestinal track, breast tissue, urogenital track, and bone. Progesterone receptors have been identified in the hypothalamus, pituitary, and vasomotor areas of the brain, as well as the heart, vascular tissues, lung, breast, pancreas, reproductive organs, and bones. As the hormone levels fluctuate and fall, symptoms develop. An individual woman's symptom experience may be related to her body size as adipose tissues store and convert androstenedione to estrogen (Speroff, Glass, & Kase, 1999).

Both the type (Table 11–2) and severity of menopausal symptoms can vary. Symptoms usually begin in the perimenopausal period and may gradually increase in severity. Postmenopausal women usually experience more symptoms with greater severity than do perimenopausal women (Avis et al., 2001). The symptoms women report most frequently are vasomotor and include hot flashes, or hot flushes, and sweats. Hot flashes are most frequent in the first five to seven years following menopause but can last for many more years in some women (Kronenberg, 1990).

Hot flashes are experienced as an intense heat sensation and may or may not be followed by sweating, which can be profuse. There is a measurable increase in skin temperature and conductance that is followed by a decrease in core body temperature. Hot flashes occur concurrently with a surge in LH levels. Although the relationship between LH secretion and body temperature change is not well understood, the same mechanisms that trigger the hypothalamic event that causes the temperature increase also stimulates GnRH secretion and causes LH elevation. Some women experience a prodrome prior to a hot flash. Many women feel cold following a hot flash due to the reduction in core temperature that is exacerbated if sweating is also present. Hot flushes are similar to hot flashes but include a flushing over the face and upper chest, most likely due to peripheral vascular dilatation. Vasomotor symptoms that occur during the night are termed night sweats.

Sleep disruptions are also common among menopausal women. Some of the sleep changes are related to normal aging, such as reduced time in sleep stages three (early deep sleep) and four (deep sleep and relaxation), more periods of brief arousal, and an overall decreased need for sleep—an average of five to seven hours for adults (Blackman, 2000). Hot flashes and sweats can further interrupt sleep (Baker, Simpson, & Dawson, 1997; Kronenberg, 1990). Sleep loss causes daytime fatigue and has been associated with irritability; emotional lability; stress; depression; headache; poor functioning at home, work, or school; and difficulty concentrating, reasoning, and remembering (NIH, 2002).

Urogenital changes leading to atrophy affect all women and may cause vaginal dryness and dyspareunia, and can predispose women to urinary incontinence. Urinary incontinence is predisposed with aging but is never normal. Lower estrogen levels are associated with urethral atrophy, which can increase the likelihood of developing incontinence further. Many normal changes of aging can also affect sexual function in women, such as needing greater time to achieve vaginal lubrication and producing fewer vaginal secretions overall; reduced vaginal elasticity, pigment, rugation and number of superficial epithelial cells leading to increased petechiae and bleeding following minor trauma; reduced lactobacilli, which increases pH and the risk of infection; and atrophy of adipose and collagen tissue in the vulva. Women may also experience lowered libido, lessened sexual activity, problems with their partner's sexual performance, or relationship problems that make them less interested in sex (Dennerstein, Dudley, & Burger, 2001). Whatever the causes of dyspareunia or sexual dysfunction may be, it is a subject that is often difficult for women to broach. Clinicians must ask about sexual function and satisfaction, and remain open to the fact that sexual expression can take many forms (see Chapters 8 and 14).

Cultural or racial background may have an effect on menopausal symptoms. The SWAN study indicated that while Caucasian and Hispanic women reported the greatest number of psychosomatic symptoms, such as moodiness, headaches, and palpitations (Avis et al., 2001), the severity of vasomotor symptoms (hot flashes, sweats) was highest among African-American women, followed by Hispanic, Caucasian, Chinese, and Japanese women (Gold et al., 2000). Vaginal dryness was more common among African-American and Hispanic women, and Hispanic women were more likely to report urine leakage, forgetfulness, and heart pounding or racing than Caucasian women. Caucasian women were more likely to have experienced difficulty sleeping than women of other races (Gold et al.). Additionally, some symptoms may be more bothersome for certain women. For example, African-American women have described a high degree of bother from vaginal and body odor, sleep changes and night sweats, weight gain, moodiness, "rage," and irritability (Alexander et al., 2003). Asian women have reported greater problems with joint pain and stiffness, especially in the neck, shoulders, and back (Gold et al.).

A woman's expectations for menopause may also affect her experience. Expectations can range from no expectations, to positive or negative expectations, to uncertainty (Woods & Mitchell, 1999). Similarly, a woman's response to menopause can affect her experience. Many women view menopause as a natural life transition and may not be interested in any treatment options besides lifestyle changes. Others see it as a disruption and a sign of aging that they want to minimize as much as possible. Many women identify menopause as a time for reflection and reevaluation of their lives and health (Alexander et al., 2003; Woods & Mitchell).

MIDLIFE HEALTH ISSUES

Health risks change for women at midlife, partly due to the changed hormonal milieu and partly due to other normal aging processes. In particular, women are at greater risk for developing heart disease, osteoporosis, and diabetes. Weight management is also a significant issue. See Chapter 7 for a full discussion of routine health screening for midlife women.

OVERWEIGHT AND OBESITY

As women age, weight management often becomes a struggle. Although women tend to associate increased weight with menopause, it is not related specifically to hormonal changes but is rather a natural part of aging. Women gain an average of five pounds at midlife (NAMS, 2002). This increase is partly due to the normal slowing in metabolism that occurs with age, and partly due to a decrease in activity that often accompanies midlife. Maintaining one's weight through midlife usually requires both a reduction in caloric intake and an increase in activity.

Not only does weight increase at midlife, but the distribution of body fat changes. Adipose tissue tends to accumulate at the hips and thighs in most younger women (the "pear" shaped body). As women age, adipose tissue is redistributed and begins to accumulate at the waist (the "apple" shaped body). Abdominal adiposity and weight gain at midlife are significant issues. This concern relates not only to the potentially negative body-image concerns for women, but also to the fact that both obesity, defined as a body mass index (BMI) greater than $30kg/m^2$ and a waist circumference larger than 35 cm, are individually associated with a greater risk for developing insulin resistance that can lead to CVD and diabetes (American Diabetes Association [ADA], 2004a). In addition, obesity is associated with osteoarthritis, cholecystic disease, urinary incontinence, and with cancers such as breast, endometrial, and colorectal (American Obesity Association, 2002; Centers for Disease Control and Prevention, 2003). Furthermore, having a BMI greater than $27kg/m^2$ was associated with a greater frequency of hot flashes, night sweats, and soreness or stiffness in the back, shoulders, and neck in the SWAN study (Gold et al., 2000).

CARDIOVASCULAR DISEASE

The number one cause of mortality for both women and men in the United States is CVD. Approximately 500,000 women die from CVD each year in the United States. This number is higher than the next seven causes of mortality in women combined and exceeds the CVD mortality rate in men (American Heart Association [AHA], 2002, 2004). Heart disease disproportionately affects women of color. After the age of 50 years, over 50% of all deaths among women are attributed to some type of CVD. CVD includes hypertension, valvular heart disease, coronary artery disease, or coronary heart disease (leading to angina or myocardial infarction), stroke, arrhythmias, congestive heart failure, and congenital heart defects.

Women are at a significantly increased risk for developing heart disease following menopause (AHA, 2004; NAMS, 2002). Some of this increased risk is due to changes in cholesterol levels that are found in postmenopausal women. Low-density lipoprotein (LDL) and very low-density lipoprotein levels increase, and LDL oxidation is enhanced. Additionally, high-density lipoprotein (HDL) levels may decrease somewhat. However, the HDL changes are far less significant than the LDL changes. Other changes, such as the reduced elasticity in the vascular system and associated hypertension, may be related to reduced levels of estrogen and progestin. Moreover, production of some precoagulation factors (e.g., fibrinogen, factor VII) and some fibrinolytic factors (e.g., plasminogen, antithrombin III) increase, and may interact with hormonal and vascular changes to further increase risk. General risk factors for CVD include cigarette smoking, a sedentary lifestyle, stress, obesity, preexisting hypertension, abnormal serum lipids, and diabetes mellitus. Women who experience premature menopause may have an even greater risk, especially if they smoke (NAMS, 2002).

DIABETES MELLITUS

The likelihood of developing type 2 diabetes mellitus increases with age and disproportionately affects women of minority racial and ethnic groups, such as Native Americans, Hispanics or Latinas, African-Americans, Asian-Americans, and Pacific-Islanders. General risk factors for developing diabetes include being overweight or obese (BMI greater than 25), having abdominal adiposity (waist circumference over 35 inches in women), a sedentary lifestyle, insulin resistance, a history of gestational diabetes or polycystic ovary syndrome, and a family history of diabetes. Hypertension and dyslipidemia also predispose an individual to developing diabetes. Individuals with impaired fasting glucose levels (100–125 mg/dl) or impaired glucose tolerance (2-hour post 75-gram glucose load of 140–199 mg/dl) are identified as having pre-diabetes, and 30% to 40% of them will develop type 2 diabetes within five years (ADA, 2004b; Mayer-Davis, D'Antonio, & Tudor-Locke, 2003). In addition to significantly increasing the risk for CVD and cerebrovascular disease, diabetes increases the risk for developing infections, foot ulcers, peripheral vascular disease, peripheral neuropathy, nephropathy, and retinopathy (ADA, 2004a; Franz, 2003).

Managing diabetes is more difficult for women during perimenopause due to fluctuations in hormone concentrations. Insulin resistance increases with reduced levels of estrogen, causing higher serum glucose levels. Progesterone changes have a converse effect on glucose, causing lower levels due to the increase in insulin sensitivity that accompanies falling progesterone concentrations. After menopause, glucose levels tend to be lower because insulin sensitivity increases and insulin use is more efficient as estrogen and progesterone concentrations stabilize (Gaspar, Gotta, & van den Brule, 1995; Godsland, 1996; Porth & Kunert, 2002). However, other midlife changes, such as weight gain and slowed metabolism, also affect glucose levels; thus, numerous adjustments in medications and regimens are often necessary to maintain adequate glucose control.

CANCER

In 2004, the leading cause of mortality from cancer among women was lung and bronchus (25%), followed by breast (15%), and colon (10%) cancers (American Cancer Society [ACS], 2004a). The risk for developing cancer increases as women age. A woman's risk for developing breast cancer is approximately 1 out of 30 at the age of 50, and increases gradually to approximately 1 out of 9 for a woman who lives into her 80s. The lifetime risk for a woman to develop breast cancer is about 1 in 7 (ACS, 2004a; National Cancer Institute, 2003). See Chapter 7 for cancer screening recommendations and Chapter 13 for further information about breast cancer.

OSTEOPOROSIS

Osteoporosis is a disorder of the skeletal system characterized by reduced bone strength that increases the risk for fracture (Hodgson & Watts, 2003; Kans, 1994). Bone strength includes both bone density and bone quality. Bone density is the volume of bone. Bone quality refers to the rate of turnover, bone architecture, mineralization, and accumulated damage. There are two types of osteoporosis: primary and secondary (Dawson-Hughes et al., 2003). Secondary osteoporosis occurs in response to medication (e.g., corticosteroids, anticonvulsants, or methotrexate) or other disease processes (e.g., hyperthyroidism, chronic liver disease, or gastrointestinal diseases, such as malabsorption) that interfere with the normal process of bone formation and can affect women or men at any age. Primary osteoporosis is associated with aging and affects women much more significantly than men. Adults achieve peak bone mass between 30 and 35 years of age, after which time the rate of bone resorption exceeds bone formation and mass slowly declines. However, due to the loss of estrogen, the rate of bone loss in the first year after menopause is rapid, between 1–5%, and then slows to a rate of about 1% per year. In contrast, bone mass is lost in men at a rate of about 0.2–0.5% per year. Risk factors for osteoporosis are presented in Table 11–4. Screening recommendations can be found in Chapter 7.

The gold standard for diagnosing osteopenia or osteoporosis is bone mineral density (BMD) measurement by dual-energy x-ray absorptiometry, which is used to evaluate BMD at the spine, hip, or wrist. Quantitative computed tomography can be used for spine measurements and is particularly useful for testing individuals with arthritis, as it is less likely to reflect osteocytes. BMD results are reported as T-scores and Z-scores. The T-score identifies the number of standard deviations the patient's BMD is above or below a young adult norm. Osteopenia is present when the T-score is -1 to -2.5. Osteoporosis is present when the T-score is -2.5 or less. Severe or established osteoporosis is present when the T-score is -2.5 or less and fragility fractures are present. The Z-score provides a comparison in BMD for the patient to an age-matched mean and is usually used only for diagnosis in children (Kans, 1994).

Women with osteoporosis, and to a lesser extent osteopenia, are at increased risk for fracture (Kans, 1994). Although osteoporosis and osteopenia by themselves are painless

TABLE 11-4   Risk Factors for Osteoporosis

Potentially Modifiable Risk Factors	Nonmodifiable Risk Factors
Body weight <127 pounds	Advanced age
BMI <22–24	Female gender
Amenorrhea (due to eating disorder or excessive exercise)	Race (Caucasian and Asian women at greatest risk, then Hispanic and African-American)
Nulliparity	Personal history of fracture during adulthood
Low estrogen (e.g., menopause)	Family history of osteoporosis
Lifestyle factors (e.g., cigarette smoking, excessive alcohol or caffeine intake, sedentary activity level, or inadequate calcium/vitamin D intake)	First degree relative with history of fracture
Medications (e.g., thyroid hormone, corticosteroids, anticonvulsants, aluminum-containing antacids, lithium, methotrexate, gonadotropin-releasing hormone, cholesteramine, heparin, warfarin)	
Chronic diseases (e.g., endocrine disorders, gastrointestinal disorders, connective tissue diseases, bone disorders, chronic liver disease, cystic fibrosis, seizure disorders, hematologic malignancies, prolonged immobility, eating disorders, chronic renal failure, or frailty)	

Sources: Dawson-Hughes et al., 2003; Hodgson & Watts, 2003.

and not functionally problematic, the risk for fractures puts a patient at significant risk. Following a hip fracture, there is a 10–20% increase in mortality. Of survivors, 30% to 40% sustain some degree of permanent disability and 24% to 50% never return to independent living (Dawson-Hughes et al., 2003; Hodgson & Watts, 2003).

Prevention is a key factor in osteoporosis management. For perimenopausal and postmenopausal women, prevention strategies focus on adequate intake of calcium (1000 mg/day for premenopausal women and postmenopausal women on HT, 1200 mg/day for perimenopausal or premenopausal women over the age of 50, 1500 mg/day for postmenopausal women not taking HT and women older than 65 years) and vitamin D (400-800 IU/day), weight bearing and resistance exercise, fall prevention, avoiding tobacco, and moderating alcohol intake (Dawson-Hughes et al., 2003; Hodgson & Watts, 2003; NIH, 1994). Exercise is site specific and needs to be continued to maintain bone strength, and assists in maintaining balance to reduce falls. Forward bending at the waist is discouraged for women with established osteoporosis due to the possible risk of vertebral compression fractures. Exercises such as modified yoga (no forward bending), tai-chi, jogging, walking, dancing, weight lifting, and resistive exercises such as swimming and bicycling should be encouraged. Fall-prevention assessments should also be completed to identify fall risks, such as visual or hearing impairments, neurological impairments, other medical conditions or medications that increase the risk for falls, and possible risks at home, such as loose rugs and cords.

Medication management is also recommended for women with T-scores of −2.0 or lower, T-scores of −1.5 who also have one or more risk factors, and those with previous hip or vertebral fractures. Repeat BMD testing is recommended one year after treatment is initiated, and then every two to five years after levels stabilize, two satisfactory BMD results have been obtained, and the woman's medical condition is stable (Dawson-Hughes et al., 2003; Hodgson & Watts, 2003). Table 11–5 summarizes the available pharmacologic treatment options for osteoporosis in postmenopausal women. Combination therapy is also possible; usually a bisphosphonate (alendronate or risedronate) is combined with another class (e.g., estrogen or raloxifene).

THYROID DISEASE AND DEPRESSION

Thyroid disease and depression are other health issues that must be considered at midlife. Thyroid disease affects women more than men and increases with age (Baskin, 2002). Symptoms of hyperthyroidism or hypothyroidism can mimic perimenopause and menopause symptoms. Depression also can increase during midlife both due to symptoms caused by hormonal fluctuations and midlife stresses such as financial concerns, employment issues, relationship problems, family changes, or health issues of self or family members (NAMS, 2002). Depression rates are about three times as high in perimenopausal women as they are in premenopausal women (Cohen, 2004). These problems and other differential diagnoses (Table 11–3) must be considered when a woman presents with menopausal symptoms.

LIFESTYLE APPROACHES FOR SYMPTOM MANAGEMENT

Several lifestyle alterations can be implemented to reduce menopausal symptoms. Some of these interventions also afford additional health benefits such as reducing risk for CVD or osteoporosis. Lifestyle management may encompass dietary changes, exercise, vitamins or supplements, vaginal lubricants and moisturizers, changes in clothing, smoking cessation, stress management techniques, sleep aids, and activities to enhance memory function.

DIETARY CHANGES

Several dietary substances have been linked with more frequent or more severe hot flashes. Such substances include sugar (especially refined), caffeine (including hot and cold beverages and other foods, such as chocolate, that contain caffeine), spicy foods, and alcohol (Alexander et al., 2003; NAMS, 2002). Avoidance or moderate intake of these substances should be recommended.

Increased water intake is also recommended because of the augmented insensible loss of fluids through sweating. Water intake, especially cold water, has been reported to help with

TABLE 11–5   Pharmacologic Treatment Options for Osteoporosis in Postmenopausal Women*

Medication	FDA Approved for	Considerations
Alendronate (Fosamax)	Prevention—5 mg orally daily or 35 mg orally weekly	• Caution if upper gastrointestinal disease, clinical association with dysphagia, esophagitis, or ulceration
	Treatment—10 mg orally daily or 70 mg orally weekly	• Take first thing in the morning on an empty stomach with 8 oz. glass of water, remain upright and take no other food or drink for at least 30 minutes
Risedronate (Actonel)	Prevention or treatment—5 mg orally daily or 35 mg orally weekly	• Take 2 hours before antacids/calcium
Calcitonin (Miacalcin)	Treatment—200 IU intranasal spray daily or 100 IU IM or SC every other day	• Usually administered as nasal spray • Has analgesic effect on osteoporotic fractures
Estrogen (i.e., Premarin, Estratab, Menest, Alora, Climara, Estraderm, Menostar, Vivelle, Vivelle Dot, Estrace, Femhrt*, Activella**, Ortho-prefest**, Prempro**, others)	Prevention—Doses and routes vary***	• Also effective in alleviating most symptoms of menopause • Comes in several forms, including pills, patch, ring, and cream
Raloxifene (Evista)	Prevention or treatment—60 mg orally daily	• May cause hot flashes • Not recommended if taking ET or EPT
Teriparitide (Forteo)	Treatment—20 μg subcutaneously daily	• Reserved for use after failure of first-line agents

*See prescribing reference for full information on doses, side effects, contraindications, and cautions.

**Also contain progesterone compounds.

***Lowest effective dose should be used. The FDA recommends considering non-estrogen osteoporotic agents when ET/EPT use is solely for the purpose of osteoporosis prevention.

Sources: Dawson-Hughes et al., 2003; Hodgson & Watts, 2003.

reducing symptoms such as skin dryness, and reduces discomfort with hot flashes and sweating (Alexander et al., 2003; NAMS, 2004). The usual water intake of six to eight glasses per day should be recommended. However, for women who experience urinary incontinence, water consumption may need to be restricted for social occasions when there is no easy access to a bathroom, or limited to the morning for women who experience nocturia.

EXERCISE

Lower levels of physical activity have been linked with a higher frequency of menopausal symptoms, especially forgetfulness, difficulty sleeping, heart pounding or racing, and stiffness or soreness (Gold et al., 2000). Similarly, higher levels of physical activity have been associated with reduced severity of menopausal symptoms such as vasomotor symptoms, depression, and forgetfulness (Alexander, Ruff, & Udemezue, n.d.; NAMS, 2004). In addition to mediating menopause symptoms, exercise reduces cardiovascular and osteoporosis risks, improves sleep, and assists with maintaining a healthy weight, relieving stress, reducing moodiness, and improving mental function.

VITAMINS AND SUPPLEMENTS

Several vitamins and supplements may also be useful for minimizing menopausal symptoms and improving overall health. Calcium (1200–1500 mg/day) and vitamin D (400–800 IU/day) are needed for postmenopausal women to maintain bone strength (NIH, 1994). Vitamin E in doses up to 800 IU/day has shown either small improvements or no changes in hot flashes in clinical trials (Barton et al., 1998; Blatt, Weisbader, & Kupperman, 1953). A recent meta-analysis indicated that vitamin E did not provide a reduction in overall mortality, cerebrovascular accident, or cardiovascular death (Vivekananthan, Penn, Sapp, Hsu, & Topol, 2003). In the same meta-analysis, beta-carotene was shown to have a slightly increased risk for all-cause mortality. Vitamin E has, however, been linked with a reduced risk for developing Alzheimer's disease (Klatte, Scharre, Nagaraja, Davis, & Beversdorf, 2003; Onofrj et al., 2002; Thomas, Iacono, Bonanni, D'Andreamatteo, & Onofrj, 2001). The B vitamins are known to reduce homocysteine levels, high levels of which are associated with cerebrovascular accident, CVD, Alzheimer's disease, and osteoporotic fracture. For reduction of homocysteine and to partly compensate for the lack of fruits and vegetables usually found in the American diet, daily supplementation with a multivitamin containing the B vitamins (folate, B_6, and B_{12}) is recommended (Fairfield & Fletcher, 2002; Fletcher & Fairfield, 2002; McLean et al., 2004; van Meurs et al., 2004). Formulations that include iron should be avoided unless there is a documented need for iron supplementation, as excess iron can cause negative effects on the cardiovascular system or liver over time.

VAGINAL LUBRICANTS AND MOISTURIZERS

Vaginal lubricants can be used to relieve vaginal dryness and dyspareunia caused by reduced vaginal secretions. Several nonhormonal water-based preparations are available over-the-counter (e.g., K-Y Personal Lubricant, Astroglide, Lubrin, and Moist Again). These can be used for daily comfort for vaginal dryness and during sexual activity. Longer-acting vaginal moisturizers (e.g., Replens, K-Y Long-Lasting Vaginal Moisturizer) may be more appropriate for some women. The moisturizers replenish and maintain fluids in the vaginal epithelial cells and provide longer relief. Moisturizers may be particularly beneficial for women who experience daily discomfort and can reduce vaginitis by supporting a normal pH (Nachtigall, 1994).

Women must be cautioned against using any oil-based products, such as petroleum jelly (Vaseline), as these can injure vaginal tissue and are not easily removed. Vitamin E oil, applied topically to the vaginal walls, is an exception to this caution. It can provide relief for vaginal dryness without interfering with condom or diaphragm function, and does not tend to irritate. Other products that contain oils or fragrances should also be discouraged as they often cause vaginitis or irritation. Douching is not effective for moisturizing and will remove normal flora, thus increasing the risk for infection (NAMS, 2002; Willhite, 2001).

CLOTHING AND ENVIRONMENT

Wearing layered clothes, breathable fabrics such as cotton or linen, or wicking fabrics, such as those worn by runners, is recommended to reduce discomfort with hot flashes and sweats (Alexander et al., 2004; NAMS, 2002). Avoiding turtlenecks, fabrics that do not allow circulation or absorb sweat (e.g., polyester and silk), and extra layers (e.g., slips and full-length stockings) are also recommended. Keeping the room temperature cool, having an open window or using a fan to circulate air, and ingesting cold foods or beverages can reduce core body temperature and are also helpful (NAMS, 2004).

SMOKING CESSATION

Smoking is associated with increased morbidity and mortality, especially related to CVD and cancers, earlier age at menopause, increased rate of bone loss, and an increased prevalence of all menopausal symptoms with the exception of vaginal dryness (Gold et al., 2000, 2001; NAMS, 2002). Various smoking cessation programs are available. The most successful program is the one that is of interest to a specific woman. She needs to be both interested in quitting and motivated to quit. Support from a clinician and use of medications or patches can significantly improve cessation rates (ACS, 2004b).

STRESS MANAGEMENT

Stress has been reported to increase menopause symptoms (Alexander et al., 2003). Additionally, stress is associated with poor sleep and can increase depression or moodiness. Midlife women may face multiple stressors such as health changes for themselves or family members, financial concerns, loss of a parent, children leaving home, or relationship struggles with a partner, child, or parent.

Managing stress must be individualized as each woman may find different tactics helpful. Some suggestions include regular exercise, meditation, relaxation techniques like deep breathing, yoga, tai-chi, taking a bath, reading, having a massage, seeking support from friends, or through spirituality or religion. Few studies have evaluated the effects of such techniques on menopausal symptoms; however, reports indicate that avoiding and effectively managing stress are associated with less intense and fewer hot flashes (Alexander et al., 2003). While progressive muscle relaxation and biofeedback control showed no significant change in hot flashes, paced respiration has been linked with a significant reduction in hot flashes (Freedman & Woodward, 1992; Freedman, Woodward, Brown, Javaid, & Pandy, 1995; Irvin, Domar, Clark, Zuttermeister, & Freidman, 1996). Women can use yoga breathing, a variation of paced respiration, to enhance relaxation and reduce hot flashes. Yoga breathing consists of a deep inhalation for the count of four, holding the breath for a count of seven, and slowly exhaling over a count of eight.

SLEEP

Evaluating the cause of sleep disruptions is important for developing a plan of management. If sleep disruption is related to hot flashes or other menopausal symptoms, control of those symptoms will usually restore normal sleep patterns. Light blankets, cotton sleep wear or wicking pajamas, and a well-ventilated room are recommended for reducing nocturnal hot flashes. However, as is often the case, if sleep disruption is unrelated to hot flashes, a more generalized approach is needed.

Developing good sleep hygiene is especially important for perimenopausal and menopausal women. Sleep hygiene refers to actions that cue the mind that it is time for sleep and allows the part of the brain that controls the body during sleep to take over. Developing regular routines prior to bedtime, such as brushing the teeth or changing into sleepwear; doing something relaxing, such as paced respirations, progressive relaxation, guided imagery, taking a warm bath, reading a relaxing book, or drinking a warm beverage without caffeine can help cue the mind that it is time to sleep. Similarly, avoiding activities that tend to stimulate the mind should be avoided just before bed, such as watching television, reading a fast-paced or stimulating book, doing work, or exercise. The bedroom should be reserved for sleep and sexual activities. This is especially important for individuals who have difficulty falling asleep, as doing work or watching television in bed can have a stimulating effect. Establishing regular times for sleep and waking is also important for developing good sleep patterns as this will help in developing normal daily routines.

Lifestyle changes that can help restore sleep patterns include avoiding use of stimulants, such as caffeine, alcohol, or nicotine, and engaging in exercise. Effects of caffeine can last up to 20 hours in some individuals, so total elimination is preferable (Landolt, Werth, Borbely, & Dijk, 1995). Although alcohol initially can have a sedative effect, it can cause interruptions in normal sleep patterns after falling asleep, including fragmented sleep and rebound awakening (Landolt, Rioth, Dijk, & Borbely, 1996). Similarly, nicotine can cause increased sleep latency and reduces overall sleep duration. Exercise can benefit sleep quality, reduce sleep latency, and increase the time spent in deep sleep. However, timing for exercise is important as exercise right before bedtime will increase sleep latency.

For those with short sleep duration, sleep-restriction therapy can be tried (Morin et al., 1999). First the current average duration of sleep is identified along with a needed and consistent time for awakening. The woman is instructed to go to bed four hours prior to the determined time for wakening, and to get up at the pre-determined wake time. She needs to stay awake except for the determined sleep time (no napping). After she is sleeping more than 95% of this time for several nights consistently, the time to go to bed is moved to one half hour earlier. This pattern is continued until the desired sleep time is achieved.

MENTAL FUNCTION

A slow decline in mental function is expected with aging. However, some women experience bothersome cognitive changes that develop as menopausal symptoms occur. Poor mental functioning is often associated with lack of sleep or high levels of stress. Cognitive impairment can also be related to a myriad of medical problems. Thus, the first step in evaluating mental function is to complete a comprehensive assessment to identify potential causes of the cognitive problems.

For women who are experiencing reduced cognitive function that is unrelated to other organic problems, several simple memory aids may be of use. Noting appointments and dates of importance in a calendar, or writing lists to use for completing tasks, work activities, or shopping, can help reduce stress associated with forgetting these items. Participating in activities that keep the mind engaged, such as intellectually stimulating work, puzzles, or other activities can also help to maintain cognitive function.

PHARMACOLOGIC OPTIONS FOR MENOPAUSE SYMPTOM MANAGEMENT

Although the NAMS (2004) recommends lifestyle changes alone or in combination with nonprescription remedies for women with mild vasomotor symptoms, prescription systemic hormone products remain the standard for women with moderate to severe symptoms. The US Food and Drug Administration (FDA) defines moderate to severe hot flashes as seven to eight episodes per day or at least 60 per week. It is important to note that hot flashes will eventually resolve over time without medication in most women.

The Cochrane Group conducted a meta-analysis of 21 randomized, double-blind, placebo-controlled clinical trials enrolling 2511 women. They reported that systemic ET/EPT reduced hot flash severity and frequency significantly more than placebos. Some antidepressants, antihypertensives, and anticonvulsants also reduce vasomotor symptoms (NAMS, 2004). Table 11–6 lists currently recommended estrogen and estrogen/progestogen products. Note that in their review of efficacy of various preparations, the NAMS concluded that there is no evidence to claim that one product is superior to another for

TABLE 11-6 Hormone Therapy Options*

Type	Product Name (Manufacturer)	Active Ingredient	Dosage
Estrogens, oral	Cenestin (Duramed)	Conjugated estrogens	0.3 mg, 0.625 mg, 0.9 mg, or 1.25 mg once daily
	Estrace (Warner Chilcott)	Micronized estradiol	0.5 mg, 1 mg, or 2 mg once daily
	Estratab (Solvay)	Esterified estrogens	0.3 mg, 0.625 mg, or 2.5 mg once daily
	Menest (Monarch)	Esterified estrogens	0.3 mg, 0.625 mg, 1.25 mg, or 2.5 mg once daily
	Ogen (Pharmacia)	Estropipate	0.625 mg, 1.25 mg, or 2.5 mg once daily
	Ortho-est (Women First)	Estropipate	0.625 mg or 1.25 mg once daily
	Premarin (Wyeth)	Conjugated equine estrogens (CEE)	0.3 mg, 0.45 mg, 0.625 mg, 0.9 mg, 1.25 mg, or 2.5 mg once daily
Estrogens, transdermal	Climara (Berlex)	Estradiol	0.025 mg, 0.0375 mg, 0.05 mg, 0.60 mg, 0.075 mg, or 0.1 mg once weekly
	Esclim (Women First), Vivelle, Vivelle-Dot (Novartis)	Estradiol	0.025 mg, 0.0375 mg, 0.05 mg, 0.075 mg, or 0.1 mg twice weekly
	Alora (Watson)	Estradiol	0.025 mg, 0.05 mg, 0.075 mg, or 0.1 mg twice weekly
	Estrogel (Solvay)	Estradiol	1.25 gm apply once daily to arm from shoulder to wrists
	Estraderm (Novartis)	Estradiol	0.05 mg or 0.1 mg twice weekly
	Estrasorb Cream (Novavax)	Estradiol	4.35 mg (one pouch) rubbed into each thigh every morning (total 8.7 mg daily)
Progestogens	Provera (Pharmacia)	Medroxyprogesterone acetate (MPA)	2.5 mg, 5 mg, or 10 mg continuously or on set cycle schedule
	Prometrium (Solvay)	Micronized progesterone	100 mg or 200 mg continuously or on set cycle schedule
	Aygestin (Barr)	Norethindrone acetate	5 mg or 10 mg continuously or on set cycle schedule

Category	Brand (Manufacturer)	Composition	Dosing
Progestogens	Amen (Carnick), Cycrin (Wyeth-Ayerst)	MPA	2.5 mg, 5 mg, or 10 mg continuously or on set cycle schedule
Combination estrogen + progestogen, oral preparations	Prempro (Wyeth)	CEE + MPA	0.3 mg + 1.5 mg once daily; 0.45 mg + 1.5 mg once daily; 0.625 mg + 2.5 mg once daily, or; 0.625 mg + 5 mg once daily continuously
	Premphase (Wyeth)	CEE (14 tabs), then CEE + MPA (14 tabs)	0.625 mg, then 0.625 mg + 5 mg once daily sequentially
	Femhrt (Warner Chilcott)	Norethindrone acetate + ethinyl estradiol	1 mg + 5 mcg once daily, continuously
	Prefest (Monarch)	Estradiol 3 tabs then estradiol + norgestimate 3 tabs	1 mg, then 1 mg + 0.9 mg, once daily sequentially
	Activella (Novo Nordisk)	Estradiol + norethindrone acetate	1 mg + 0.5 mg once daily
Combination estrogen + progestogen transdermals	Climara Pro (Berlex)	Estradiol + levonorgestrel	0.045 mg + 0.015 mg once weekly
	Combipatch (Novartis)	Estradiol + norethindrone acetate	0.05 mg + 0.14 mg per day; 0.05 mg + 0.25 mg per day twice weekly
Combination estrogen + androgens	Estratest HS (Solvay)	Esterified estrogens + methytestosterone	0.625 mg + 1.25 mg once daily
	Estratest (Solvay)	Esterified estrogens + methytestosterone	1.25 mg + 2.5 mg once daily

*See prescribing reference for full information on doses, side effects, contraindications, and cautions.

symptom relief. Table 11–7 lists nonhormonal prescription options and Table 11–8 lists vaginal preparations.

There is no FDA-approved therapy for treating hot flashes in women at high risk for or who have been diagnosed with breast cancer. Nonhormonal agents may provide hot flash relief for women who have had breast cancer. Herbal alternatives to HT should be used with caution because they can have estrogen-like activity.

THERAPY CONSIDERATIONS

Prior to prescribing HT, it is imperative that clinicians and their patients review any cautions or contraindications to hormone use (Table 11–9). Clinicians must engage the patient in the decision-making process and weigh the risks, benefits, and scientific uncertainty with each patient in order to individualize treatment options. Data from the WHI and the HERS support the increased risk for breast cancer, coronary heart disease, thromboembolism, stroke, and dementia when HT is used. As mentioned previously, however, these data must be extrapolated with caution to women under the age of 50 who begin HT. Breast cancer risk is increased after five years of use, and progestogens may contribute to that risk (NAMS, 2004).

Women considering using HT should have the recommended screening tests for health promotion and disease prevention in addition to a complete history and physical examination (see Chapter 7 for screening recommendations). Special attention should be paid to any personal or family history of health problems that would contraindicate ET or EPT use. Once they are considered appropriate candidates, the clinician explains the various protocols for administering HT: ET alone (for women without an intact uterus), EPT continuously or sequentially, local ET, or estrogen–androgen therapy.

HT PROTOCOLS AND FORMULATIONS

Estrogen therapy   ET has been prescribed exclusively for women who have had a hysterectomy since the documentation in 1975 that unopposed estrogen increases risk for endometrial hyperplasia and cancer. Side effects of ET are listed Table 11–10.

Estrogen–progestogen therapy   Combination estrogen and progestogen therapy can be taken either sequentially (CS-EPT) or continuously (CC-EPT). In the sequential regimen, an estrogen is taken daily with the addition of a progestogen in a cyclic fashion, usually on days 1 to 12 of the month. One frequent side effect is that most women will have a withdrawal bleed monthly. To avoid this, the continuous regimen was developed in which the estrogen and progestogen are taken on a daily basis. Another option includes pulsed combination therapy wherein the progestogen is taken for two days followed by a day off in a repeating pattern. The idea was to reduce potential side effects from the progestogen; however, breakthrough bleeding is usually more problematic with this regimen. A less frequently used regimen is the cyclic regimen, where estrogen is taken daily for the first 21 days of the cycle and progestogen is added for days 12 to 21. A withdrawal bleed usually occurs between days 22 and 28, during which neither estrogen nor

TABLE 11-7 Nonhormonal Pharmacologic Options for Vasomotor Symptoms*

Category	Drug	Dosage	Comments	Side Effects	Contraindications
Antidepressants	Venlafaxine (Effexor)	37.5–75 mg/day; up-titrate when starting therapy	Response is immediate	Nausea, vomiting, mouth dryness, decreased appetite	Concomitant use of MAO inhibitors; taper when discontinuing
	Fluoxetine (Prozac)	20 mg/day; up-titrate when starting therapy	Response is immediate	Asthenia, sweating, nausea, somnolence, anorgasmia, decreased libido	Concomitant use of MAO inhibitors or thioridazine; caution with warfarin; taper when discontinuing
	Paroxetine (Paxil)	12.5–25 mg/day; up-titrate when starting therapy	Response is immediate	See fluoxetine	See fluoxetine; taper when discontinuing
Anticonvulsants	Gabapentin (Neurontin)	Initial dose 300 mg/day, increasing to 300 mg three times per day at 3–4 day intervals		Somnolence, dizziness, ataxia, fatigue	Avoid antacids within 2 hours of use
Antihypertensives	Clonidine	0.05–0.1 mg twice daily	Available as a patch, less effective than antidepressants or gabapentin	Dry mouth, drowsiness, dizziness, weakness, constipation, rash, myalgia, urticaria, insomnia, nausea, agitation, orthostatic hypotension, impotence, arrhythmias	Taper when discontinuing

(continues)

TABLE 11-7 (continued)

Category	Drug	Dosage	Comments	Side Effects	Contraindications
Antihypertensives	Methyldopa and Bellergal		NAMS does not recommend due to toxicity		
Breast cancer agent	Megestrol (Megace)	20 mg daily (divided doses)		Intestinal disturbance, weight gain, chest pain, edema, hypertension, hyperglycemia, rash, fever, insomnia, urinary frequency, asthenia, decreased libido, dyspepsia	Caution in diabetes, history of thromboembolic disease

*See prescribing reference for full information on doses, side effects, contraindications, and cautions.

Sources: Grady, 2002; NAMS, 2004.

TABLE 11-8   Vaginal Hormone Products*

Type	Product Name	Active Ingredient	Dose
Estrogen			
Vaginal hormone creams	Estrace (Warner Chilcott)	Micronized 17-beta-estradiol	2–4 gm daily for 1–4 weeks, then 1 gm daily 1–3 times per week for 1–3 weeks. Maintenance: 1 gm 1–3 times a week, cyclically (3 weeks on, 1 week off). Taper dosage or discontinue at 3–6 month intervals
	Premarin (Wyeth)	Conjugated equine estrogen	0.5–2 g intravaginally daily cyclically (3 weeks on, 1 week off). Reevaluate periodically. Tapering is frequently appropriate but not specified in product information
Vaginal tablets	Vagifem (Novo Nordisk)	Estradiol hemihydrate	25 mcg once daily for two weeks then twice weekly
Ring	Estring (Pharmacia)	Micronized 17-beta-estradiol	7.5 mcg/24 hours once every 90 days
	Femring (Warner Chilcott)	Estradiol acetate	0.05 mg/day or 0.1 mg/day once every 3 months
Progestogen			
Gel	Crinone (Serono)	Progesterone	4% gel–45 mg, 1 applicator every other day, give 6 doses; increase to 8% if no response
IUD	Mirena (Berlex)	Evonorgestrel	20 mcg daily

*See prescribing reference for full information on doses, side effects, contraindications, and cautions.

TABLE 11-9   Contraindications to HT and Adverse Effects

Absolute Contraindications to Estrogen Use Include:	Adverse Effects of ET
• Known or suspected cancer of the breast • Known or suspected estrogen-dependent neoplasia • History of uterine or ovarian cancer • History of coronary heart disease or stroke • History of biliary tract disorder • Undiagnosed, abnormal genital bleeding • History of or active thrombophlebitis or thromboembolic disorders	• Uterine bleeding • Breast tenderness • Nausea • Abdominal bloating • Fluid retention in extremities • Headache • Dizziness • Hair loss

Absolute Contraindications to Progestogen Use Include:	Adverse Effects of EPT
• Active thrombophlebitis or thromboembolic disorders • Liver dysfunction or disease • Known or suspected cancer of the breast • Undiagnosed abnormal vaginal bleeding • Pregnancy	• Mood changes • Possible increased uterine bleeding than if taking ET alone

TABLE 11-10   Management of HT Side Effects

Side Effect	Strategy
Fluid retention	Decrease salt intake, maintain adequate water intake, exercise, recommend an herbal diuretic or mild prescription diuretic
Bloating	Change to low-dose transdermal estrogen, lower the progestogen dose to a level that still protects the uterus, change progestogen or try micronized progesterone
Breast tenderness	Decrease estrogen, change estrogen, decrease salt intake, change progestogen, decrease caffeine and chocolate consumption
Headaches	Change to transdermal estrogen, decrease estrogen and/or progestogen, change to a CC-EPT regimen, ensure adequate water intake, decrease salt, caffeine, and alcohol use
Mood changes	Lower the progestogen dose, change to a CC-EPT regimen, ensure adequate water intake, restrict salt, caffeine, and alcohol consumption
Nausea	Take hormones with meals, change estrogen, change to transdermal estrogen, decrease estrogen or progestogen

Source: Adapted with permission from North American Menopause Society. (2002). *Menopause Core Curriculum Study Guide* (2nd ed.). Cleveland, OH: Author.

progestogen is taken. However, menopausal symptoms usually rebound when the estrogen is not taken; therefore, few women opt for the cyclic regimen.

Estrogens   There are a variety of estrogen compounds: estrogens that are bioidentical and transformed into human estrogens, such as 17-Beta Estradiol, estriol, and estrone; synthetic estrogen analogs, such as ethinyl estradiol; and nonhuman estrogens, such as CEE. CEE is the most widely used estrogen and has been the product used in the majority of clinical trials, including the WHI and HERS.

Estrogens differ in target tissue response and in dose equivalency. They can be administered either systemically or locally. Systemic preparations are available as oral tablets or transdermal patches. Local preparations are available as creams, tablets, or rings. The vaginal ring containing 0.5mg or 0.1 mg/day of estradiol acetate over three months is the only local treatment that has been effective in treating hot flashes (NAMS, 2004). Local treatment with estrogen theoretically avoids systemic absorption; however, in a review of the studies on vaginal preparations, Crandall (2002) found that the ring has slightly more systemic absorption. Women who want to avoid systemic effects, such as breast cancer survivors, should probably use a different preparation until more evidence is available.

Progestogens   Progestogens are hormones that possess progestational properties. The most commonly prescribed progestogen has been MPA, but others are being used with more regularity, such as micronized progesterone (which is bioidentical), norgestimate, and norethindrone acetate. Side effects of adding progestogens to estrogens are listed in Table 11–9.

Estrogen–androgen therapy   Therapy combining androgens and estrogens has been theorized to improve loss of libido in postmenopausal women; however, there are too few randomized clinical trials to prove that testosterone plus estrogen is more effective than estrogen alone. One older study of 40 women showed no significant differences in levels of self-reported sexual enjoyment and desire (Dow, Hart, & Forrest, 1982). Another crossover study from the same era compared estrogen alone, estrogen plus testosterone, testosterone, and placebo. These researchers found that women reported significantly improved levels of sexual desire, arousal, and fantasies, while taking both testosterone and estrogen plus testosterone (Sherwin, Gelfand, & Brender, 1985). Additional clinical trials are currently being conducted. Side effects of androgens include alopecia, acne, deepening of the voice, and hirsutism.

PLAN OF CARE AND PATIENT EDUCATION

NAMS recommends initiating ET and EPT at lower than standard doses, such as 0.3 mg CEE, 0.25–0.5 mg 17-beta estradiol patch, or the equivalent. Studies have shown adequate vasomotor relief, but endometrial protection has not been evaluated in long-term clinical trials. Vasomotor symptoms usually begin to resolve in two to six weeks after initiating HT.

Patients should be offered anticipatory guidance about management of side effects, should they occur. Research evidence has absolved HT from contributing to weight gain; however, fluid retention may make women feel as if they are gaining weight. Table 11–10 lists possible side effects and strategies.

Patients should return for a follow-up visit in six to eight weeks to evaluate their progress; if the initial dose of ET/EPT is not adequate, it can be increased or taken on a daily divided dose schedule. The decision to continue or discontinue HT should be revisited at least annually. Some women will have symptoms for a short time, such as a few months to a year. Others are symptomatic for years and may need to continue HT up to five years (Wysocki et al., 2003).

When discontinuing, HT should be tapered to avoid rebound symptoms. While there are no particular guidelines for weaning patients, NAMS (2004) advises gradually decreasing the dose or gradually lengthening the time between doses.

COMPLEMENTARY AND ALTERNATIVE MEDICINE OPTIONS FOR MENOPAUSE SYMPTOM MANAGEMENT

The use of complementary and alternative medicine (CAM) is on the rise in the United States (Eisenberg, Kessler, et al., 1993; Eisenberg, Davis, et al., 1998; Kessler et al., 2001). Visits to alternative providers now exceed visits to primary care clinicians, and most patients who use CAM do not report this usage to their primary care clinicians. Furthermore, women are the largest group of CAM users. It is imperative for clinicians to ask patients about the use of CAM and to become knowledgeable about the CAM therapies that women are using.

NATURAL VERSUS BIOIDENTICAL HORMONES

Many women seek "natural" hormones, believing that they are less likely to cause harmful side effects than manufactured hormones. However, "natural" actually refers to any product with principal components that originate from plant, animal, or mineral sources. This then also encompasses pharmaceutically manufactured hormones, as these are derived from animal, plant, or mineral substances. "Natural" hormones are not necessarily identical to what a woman's body produces.

There are, however, several hormones available that are "bioidentical" to the hormones produced in women's bodies. Frequently women requesting "natural hormones" are actually seeking "bioidentical" formulations. Bioidentical hormones are available through prescription from usual and compounding pharmacies. Several forms of estrogen are available in bioidentical formulations such as estrone, estriol, and 17-beta estradiol. Bioidentical progesterone is also available in micronized form.

Estrogens can be prescribed through compounding pharmacies. Two commonly available preparations that contain bioidentical estrogens are Tri-est and Bi-est. Bi-est contains 2 mg estriol (80%) and 0.5 mg estradiol (20%). Tri-est contains 2 mg estriol (80%), 0.25 mg estrone (10%), and 0.25 mg estradiol (10%). These products are advertised as containing 80% estriol, which is correct. However, they contain significant amounts of estradiol and therefore may require progesterone for endometrial protection (Gaudet, 2004). Estriol also can be compounded as a vaginal cream.

HERBALS

Although many women seek relief of menopausal symptoms, especially hot flashes, from herbal preparations, few studies exist to offer information regarding their efficacy or safety. Because these products are generally identified as diet supplements, rather than medications, they are not regulated by the FDA in the same way as prescription medications and other over-the-counter products. Federal regulations do exist; however, they are poorly enforced. This raises questions regarding purity, contents, and consistency from package to package or tablet to tablet. Various preparations of the same herbal product can have dramatically different amounts of active ingredients (e.g., extract versus tincture), and many products come with mixtures of various different herbs in a single preparation, making dosing difficult. Furthermore, little is known regarding interaction between various herbal products and prescription medications or other herbal products.

Despite these concerns, herbal products are widely used for menopausal symptom relief. Several of these are commonly used in combination products or in Chinese herb mixtures. Table 11–11 provides information regarding some of these preparations.

ISOFLAVONES

Isoflavones are compounds derived from plants that have both estrogenic and nonestrogenic properties. They are present in foods, such as soy and red clover, as well as commercial preparations. Isoflavones are often referred to as phytoestrogens because of their ability to bind weakly with estrogen receptors, especially the beta receptors, and have been extensively studied for reducing hot flashes. Several recent placebo-controlled trials show little or no statistically significant differences in hot flash reduction in treatment versus control groups (Nikander et al., 2003; Penotti et al., 2003; Tice et al., 2003).

Despite these disappointing findings, soy is a healthy food that the FDA has allowed to be identified as one that reduces the risk of heart disease. There is no evidence that soy is harmful nor that it predisposes women to breast cancer nor is it problematic for breast cancer survivors. Women who choose to add soy to their diets need to be educated to use the soy to replace something else, rather than adding extra calories through soy nuts, shakes, or cereals.

Other classes of phytoestrogens include flavonoids, lignans, and coumestrans. These classes have much lower hormonal affinity and are generally not thought to be useful for menopausal symptom management. They are found in some foods and food products and carry some of the cardioprotective properties of isoflavones. Lignans are found in flaxseed

TABLE 11-11 Herbals Commonly Used for Menopausal Symptom Relief*

Product	Usual Dosage**	Purpose in Menopause	Comments
Black cohosh (*Cimicifuga racemosa*)	20 mg twice daily (proprietary standardized extract)	• Vasomotor symptoms	• Multiple products and formulations available • Research evidence suggests beneficial effect on menopausal symptoms, benefit similar to estrogen for hot flash relief • Safety for use > 6 months not established • Product labels frequently recommend much higher doses • Can potentiate antihypertensives • Wide variations in product ingredients, extraction processes, and purity • Side effects rare, usually intestinal upset, headache, dizziness, hypotension, or painful extremities; more common with higher doses
Chastetree berry (*Vitex agnus castus*)	Effective dose unknown, hard to find standardized extract	• Menstrual irregularity	• More popular in Europe than the US; approved in Germany for PMS, mastalgia, and menopause symptoms • Often found in combination products • Research focuses on PMS symptoms, no data on relief of menopause symptoms • Side effects rare, usually headache, intestinal upset
Dong quai (*Angelica sinensis*)	2 capsules two to three times per day; usually in combination products	• Gynecologic conditions	• Widely used in Asia • Research found no benefit for menopause symptoms • Often in Chinese herb combination products (*Chinese Materia Medica* advises against giving it alone) • A "heating" herb, can cause a red face, hot flashes, sweating, irritability, or insomnia • Contains coumarin derivatives, contraindicated in those taking warfarin • Can cause photosensitivity, hypotension

Evening primrose oil (*Oenothera biennis*)	3–4 gms daily in divided doses	• Hot flashes • Mastalgia	• Data show no benefit in treatment versus controls • Potentiates risk for seizure if taken with seizure disorder, phenothiazines, and other medications that lower the seizure threshold • Side effects include diarrhea and nausea
Ginkgo (*Ginkgo biloba*)	40–80 mg of standardized extract three times daily	• Memory changes	• Insufficient research on safety and efficacy • Memory changes often related to sleep disturbances, menopausal sleep disturbances frequently related to vasomotor symptoms or other life stressors • Side effects include gastrointestinal distress, hypotension; chronic use had been linked with subarachnoid hemorrhage, subdural hematoma, and increased bleeding times
Ginseng (*Panax ginseng*)	1–2 gm root daily in divided doses	• General "tonic" • Improved mood, fatigue	• Heavily adulterated • Research showed no benefit on menopausal symptoms; showed benefits on well-being, general health, and depression • Can cause uterine bleeding, mastalgia • Contraindicated with breast cancer, and with monoamine oxidase inhibitors, stimulants, or anticoagulants; may potentiate digoxin and others (multiple drug interactions) • Side effects include rash, nervousness, insomnia, hypertension
Kava (*Piper methysticum*)	150–300 mg of root extract daily in divided doses	• Irritability • Insomnia	• Banned in several countries due to hepatotoxicity, thus not recommended • Contraindicated with depression • Side effects include gastrointestinal discomfort, impaired reflexes and motor function, weight loss, hepatotoxicity, rash

(continues)

TABLE 11-11 (continued)

Product	Usual Dosage*	Purpose in Menopause	Comments
Licorice root (*Glycyrrhiza glabra*)	5–15 mg of root equivalent daily in divided doses	• Menopause-related symptoms	• Found in many Chinese herb mixtures • No data supporting relief of hot flashes • High doses can lead to primary aldosteronism cardiac arrhythmias, cardiac arrest • Contraindicated if hepatic or renal disease, diabetes, hypertension, arrhythmia, hypokalemia, hypertonis, pregnancy, or on diuretics
Passion flower (*Passiflora incarnata*)	3–10 grains daily in divided doses	• Sedative	• Research shows mixed results in sleep improvement • Menopausal sleep disturbances frequently related to vasomotor symptoms or other life stressors
St. John's wort (*Hypericum perforatum*)	300 mg three times daily (standardized extract)	• Vasomotor symptoms • Irritability • Depression	• No data supporting vasomotor relief • Research findings support use for depression, there are no clinical trials for menopause • Often combined with black cohosh for menopause symptom treatment • Interferes with metabolism of many medications that are metabolized in the liver (C 450) (e.g., estrogen, digoxin, theophylline), reduces international normalized ratio (INR) levels, not to be used concomitantly with antidepressants, monoamine oxidase inhibitors, or immunosuppressants • Side effects include photosensitivity, rash, constipation, cramping, dry mouth, fatigue, dizziness, restlessness, insomnia

Valerian root (*Valeriana officinalis*)	300–600 mg aqueous extract ½–1 hour before bed (insomnia); 150–300 mg aqueous extract each morning and 300–400 mg each evening (anxiety)	• Sedative • Antianxiety	• Used for insomnia in intermittent dosing, for anxiety with chronic dosing • Research showed improvement in sleep and depression/mood scales • Side effects include headache, uneasiness, excitability, arrhythmias, morning sedation, gastrointestinal upset, cardiac function disorders (with long-term use)
Wild yam (*Dioscorea villosa*)	Unknown	• Menopausal symptoms	• Products claim that creams are converted to progesterone; however, the human body cannot convert topical or ingested wild yam into progesterone • Research showed no benefit on menopausal symptoms

*See prescribing reference for full information on doses, side effects, contraindications, and cautions.
**Dosages vary and differ according to form (e.g., tincture, liquid extract, drops, essential oil, standardized extract).
Sources: Decker & Meyers, 2001; Gaudet, 2004; Low Dog, 2004; NAMS, 2004.

oil, whole grains, and some fruits and vegetables. Flavonoids are in oils, spices, wine, tea, and some vegetables. Coumestrans are found in alfalfa sprouts, red beans, split peas, spinach, and some species of clover. Coumestrans can interfere with bleeding profiles and may have interactions with warfarin.

PROGESTERONE CREAMS

Several different progesterone creams are available over-the-counter. FDA regulations are not currently enforced for these products, again raising concerns about purity and content. Progesterone creams include products such as PhytoGest, Progest, Endocreme, and Pro-Dermex, and progesterone content varies from under 2 mg to 700 mg. These creams can also be prescribed using compounding pharmacies.

Although some women taking systemic estrogens may want to use progesterone creams for endometrial protection to avoid systemic progesterone effects, there are no data that support the use of progesterone creams for endometrial protection. At least one randomized, controlled study identified improvement in vasomotor symptoms for women using transdermal progesterone cream as compared with controls (Leonetti, Longo, & Anasti, 1999). Topical progesterone creams may be a promising option if future research supports these findings.

ACUPUNCTURE

Research findings evaluating acupuncture for the relief of menopause-related hot flashes have been contradictory. One small study of 24 women identified no differences in subjects treated with electroacupuncture versus controls (Wyon, Lindgren, Lundberg, & Hammar, 1995). However, a more recent study (N=17) identified significant reductions in hot flashes and sleep disturbances in women treated over a six-week period with acupuncture at menopause symptom-specific sites as compared with controls who were treated with a general tonic acupuncture (Cohen, Rousseau, & Carey, 2003). Acupuncture may prove to provide some benefit but further research is needed.

CONCLUSION

Menopause is a marker in the lives of middle-aged women. While a normal developmental stage, it gives women the opportunity to evaluate their health and risks for diseases of aging, thereby instituting lifestyle changes that prevent disease and promote health. Although many women will transition through perimenopause to postmenopause without incident, many will also experience mild to severe vasomotor symptoms. Treatments for these problems can decrease symptoms and improve women's quality of life. As the numbers of posmenopausal women increase, clinicians are in a prime position to counsel their patients about healthy aging.

REFERENCES

Administration on Aging. (2004). *Statistics on the aging population.* Washington, DC: Author. Retrieved May 30, 2004, from www.aoa.gov/prof/Statistics/statistics.asp.

Alexander, I. M., Ruff, C., Rousseau, M. E., White, K., Motter, S., McKie, C., et al. (2003). Menopause symptoms and management strategies identified by black women [Abstract]. *Menopause, 10*(6), 601.

Alexander, I. M., Ruff, C., Rousseau, M. E., White, K., Motter, S., McKie, C., et al. (2004, April). *Experiences and perceptions of menopause and midlife health among black women.* Paper presented at the meeting of the Eastern Nursing Research Society 16th Annual Scientific Sessions, Quincy, MA.

Alexander, I. M., Ruff, C. C., & Udemezue, C. (n.d.). *Correlation between lifestyle behaviors and severity of menopausal symptoms in black women.* [Unpublished data.] P20 pilot study in the Yale-Howard Center for reducing health disparities through self- and family-management, (Grant No. 1P20NR08349-01). Bethesda, MD: National Institute of Nursing Research.

American Cancer Society. (2004a). *Cancer statistics 2004.* Retrieved May 7, 2004, from www.cancer.org.

American Cancer Society. (2004b). *Smoking cessation.* Retrieved May 20, 2004, from www.cancer.org.

American Diabetes Association. (2004a). Position statement: Diagnosis and classification of diabetes mellitus. *Diabetes Care, 27*(Suppl. 1), S5–S10.

American Diabetes Association. (2004b). Position statement: Screening for type 2 diabetes. *Diabetes Care, 27*(Suppl. 1), S11–S14.

American Heart Association. (2002). *Heart disease and stroke statistics: 2003 update.* Dallas, TX: Author.

American Heart Association. (2004). *Women and cardiovascular disease.* Retrieved May 7, 2004, from www.americanheart.org.

American Obesity Association. (2002). *Obesity fact sheets* (Updated March 24, 2004). Retrieved May 7, 2004, from www.obesity.org.

Anderson, G. L., Limacher, M., Assaf, A. R., Bassford, T., Beresford, S. A., Black, H., et al. (2004). Effects of conjugated equine estrogen in postmenopausal women with hysterectomy: The Women's Health Initiative randomized controlled trial. *Journal of the American Medical Association, 291*(14), 1701–1712.

Andrist, L. C., & MacPherson, K. I. (2001). Conceptual models for women's health research: Reclaiming menopause as an exemplar of nursing's contributions to feminist scholarship. In D. Taylor & N. F. Woods (Eds.), *Annual Review of Nursing Research* (Vol. 19, pp. 29–60). New York: Springer.

Avis, N. E., Stellato, R., Crawford, S., Bromberger, J., Ganz, P., Cain, V., et al. (2001). Is there a menopausal syndrome? Menopausal status and symptoms across racial/ethnic groups. *Social Science and Medicine, 52*(3), 345–356.

Baker, A., Simpson, S., & Dawson, D. (1997). Sleep disruption and mood changes associated with menopause. *Journal of Psychosomatic Research, 43*(4), 359–369.

Ballard, K. D., Kuh, D. J., & Wadsworth, M. E. J. (2001). The role of the menopause in women's experiences of the 'change of life.' *Sociology of Health and Illness, 23*(4), 397–424.

Barton, D. L., Loprinzi, C. L., Quella, S. K., Sloan, J. A., Veeder, M. H., Egner, J. R., et al. (1998). Prospective evaluation of vitamin E for hot flashes in breast cancer survivors. *Journal of Clinical Oncology, 16*(2), 495–500.

Baskin, H. J. (2002). American Association of Clinical Endocrinologists' medical guidelines for clinical practice for the evaluation and treatment of hyperthyroidism and hypothyroidism. *Endocrine Practice, 8*(6), 457–469.

Bastian, L. A., Smith, C. M., & Nanda, K. (2003). Is this woman perimenopausal? *Journal of the American Medical Association, 289*(7), 895–902.

Blackman, M. R. (2000). Age-related alterations in sleep quality and neuroendocrine function: Interrelationships and implications. *Journal of the American Medical Association, 284*(7), 879–881.

Blatt, M. H. G., Weisbader, H., & Kupperman, H. S. (1953). Vitamin E and the climacteric syndrome. *Archives of Internal Medicine, 91,* 792–796.

Bromberger, J. T., Matthews, K. A., Kuller, L. H., Wing, R. R., Meilahn, E. N., & Plantinga, P. (1997). Prospective study of the determinants of age at menopause. *American Journal of Epidemiology, 145*(2), 124–133.

Busch, H., Barth-Olofsson, A. S., Rosenhagen, S., & Collins, A. (2003). Menopause transition and psychological development. *Menopause, 10*(2), 179–187.

Centers for Disease Control and Prevention. (2003). *Nutrition and physical activity: Overweight & obesity.* (Updated December 8, 2003.) Retrieved May 7, 2004, from www.cdc.gov.

Cohen, L. (2004, April). *Depression rates in perimenopausal and premenopausal women: A longitudinal study.* Paper presented at the meeting of the American Psychiatric Association, New York.

Cohen, S. M., Rousseau, M. E., & Carey, B. (2003). Can acupuncture ease the symptoms of menopause? *Holistic Nursing Practice, 17*(6), 295–299.

Collins, P. H. (1990). *Black feminist thought: Knowledge, consciousness, and the politics of empowerment.* Boston: Unwin Hyman.

Cooper, G. S., Sandler, D. P., & Bohlig, M. (1999). Active and passive smoking and the occurrence of natural menopause. *Epidemiology, 10*(6), 771–773.

Cramer, G., Xu, H., & Harlow, B. L. (1995). Family history as a predictor of early menopause. *Fertility and Sterility, 64,* 740–745.

Crandall, C. (2002). Vaginal estrogen preparations: A review of safety and efficacy for vaginal atrophy. *Journal of Women's Health, 11*(10), 857–877.

Dawson-Hughes, B., Gold, D. T., Rodbard, H. W., Bonner, F. J., Khosla, S., & Swift, S. (2003). *Physician's guide to prevention and treatment of osteoporosis* (2nd ed.). Washington, DC: National Osteoporosis Foundation.

de Bruin, J. P., Bovenhuis, H., van Noord, P. A. H., Pearson, P. L., van Arendonk, J. A. M., te Velde, E. R., et al. (2001). The role of genetic factors in age at natural menopause. *Human Reproduction, 16*(9), 2014–2018.

Decker, G. M., & Meyers, J. (2001). Commonly used herbs: Implications for clinical practice [insert]. *Clinical Journal of Oncology Nursing, 5*(2).

Dennerstein, L., Dudley, E., & Burger, H. (2001). Are changes in sexual functioning during midlife due to aging or menopause? *Fertility & Sterility, 76*(3), 456–460.

Dow, M. G., Hart, D. M., & Forrest, C. A. (1982). Hormonal treatments of sexual unresponsiveness in postmenopausal women: A comparative study. *British Journal of Obstetrics and Gynaecology, 90,* 361–366.

Eisenberg, D. M., Davis, R. B., Ettner, S. L., Appel, S., Wilkey, S., Van Rompay, M., et al. (1998). Trends in alternative medicine use in the United States, 1990–1997: Results of a follow-up national survey. *Journal of the American Medical Association, 280*(18), 1569–1575.

Eisenberg, D. M., Kessler, R. C., Foster, C., Norlock, F. E., Calkins, D. R., & Delbanco, T. L. (1993). Unconventional medicine in the United States. Prevalence, costs, and patterns of use. *New England Journal of Medicine, 328*(4), 246–252.

Fairfield, K. M., & Fletcher, R. H. (2002). Vitamins for chronic disease prevention in adults: Scientific review. *Journal of the American Medical Association, 287*(23), 3116–3126.

Fletcher, R. H., & Fairfield, K. M. (2002). Vitamins for chronic disease prevention in adults: Clinical applications. *Journal of the American Medical Association, 287*(23), 3127–3129.

Franz, M. J. (Ed.). (2003). *A CORE curriculum for diabetes education: Diabetes and complications* (5th ed.). Chicago: American Association of Diabetes Educators.

Freedman, R. R., & Woodward, S. (1992). Behavioral treatment of menopausal hot flashes: Evaluation by ambulatory monitoring. *American Journal of Obstetrics and Gynecology, 167,* 436–439.

Freedman, R. R., Woodward, S., Brown, B., Javaid, J. I., & Pandy, G. N. (1995). Biochemical and thermoregulatory effects of treatment for menopausal hot flashes. *Menopause, 2,* 211–218.

Gaspar, U. J., Gotta, J. M., & van den Brule, F. A. (1995). Post menopausal changes of lipid and glucose metabolism: A review of the main aspects. *Maturitas, 21,* 171–178.

Gaudet, T. W. (2004). CAM approaches to menopause management: Overview of the options. *Menopause Management: Women's Health Through Midlife & Beyond, 13*(Suppl. 1), 48–50.

Gilligan, C. (1982). *In a different voice: Psychological theory and women's development.* Cambridge, MA: Harvard University Press.

Godsland, I. F. (1996). The influence of female sex steroids on glucose metabolism and insulin action. *Journal of Internal Medicine, 738*(Suppl.), 1–60.

Gold, E. B., Bromberger, J., Crawford, S., Samuels, S., Greendale, G. A., Harlow, S. D., et al. (2001). Factors associated with age at natural menopause in a multiethnic sample of midlife women. *American Journal of Epidemiology, 153*(9), 865–874.

Gold, E. B., Sternfeld, B., Kelsey, J. L., Brown, C., Mouton, C., Reame, N., et al. (2000). Relation of demographic and lifestyle factors to symptoms in a multi-racial/ethnic population of women 40–55 years of age. *American Journal of Epidemiology, 152*(5), 463–473.

Grady, D. (2002). A 60-year-old woman trying to discontinue hormone replacement therapy. *Journal of the American Medical Association, 287*(16), 2130–2137.

Grady, D. (2004, April 17). Study plans to retest use of hormones in menopause. *New York Times*, A11.

Greendale, G. A., Lee, N. P., & Arriola, E. R. (1999). The menopause. *Lancet, 353*(9152), 571–580.

Hodgson, S. F., & Watts, S. F. (2003). American Association of Clinical Endocrinologists medical guidelines for clinical practice for the prevention and treatment of postmenopausal osteoporosis: 2001 edition with selected updates for 2003. *Endocrine Practice, 9*(6), 544–564.

Irvin, J. H., Domar, A. D., Clark, C., Zuttermeister, P. C., & Freidman, R. (1996). The effects of relaxation response training on menopausal symptoms. *Journal of Psychosomatic Obstetrics and Gynaecology, 17*, 202–207.

Jacobs Institute on Women's Health. (2003). *Expert panel on menopause counseling*. Retrieved June 30, 2003, from www.jiwh.org/menodownload.htm.

Johnson, J., Canning, J., Kaneko, T., Pru, J. K., & Tilly, J. L. (2004). Germline stem cells and follicular renewal in the postnatal mammalian ovary. *Nature, 428*(6979), 145–150.

Jordan, J. V., Kaplan, A. G., Miller, J. B., Stiver, I. P., & Surrey, J. L. (1991). *Women's growth in connection*. New York: Guilford Press.

Kans, J. A. (1994). World Health Organization study group: Assessment of fracture risk and its application to screening for postmenopausal osteoporosis. A synopsis of the WHO report. *Osteoporosis International, 4*, 368–381.

Kessler, R. C., Davis, R. B., Foster, D. F., Van Rompay, M. I., Walters, E. E., Wilkey, S. A., et al. (2001). Long-term trends in the use of complementary and alternative medical therapies in the United States. *Annals of Internal Medicine, 135*(4), 262–268.

Klatte, E. T., Scharre, D. W., Nagaraja, H. N., Davis, R. A., & Beversdorf, D. Q. (2003). Combination therapy of donepezil and vitamin E in Alzheimer disease. *Alzheimer Disease & Associated Disorders, 17*(2), 113–116.

Kronenberg, F. (1990). Hot flashes: Epidemiology and physiology. *Annals of the New York Academy of Sciences, 592*, 52–86, 123–133.

Landolt, H. P., Rioth, C., Dijk, D. J., & Borbely, A. A. (1996). Late-afternoon ethanol intake affects nocturnal sleep and the sleep EEG in middle-aged men. *Journal of Clinical Psychopharmacology, 16*, 428–436.

Landolt, H. P., Werth, E., Borbely, A. A., & Dijk, D. J. (1995). Caffeine intake (200 mg) in the morning affects human sleep and EEG spectra at night. *Brain Research, 675*, 67–74.

Leonetti, H. B., Longo, S., & Anasti, J. N. (1999). Transdermal progesterone cream for vasomotor symptoms and postmenopausal bone loss. *Obstetrics & Gynecology, 94*(2), 225–228.

Liu, J. (2004). Use of conjugated estrogens after the Women's Health Initiative. *The Female Patient, 29*, 8–13.

Low Dog, T. (2004). CAM approaches to menopause management: The role for botanicals in menopause. *Menopause Management: Women's Health Through Midlife & Beyond, 13*(Suppl. 1), 51–53.

MacPherson, K. I. (1981). Menopause as disease: The social construction of a metaphor. *Advances in Nursing Science, 3*, 95–113.

Mayer-Davis, E. J., D'Antonio, A., & Tudor-Locke, C. (2003). Lifestyle for diabetes prevention. In M. J. Franz (Ed.), *A core curriculum for diabetes education: Diabetes in the life cycle and research* (5th ed.). Chicago: American Association of Diabetes Educators.

McKinlay, S. M. (1996). The normal menopause transition: An overview. *Maturitas, 23*(2), 137–145.

McLean, R. R., Jacques, P. F., Selhub, J., Tucker, K. L., Samelson, E. J., Broe, K. E., et al. (2004). Homocysteine as a predictive factor for hip fracture in older persons. *New England Journal of Medicine, 350*(20), 2042–2049.

Morin, C. M., Hauri, P. J., Espie, C. A., Speilman, A. J., Buysse, D. J., & Bootzin, R. R. (1999). Nonpharmacologic treatment of chronic insomnia: An American Academy of Sleep Medicine review. *Sleep, 22*, 1134–1156.

Nachtigall, L. E. (1994). Comparative study: Replens versus local estrogen in menopausal women. *Fertility & Sterility, 61*, 178–180.

National Cancer Institute. (2003). *Probability of developing or dying of cancer.* Retrieved May 7, 2004, from http://srab.cancer.gov/devcan.

National Institutes of Health. (1994). *Optimal calcium intake. NIH consensus statement.* Retrieved September 25, 1998, from text.nlm.nih.gov/nih/cdc/www/97txt.html.

National Institutes of Health. (2002). *National Center on Sleep Disorder Research and Office of Prevention, Education, and Control.* Retrieved January 16, 2002, from www.nhlbi.nih.gov/health/prof/sleep/pslp_pat.htm.

National Institutes of Health. (2004). *NIH asks participants in Women's Health Initiative Estrogen-Alone Study to stop study pills, begin follow-up phase.* Retrieved April 30, 2004, from www.nhlbi.nih.gov.

National Women's Health Network. (2000). *Taking hormones and women's health: Choices, risks, and benefits.* Washington, DC: Author.

Nikander, E., Kilkkinen, A., Metsa-Heikkila, M., Adlercreutz, H., Pietinen, P., Tiitinen, A., et al. (2003). A randomized placebo-controlled crossover trial with phytoestrogens in treatment of menopause in breast cancer patients. *Obstetrics & Gynecology, 101*(6), 1213–1220.

North American Menopause Society. (2002). *Menopause core curriculum study guide* (2nd ed.). Cleveland, OH: Author.

North American Menopause Society. (2003). Estrogen and progestogen use in peri- and postmenopausal women: September 2003 position statement of The North American Menopause Society. *Menopause, 10*(6), 497–506.

North American Menopause Society. (2004). Treatment of menopause-associated vasomotor symptoms: Position statement of the North American Menopause Society. *Menopause, 11*(1), 11–33.

Onofrj, M., Thomas, A., Luciano, A. L., Iacono, D., Di Rollo, A., D'Andreamatteo, G., et al. (2002). Donepezil versus vitamin E in Alzheimer's disease: Part 2: Mild versus moderate-severe Alzheimer's disease. *Clinical Neuropharmacology, 25*(4), 207–215.

Palmer, J. R., Rosenberg, L., Wise, L. A., Horton, N. J., & Adams-Campbell, L. L. (2003). Onset of natural menopause in African American women. *American Journal of Public Health, 93*(2), 299–306.

Penotti, M., Fabio, E., Modena, A. B., Rinaldi, M., Omodei, U., & Vigano, P. (2003). Effect of soy-derived isoflavones on hot flushes, endometrial thickness, and the pulsatility index of the uterine and cerebral arteries. *Fertility & Sterility, 79*(5), 1112–1117.

Porth, C. M., & Kunert, M. P. (Eds.). (2002). *Pathophysiology concepts of altered health states* (6th ed.). Philadelphia: Lippincott Williams & Wilkins.

Quinn, A. A. (1991). A theoretical model of the perimenopausal process. *Journal of Nurse-Midwifery, 36*(1), 25–29.

Rossouw, J. E., Anderson, G. L., Prentice, R. L., LaCroix, A. Z., Jackson, R. D., Beresford, S. A. A., et al. (2002). Risks and benefits of estrogen plus progestin in healthy postmenopausal women: Principal results from the Women's Health Initiative Randomized Controlled Trial. *Journal of the American Medical Association, 288*(3), 321–333.

Sampselle, C. M., Harris, V. H., Harlow, S. D., & Sowers, M. (2002). Midlife development and menopause in African American and Caucasian women. *Health Care for Women International, 23*(4), 351–363.

Sheehy, G. (1976). *Passages: Predictable crises of adult life.* New York: Dutton.

Sheehy, G. (1995). *New passages: Mapping your life across time.* New York: Random House.

Sherwin, B. B., Gelfand, M. M., & Brender, W. (1985). Androgen enhances sexual motivation in females: A prospective crossover study of sex steroid administration in the surgical menopause. *Psychosomatic Medicine, 47*, 339–351.

Soules, M. R., Sherman, S., Parrott, E., Rebar, R., Santoro, N., Utian, W., et al. (2001). Executive summary: Stages of Reproductive Aging Workshop (STRAW). *Fertility & Sterility, 76*(5), 874–878.

Speroff, L., Glass, R. H., & Kase, N. G. (1999). *Clinical gynecologic endocrinology and infertility* (6th ed.). Philadelphia: Lippincott Williams & Wilkins.

Thomas, A., Iacono, D., Bonanni, L., D'Andreamatteo, G., & Onofrj, M. (2001). Donepezil, rivastigmine, and vitamin E in Alzheimer disease: A combined P300 event-related potentials/neuropsychologic evaluation over 6 months. *Clinical Neuropharmacology, 24*(1), 31–42.

Tice, J. A., Ettinger, B., Ensrud, K., Wallace, R., Blackwell, T., & Cummings, S. R. (2003). Phytoestrogen supplements for the treatment of hot flashes: The Isoflavone Clover Extract (ICE) Study: A randomized controlled trial. *Journal of the American Medical Association, 290*(2), 207–214.

US Department of Health, Education, and Welfare, National Institute on Aging. (1979). *Summary of conclusions of the NIH Conference on Estrogen Use and Postmenopausal Women.* Washington, DC: Author.

US Department of Health and Human Services. (1998). *Clinician's handbook of preventive services* (2nd ed.). Washington, DC: GPO.

US Preventive Services Task Force. (1996). *Guide to preventive services.* Rockville, MD: Agency for Healthcare Research and Quality.

US Preventive Services Task Force. (2003). *Guide to preventive services* (2nd ed.). (Publication No. 00-P046). Rockville, MD: Agency for Healthcare Research and Quality.

Utian, W. H. (1987). Overview on menopause. *American Journal of Obstetrics and Gynecology, 156,* 1280–1283.

Utian, W. (1999a). The International Menopause Society: Menopause-related terminology definitions. *Climacteric, 2,* 284–286.

Utian, W. H. (1999b). An historical perspective of natural and surgical menopause. *Menopause, 6*(2), 83–86.

Utian, W. H. (2001). Semantics, menopause-related terminology, and the STRAW reproductive aging staging system. *Menopause, 8*(6), 398–401.

van Meurs, J. B. J., Dhonukshe-Rutten, R. A. M., Pluijm, S. M. F., van der Klift, M., de Jonge, R., Lindemans, J., et al. (2004). Homocysteine levels and the risk of osteoporotic fracture. *New England Journal of Medicine, 350*(20), 2033–2041.

van Noord, P. A., Dubas, J. S., Dorland, M., Boersma, H., & te Velde, E. (1997). Age at natural menopause in a population-based screening cohort: The role of menarche, fecundity, and lifestyle factors. *Fertility & Sterility, 68*(1), 95–102.

Vivekananthan, D. P., Penn, M. S., Sapp, S. K., Hsu, A., & Topol, E. J. (2003). Use of antioxidant vitamins for the prevention of cardiovascular disease: Meta-analysis of randomized trials. *Lancet, 361*(9374), 2017–2023.

Weiss, N. S., Ure, C. L., Ballard, J. H., William, A. R., & Daling, J. R. (1980). Decreased risk of fractures of the hip and lower forearm with postmenopausal use of estrogen. *New England Journal of Medicine, 303,* 1195–1198.

Willhite, L. A. (2001). Urogenital atrophy: Prevention and treatment. *Pharmacotherapy, 21,* 464–480.

Wilmoth, M. C. (1996). The middle years: Women, sexuality, and the self. *Journal of Obstetric, Gynecologic, and Neonatal Nursing, 25*(7), 615–621.

Wilson, R. (1966). *Feminine forever.* New York: Evans.

Woods, N. F., & Mitchell, E. S. (1999). Anticipating menopause: Observations from the Seattle Midlife Women's Health Study. *Menopause, 6*(2), 167–173.

Wyon, Y., Lindgren, R., Lundberg, T., & Hammar, M. (1995). Effects of acupuncture on climacteric vasomotor symptoms, quality of life, and urinary excretion of neuropeptides among postmenopausal women. *Menopause, 2,* 3–12.

Wysocki, S., Alexander, I., Schnare, S. M., Moore, A., & Freeman, S. B. (2003). Individualized care for menopausal women: Counseling women about hormone therapy. *Women's Health Care: A Practical Journal for Nurse Practitioners, 2*(12), 8–16.

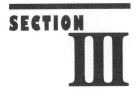

SECTION

III

WOMEN'S GYNECOLOGIC
HEALTH CARE MANAGEMENT

INTIMATE PARTNER VIOLENCE AND SEXUAL ASSAULT

DANIEL J. SHERIDAN

LINDA A. FERNANDES

ALIDA D. ALDEN

DAWN M. VAN PELT

JACQUELYN C. CAMPBELL

An overall goal of this textbook is to explore women's health from a feminist perspective. Most certainly, any woman who experiences intimate partner violence (IPV) and sexual assault, either by a stranger or someone known to her, has personally experienced a crime embedded in male power and control. Health care of women who report being assaulted needs to be thorough and objective, but does not need to be emotionally distant. Douglas and Olshaker (2001), a retired Federal Bureau of Investigation profiler and a forensic writer respectively, state that besides excellent medical care, caring and empathy are the two most important attributes to bring to the examination process.

Throughout this chapter, the word "patient" will be used much more frequently than the words "victim" or "survivor." The criminal justice system primarily uses the word "victim" when describing individuals who have experienced a reported assault. Community-based women's advocacy programs often refer to women who have experienced an assault as "survivors" to promote their empowerment. During discussions at the International Association of Forensic Nurses (IAFN) Annual Scientific Assembly held October 2004 in Chicago, Illinois, there was consensus among most of the IAFN leaders interviewed by the primary author of this chapter to use the word "patient" when discussing or documenting health care provided to individuals who report being assaulted. Clinicians are trained to provide care to patients, not to victims, nor to survivors. It is the language of our profession.

The IPV and sexually assaulted patients served by clinicians have been criminally victimized and, unless murdered in the process, are survivors of the assaults. However, clinicians providing forensic-related care to IPV and sexually assaulted patients should keep the boundaries between the criminal justice, advocacy, and health care systems separate. Clinicians need to provide excellent evidence-based patient care with caring and empathy.

INTIMATE PARTNER VIOLENCE

Health care providers working in primary care settings can be instrumental in providing comprehensive, ongoing assessments and intervention for patients abused in intimate relationships. Women seek primary health care for a variety of routine health issues, such as gynecologic and women's health care, contraception, and prenatal care. Primary care settings afford a unique opportunity for assessment of violence and abuse in the lives of all female patients because women are often seen in these settings for episodic health care, and often return for periodic health maintenance and routine screening (King, 1998).

Most women who are abused say that they have had some contact with the health care system either for a routine examination or for treatment of one of the long-term health problems associated with IPV. This section identifies the most common health consequences of living in intimate partner abusive relationships and highlights the importance of IPV screening and forensic documentation.

DEFINITIONS

The Centers for Disease Control and Prevention (CDC) define IPV as "an escalating pattern of abuse where one partner in an intimate relationship controls the other through force, intimidation, or threat of violence" (Saltzman, Fanslow, McMahon, & Shelley, 1999). IPV is actual or threatened physical, sexual, psychological, or emotional abuse, by a current or former spouse, dating partner, boyfriend, or girlfriend. Intimate partners can be of the same or opposite sex. Physical violence includes acts such as hitting, slapping, kicking, punching, shoving, strangulation, and injuries from weapons. Emotional abuse is characteristic of most abusive relationships and often precedes the use of physical violence (King, 1998). Emotional abuse includes yelling, screaming, name-calling, insulting comments, harassment, and public humiliation.

EPIDEMIOLOGY

In the National Violence Against Women Survey, cosponsored by the CDC and the National Institute of Justice, 25% of a nationally representative sample of 8,000 US women said an intimate partner had assaulted them at some time in their lives (Tjaden & Thoennes, 1998). Coker, Smith, McKeown, and King (2000) found that 55.1% of 1,401 women attending family practice clinics in Canada had experienced some type of violence at the hands of a male partner, and that 20.2% of participants were currently experiencing IPV. In prenatal settings, studies have identified the prevalence of abuse during pregnancy as ranging from 18.1% in a sample of adolescents and adult women (Parker, McFarlane & Soeken, 1994), to as high as 37.6% in a sample of pregnant adolescents (Curry, 1998).

HEALTH EFFECTS

Gynecologic and Chronic Health Conditions   Gynecologic problems are the most consistent, long-lasting, and widespread physical health problems experienced by women who are battered (Campbell, 2002). Increased rates of pelvic inflammatory disease (PID), heightened risks of sexually transmitted infections (STIs) including human immunodeficiency virus (HIV) and acquired immune deficiency syndrome (AIDS), unexplained vaginal bleeding, fibroids, pelvic pain, urinary tract infections, painful intercourse, decreased sexual desire, genital irritation, and other health problems that are genitourinary related have been documented for women who have been battered in several population-based heath care setting studies (Bergman & Brismar, 1991; Campbell et al., 2002; Campbell & Soeken, 1999; Chapman, 1989; Coker, Smith, Bethea, King, & McKeown, 2000; Ebby, Campbell, Sullivan, & Davidson, 1995; McCauley et al., 1995; Plichta, 1996; Plichta & Abraham, 1996). Anytime a woman presents with one or more of these gynecologic conditions, it is crucial she be screened for IPV. Additionally, women who are abused are at a significantly higher risk for chronic health problems such as neurologic, gastrointestinal, and chronic pain symptoms (Campbell, 2002; Campbell et al., 2002; Coker, Smith, Bethea, King, & McKeown; McCauley et al.; Plichta; Plichta & Abraham, 1996).

Mental Health Conditions   Post-traumatic stress disorder (PTSD) can occur when a person has experienced or witnessed a traumatic or life-threatening event. Repeated domestic assault is very traumatic and can lead to PTSD. Many IPV patients experience the four major criteria for diagnosing PTSD: (a) experiencing a traumatic event, (b) reexperiencing the traumatic event, (c) numbness and avoidance, and (d) hypervigilance (Woods & Campbell, 1993). Campbell (2002) reports that women who have been battered experience PTSD more frequently than women who have not been in a violent relationship.

Campbell (2002) states that women who have experienced PTSD may use drugs and alcohol as coping mechanisms to deal with certain symptoms of PTSD, namely, intrusion, avoidance, and hyperarousal. Substance abuse may also begin during the abusive relationship, as the woman seeks a way to escape the reality of her situation. Substance abuse creates additional problems for IPV patients because they are more likely to experience repeated patterns of partner abuse (Schornstein, 1997). In addition, it can often be difficult to find a women's shelter willing to admit a patient with a substance abuse problem. This creates difficulties when a clinician is assisting a woman to arrange a safety plan.

Depression is also commonly experienced by women who have been battered (Campbell, Kub, & Rose, 1996). Physical, emotional, and sexual abuse are strongly associated with depression (Hegarty, Gunn, Chondros, & Small, 2004). All women with depression should be screened for IPV, and all women experiencing IPV should be evaluated for depression.

SCREENING

Guidelines developed by an interdisciplinary team of health care experts in IPV recommend that women be screened for IPV in primary care settings during their periodic examinations, especially gynecologic visits, and at all visits for a new concern (Family Violence Prevention Fund, 1999). Providers should routinely consider IPV as a possible diagnosis for women who present with gynecologic problems, especially multiple problems, chronic stress-related symptoms, and central nervous system (CNS) symptoms. In addition to the effects of stress and mental distress, IPV patients usually present with physical health problems as well.

Most women who have been battered do not come to health care facilities with obvious trauma or injuries, although women who have been battered and who present to an emergency department usually have more injuries to the head, neck, face, thorax, breasts, and abdomen than women who have not been physically abused (Campbell, 2002). When there is a question of IPV, either past or present, it is important for clinicians to obtain a focused history and perform a systematic physical examination to assess the severity and timing of trauma, injuries, gynecologic conditions, CNS disorders, and chronic stress-related problems.

With a general understanding of the relationships and patterns associated with partner violence, the provider can begin to understand the development of stress-related illnesses and mental disorders in women who have been battered. When a woman presents for health care, symptoms can be very general and vague. These can include generalized concerns, such as unexplained pain or malaise. Clinicians often have preconceived notions that these women may have some other psychological disorder, or are perhaps displaying drug-seeking behaviors. Based on the authors' extensive clinical experiences, this behavior can many times be attributed to the woman's cry for help, or as an attempt to prove to her batterer that she is afflicted with some medical disorder as a way to prevent future violence or receive sympathy. For a variety of reasons, including fear of further abuse and embarrassment, an abused woman is not always up front about her abuse. Therefore, it is important for providers to identify signs of IPV.

THEORIES

Lenore Walker (1979) was the first researcher to recognize the patterns or cycles in abusive relationships. Walker developed a basic three-part cycle of violence theory to describe the patterns of violence that occur in IPV. The first part of the cycle is the tension-building phase, the second is the acute-battering incident, and the final phase is the calm or loving phase. The tension-building phase often includes verbal put-downs by the batterer, increased arguing, and in some cases the woman trying to appease her batterer. The acute battering phase can include sexual assault, hitting, kicking, strangulation, and use of weapons. During the calm phase, often referred to as the "honeymoon phase," the batterer may apologize, promise it will never happen again, or even deny the violence occurred. As time goes on, the calm phase may disappear altogether. As early as 1980, clinicians were beginning to recognize that women were often seeking treatment during the tension-building phase for stress-related symptoms or immediately after the battering phase for physical injuries (Schornstein, 1997).

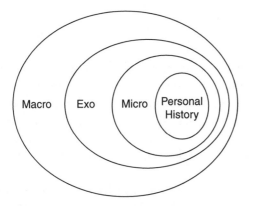

FIGURE 12-1   Heise's Framework of Violence *Source:* Reprinted by permission of Sage Publications, Inc. from Heise, L. L. (1998). Violence against women: An integrated, ecological framework. *Violence Against Women, 4*(3), 262–290.

While Walker's cycle of violence theory is useful in understanding some IPV situations, it is not viewed as the best model of IPV. To better understand the dynamics associated with the intimate partner cycle of violence, a brief discussion of Heise's (1998) framework of violence is helpful. Heise's theory is based on a social-ecological framework and includes the following four categories to describe factors that contribute to a violent relationship: personal history, microsystem, exosystem, and macrosystem. This framework is illustrated as four concentric circles with personal history in the center, followed outward by the micro-, exo-, and macrosystems (Figure 12–1).

The factors influencing the first category include personal history, witnessing marital violence as a child, being abused oneself as a child, and an absent or rejecting father. The second category, the microsystem, involves male dominance in the family, male control of wealth in the family, use of alcohol, and marital and verbal conflicts. The factors influencing the third category, the exosystem, or formal and informal social structures, are low socioeconomic status or unemployment, isolation of the woman and family, and delinquent peer associations. The fourth category, the macrosystem, encompasses the attitude and view of the public, includes male entitlement or ownership of women, masculinity linked to aggression and dominance, rigid gender roles, acceptance of interpersonal violence, and acceptance of physical chastisement (Heise, 1998). These factors can be attributed to both the batterer and the victim in some circumstances.

SCREENING TOOLS

Routine screening for IPV in clinical settings is no longer an option. It is viewed as a standard of care, with failure to screen and document one's findings grounds for litigation (Sheridan, 2003). In 1992 the American Medical Association published guidelines that indicates physicians must be willing to routinely ask all women about IPV and screen for abuse, because of the prevalence of IPV (Schroeder & Weber, 1998). The Surgeon Generals of the United States, and the public health objectives for *Healthy People 2000* and *2010*, have identified family violence as an epidemic, and have called for an organized approach to screen, treat, and prevent further violence (Poirier, 1997).

There are numerous reliable and valuable IPV screening tools that are effective in a variety of clinical settings. Versions of the Abuse Assessment Screen (AAS) are the screening tools used most often in published research (Helton, 1987; McFarlane, Greenberg, Weltge, & Watson, 1995; McFarlane, Parker, Soeken, & Bullock, 1992; Parker & McFarlane, 1991; Soeken, McFarlane, Parker, & Lominack, 1998). Helton developed the original nine-question AAS (Table 12–1) in an effort to determine if a link existed between IPV health effects on women and fetal health.

Six, then three, and then two-question versions of the AAS have been tested with good reliability and validity (Parker & McFarlane, 1991; McFarlane et al., 1992; McFarlane et al., 1995, respectively) (Tables 12–2, 12–3, and 12–4, respectively). Based on extensive clinical experiences, the primary author of this chapter prefers to use a six-question version of the AAS, with a preface that generalizes violence in society, and the fact that all patients are routinely screened. With any "yes" answer on any IPV screen, the primary author recommends the interviewer respond with the following: "Thank you for sharing. Can you give me an example? When was the last time?"

TABLE 12–1 Original 9-Question Abuse Assessment Screen

1. Do you know where you would go or who could help you if you were abused or worried about abuse?

   Yes _____ No _____

   If yes, where _____

2. Are you in a relationship with a man who physically hurts you?

   Yes _____ No _____ Sometimes _____

3. Does he threaten you with abuse?

   Yes _____ No _____ Sometimes _____

4. Has the man you are with hit, slapped, kicked, or otherwise physically hurt you?

   Yes _____ No _____ Sometimes _____

5. If yes, has he hit you since you've been pregnant?

   Yes _____ No _____ Sometimes _____

6. If yes, did the abuse increase since you've been pregnant?

   Yes _____ No _____ Sometimes _____

7. Have you ever received medical treatment for any abuse injuries?

   Yes _____ No _____ Sometimes _____

8. If you have been abused, remembering the last time he hurt you, mark the places on the body map where he hit you (see map in Figure 12–2).

9. Were you pregnant at the time?

   Yes _____ No _____ Not Applicable _____

Source: Reprinted with permission from the Nursing Research Consortium on Violence and Abuse. Adapted from Helton, 1987.

**MARK THE AREA OF INJURY ON THE BODY MAP. SCORE EACH INCIDENT
ACCORDING TO THE FOLLOWING SCALE:**

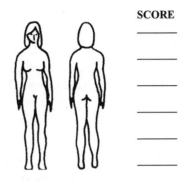

SCORE

1 = Threats of abuse including use of a weapon   _____

2 = Slapping, pushing; no injuries and/or lasting pain   _____

3 = Punching, kicking, bruises, cuts and/or continuing pain   _____

4 = Beating up, severe contusions, burns, broken bones   _____

5 = Head injury, internal injury, permanent injury   _____

6 = Use of weapon; wound from weapon   _____

If any of the descriptions for the higher number apply, use the higher number.

FIGURE 12–2   Body Map. *Source:* Reprinted with permission from the Nursing Research Consortium on Violence and Abuse. Adapted from Parker & McFarlane, 1991.

TABLE 12–2   Six-Question Abuse Assessment Screen

1. When you and your partner argue, are you ever afraid of him (her)?

2. When you and your partner verbally argue, do you think he (she) tries to emotionally hurt/abuse you?

3. Does your partner try to control you? Where you go? Who you see? How much money you can have?

4. Has your partner (or anyone) ever slapped you, pushed you, hit you, kicked you, or otherwise physically hurt you?

5. Since you have been pregnant (when you were pregnant), has your partner ever hit you, slapped you, pushed you, hit you, kicked you, or otherwise physically hurt you?

6. Has your partner ever forced you into sex when you did not want to participate?

Source: Reprinted with permission from the Nursing Research Consortium on Violence and Abuse. Adapted from Parker & McFarlane, 1991.

TABLE 12–3   Three-Question Abuse Assessment Screen

1. Within the last year have you been hit, slapped, kicked, or otherwise physically hurt by someone?

   a. Yes _____

   b. No _____

   If YES, by whom? _____

   Total number of times _____

2. Since you have been pregnant, have you been hit, slapped, kicked, or otherwise physically hurt by someone?

   a. Yes _____

   b. No _____

   If YES, by whom? _____

   Total number of times _____

3. Within the last year has anyone forced you to have sexual activities?

   a. Yes _____

   b. No _____

   If YES, by whom? _____

   Total number of times _____

Source: Reprinted with permission from the Nursing Research Consortium on Violence and Abuse. Adapted from McFarlane, Parker, Soeken, & Bullock, 1992.

TABLE 12–4   Two-Question Abuse Assessment Screen

1. Have you ever been hit, slapped, kicked, or otherwise physically hurt by your male partner?

2. Have you ever been forced to have sexual activities?

Source: Reprinted with permission from the Nursing Research Consortium on Violence and Abuse. Adapted from McFarlane, Greenberg, Weltge, & Watson, 1995.

The three-question AAS (McFarlane et al., 1992) is probably the most widely used IPV screen. However, it does not include questions about being afraid of one's partner, nor about being emotionally abused or controlled. It is very common to hear from women who have been battered that the pain and scars from being emotionally abused take longer to heal than the pain of physical abuse. Therefore, the clinical pressures to keep IPV screens short have to be weighed against failing to assess the significant emotional abuse and fear of a partner that could be linked to an increased risk of intimate partner homicide.

Many providers are reluctant to screen for IPV because they are uncertain as to what to do with a "yes" response (Sheridan, 2003). Patients who give a positive response to being involved in ongoing IPV need to complete Campbell's Danger Assessment (DA, Table 12–5) and Sheridan's Harassment in Abusive Relationships: A Self-report Scale (HARASS, Table 12–6) tools. All of the items on these screening tools have been linked to an increased risk of domestic homicide. The DA is best completed in conjunction

TABLE 12-5   Danger Assessment

DANGER ASSESSMENT

Jacquelyn C. Campbell, Ph.D., R.N.
Copyright, 2003

Several risk factors have been associated with increased risk of homicides (murders) of women and men in violent relationships. We cannot predict what will happen in your case, but we would like you to be aware of the danger of homicide in situations of abuse and for you to see how many of the risk factors apply to your situation.

Using the calendar, please mark the approximate dates during the past year when you were abused by your partner or ex partner. Write on that date how bad the incident was according to the following scale:
1. Slapping, pushing; no injuries and/or lasting pain
2. Punching, kicking; bruises, cuts, and/or continuing pain
3. "Beating up"; severe contusions, burns, broken bones
4. Threat to use weapon; head injury, internal injury, permanent injury
5. Use of weapon; wounds from weapon

(If **any** of the descriptions for the higher number apply, use the higher number.)

Mark **Yes** or **No** for each of the following. ("He" refers to your husband, partner, ex-husband, ex-partner, or whoever is currently physically hurting you.)

_____   1.   Has the physical violence increased in severity or frequency over the past year?
_____   2.   Does he own a gun?
_____   3.   Have you left him after living together during the past year?
            3a. (If have *never* lived with him, check here___)
_____   4.   Is he unemployed?
_____   5.   Has he ever used a weapon against you or threatened you with a lethal weapon?
            (If yes, was the weapon a gun?____)
_____   6.   Does he threaten to kill you?
_____   7.   Has he avoided being arrested for domestic violence?
_____   8.   Do you have a child that is not his?
_____   9.   Has he ever forced you to have sex when you did not wish to do so?
_____   10.   Does he ever try to choke you?
_____   11.   Does he use illegal drugs? By drugs, I mean "uppers" or amphetamines, speed, angel dust, cocaine, "crack", street drugs or mixtures.
_____   12.   Is he an alcoholic or problem drinker?
_____   13.   Does he control most or all of your daily activities? For instance: does he tell you who you can be friends with, when you can see your family, how much money you can use, or when you can take the car? (If he tries, but you do not let him, check here: ____)
_____   14.   Is he violently and constantly jealous of you? (For instance, does he say "If I can't have you, no one can.")
_____   15.   Have you ever been beaten by him while you were pregnant? (If you have never been pregnant by him, check here: ____)
_____   16.   Have you ever threatened or tried to commit suicide?
_____   17.   Has he ever threatened or tried to commit suicide?
_____   18.   Does he threaten to harm your children?
_____   19.   Do you believe he is capable of killing you?
_____   20.   Does he follow or spy on you, leave threatening notes or messages on answering machine, destroy your property, or call you when you don't want him to?

_____   Total "Yes" Answers

**Thank you. Please talk to your nurse, advocate or counselor about
what the Danger Assessment means in terms of your situation.**

Source: Reprinted with permission of Jacquelyn C. Campbell, PhD, RN.

TABLE 12–6 HARASS

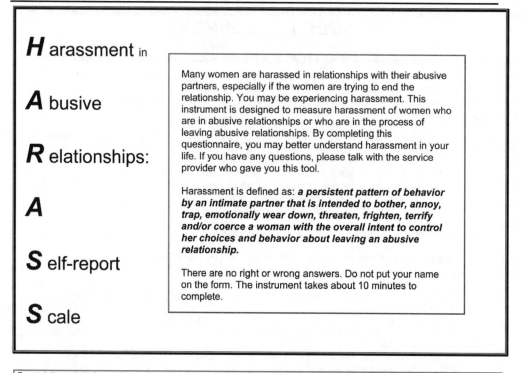

H arassment in

A busive

R elationships:

A

S elf-report

S cale

Many women are harassed in relationships with their abusive partners, especially if the women are trying to end the relationship. You may be experiencing harassment. This instrument is designed to measure harassment of women who are in abusive relationships or who are in the process of leaving abusive relationships. By completing this questionnaire, you may better understand harassment in your life. If you have any questions, please talk with the service provider who gave you this tool.

Harassment is defined as: *a persistent pattern of behavior by an intimate partner that is intended to bother, annoy, trap, emotionally wear down, threaten, frighten, terrify and/or coerce a woman with the overall intent to control her choices and behavior about leaving an abusive relationship.*

There are no right or wrong answers. Do not put your name on the form. The instrument takes about 10 minutes to complete.

For each item, circle the number that best describes how often the behavior occurred. Next, rate how distressing the behavior is to you. If the behavior has never occurred, circle 0 (NEVER) and go to the next question. If the question does not apply to you, circle NA (NOT APPLICABLE). If you are still in the relationship please circle below MY PARTNER. If you have left the relationship, please circle below MY FORMER PARTNER.

THE BEHAVIOR MY PARTNER MY FORMER PARTNER (circle one)	0 = Never 1 = Rarely 2 = Occasionally 3 = Frequently 4 = Very Frequently NA = Not applicable **How often does it occur?**	0 = Not at all distressing 1 = Slightly distressing 2 = Moderately distressing 3 = Very distressing 4 = Extremely distressing NA = Not applicable **How distressing is this behavior to you?**
1. Frightens people close to me	0 1 2 3 4 NA	0 1 2 3 4 NA
2. Pretends to be someone else in order to get to me	0 1 2 3 4 NA	0 1 2 3 4 NA
3. Comes to my home when I don't want him there	0 1 2 3 4 NA	0 1 2 3 4 NA
4. Threatens to kill me if I leave or stay away from him	0 1 2 3 4 NA	0 1 2 3 4 NA
5. Threatens to harm the kids if I leave or stay away from him	0 1 2 3 4 NA	0 1 2 3 4 NA
6. Takes things that belong to me so I have to see him to get them back	0 1 2 3 4 NA	0 1 2 3 4 NA
7. Tries getting me fired from my job	0 1 2 3 4 NA	0 1 2 3 4 NA
8. Ignores court orders to stay away from me	0 1 2 3 4 NA	0 1 2 3 4 NA
9. Keeps showing up wherever I am	0 1 2 3 4 NA	0 1 2 3 4 NA
10. Bothers me at work when I don't want to talk to him	0 1 2 3 4 NA	0 1 2 3 4 NA
11. Uses the kids as pawns to get me physically close to him	0 1 2 3 4 NA	0 1 2 3 4 NA
12. Shows up without warning	0 1 2 3 4 NA	0 1 2 3 4 NA

TABLE 12–6   continued

THE BEHAVIOR	0 = Never 1 = Rarely 2 = Occasionally 3 = Frequently 4 = Very Frequently NA = Not applicable	0 = Not at all distressing 1 = Slightly distressing 2 = Moderately distressing 3 = Very distressing 4 = Extremely distressing NA = Not applicable
MY PARTNER MY FORMER PARTNER (circle one)	How often does it occur?	How distressing is this behavior to you?
13. Messes with my property (For example: sells my stuff, breaks my furniture, damages my car, steals my things)	0 1 2 3 4 NA	0 1 2 3 4 NA
14. Scares me with a weapon	0 1 2 3 4 NA	0 1 2 3 4 NA
15. Breaks into my home	0 1 2 3 4 NA	0 1 2 3 4 NA
16. Threatens to kill me if I leave or stay away from him	0 1 2 3 4 NA	0 1 2 3 4 NA
17. Makes me feel like he can again force me into sex	0 1 2 3 4 NA	0 1 2 3 4 NA
18. Threatens to snatch or have the kids taken away from me	0 1 2 3 4 NA 0 1 2 3 4 NA	0 1 2 3 4 NA 0 1 2 3 4 NA
19. Sits in his car outside my home	0 1 2 3 4 NA	0 1 2 3 4 NA
20. Leaves me threatening messages (for example: puts scary notes in the car, sends me threatening letters, sends me threats through family and friends, leaves threatening messages on the telephone answering machine)		
21. Threatens to harm our pet	0 1 2 3 4 NA	0 1 2 3 4 NA
22. Calls me on the telephone and hangs up	0 1 2 3 4 NA	0 1 2 3 4 NA
23. Reports me to the authorities for taking drugs when I don't.	0 1 2 3 4 NA	0 1 2 3 4 NA
Additional harassing behaviors not listed above:		
24. _____	0 1 2 3 4 NA	0 1 2 3 4 NA
25. _____	0 1 2 3 4 NA	0 1 2 3 4 NA

Please answer a few additional questions:

_____ Your age in years

Check the statement that best describes you:

__ Married, living with an abusive partner

__ Single, living with an abusive partner

__ Married, living apart from an abusive partner

__ Single, living apart from an abusive partner.

How long were you in the above relationship? _____

Are you still in the relationship?   __ Yes __ No

If you have left the relationship, how long have you been out? _____

What is your approximate annual income? _____

How many years of school have you completed? _____

Check the statement that best describes you:

__ Asian / Pacific Islander

__ Black/African American

__ Caucasian/White

__ Hispanic

__ Native American/American Indian

__ Other _____

Source: Reprinted with permission of Daniel J. Sheridan, PhD, RN.

*The HARASS instrument can be used without copyright permission in any clinical setting. Anyone interested in using the HARASS instrument in a research project is requested to contact the author at dsheridan@son.jhmi.edu.

with a calendar that serves as a prompt to remind women of abusive events around certain dates. The DA and HARASS take about five to ten minutes each to complete. They are self-report scales that can be completed by the patient. Both instruments can be read to patients who are illiterate, have language barriers, or are unable to read secondary to the nature of their injuries.

While the DA has some preliminary data to suggest cut-off scores related to risk of homicide, the DA and HARASS are best used as guides to structure safety planning. In general, the more "yes" responses on the DA tool, and the more positive responses to some form of harassment, the more dangerous and potentially deadly the relationship.

HISTORY

Interviewing women about IPV requires that questioning be done in a sympathetic and nonjudgmental manner. Not only is this approach therapeutic, but it can also signal that someone is interested, that the woman is not alone, and that there is a safe place in which she can talk about the problem, if and when she wishes to do so. Express the belief that violence is not acceptable, no matter what she has been told by the batterer. Privacy and confidentiality must be guaranteed when asking questions about IPV. The most effective means of obtaining the history of abuse is to use a communication model that allows the woman to talk about the problem from her perspective, without interruption, and with enough time to relate, emphasize, and even repeat her full story (Campbell, McKenna, Torres, Sheridan, & Landenburger, 1993).

Another issue for consideration by clinicians when interviewing women about IPV is the presence of their children. IPV screening in front of children raises a variety of safety concerns. If the child talks afterward to the perpetrator about the disclosure of IPV to the clinician, it may result in retaliation for the patient, such as further abuse or prohibiting further contact with the clinician. In addition, the child may be exposed to new information or retraumatized by painful memories (Zink & Jacobson, 2003). Guidelines in the literature support that screening in front of children older than three years of age should be done only with prior permission from the mother, or with only general IPV screening questions and sensitivity to the mother's nonverbal behaviors and comfort (Zink & Jacobson, 2003). General questions should avoid charged words such as "hit," "hurt," "harm," and "afraid." Clinicians need to be sensitive to the unique privacy, safety, and protection issues of mothers who are survivors of IPV.

PHYSICAL EXAMINATION

The physical examination of women suspected of being abused or battered should be conducted as any other physical assessment of an adult female. Careful attention must be directed to any signs of injury, past and present, with exact measurement taken of even the most insignificant-looking bruise (Campbell, McKenna, Torres, Sheridan, & Landenburger, 1993). Because most injuries are to the face, chest, breasts, and abdomen, special attention should be paid to these areas. The general examination of the woman should include observations about her behavior as well as physical appearance.

Offer all patients with visible injuries photographic documentation in the medical record after obtaining consent to photograph (Sheridan, 2003). There are a few principles of forensic photography that should be followed when using any photographic system. The first photograph needs to be a facial image of the patient as an identifier (Sheridan). Photographs of each injured area need to be taken in a series from furthest away (about six feet), to a middle distance (about four feet), to close up (about two feet) (Sheridan). There should be a scale in each photograph to assist in determining the relative size of the injury. If a scale used in the photograph shields any part of the body, an additional photograph is needed of the part of the body without the scale. The photograph should be labeled on the back with a white adhesive label that includes the patient's name, date of birth, hospital chart or number, date of photograph, body part location, and the photographer's name.

Using body maps and diagrams is also recommended to accurately portray the patient's physical condition. Body maps provide pictoral diagrams of all body surfaces, including separate diagrams for external genitalia, vagina, cervix, anus, and rectum. Areas of injury should be drawn on the body maps or diagrams of the corresponding location. A description of the injury should be included with each drawing.

DOCUMENTATION

It is critical that the provider accurately document her or his findings in the patient's record using the correct medical forensic terms. Misuse of common forensic terms in the medical record can lead to questioning the overall accuracy and competence of the provider should legal proceedings ensue. The terms "laceration," "ecchymosis," and "hematoma" are among the most commonly misused medical forensic terms (Brockmeyer & Sheridan, 1998; Campbell & Sheridan, 2004; Sheridan, 2001; Sheridan, 2003). A laceration is a tear in the skin or organ caused by blunt or shearing force trauma, while a cut or incision is sharp injury caused by the cutting of skin or an organ with a sharp object such as a scalpel, razor, or knife. Ecchymoses are not bruises, but rather discolorations under the skin from a leakage or oozing of blood. Ecchymoses are not caused directly by blunt force trauma. A bruise or contusion is bleeding under the skin or organ caused by trauma. A hematoma is a collection of blood that can be caused by blunt force trauma or by spontaneous bleeding. Do not use hematoma as a synonym for bruise.

The following is a useful summary of the correct usage of common terms:

- Bruise can be used interchangeably with contusion.
- Laceration is related to a partial avulsion.

- Ecchymosis is related to (senile) purpura.
- Petechia is related to purpura.
- "Rug burn" is more accurately described as a friction abrasion.
- "Incision" can be used interchangeably with "cut."
- "Cut" can be used interchangeably with "sharp injury."
- Stab wounds are penetrating, deep, sharp injuries.
- Hematoma is a collection of blood that is often, but not always, caused by blunt force trauma (Campbell & Sheridan, 2004, p. 77).

Documentation in the medical record of IPV histories needs to be as thorough and objective as possible. When quoting the patient, the provider should use such words as "states," "says," and "reports," instead of "claims" or "alleges," which can be interpreted to mean that the patient is not a credible historian (Sheridan, 2003). If a patient gives an extremely informative and powerful statement concerning the reported abuse, quote it directly in the progress note. Avoid biased documentation by avoiding words or phrases like "refuses," "uncooperative," or "noncompliant." For example, do not chart: "Patient refused to talk with the police." Instead chart: "Patient said she did not want to talk with the police."

MANAGEMENT

Clinical interventions for IPV patients should be based on four important principles: empowerment, childbearing cycle-stage specificity, abuse-stage specificity, and cultural competence (Campbell & Campbell, 1996). Abusers take power and control away from victims by isolating them from the people and information that can help them make thoughtful choices. Therefore, it is crucial that clinicians use an empowerment model of offering information, options, and support. Clinicians must not judge an abused woman's choices, nor use any kind of tactics to get her to cooperate. An empowerment model should include the information given in the following list. Use the mnemonic device of EMPOWER to help remember these items:

- **E**mpathic listening
- **M**aking time to properly document
- **P**roviding information about domestic violence (including in later life)
- **O**ffering options and choices
- **W**orking with a domestic abuse specialist (including elder domestic abuse)
- **E**ncouraging planning for safety and support
- **R**eferring to local services (Brandl & Raymond, 1997, p. 65)

Women in ongoing abusive relationships choose to return to the abusive home for many reasons. Prior to leaving the provider's office, all patients need to know where they can find an IPV hotline and shelter information. Wallet-sized referral cards and information posters with tear-off numbers have been effective ways for women who have been abused to access helpful numbers in a manner more easily hidden from perpetrators (Sheridan & Taylor, 1993). Abused patients need to be shown the pages of telephone books that list hotline and shelter-referral numbers. The employees and volunteers who staff the IPV hotlines and women's service programs are experts at safety planning, and should be called not only by the victims of abuse, but also by providers for guidance.

Minimum safety planning by a provider should include a brief discussion about having the patient pack an emergency bag containing some money, clothing for the patient and her children, copies of bank records, immunization records, birth certificates, and protective legal orders. Patients should be encouraged to call the police *before* actual abuse occurs, and most definitely after any abusive act (Sheridan, 2003). Finally, every abused patient should be encouraged to use any 24-hour health setting as a safety net if she does not have access to any other safe place (Sheridan).

SPECIAL POPULATIONS

Pregnant Women   Many think of pregnancy as a time of celebration and planning for the unborn child's future. However, health professionals have known for years that pregnancy can be a time of escalating violence in an already troubled relationship (Campbell, 1989; Campbell & Alford, 1989; McFarlane et al., 1992). Bohn and Parker (1993) report that violence during pregnancy affects more women than hypertension, gestational diabetes, or almost any other serious antepartum complication. On the other hand, pregnancy can provide a period of protection for some women who suffer the ill effects of IPV (Fagen, Stewart, & Hanson, 1983; Stacey & Schupe, 1983). Despite this period of protection during pregnancy, women need to be aware that the abuse may resume, and the implications this can have for her and the child born into the abusive relationship (Campbell, Oliver, & Bullock, 1993). Even if the violence does not escalate, but continues at the rate prior to pregnancy, there are negative health effects associated with the violence for both the woman and her unborn fetus.

Complications associated with abuse during pregnancy can be the result of trauma or side effects of the psychological or controlling effects of the abuse. Mechanisms of injury are related to direct trauma to the pregnant abdomen, leading to premature labor due to rupture of membranes, placental abruption, and uterine rupture. Abusive environments are associated with indirect mechanisms leading to low birth weight infants. Women in abusive situations are more likely than women not in abusive relationships to use alcohol, nicotine, prescription, over-the-counter, and illicit drugs to help deal with the stress (Curry, 1998). Low birth weight may also be due to poor maternal weight gain, anemia, an unhealthy diet, STIs, and lack of social support, all stemming from the effects of stress related to an abusive relationship. Through these mechanisms, Murphy and colleagues (2001) state that abuse should be recognized as a factor contributing to low birth weight infants.

Adolescents   All young women should be routinely questioned about IPV during health encounters because one out of every eight adolescents will be involved in some form of dating violence (Furniss, 1998). Dating violence results in serious and negative health outcomes, with lifelong implications for adolescent victims, including depression, unhealthy weight control behavior, sexually risky behavior, and substance abuse (Coker, Smith, Bethea, King, & McKeown, 2000; Sells & Blum, 1996; Silverman, Raj, Mucci, & Hathaway, 2001). Plichta (1996) reported that rates of depression, eating disorders, and drug, alcohol, and tobacco use were more than twice as high in girls who reported physical or sexual dating violence than in girls who had not been abused.

The simple act of asking adolescents in a private and safe location about dating violence victimization and perpetration may be an important initial step toward effective intervention and prevention strategies. Questioning teenagers in a family planning clinic, emergency department, or pediatric setting about jealous or possessive partners could provide clues to the existence of dating violence. Teenagers are often uncomfortable disclosing violence to a health care provider and may present with headaches, weight loss, or other somatic clues that may signal distress (Furniss, 1998). Because many adolescents accept physical and sexual aggression as normal in dating and partner relationships, clinicians can be invaluable in providing an alternative view by talking with them about types of behavior that are appropriate in an intimate relationship.

Older Women   Family violence involving the elderly has been addressed by laws in all 50 states requiring the reporting of elder or vulnerable person abuse (Fulmer & Wetle, 1986). Providers are mandated by law to report a case if there is reasonable cause to suspect that an elderly patient has been the victim of abuse, neglect, or mistreatment. Estimates suggest that 500,000 to 1.5 million cases of elder abuse and neglect occur annually in the United States (Brandl, 1997; Jogerst, Daly, Brinig, Dawson, Schmuch, & Ingran, 2003). Accurate detection and assessment of elder abuse patients are critical duties of all clinicians, especially those in ambulatory care settings.

IPV affects women of all ages, but often the literature focuses on women in the childbearing years, ignoring the unique problems of aging women who are experiencing IPV. Often elder abuse and mistreatment is viewed from an inadequate care perspective, and this view obscures important issues. Some forms of elder abuse and mistreatment are from inadequate care and are rooted in the dynamics of caregiving. Other forms of elder abuse and mistreatment, especially physical assaults, are in fact, domestic violence (Phillips, 2000). Also, it makes unclear the gender issues and power dynamics inherent in IPV as they apply to older women. Serious physical and emotional harm, and even death, may result from wife or partner abuse at any age, but among older women, because of their physical vulnerability that increases with age, even so-called "low-severity violence" can cause serious injury or death (Phillips).

Although injury may be the reason an older woman seeks health care, it is important to remember that the physical and mental sequelae of IPV could be more subtle, including depression, sleeplessness, chronic pain, atypical chest pain, and other kinds of somatic symptoms (Phillips, 2000). Cognitively impaired or unresponsive elderly women require that the clinician assess for nonverbal cues and focus assessment on the caregiver. Characteristics of batterers that might trigger suspicion include showing possessiveness and jealousy of the victim, denying or minimizing the seriousness of the violence, refusing to take responsibility for the violence, and holding a rigid view of sex roles, or negative attitudes toward women.

Influences of Culture   Cultural awareness is the process that allows the provider to interact sensitively with persons from other cultures. It requires self-examination for biases and prejudices toward other cultures, and assists the clinician in avoiding cultural imposition or the tendency to impose one's own beliefs, values, and patterns of behavior on persons from other cultures (Campbell & Campbell, 1996). Cultural skill is a process in which the provider learns how to assess the woman's cultural values, beliefs, and practices without solely relying on written "facts" about a specific cultural group. It enables the provider to learn systematically from the woman her perception of her situation and what she believes can be done about it (Campbell & Campbell).

The IPV patient may assume that a clinician from a majority ethnic group will further stigmatize her or her whole cultural group if the clinician learns of the family violence. Women of color who have been battered may be particularly afraid that a clinician from another ethnic group will call the police, who have historically physically assaulted men of minority ethnic groups (Campbell & Campbell, 1996). Further, women of color who have been battered may consider IPV to be a relatively unimportant issue in comparison to a serious health problem or issues of economic survival (Campbell & Campbell). Minority cultural groups often perceive IPV to be merely an outgrowth of other community problems, such as joblessness, prejudice, or substance abuse. They may consider IPV not a particularly important problem in comparison to others, or one not to be addressed in isolation (Campbell & Campbell). The IPV patient may not see the health care provider as one who understands the complexities of family violence in her cultural context, and therefore may prefer that the clinician concentrate on other areas of care (Campbell & Campbell).

When the clinician does not speak the primary language of the patient, assessing and intervening in the area of IPV may become very difficult. To ensure that there is not a breakdown in communication, clinicians should ask the meaning of unfamiliar words. This demonstrates a willingness to learn and appreciate cultural nuances rather than pretending such differences do not exist or are related to a lack of education (Campbell & Campbell, 1996). The clinician must learn to listen with a sensitive ear and must accept the challenges and rewards inherent in effective cultural communications as the patient from a different ethnic group discloses her experiences.

SEXUAL ASSAULT

Sexual violence is a crime that crosses all races and spans all ages. Clinicians in primary care settings may provide the initial or follow-up examination, treatment, and support for sexual assault patients. This section describes a systematic approach to the care of women who have been sexually assaulted and draws attention to the frequency of intimate partner sexual violence.

DEFINITIONS

Sexual violence is committed by an intimate or nonintimate perpetrator such as a spouse, family member, person in position of power or trust, friend, acquaintance, or stranger. Note that there are no standardized clinical definitions for such terms as "sexual abuse" and "sexual assault," and legal definitions often vary from state to state. The legal definitions of rape and penetration typically involve: (1) forced sexual intercourse; (2) psychological coercion, verbal threats, and physical force; and (3) lack of consent (Bureau of Justice Statistics, 1995). A commonly used clinical definition of sexual assault, and the one that will be used for this chapter, defines sexual assault as penetration of the vagina, oral cavity, or anus, occurring with the penis, fingers, or foreign objects, to both females and males, between marriage partners, persons of the same gender, acquaintances, and strangers (Burgess, Fehder & Hartman, 1995; Kempthorne, 2001).

EPIDEMIOLOGY

Sexual assault represented 6.3% of all violent crimes reported in the United States during 2001 (US Census Bureau, 2003). There were 90,000 forcible rapes reported in 2001 in the United States, although sexual assault is well-known to be underreported (US Census Bureau). A 1996 National Violence Against Women telephone survey of 8,000 women aged 18 years or older, found that 17.6% of women reported being raped in their lifetime, and 74% of the women who had been sexually assaulted knew their assailant (McConkey, Sole, & Holcomb, 2001).

INTIMATE PARTNER SEXUAL VIOLENCE

Clinicians should not ignore the possibility of marital sexual assault during the examination of female patients. Approximately 10–14% of all married women, and at least 40% of battered wives in the United States, have been sexually assaulted by their husbands (Campbell & Alford, 1989). Despite advances in women's rights, archaic attitudes of women and wives as possessions persist. The emotional and psychological trauma of spousal sexual assault can be more devastating because trust, the most basic marital bond, is shattered (Dupre, Hampton, Morrison, & Meeks, 1993). Spousal sexual assault is often more violent, repetitive, and less commonly reported, because of economic considerations as well as the humiliation and sense of marital failure that may accompany this form of sexual violence (Dupre et al.). Marital sexual assault meets the legal criteria for criminal sexual conduct in most states, but unfortunately, because the rapist and victim are married, the rapist is immune from prosecution in some states.

   A US population-based study of self-reported data found the odds of having a gynecologic problem were three times higher for IPV patients (McCauley et al., 1995). Gynecologic health problems could stem from forced anal, vaginal, or other abusive sex practices, such as unsafe sex by partners outside of the relationship (Campbell et al., 2002; Ebby et al., 1995). Forced sex has been defined in the literature as sexual activity that includes unwanted roughness, painful, or particular sexual acts; threatened violence if sexual demands are not met; actual beatings prior, during, or after sex; and painful sex by penetration with objects (Campbell & Alford, 1989). The results of two different empirical studies reported an estimated 40–45% of all women experiencing IPV are forced to have sex by their male partners (Campbell, 1989; Campbell & Soeken, 1999; Finkelhor & Yllo, 1997). An additional smaller percentage of women are sexually abused by their intimate partner without any physical abuse (Campbell; Campbell & Soeken).

Providers should explore the possibility of sexual assault or forced sexual intercourse for all women presenting with gynecologic symptoms. This is especially true for women who present with multiple or persistent gynecologic symptoms. Campbell et al. (2002) found that 30% of women who were sexually abused as an adult, either with or without other forms of physical abuse, reported three or more gynecologic health problems, compared with 8% of women who experienced only physical abuse, and 6% of those never abused. Asking a patient about forced sex from her partner or her partner's sexual practices has to be conducted in a very professional, nonjudgmental, caring, sensitive manner, and in a private and safe environment. Women are often too embarrassed or afraid to volunteer such information, or they may not link their health problems to the abuse in their lives.

SCREENING

Numerous barriers exist that could cause a patient to delay reporting sexual assault. Delays can be hours, days, weeks, months, or years. Barriers to reporting include fear of retaliation by the assailant, self-blaming, feeling humiliated, or inability to remember details of the assault due to drugs or alcohol. The usual legal time limit for collection of evidence is 72 hours from the time of the assault (Groleau & Jackson, 2001). However, there are a growing number of anecdotal clinical cases in which DNA evidence has been found during a sexual assault examination well beyond 72 hours. Because of this, the State of Maryland Crime Lab recently released a memo recommending sexual assault examinations be conducted up to 120 hours following a vaginal assault. If more than 72 hours (or up to 120 hours) have passed since the assault, a complete physical examination should still be conducted to examine the patient for injuries to the body and the genitalia, and to assess for emotional and psychological injuries (Groleau & Jackson).

The following description of the sexual assault evidentiary examination will primarily focus on the areas of the examination that all practitioners would want to perform, regardless of whether evidence collection with a "sexual assault kit" will be completed. This would include acute events of sexual assault as well as those situations in which there has been a delay in reporting. Ideally, the forensic evidentiary examination should be completed by a trained Sexual Assault Nurse Examiner (SANE); however, for numerous reasons, this is not always feasible. It should be noted that the collection of evidence such as clothing, swabs, hair combings, and foreign debris is not applicable if the facility or clinic is not able to maintain a "chain of custody." Chain of custody means handling the evidence in a way that is accurately documented, so as to establish and safeguard the integrity and competence of the evidence (Brockmeyer & Sheridan, 1998). The clinician must demonstrate that the gathering, preservation, sealing, and storage of collected evidence were done in a manner that prevents tampering. Chain of custody requires that the evidence collected be stored in a locked or secured cabinet or closet (Brockmeyer & Sheridan).

Regardless of whether evidence is collected, practitioners will always want to document a detailed history, perform a complete physical and pelvic examination, provide injury documentation either through photographs or the use of body maps, provide treatment and follow-up for pregnancy and STIs, and provide the necessary care or referral for psychosocial issues (Brockmeyer & Sheridan, 1998). Consent should be obtained from the sexual assault patient during each step of the medical investigation, including the history, physical examination, evidence collection, and photography (Petter & Whitehill, 1998). Asking consent for each aspect of the examination serves to help assaulted patients regain control and establish trust between the clinician and the patient.

HISTORY

Obtaining a history from a sexual assault patient requires collecting specific and detailed information with attention to the location and manner of the interview. Provide a quiet and private environment. Listen carefully, do not hurry, and do not place blame—the provider should remain objective throughout the examination. A tailored medical history should include the following information:

- Age and identifying information for both the patient and the reported assailant (if available)
- Date, time, and location of the reported assault
- Circumstances of the assault
- Details of the sexual contact—whether it was penile, digital, or object penetration of the vagina, oral cavity, or anus—as well as documentation of any ejaculation or urination by the assailant
- Type of physical restraint used, such as weapons, drugs, or alcohol
- Activities of the patient after the assault, such as change of clothing, bathing, douching, dental hygiene, urination, or defecation
- Focused gynecologic history—last menstrual period, contraceptive use, pregnancy history, last voluntary sexual encounter, and any recent episode of gynecologic infection or pelvic surgery (Petter & Whitehill, 1998)

PHYSICAL EXAMINATION

The purpose of the physical examination is twofold: to assess the woman for physical injuries, and to collect evidence for the forensic evaluation. Physical examination and evidence collection are done congruently. However, evidence collection can only be completed if within the 72 to 120 hour time frame and, in some jurisdictions, only if the case is reported to law enforcement. The clinician should be familiar with the guidelines within her or his state and jurisdiction. In addition to the clinician, the police and an advocate for the victim may be present during the evidentiary examination. Standardized sexual assault kits are available from state police crime labs, emergency departments, and sometimes from state attorneys' offices.

Evidence collection, preservation, and chain-of-custody procedures are best developed in collaboration with representatives from the health care setting, local law enforcement officers, the local crime lab staff, and local prosecutors. In general, each piece of evidence that is going to be saved needs to be packaged in its own paper bag and labeled with the patient's name, date of birth, and clinic or hospital number. In addition, each bag needs a label listing the item of evidence it contains, the date and time of collection, and who collected the evidence. Each bag needs to be sealed with either typical hospital tape or special tamper-proof evidence tape that is often provided by the criminal justice system to the health care setting. The sealed bags need to be stored in a locked, well-ventilated evidence locker to maintain chain of custody and promote air-drying of the contents to prevent mold and bacterial growth (Sheridan, 2003).

In addition to saving clothing, the clinician should consider saving trace physical evidence that might be discovered on or in a patient. This may include exudates, soil, loose hairs, miscellaneous fibers, grass, and leaves. Each unique piece of trace physical evidence needs to be placed in a paper envelope, bag, or cardboard box; labeled as described previously; allowed to air-dry; and secured in an appropriate storage locker. Every packaged piece of evidence needs to be logged in an evidence inventory log. The evidence log needs to list at what time the evidence was placed in the locker and by whom. When law enforcement personnel pick up the evidence, the log should list the officer's name, badge, or identification number; date and time of removal; and who from the health setting witnessed the removal. More detailed information about evidence collection after sexual assault can be found in selected references for this chapter (American College of Emergency Physicians, 1999; Crowley, 1999; Girardin, Faugno, Seneski, Slaughter, & Whelan, 1997; US Department of Justice, 2004).

The general examination must place emphasis on areas of trauma such as bruises, linear abrasions, scratches, and cuts, regardless of degree of injury. Start with a nonthreatening portion of the physical examination, such as the eyes, ears, nose, and throat, to help in gaining the patient's trust. Throughout the examination, observe the patient for signs of extragenital trauma. The most commonly injured extragenital areas are the mouth, throat, wrist, arms, breasts, and thighs (Brockmeyer & Sheridan, 1998). Document the presence, size, and location of bruises, lacerations, bite marks, and scratches (Brockmeyer & Sheridan). If the patient consents, photograph the areas of trauma. Photographic documentation and the use of body maps should follow the same guidelines as outlined in the IPV section.

Pelvic Examination   In addition to the standard pelvic examination, an evaluation should be attempted to identify more subtle signs of recent sexual activity. Engorgement of the labia or clitoris may last for one to two hours after injury. Note the condition of the hymen and document any perineal trauma. If an alternate light source is available, the patient's body and clothing can be examined for areas of fluorescence that can occur where semen is present. When applicable, these areas should be documented on the body map and swabbed for evidence.

When performing the internal vaginal examination as part of the forensic evidentiary examination, the speculum should only be lubricated with sterile water to facilitate examination. The use of saline or lubricant can contaminate vaginal secretions, destroy DNA evidence, and interfere with the forensic evaluation. Examine the vaginal walls and cervix for abrasions, ecchymoses, and lacerations. Injuries should be documented on the appropriate body maps. If a colposcope with photographic capabilities is available, photographic documentation of cervical-vaginal microtrauma should be obtained. Cultures or nucleic acid-amplification testing for gonorrhea and chlamydia, and a vaginal sample for wet prep or culture testing for trichonomiasis, should be obtained (CDC, 2002). A culture for herpes simplex virus is not routinely obtained.

Lastly, a bimanual and rectal examination should be performed to assess uterine size and to check for masses and tenderness. Anorectal samples for semen, chlamydia, and gonorrhea testing should be performed only if indicated by the history. In patients who have experienced an anal assault, digital examination is recommended to assess for sphincter laxity or spasm.

DOCUMENTATION

The role of women's health clinicians in documenting sexual abuse and collecting and preserving evidence in ambulatory settings is just as critical as documentation and evidence collection in emergency department settings. Comprehensive medical documentation includes a thorough history and physical, body maps, and photographic wound documentation. Document with the phrase "reported sexual assault," (Sheridan, 2003) or "sexual assault by history," not "she was sexually assaulted" (Petter & Whitehill, 1998). Additionally, be specific and state the facts as reported by the patient. Confine yourself to the medically relevant history. It is also critical to document the patient's affect as she shares her history; however, it is important to remember that women respond to sexual violence with a wide range of behaviors. Emotions can range from an unexpected calm and appearing emotionally detached, to tearful and self-blaming, to screaming and yelling.

MANAGEMENT

Acute Treatment of sexual assault patients should include care of the physical injuries, pregnancy prophylaxis with emergency contraception, STI testing and prophylaxis, and anticipation of psychosocial consequences. Approximately 1–5% of sexual assaults result in pregnancy (Petter & Whitehill, 1998). A pregnancy test is performed to rule out pregnancy prior to the administration of any medications. Emergency contraception is provided as described in Chapter 9.

The overall risk of acquiring an STI from a single sexual encounter is 5–10%, and the risk of acquiring hepatitis B or HIV from a one-time sexual encounter is less than 1% (Katz & Gerberding, 1997; Petter & Whitehill, 1998). Serum testing for syphilis, hepatitis, and HIV should be performed after pretest HIV counseling (CDC, 2002). Empiric STI treatment is routinely administered due to the low rate of follow-up among sexually assaulted patients, and for the reassurance they may receive from prophylaxis (CDC; Holmes, Resnick, & Frampton, 1998). Recommended preventive therapy includes hepatitis B vaccine if not previously immunized, and a regimen that includes prophylaxis for gonorrhea, chlamydia, trichonomiasis, and bacterial vaginosis, which are the infections most commonly diagnosed after sexual assault. Single-dose therapies that can be administered at the initial examination (e.g., a regimen of ceftriaxone 125 mg by intramuscular injection, metronidazole 2 g orally, and azithromycin 1 g orally) are recommended (CDC).

The probability of HIV transmission increases depending on the local prevalence rates, the assailant's serologic status (if known), the number of assailants, the type of exposure (vaginal, anal, or oral), whether and where ejaculation occurred, the vaginal pH, and the presence of other STIs (CDC, 2002; Royce, Sena, Cates, & Cohen, 1997). Antiretroviral prophylaxis for HIV needs to be decided on a case-by-case basis, weighing the likelihood of exposure against cost and potential drug toxicity of therapy (Petter & Whitehill, 1998). Repeat testing for syphilis and HIV should be performed at 6, 12, and 24 weeks after the assault (CDC, 2002).

Psychological Sequlae   In addition to the previously listed follow-up testing, patients need to be assessed for psychological trauma related to the sexual assault. The psychological sequelae of sexual assault can be profound and long term. Rape trauma syndrome (RTS), depression, and PTSD may follow sexual assault. The short-term effects include denial, shock, disbelief, disruption, and feelings of guilt, shame, blame, and hostility (Burgess et al., 1995). The long-term effects may be more deeply rooted, causing phobias and sexual problems, and affecting the patient's ability to function (Burgess et al.). Referral to agencies or professionals specializing in psychological sequelae after sexual assault is recommended.

Rape trauma syndrome is a cluster of varying degrees of biopsychosocial and behavioral responses with the sole purpose of the symptoms being self-preservation by the patient. All the symptoms are appropriate and should be validated by the clinician. RTS is usually divided into an acute phase, which may last from a few days to a few weeks, and a reorganization phase, which can last years. During the acute phase, RTS patients can experience a wide range of emotions varying from anger, fear, anxiety, and sobbing, to being calm, composed, and subdued (Girardin et al., 1997). Physical responses during the acute phase can include muscle tension and general soreness; gastrointestinal irritability and genitourinary disturbances; sleeping, eating, and sexual disruptions; and nightmares (Giradin et al.). Emotional and physical responses during the reorganization phase center around the patient's attempt to reorganize her life after the assault. Symptoms can range from withdrawing socially to wanting to be with other people constantly, increased motor activity, repeated and disturbing nightmares, and development of fears and phobic reactions (Giradin et al.).

Approximately 50% of sexually assaulted patients experience depression during the first year following a sexual assault, and sexual dysfunction has been reported in 24–40% of these patients for up to six years after the incident (Moscarello, 1990). One hundred percent of the sexually assaulted patients surveyed in one study reported that the experience continued to affect their lives five years later. Also of notable interest are findings that visits to primary care providers increased by 18% during the first year after the sexual assault, and to 56% by the second year before declining to 31% after the third year (Ruckman, 1993).

SPECIAL POPULATIONS

Adolescents   Adolescent sexual assault is a unique and complex situation. The adolescent patient is vulnerable to sexual victimization in ways that differ from both the child and the adult. The process of puberty heightens the adolescent's interest in sex and in forming his or her sexual identity (Kempthorne, 2001). Sexual curiosity and some sexual experimentation are natural consequences that can increase adolescent risk of sexual victimization (Kempthorne). Sexual encounters that start out as consensual may rapidly evolve into coercive experiences.

All states require clinicians to report sexual abuse to a child protection agency, but the laws regarding adolescent sexual victimization are not as clear. Reporting guidelines for statutory rape vary widely. In some states, statutory rape does not need to be reported unless it is due to parental neglect. In other states, this may require reporting to child protection or the police (Kempthorne, 2001). Statutory rape has been previously defined as vaginal penetration of a child less than 10 years of age, but now this age has been increased to 12 years of age in most states. Furthermore, most states have now initiated an age-differential system between the victim and assailant to aid in prosecution (Dupre et al., 1993).

During any routine history and physical, adolescents should be asked about any history of sexual victimization. When obtaining a history from the adolescent, the clinician should follow certain guidelines:

- The history should be obtained with the adolescent fully clothed and comfortable.
- The clinician should be at the same eye level as the adolescent and make good eye contact.
- Note taking should be limited to avoid distracting the adolescent.

- Limits of confidentiality should be discussed, and no promise of unconditional confidentiality should be given.
- The teen should be interviewed without the parent present for matters regarding sexuality, history of abuse, and high-risk behaviors.
- In approaching the psychosocial interview, less intimate questions, such as those pertaining to the home, education, and activities, should be asked initially, followed by questions regarding sexual activity and abuse (Kempthorne, 2001, p. 129).

The sexual history should include the following areas: (1) any consensual sexual activity, (2) any history of STIs, (3) any history of clinical signs suggesting STIs, (4) for girls, a menstrual history, and (5) any history of sexual abuse and sexual assault (Kempthorne, 2001).

Older Women   The national incidence of sexual assault in elderly females 65 years of age and older was 10 per 10,000 in 2001 (U.S. Census Bureau, 2003). Many elderly women are unaware of their vulnerability to sexual assault and perceive sexual assault as a sexually motivated crime, directed primarily at young and promiscuous women who somehow contribute to being selected as victims through their actions and behaviors (Safarik, Jarvis, & Nussbaum, 2000). National crime data in the United States indicates that many elderly victims lived alone and were assaulted in their homes in the evening by strangers with guns or sharp objects (Bureau of Justice Statistics, 1994). They are less likely to try to protect themselves during a crime and more likely to sustain injury (Safarik et al.). The motive for sexual assault in the elderly may be revenge against an authority figure, or the sexual assault may occur secondary to robbery with the elderly serving as an accessible, vulnerable target (Girardin et al., 1997).

REFERENCES

American College of Emergency Physicians. (1999). *Evaluation of the sexually assaulted or sexually abused patient.* Retrieved October 20, 2004, from http://www.acep.org/library/pdf/sxa_handbook.pdf.

Bergman, B., & Brismar, B. (1991). A 5-year follow-up study of 117 battered women. *American Journal of Public Health, 81,* 1486–1489.

Bohn, D. K., & Parker, B. (1993). In J. C. Campbell & J. Humphreys (Eds.), *Nursing care of survivors of family violence* (pp. 156–172). St. Louis, MO: Mosby.

Brandl, B. (1997). Developing services for older abused women. In *Wisconsin Coalition Against Domestic Violence,* Madison, WI: Wisconsin Coalition Against Domestic Violence.

Brandl, B., & Raymond, J. (1997). Unrecognized elder abuse victims: Older abused women. *Journal of Case Management, 6*(2), 62–68.

Brockmeyer, D. M., & Sheridan, D. J. (1998). Domestic violence: A practical guide to the use of forensic evaluation in clinical examination and documentation of injuries. In J. C. Campbell (Ed.), *Empowering survivors of abuse: Health care for battered women and their children* (pp. 23–31). Thousand Oaks, CA: Sage.

Bureau of Justice Statistics. (1994). *National crime victimization survey.* Washington, DC: Author.

Bureau of Justice Statistics. (1995*). National crime victimization survey.* Washington, DC: Author.

Burgess, A. W., Fehder, W., & Hartman, C. R. (1995). Delayed reporting of rape victims. *Journal of Psychosocial Nursing, 33,* 21.

Campbell, J. C. (1989). Women's response to sexual abuse in intimate relationships. *Women's Healthcare International, 38,* 335–347.

Campbell, J. C. (2002). Health consequences of intimate partner violence. *Lancet, 359*(9314), 1331–1336.

Campbell, J. C., & Alford, P. (1989). The dark consequences of marital rape. *American Journal of Nursing, 89,* 946–949.

Campbell, J.C., & Campbell, D. W. (1996). Cultural competence in the care of abused women. *Journal of Nurse-Midwifery, 41*(6), 457–462.

Campbell, J. C., Jones, A. S., Dienemman, J., Kub, J., Schollenberger, J., O'Campo, P., et al. (2002). Intimate partner violence and physical health consequences. *Archives of Internal Medicine, 162,* 1157–1163.

Campbell, J. C., Kub, J. E., & Rose, L. (1996). Depression in battered women. *Journal of the American Medical Women's Association, 51*(3), 106–110.

Campbell, J. C., McKenna, L. S., Torres, S., Sheridan, D., & Landenburger. (1993). In J. C. Campbell & J. Humphreys (Eds.), *Nursing care of survivors of family violence* (pp. 248–289). St. Louis, MO: Mosby.

Campbell, J. C., Oliver, C., & Bullock, L. (1993). Why battering during pregnancy? In J. C. Campbell & J. A. Lewis (Eds.), *Clinical issues in perinatal and women's health nursing* (pp. 343–349). Philadelphia: Lippincott.

Campbell, J. C., & Sheridan, D. J. (2004). Domestic violence assessments. In C. Jarvis (Ed.), *Physical examination and health assessment* (4th ed., pp. 73–82). St. Louis, MO: Saunders.

Campbell, J. C., & Soeken, K. (1999). Women's response to battering over time. *Journal of Interpersonal Violence, 14,* 21–40.

Centers for Disease Control and Prevention. (2002). Sexually transmitted diseases guidelines 2002. *Morbidity and Mortality Weekly Report, 51*(No. RR-6), 1–80.

Chapman, J. D. (1989). A longitudinal study of sexuality and gynecologic health in abused women. *Journal of the American Osteopathic Association, 89,* 946–949.

Coker, A. L., Smith, P. H., Bethea, L., King, M. R., & McKeown, R. E. (2000). Physical health consequences of physical and psychological intimate partner violence. *Archives of Family Medicine, 9,* 451–457.

Coker, A. L., Smith, P. H., McKeown, R. E., & King, M. J. (2000). Frequency and correlates of intimate partner violence by type: Physical, social and psychological battering. *American Journal of Preventive Medicine, 90,* 553–559.

Crowley, S. R. (1999). *Sexual assault: The medical-legal examination.* Stamford, CT: Appleton & Lange.

Curry, M. A. (1998). The interrelationships between abuse, substance use, and psychosocial stress during pregnancy. *Journal of Obstetric, Gynecologic, and Neonatal Nursing, 27*(6), 692–699.

Douglas, J. E., & Olshaker, M. (2001). Perpetrators. In J. S. Olshaker, M. C. Jackson, & W. S. Smock (Eds.), *Forensic emergency medicine* (pp. 1–23). Philadelphia: Lippincott Williams & Wilkins.

Dupre, A. R., Hampton, H. L., Morrison, H., & Meeks, G. R. (1993). Sexual assault. *Obstetrics and Gynecological Survey, 332,* 234–237.

Ebby, K. K., Campbell, J. C.. Sullivan, C. M., & Davidson, W. S. (1995). Health effects of experiences of sexual violence for women with abusive partners. *Health Care of Women International, 16,* 563–576.

Fagen, J., Stewart, D., & Hanson, K. (1983). Violent men or violent husbands? In D. Finkelhor, R. Gelles, G. Hotaling, & M. Straus (Eds.), *The dark side of families* (pp. 49–67). Beverly Hills, CA: Sage.

Family Violence Prevention Fund. (1999). *Preventing domestic violence: Clinical guidelines on routine screening.* San Francisco: Author.

Finkelhor, D., & Yllo, K. (1997). *License to rape: The sexual abuse of wives.* New York: Holt, Reinehart, & Winston.

Fulmer, T., & Wetle, T. (1986). Elder abuse screening and intervention. *Nurse Practitioner, 11*(5), 33–38.

Furniss, K. K. (1998). Screening for abuse in the clinical setting. In J. C. Campbell (Ed.), *Empowering survivors of abuse: Health care for battered women and their children* (pp. 190–194). Thousand Oaks, CA: Sage.

Girardin, B. W., Faugno, D. K., Seneski, P. C., Slaughter, L., & Whelan, M. (1997). *Color atlas of sexual assault.* St. Louis, MO: Mosby.

Groleau, G. A., & Jackson, M. C. (2001). Forensic examination of victims and perpetrators of sexual assault. In J. S. Olshaker, M. C. Jackson, & W. S. Smock (Eds.),

Forensic emergency medicine (pp. 85–118). Baltimore: Lippincott Williams & Wilkins.

Hegarty, K., Gunn, J., Chondros, P., & Small, R. (2004). Association between depression and abuse by partners of women attending general practice: Descriptive, cross sectional survey. *British Medical Journal, 328*, 621–624.

Heise, L. L. (1998). Violence against women: An integrated, ecological framework. *Violence Against Women, 4*(3), 262–290.

Helton, A. (1987). *A protocol of care for battered women*. White Plains, NY: March of Dimes Birth Defects Foundation.

Holmes, M. M., Resnick, H. S., & Frampton, D. (1998). Follow-up of sexual assault victims. *American Journal of Obstetric Gynecology, 179*, 336–342.

Jogerst, G. J., Daly, J. M., Brinig, M. F., Dawson, J. D., Schmuch, G. A., & Ingran, J. G. (2003). Domestic elder abuse and the law. *American Journal of Public Health, 93*(12), 2131–2137.

Katz, M. H., & Gerberding, J. L. (1997). Postexposure treatment of people exposed to the human immunodeficiency virus through sexual contact or injection drug use. *New England Journal of Medicine, 336*, 1091–1100.

Kempthorne, V. J. (2001). Forensic examination of victims and perpetrators of sexual assault. In J. S. Olshaker, M. C. Jackson, & W. S. Smock (Eds.), *Forensic emergency medicine* (pp. 119–150). Baltimore: Lippincott Williams & Wilkins.

King, M. C. (1998). Changing women's lives: The primary prevention of violence against women. In J. C. Campbell (Ed.), *Empowering survivors of abuse: Health care for battered women and their children* (pp. 177–189). Thousand Oaks, CA: Sage.

McCauley, J., Kern, D. E., Kolodner, K., Dill, L., Schroeder, A. F., DeChant, H. K., et al. (1995). The "battering syndrome": Prevalence and clinical characteristics of domestic violence in primary care internal medicine practices. *Annals of Internal Medicine, 123*(10), 737–746.

McConkey, T. E., Sole, M. L., & Holcomb, L. (2001). Assessing the female sexual assault survivor. *The Nurse Practitioner, 26*(7), 28–30, 33–34, 37–39.

McFarlane, J., Greenberg, L., Weltge, A., & Watson, M. (1995). Identification of abuse in emergency departments: Effectiveness of a two-question screening tool. *Journal of Emergency Nursing, 21*(5), 391–394.

McFarlane, J., Parker, B., Soeken, K., & Bullock, L. (1992). Assessing for abuse during pregnancy: Severity and frequency of injuries and associated entry into prenatal care. *Journal of the American Medical Association, 267*(23), 3176–3178.

Moscarello, R. (1990). Psychological management of victims of sexual assault. *Canadian Journal of Psychiatry, 35*, 25–30.

Murphy, C. C., Schei, B., Myhr, T. L., & Du Mont, J. (2001). Abuse: A risk factor for low birth weight? A systematic review and meta-analysis. *Canadian Medical Association Journal, 164*, 1567–1572.

Parker, B., & McFarlane, J. (1991). Identifying and helping battered pregnant women. *Maternal Child Nursing, 16*(3), 161–164.

Parker, B., McFarlane, J., & Soeken, K. (1994). Abuse during pregnancy: Effects on maternal complications and birthweight in adult and teenage women. *Obstetrics and Gynecology, 84*, 323–328.

Petter, L. M., & Whitehill, D. L. (1998). Management of female sexual assault. *American Family Physician, 58*, 920–926.

Phillips, L. R. (2000). Domestic violence and aging women. *Geriatric Nursing, 21*(4), 188–193.

Plichta, S. B. (1996). Violence and abuse: Implications for women's health. In M. K. Falik & K. S. Collins (Eds.), *Women's health: The Commonwealth Fund Survey*. Baltimore: Johns Hopkins University Press.

Plichta, S. B., & Abraham, C. (1996). Violence and gynecologic health in women <50 years old. *American Journal of Obstetrics and Gynecology, 174*, 903–907.

Poirier, L. (1997). The importance of screening for domestic violence in all women. *The Nurse Practitioner, 22*(5), 105–122.

Royce, R. A., Sena, A., Cates, W., & Cohen, M. S. (1997). Sexual transmission of HIV. *New England Journal of Medicine, 336*, 1072–1078.

Ruckman, L. M. (1993). Victims of rape: The physician's role in treatment. *Current Opinion in Obstetric Gynecology, 5*, 721–725.

Safarik, M. E., Jarvis, J. P., & Nussbaum, K. E. (2000). Elderly female serial sexual homicide: A limited empirical test of criminal investigative analysis. *Homicide Studies, 4*(3), 294–307.

Saltzman, L. E., Fanslow, J. L., McMahon, P. M., & Shelley, G. A. (1999). *Intimate partner violence surveillance: Uniform definitions and recommended data elements.* Atlanta, GA: Centers for Disease Control and Prevention, National Center for Injury Prevention and Control.

Schroeder, M., & Weber, J. R. (1998). Promoting domestic violence education for nurses. *Nursing Forum, 33*(4), 13–21.

Schornstein, S. L. (1997). *Domestic violence and health care: What every professional needs to know.* Thousand Oaks, CA: Sage.

Sells, C. W., & Blum, R. W. (1996). Morbidity and mortality among US adolescents: An overview of data and trends. *American Journal of Public Health, 86*(4), 513–519.

Sheridan, D. J. (2001). Treating survivors of intimate partner abuse: Forensic identification and documentation. In J. S. Olshaker, M. C. Jackson, & W. S. Smock (Eds.), *Forensic emergency medicine* (pp. 203–228). Philadelphia: Lippincott, Williams, & Wilkins.

Sheridan, D. J. (2003). Forensic identification and documentation of patients experiencing intimate partner violence. *Clinics in Family Practice, 5*(1), 113–143.

Sheridan, D. J., & Taylor, W. K. (1993). Developing hospital-based domestic violence programs, protocols, policies, and procedures. *Association of Women's Health, Obstetrics and Neonatal Nurses Clinical Issues in Perinatal and Women's Health Nursing, 4*(3), 471–482.

Silverman, J. G., Raj, A., Mucci, L. A., & Hathaway, J. E. (2001). Dating violence against adolescent girls and associated substance use, unhealthy weight control, sexual risk behavior, pregnancy, and suicidality. *Journal of the American Medical Association, 286*(5), 572–579.

Soeken, K., McFarlane, J., Parker, B., & Lominack, M. C. (1998). The Abuse Assessment Screen: A clinical instrument to measure the frequency, severity, and perpetrator of abuse against women. In J. C. Campbell (Ed.), *Empowering survivors of abuse: Health care for battered women and their children* (pp. 195–203). Thousand Oaks, CA: Sage.

Stacey, W., & Schupe, A. (1983). *The family secret: Domestic violence in America.* Boston: Beacon Press.

Tjaden, P., & Thoennes, N. (1998, November). *Prevalence, incidence, and consequences of violence against women: Findings from the national violence against women survey.* U.S. Department of Justice, National Institute of Justice, Research in Brief. Retrieved October 20, 2004, from http://www.ncjrs.org/pdffiles/172837.pdf.

US Census Bureau. (2003). *Statistical abstract of the United States: 2003* (123rd ed.). Washington, DC: Author.

US Department of Justice. (2004). *A national protocol for sexual assault medical forensic examinations: Adult/adolescent.* Retrieved October 20, 2004, from http://www.ncjrs.org/pdffiles1/ovw/206554.pdf.

Walker, L. E. (1979). *The battered woman.* New York: Harper & Row.

Woods, S. J., & Campbell, J. C. (1993). Posttraumatic stress in battered women: Does the diagnosis fit? *Issues in Mental Health Nursing, 14,* 173–186.

Zink, T. M., & Jacobson, J. (2003). Screening for intimate partner violence when children are present. *Journal of Interpersonal Violence, 18*(8), 872–890.

Chapter 13

BREAST CONDITIONS

HEATHER M. ALIOTTA
NANCY J. SCHAEFFER

Women rarely have neutral feelings about their breasts because, for most women, breasts are an important part of their self-image (Young, 1998). Breasts are an outward sign of being female and, depending on the culture, may be tabooed, worshipped, or exploited (Jones, 2004). Women may feel they are judged and evaluated by their breast size and shape, which are often associated with sexual attractiveness (Jones; Young). The importance of breast appearance is underscored by the availability of surgical procedures that offer an idealized breast size and shape. Breasts can provide both sexual pleasure and nourishment, which may cause the belief that a woman's breasts belong not only to her, but also to her sexual partner and baby (Jones). The meaning of her breasts to a woman will have a great impact on how she reacts to having a breast condition.

The presence of symptoms in the breasts causes understandable concern for many women. A woman may have an underlying fear, which may not be articulated or even conscious, that she has breast cancer. Providing adequate emotional support when a woman presents with a breast condition is as important as the necessity for accurate assessment, diagnosis, and management. The breast conditions that are the focus of this chapter are mastalgia, nipple discharge, benign breast masses, and breast cancer.

MASTALGIA

Mastalgia, or breast pain, is one of the most common breast concerns for which women seek health care. Breast pain is a significant cause of anxiety, even though mastalgia is the sole symptom of breast cancer in less than 10% of cases. When mastalgia is associated with breast cancer, it is usually related to advanced disease (Fiorica, Schorr, & Sickles, 1998). Mastalgia is classified as cyclical or noncyclical, depending on whether or not its presence is related to the menstrual cycle. The majority of breast pain is cyclical and occurs premenstrually. As many as 70% of women experience cyclical mastalgia, and 11–22% of women have moderate to severe breast pain (Ader & Browne, 1997; Ader, South-Paul, Adera, & Deuster, 2001). Noncyclical mastalgia is less common, and the exact incidence is unknown.

ETIOLOGY AND PATHOPHYSIOLOGY

The causes of mastalgia are not well understood. Breast pain is a principal component of fibrocystic breast changes, which are common among women with mastalgia. Fibrocystic breast changes were originally called fibrocystic breast disease, but the associated constellation of symptoms have become increasingly recognized as common to many women and therefore are no longer considered a disease. These changes include tender, nodular, and swollen breast tissue. As many as 85% to 90% of women with fibrocystic breast changes experience mastalgia, with the severity and frequency increasing over time until a woman is in her midforties (Fiorica et al., 1998). Hormones are thought to play a role in mastalgia because the pain is often cyclical and generally resolves at menopause, but a specific hormonal-related cause has not been identified. Other potential etiologies include inflammatory changes and nerve irritation (Lester, 2000).

CLINICAL PRESENTATION

Cyclical mastalgia typically begins in the luteal phase and subsides with menses. The pain is usually bilateral and poorly localized. The median age of onset of cyclical mastalgia is 30 years. Noncyclical mastalgia may be constant or intermittent, and is unrelated to the menstrual cycle. Noncyclical mastalgia is more likely to cause unilateral pain and occurs most frequently in women aged 40 years and older (Millet & Dirbas, 2002). Women with macromastia (very large breasts) may report shoulder grooving, neck pain, and back pain in addition to breast pain (Smith & Kent, 2002).

ASSESSMENT

History   The clinician must determine if the mastalgia is cyclical or noncyclical and eliminate nonbreast causes, such as chest wall pain. Ask the woman about the timing, location, severity, and mitigating factors of the pain. The use of an instrument to rate pain, such as a visual analog scale, may be helpful in evaluating mastalgia and monitoring the response to treatment. Prospective evaluation of pain with a daily diary has been found to be more accurate than retrospective reporting (Tavaf-Motamen, Ader, Browne, & Shriver, 1998). Ask the woman about other breast symptoms, such as nipple discharge or breast mass, and whether there is a previous history of any type of breast disease or surgery. Menstrual, pregnancy, lactation, and general medical histories are necessary for a comprehensive assessment. Note current medications, including exogenous hormones. Ask about the amount of caffeine intake. Obtain a family history, particularly of breast and ovarian

TABLE 13–1   Diagnostic Imaging Tests

Test	Source of Images	Best for Detecting	Limitations of Test
Mammogram	X-rays	Calcifications, densities, and architectural distortion	Cannot show if density is solid or cystic, lower sensitivity in younger women
Ultrasound	Sound waves	Differentiation of solid and cystic masses	Cannot show calcifications
Magnetic resonance imaging	Magnetic fields, may be enhanced with gadolinium contrast	Tissue with increased blood flow such as tumors	Expensive, limited evidence for effectiveness, false positive results

cancer. A complete review of systems is helpful in eliminating nonbreast causes (see differential diagnoses).

Physical Examination   Perform a comprehensive breast examination that includes inspection and palpation with the woman in both the upright and supine positions, and evaluate the lymph nodes (see Chapter 6). Assess for skin changes, nipple discharge, and breast masses. If the pain can be reproduced with examination, note the location. The chest wall structures should also be examined for nonbreast causes of pain.

Diagnostic Testing   Pregnancy testing should be performed if indicated by the woman's history because mastalgia can be a sign of pregnancy. Diagnostic imaging is frequently used in the evaluation of breast conditions, and information about these tests is provided in Table 13–1. A mammogram can be ordered if the woman is of appropriate age for screening with mammography; however, diagnostic imaging is not particularly helpful unless a woman has a palpable abnormality in addition to mastalgia (Cady et al., 1998). Mammography should also be considered for women with focal breast pain who have a family history of early breast cancer or other breast cancer risk factors (Smith, Pruthi, & Fitzpatrick, 2004). If a breast mass is discovered during the evaluation of mastalgia, it needs to be evaluated appropriately as described later in this chapter.

DIFFERENTIAL DIAGNOSES

Extramammary or nonbreast causes of pain are important differential diagnoses. If the pain is reproducible with palpation of the chest wall, costochondritis or Tietze Syndrome should be suspected (Smith et al., 2004). Costochondritis is inflammation of the costochondral or chondrosternal joints. The second through the fifth costochondral junctions are most likely to be affected. Tietze syndrome is differentiated from costochondritis by the presence of swelling with or without erythema. Nonsteroidal anti-inflammatory drugs

(NSAIDs) can be helpful for both conditions. Other causes of chest wall pain should also be considered, including trauma and gastrointestinal, pulmonary, and cardiac etiologies (Gumm, Cunnick, & Mokbel; Millet & Dirbas).

Mastalgia is rarely the principal sign of a developing breast cancer, but the possibility of cancer increases when the mastalgia is accompanied by certain findings. These situations include a woman with mastalgia who is postmenopausal and not taking hormone therapy (HT, see Chapter 11), or breast pain that is accompanied by skin changes or a palpable abnormality (Smith & Souba, 1995). Mastalgia related to breast cancer is usually in only one area of one breast and is unrelated to a cyclic pattern (Fiorica et al., 1998; Smith et al., 2004).

MANAGEMENT

Once a clinician has ruled out malignancy and nonbreast causes of mastalgia, attention turns to reassuring the woman that she does not have a serious illness and relieving her symptoms. Nonpharmacologic, complementary, and alternative therapies are often successful in the treatment of mastalgia. Severe breast pain can be chronic and relapsing, and may require pharmacologic treatment.

Nonpharmacologic   Reassurance is the first-line treatment for mastalgia, and has been found to be effective for up to 85% of women, with more success in women with mild or moderate symptoms than those with severe mastalgia (Barros, Mottola, Ruiz, Borges, & Pinotti, 1999). Wearing a supportive bra is frequently recommended and was shown to be more effective than pharmacologic therapy in one study (Hadi, 2000). Reductions in caffeine and dietary fat have been effective in some studies, but not others (Gumm et al., 2004; Millet & Dirbas, 2002). However, neither of these dietary recommendations is likely to be harmful. Supplementation with vitamins A, B, or E has not consistently demonstrated effectiveness (Gumm et al., 2004; Millet & Dirbas, 2002).

Pharmacologic   Modifying the dose or route of HT may be helpful in reducing breast pain in a woman who is postmenopausal. Some women report increased mastalgia with hormonal contraception. Trying a different contraceptive method or delivery system, such as changing from combined oral contraceptives to a nonoral combined method (i.e., the ring or patch), may be useful. Alternately, some women report an improvement in mastalgia with hormonal contraception.

Danazol, tamoxifen, and bromocriptine are the primary pharmacologic therapies for mastalgia. All three of these medications can produce significant side effects, and relapses after discontinuation of therapy are common (Gumm et al., 2004; Millet & Dirbas, 2002). Danazol is the only medication approved by the Food and Drug Administration (FDA) for the treatment of mastalgia as of this writing. Two recent studies have identified localized therapies that appear promising for the treatment of mastalgia. Topical use of the NSAID diclofenac diethylammonium gel three times daily for six months was found to be superior to a placebo for relieving the pain of both cyclical and noncyclical mastalgia in one study (Colak, Ipek, Kanik, Ogetman, & Aydin, 2003). In another study, women with noncyclical mastalgia were offered injection of 1 ml of 2% lidocaine and 40 mg of methyl prednisone at the area of maximum tenderness. Participants who were given an injection had greater relief of symptoms than those who were treated with reassurance, or oral or topical NSAIDs. Recurrence of symptoms occured in 16% of the women who had an injection, and all elected for a second injection (Khan, Rampaul, & Blamey, 2004).

Complementary and Alternative   The herbal evening primrose oil (EPO) is frequently recommended for the treatment of mastalgia. EPO is more likely to be effective as a first-line therapy for women with cyclical mastalgia than when medications have failed or for those with noncyclical mastalgia (Millet & Dirbas, 2002). EPO has fewer side effects than the prescription medications that are used to treat mastalgia and is a reasonable therapy to try if nonpharmacologic treatments have been unsuccessful. Response to EPO may take several months (Millet & Dirbas). Isoflavones, naturally occurring phytoestrogens, have also been proposed as a treatment for mastalgia. A small, randomized, controlled trial found that women taking isoflavones had a greater reduction in pain than women taking a placebo (Ingram, Hickling, West, Mahe, & Dunbar, 2002).

Surgical   Surgery is rarely indicated in the treatment of mastalgia (Davies, Cochrane, Stansfield, Sweetland, & Mansel, 1999). The exception is the woman with macromastia whose symptoms warrant reduction mammoplasty. As with any surgery, the risks and benefits of the procedure must be considered.

SPECIAL CONSIDERATIONS

Pregnant Women   Mastalgia is common during pregnancy and lactation. The pain is attributed to the proliferation of breast tissue and hormonal influences on that tissue (Fiorica et al., 1998). Mastitis is the most likely diagnosis when breast pain in a lactating woman is accompanied by inflammation, chills, myalgia, and fever. Mastitis is estimated to occur in as many as 33% of breast-feeding mothers (Barbosa-Cesnik, Schwartz, & Foxman, 2003). Abscesses can also develop and should be suspected when mastitis is unresponsive to antibiotic therapy and the breast pain is worsening.

NIPPLE DISCHARGE

Nipple discharge is another breast symptom that causes women to seek care, although its incidence in the general population is unknown. Concern can range from minor embarrassment to fear and anxiety about underlying pathology. Nipple discharge is often classified as physiologic, pathologic, or galactorrhea. The term "physiologic nipple discharge" can be misleading because the discharge may result from nonmalignant breast pathology. Characteristics of pathologic discharge are those associated with malignancy. Galactorrhea is milky nipple discharge. The clinician's ability to differentiate whether the nipple discharge represents a benign or malignant process is of greater importance than the terminology used. Discharge that is spontaneous, unilateral, from a single duct, and clear or bloody in color, is more likely to be associated with cancer than discharge that occurs with nipple manipulation (squeezing the nipple), is bilateral, comes from multiple ducts (multiductal), and is white, yellow, green, brown, or black in color. Nipple discharge is usually the result of a benign process, but malignancy must always be considered in the evaluation.

ETIOLOGY, PATHOPHYSIOLOGY, AND CLINICAL PRESENTATION

There are numerous etiologies of nipple discharge including pregnancy and lactation, fibrocystic breast changes, mammary duct ectasia, intraductal papilloma, galactorrhea, and cancer. Clear nipple discharge during pregnancy, particularly in the third trimester, is usually colostrum. Bloody nipple discharge during pregnancy or lactation is not uncommon and results from irritation of the proliferating tissue lining the ducts (Fiorica et al., 1998; Harris, Lippman, Morrow, & Hellman, 2000). Approximately one-third of women with fibrocystic breast tissue experience nipple discharge that is typically serous, or light green, multiductal, and occurs only with manipulation of the nipple or breast (Falkenberry, 2002; Fiorica et al.). Mammary duct ectasia results from dilation of the ducts with surrounding inflammation and fibrosis. Nipple discharge with mammary duct ectasia is typically bilateral, multiductal, and green, brown, or black in color (Falkenberry, 2002). Intraductal papilloma is the most common cause of bloody nipple discharge, and results from a small, benign growth in the duct. The discharge is typically uniductal, and a single intraductal papilloma is more common than multiple papillomas (Fiorica et al.; Harris et al.).

Galactorrhea is milky nipple discharge in a woman who has not been pregnant or lactated in the last 12 months. Galactorrhea is usually bilateral and multiductal, and it may occur spontaneously or only with nipple or breast manipulation. Galactorrhea results from hyperprolactinemia, which may be caused by pituitary prolactin-secreting tumors, medications, hypothyroidism, stress, trauma, chronic renal failure, hypothalamic lesions, previous thoracotomy, and herpes zoster. In addition to galactorrhea, pituitary tumors can cause headaches and visual disturbances. Numerous medications can cause galactorrhea, including combined contraceptives containing estrogen and progestin, phenothiazines, tricyclic antidepressants, metoclopramide, opiates, methyldopa, cimetidine, calcium channel blockers, and amphetamines (Falkenberry, 2002; Fiorica et al., 1998). Hyperprolactinemia can also interfere with the normal menstrual cycle, resulting in anovulation, oligomenorrhea or amenorrhea, and infertility (Speroff & Fritz, 2005).

Nipple discharge without an associated palpable mass or abnormal mammogram is rarely caused by malignancy (Falkenberry, 2002). Approximately 4–12% of women undergoing surgical evaluation for nipple discharge have breast cancer according to recent studies (Dietz, Crowe, Grundfest, Arrigain, & Kim, 2002; Sauter, Schlatter, Lininger, & Hewett,

2004; Simmons et al., 2003). Traditionally bloody discharge was felt to be significant for malignancy, but cancer can be present with nonbloody discharge (Sauter et al., 2004).

ASSESSMENT

History   Ask the woman about the color of her nipple discharge, whether it occurs spontaneously or only with manipulation of the nipple or breast, if it is unilateral or bilateral, and whether it comes from one or more ducts. Review the medications she is taking and determine if any could be causing galactorrhea. Note other breast symptoms, such as mastalgia or breast mass, and if there is a history of any type of breast disease or surgery. Ask about symptoms of hypothyroidism (e.g., fatigue, weight gain, cold intolerance), headaches, and visual problems. Menstrual, pregnancy, lactation, general medical, and family histories should be obtained. Any family history of breast and ovarian cancer should be noted.

Physical Examination   Perform a comprehensive breast examination that includes inspection and palpation with the woman in both the upright and supine positions, and palpation of the lymph nodes (see Chapter 6). If the nipple discharge is able to be reproduced, note the color, consistency, whether it is unilateral or bilateral, and the number of ducts involved. Assess for skin changes, breast masses, and tenderness.

Diagnostic Testing   Laboratory tests used in the evaluation of nipple discharge include serum prolactin level, thyroid stimulating hormone (TSH) measurement, and hemoccult testing. Women with galactorrhea should have prolactin and TSH tests. If hyperprolactinemia is present, imaging of the sella turcica with computed tomography (CT) or magnetic resonance imaging (MRI) should be performed to rule out a pituitary prolactin-secreting tumor (Falkenberry, 2002). Hemoccult testing can be used to detect occult blood in nipple discharge, although its predictive value for malignancy may be limited (Simmons et al., 2003). Cytological evaluation of nipple discharge is no longer performed because this test is unreliable and will not change management.

   If the discharge has characteristics associated with malignancy or a palpable mass is present, diagnostic imaging tests (Table 13–1) should be performed. A normal mammogram does not rule out breast cancer in women who have nipple discharge (Dietz et al., 2002). When a palpable mass is present, it should be evaluated as described later in this chapter.

   Additional diagnostic modalities that assist in ruling out malignancy include duct excision, ductoscopy, and ductography. Excision of the affected duct or ducts allows for definitive evaluation and may also be therapeutic. A fiber-optic ductoscope can be used to visualize the ducts and may be helpful in both the diagnosis and to guide duct excision (Dietz et al., 2002). Ductography allows visualization of the ductal pattern through the use of dye instilled into the nipple. This test shows a filling defect that may be due to carcinoma, papilloma, or other blockage. Although visualization of a filling defect in the duct may be helpful, the information does not significantly change the management of nipple discharge (Cady et al., 1998). Limited availability of ductoscopy and ductography may preclude their use.

DIFFERENTIAL DIAGNOSES

In addition to the conditions already described, sexual stimulation, infection, and Paget's disease (described in the section on breast cancer) can cause nipple discharge.

MANAGEMENT

Women who have colostrum during pregnancy, or nipple discharge related to fibrocystic breast changes, should be reassured that their discharge is benign and should be advised that avoiding nipple stimulation will generally cause the discharge to resolve. Mammary duct ectasia can be expectantly managed or surgically treated with removal of the subareolar duct system, if symptoms are severe. Intraductal papilloma is treated with duct excision (Falkenberry, 2002; Osuch, 2002). If breast cancer is diagnosed, appropriate management should be initiated according to the disease stage, as is discussed in the breast cancer section.

The treatment of galactorrhea depends on the etiology. Pituitary tumors may be treated surgically, with medications, or expectantly managed in certain circumstances (Speroff & Fritz, 2005). Discontinuing a medication that causes galactorrhea or treating hypothyroidism if it is present may resolve the galactorrhea. Bromocriptine can be used to treat galactorrhea, but one-third of patients cannot tolerate the side effects of this medication. Cabergoline can be used as an alternative to bromocriptine, as it may have less side effects. Bilateral total duct ligation is an option for women when medical therapy causes intolerable side effects or does not relieve symptoms (Harris et al., 2000).

BENIGN BREAST MASSES

A breast mass can be alarming for the woman as well as her clinician. Fortunately, approximately 90% of breast masses are benign; however, malignancy must always be considered in the evaluation of a breast mass (Kerlikowske, Smith-Bindman, Ljung, & Grady, 2003). The likelihood of malignancy increases with age and other associated risk factors, which are detailed in the breast cancer section.

INCIDENCE, ETIOLOGY, AND CLINICAL PRESENTATION

The most common benign breast masses are fibroadenomas and cysts. Lipomas, fat necroses, hamartomas, and galactoceles may also be encountered. Fibrodenomas are found in 10% of all women. They usually occur in women aged 20 to 40 years, and the incidence decreases with increasing age. Bilateral fibroadenomas occur in up to

20% of cases (Fiorica et al., 1998). A proposed etiology is the effect of estrogen on susceptible tissue (Marchant, 2002). Cysts are fluid-filled masses that are most common among women 35–50 years of age. They are thought to result from cystic lobular involution (Harris et al., 2000; Marchant). A lipoma is an island of fatty tissue that may occur in the breast or other areas of the body, including the arms, legs, and abdomen. Lipomas typically occur in the later reproductive years (Marchant). Fat necrosis is usually the result of trauma to the breast, whether by external force on the tissue, or subsequent to surgical manipulation of tissue, and is most common in women over 40 years old (Harris et al.). Hamartomas are most often seen after menopause and are composed of glandular tissue, fat, and fibrous connective tissue (Harris et al., 2000). Galactoceles are milk-filled cysts that usually occur during or after lactation. Galactoceles probably result from an obstructed duct (Fiorica et al.). A woman may present with a breast mass found on self-examination, or a mass may be discovered on clinical breast examination.

ASSESSMENT

History   If the woman found the mass, determine when she first noticed it and any changes she has noticed since that time. Ask about other breast symptoms, such as mastalgia or nipple discharge, and whether there is a history of any type of breast disease or surgery. Menstrual, pregnancy, lactation, and general medical histories should be taken. A family history of breast and ovarian cancer is particularly important.

Physical Examination   Perform a comprehensive breast examination that includes inspection and palpation with the woman in both the upright and supine positions, and evaluation of the lymph nodes (see Chapter 6). If a mass is palpable, identify the size in centimeters, shape, and consistency or texture. Determine whether the mass is discrete (well-delineated, distinct edges) or poorly differentiated, tender to palpation, and mobile or fixed. Assess for skin changes, nipple discharge, and lymphadenopathy. When documenting the location of a mass, it may be helpful to draw a sketch of the breast with the site of the mass marked or to describe the position of the mass on the breast relative to a clock face, such as "at seven o'clock." Typical physical examination findings for benign breast masses are described in Table 13–2.

Diagnostic Testing   Ultrasound helps to distinguish a cystic from a solid mass but is not as accurate as tissue sampling. Mammography can be used to detect nonpalpable abnormalities if a woman is of appropriate screening age or has a solid mass. Palpable breast masses may not be visible with diagnostic imaging tests, and therefore these tests cannot rule out malignancy. Biopsy is required to definitively ascertain whether a mass is solid or cystic, and benign or malignant. A fine-needle aspiration (FNA) biopsy is a minimally invasive

TABLE 13-2 Features of Benign Breast Masses

Type of Mass	Typical Physical Examination Findings	Tissue Sampling Findings
Fibroadenoma	Discrete, smooth, round or oval, nontender, mobile	Ductal epithelium, dense stroma, numerous elongated nuclei without fat
Cyst	Discrete, tender, mobile	Cyst fluid and inflammation
Lipoma	Discrete, soft, nontender, may or may not be mobile	Fatty tissue
Fat necrosis	Ill-defined, firm, nontender, nonmobile	Necrotic fat with inflammation
Hamartoma	Discrete, nontender, nonmobile, may be nonpalpable with incidental diagnosis on imaging studies	Glandular tissue, fat, and fibrous connective tissue
Galactocele	Discrete, firm, sometimes tender	Fat globules

way to differentiate solid and cystic masses, and provides cytologic evaluation of a palpable mass. FNA biopsy may also be therapeutic if the mass is fluid filled. If cytologic evaluation is not definitive, a more invasive method of tissue sampling (Table 13–3) is required to rule out breast cancer or to determine the type of tumor if the mass is benign (Kerlikowske et al., 2003). Tissue sample findings for benign breast masses are described in Table 13–2.

DIFFERENTIAL DIAGNOSES

In addition to the types of breast masses already discussed, the differential diagnosis of breast masses includes fibrocystic changes, infection or abscess, cytosarcoma phyllodes, and malignancy. Women with fibrocystic breast tissue may present having found what is perceived as a mass, though these changes are typically associated with nodularity or thickening rather than a discrete mass. Cytosarcoma phyllodes is a rare, rapidly growing tumor that is usually benign, but can be malignant.

MANAGEMENT

Management of benign breast masses depends upon the type of mass. Often a breast mass proven to be a fibroadenoma by cytologic analysis does not need to be removed. Excision is recommended if the mass increases in size or tenderness; however, as many as 20% of fibroadenomas recur (Fiorica et al., 1998; Harris et al., 2000). Asymptomatic cysts do not require intervention. FNA can be used to treat large or painful cysts. Ultrasound guidance can be helpful to ensure complete aspiration of a large cyst (Marchant, 2002). Excision of a lipoma is not required if a breast mass is consistent with lipoma on clinical examination and tissue sampling, and if there are no suspicious findings at the site on mammography and ultrasound. If these conditions are not met, excision should be performed (Lanng,

TABLE 13-3 Breast Tissue Sampling Procedures

Procedure	Description	Breast Target
Fine-needle aspiration biopsy	• Tissue for cytologic evaluation aspirated with a small needle • Differentiates solid and cystic masses	Palpable breast mass or thickening
Stereotactic core needle biopsy	• Large-bore needle used to obtain cores of tissue for histologic examination • Stereotactic mammography used for localization and targeting	Density or calcification seen on mammogram
Ultrasound-guided core needle biopsy	• Large-bore needle used to obtain cores of tissue for histologic examination • Ultrasound used for localization and targeting	Solid lesion seen on ultrasound
Needle-localized breast biopsy	• Use of a wire to localize an occult mammographic abnormality prior to excisional biopsy	Density or calcification seen on mammogram in a location that cannot be effectively core biopsied
Excisional breast biopsy	• Surgical procedure that requires a skin excision • Mass or mammographic abnormality is removed with a surrounding margin of normal-appearing tissue	Palpable breast mass, thickening or skin change

Eriksen, & Hoffman, 2004). Fat necroses and hamaratomas may require excision for diagnosis, but otherwise do not have to be removed, and may be expectantly managed. A galactocele will spontaneously resolve, but aspiration can be attempted if it is painful, although this procedure is not always successful for these masses (Marchant). When benign breast masses are expectantly managed, the patient should be advised to report any new symptoms and encouraged to follow up for clinical examinations and diagnostic testing as recommended.

SPECIAL CONSIDERATIONS

Adolescents   In 70–80% of adolescents presenting with a breast mass, the diagnosis is a fibroadenoma. Evaluation of breast masses in this age group does not include mammography (Osuch, 2002). Breast cancer in women under 20 years of age is very rare (Cady et al., 1998).

Pregnant and Lactating Women   Evaluation of palpable findings in pregnant and lactating women is complicated by the complex breast parenchyma. However, appropriate diagnostic imaging and breast tissue sampling should not be deferred, with the exception of mammography, which is not generally used during pregnancy. Fibroadenomas may increase in size and become symptomatic during pregnancy (Osuch, 2002).

Older Women   The likelihood of malignancy increases with age. Among women aged 55 years and older, 85% of breast masses are malignant. Masses in postmenopausal women are presumed malignant until proven otherwise (Osuch, 2002).

BREAST CANCER

Breast cancer is one of the most feared diseases among women, yet breast cancer treatment has become increasingly successful in prolonging women's lives after diagnosis. From the Halsted radical mastectomy of the 1890s to breast-sparing surgery in conjunction with other treatment modalities, the management of breast cancer has evolved dramatically over time. With increased public awareness and earlier detection, comprehensive treatment can be initiated promptly for this disease process.

INCIDENCE

Over 200,000 cases of invasive breast cancer are diagnosed in the United States each year (American Cancer Society). The lifetime risk of being diagnosed with breast cancer is 12.8%, or 1 in 8 women (Donegan & Spratt, 2002). Breast cancer is the second leading cause, after lung cancer, of cancer deaths in women (American Cancer Society).

ETIOLOGY

Two challenging aspects of breast cancer are that many of the risk factors are nonmodifiable, and many women with breast cancer have no risk factors. Known risk factors for developing breast cancer include the following:

- Being female
- Advancing age
- Prior personal history of breast cancer
- Nulliparity
- First pregnancy after the age of 30 years
- Early menarche (before age 12)
- Late menopause (after age 55)
- Family history, particularly in a first-degree relative (mother, sister, or child)
- BRCA1 and BRCA 2 genetic mutations
- Previous breast biopsy revealing atypical, ductal, or lobular hyperplasia
- Ductal or lobular carcinoma in situ

- Exposure to chest radiation (Harris et al., 2000; Winer, Morrow, Osborne, & Harris, 2001)

The discovery of BRCA1 and BRCA2 genetic mutations was monumental because mutations of these genes account for 20–30% of breast cancer cases. These mutations are also associated with a 10–20% risk of developing ovarian cancer (Donegan & Spratt, 2002). As a result of the increasing significance of the genetic link to the development of breast cancer, the role of the genetic counselor working in collaboration with the medical team in the care of women with breast cancer has become significant.

Risk factors for breast cancer that have been debated include oral contraceptives, HT, alcohol, diet, weight, tobacco, and abortion. Oral contraceptives slightly increase breast cancer risk during or within 10 years after their use. This is thought to be related to increased detection rather than a causative effect (Collaborative Group on Hormonal Factors in Breast Cancer, 1996; Westhoff, 1999). HT also increases the risk of breast cancer with higher risk associated with longer usage (Collaborative Group on Hormonal Factors in Breast Cancer, 1997; Rossouw et al., 2002). The exact extent of increased risk with HT is unclear (Garbe, Levesque, & Suissa, 2004). Alcohol use also increases the risk of breast cancer, and risk is greater with larger amounts of alcohol consumption (Collaborative Group on Hormonal Factors in Breast Cancer, 2002a). Dietary factors that influence breast cancer risk are unresolved, but it appears that high dietary fat intake does not increase risk, while weight gain during midlife does increase risk (Holmes & Willett, 2004). Although frequently cited as risk factors, cigarette smoking and spontaneous or elective abortion do not increase the risk of breast cancer (Collaborative Group on Hormonal Factors in Breast Cancer, 2002a; Beral et al., 2004). Breast-feeding protects a woman from developing breast cancer, and this effect increases with longer duration of lactation (Collaborative Group on Hormonal Factors in Breast Cancer, 2002b).

PATHOPHYSIOLOGY

Breast cancer occurs when there is erratic cell growth and proliferation in the breast tissue. It is not well understood what hormones are most critical in the development of breast cancer and why a large percentage of women who develop breast cancer have no identified risk factors (Donegan & Spratt, 2002). While genetic factors have clarified the predisposition toward developing breast cancer in some women, there remains a significant amount of ongoing research dedicated to understanding more about the development of this disease.

CLINICAL PRESENTATION AND TYPES OF BREAST CANCER

Breast cancer may be detected by a palpable lesion or by screening mammography. Skin changes can also be the initial manifestation of breast cancer. The types of breast cancer include carcinoma in situ, invasive breast cancer, Paget's disease, and inflammatory carcinoma. Breast cancer is further classified by whether it originated in the ducts or lobules (see Chapter 5 for breast anatomy and physiology).

Carcinoma in Situ   Ductal carcinoma in situ (DCIS), or intraductal carcinoma, is the earliest manifestation of breast cancer and involves abnormal cells that are confined to the ducts. DCIS is usually diagnosed in association with microcalcifications seen on mammography. It is rare to find a palpable mass. DCIS is sometimes referred to as a precancerous condition, although the likelihood of DCIS progressing to invasive cancer is unknown. With lobular carcinoma in situ (LCIS), the abnormal cells are limited to the breast lobules. LCIS is a noninvasive lesion that does not clearly progress to invasive cancer; thus the term lobular neoplasia is often recommended. LCIS may be bilateral and is often an incidental finding noted during biopsy for another lesion (Donegan & Spratt, 2002; National Cancer Institute, 2004). Atypical ductal hyperplasia (ADH) and atypical lobular hyperplasia (ALH) are benign findings that are similar histologically to DCIS and LCIS respectively. ADH and ALH are associated with an increased risk of breast cancer as noted previously.

Invasive Breast Cancer   Invasive or infiltrating ductal carcinoma is the most common malignancy of the breast. Invasive ductal carcinoma usually presents as a discrete, solid mass with malignant cells escaping the confines of the ducts and infiltrating the breast parenchyma. The most common sites of metastatic spread of invasive breast cancer are the lymph nodes, bones, liver, lungs, and brain (Entrekin, 1992).

Invasive or infiltrating lobular carcinoma is much less common and may present as a discrete mass, usually found in the upper-outer quadrant of the breast. The mass may be characterized only by thickening or induration, with margins that are diffuse and ill defined, both on physical examination and on mammogram. Women with infiltrating lobular carcinoma have an increased risk of developing bilateral breast cancer (Harris et al., 2000). Invasive lobular cancer is associated with the unusual spread of metastases, including carcinomatous meningitis, intra-abdominal metastases with intestinal and ureteral obstruction, and those spreading to the uterus and ovaries.

Paget's Disease   Paget's disease is a rare form of breast cancer that causes eczematous nipple changes as well as itching, erythema, and nipple discharge. Approximately 45% of women with Paget's disease present with a palpable underlying breast carcinoma that may be intraductal or invasive ductal carcinoma. Controversy exists regarding whether the nipple involvement arises from infiltration from an underlying breast tumor or is a separate process involving the nipple epidermis (Harris et al., 2000; Winer et al., 2001).

Inflammatory Carcinoma   Inflammatory breast carcinoma is the most aggressive type of breast cancer (Donegan & Spratt, 2002). This type of carcinoma causes diffuse inflammatory changes of the breast skin with erythema, warmth, skin thickening, and peau d'orange (edema that makes the breast skin similar in appearance to the skin of an orange). There may or may not be an underlying invasive malignancy (Donegan & Spratt, 2002; Harris et al., 2000).

ASSESSMENT

History The initial history for a woman with a breast mass is the same as previously described in the section on benign breast masses. If the cancer is already diagnosed and classified as a T3 or T4 lesion (Table 13–4), the woman should be asked about symptoms of metastases such as bone pain, arthralgias, cough, jaundice, abdominal pain, headaches, visual disturbances, malaise, loss of appetite, weight loss, fever, and fatigue. Clinicians should remain vigilant for symptoms of metastases in any woman with a history of breast cancer.

TABLE 13–4 TNM Classification of Breast Cancers

Primary Tumor (T)

TX	Primary tumor cannot be assessed
T0	No evidence of primary tumor
Tis	Carcinoma in situ: ductal carcinoma in situ, lobular carcinoma in situ, or Paget's disease of the nipple with no tumor (Paget's disease with a tumor is classified according to tumor size)
T1	Tumor 2 cm or smaller in greatest dimension (may be subdivided to T1mic, T1a, T1b, and T1c depending on exact size of the tumor)
T2	Tumor larger than 2 cm but not larger than 5 cm in greatest dimension
T3	Tumor larger than 5 cm in greatest dimension
T4	Tumor of any size with direct extension to chest wall (T4a), skin (T4b), or both (T4c); inflammatory carcinoma (T4d)

Regional Lymph Nodes (N)

NX	Regional lymph nodes cannot be assessed (e.g., previously removed)
N0	No regional lymph node metastases
N1	Metastasis in movable ipsilateral axillary node(s)
N2	Metastasis in ipsilateral axillary lymph node(s) fixed or matted, or in clinically apparent (detected by imaging studies or clinical examination) ipsilateral internal mammary nodes in the absence of clinically evident axillary lymph node metastasis
N3	Metastasis in ipsilateral infraclavicular lymph node(s), or in clinically apparent ipsilateral internal mammary lymph node(s), and in the presence of clinically evident axillary lymph node metastasis; or metastasis in ipsilateral supraclavicular lymph node(s), with or without axillary or internal mammary lymph node involvement

Distant Metastases (M)

MX	Distant metastases cannot be assessed
M0	No distant metastasis
M1	Distant metastasis

Source: Adapted from American Joint Committee on Cancer, 2002.

Physical Examination   Perform a comprehensive breast examination (see Chapter 6). Note any skin changes, palpable masses, and nipple discharge. A suspicious lesion is usually hard, painless, and has irregular borders that may be immobile and fixed to the skin or surrounding breast tissue. Palpate for the axillary, cervical, and supraclavicular lymph nodes. Enlargement of any of these nodes is suspicious. Examination of the lungs, abdomen, and neurologic system should also be performed to detect signs of metastases.

Diagnostic Testing   Diagnostic testing for breast cancer includes imaging studies and tissue sampling. The diagnostic imaging tests most frequently used in the evaluation of breast cancer are mammography and ultrasound (Table 13–1). Mammography can identify breast cancers that are too small to palpate on physical examination. Mammograms can also detect both benign and malignant calcifications. Benign calcifications are identified by their large, coarse, and scattered appearance. Malignant appearing calcifications are much smaller, appearing as grains of sand. With digital mammography, a wider range of tissue contrast can be seen, subtle contrast differences can be amplified, and the images are immediately available. Mammography also identifies densities that ultrasound can further characterize as solid or fluid filled. Solid masses require further intervention while simple fluid-filled cysts generally do not.

MRI is helpful in identifying occult breast cancer when there are axillary node metastases but no visible carcinoma on mammogram or ultrasound. MRI can also differentiate cancer from scars, and is useful when women have had previous breast procedures (National Cancer Institute, 2004). Breast tissue sampling procedures are described in Table 13–3. If pathologic evaluation after excisional biopsy confirms that the tissue margins are negative and not infiltrated with tumor cells, no further surgery is necessary (Donegan & Spratt, 2002; Harris et al., 2000).

Further Assessment When Breast Cancer Is Diagnosed   There are several factors that guide appropriate treatment options and also serve as prognostic indicators when breast cancer is diagnosed. Malignancies are staged using the TNM system, which refers to the size of tumor, lymph node involvement, and metastatic spread (Table 13–4). Tumors can be graded and are also assessed for estrogen and progesterone receptors (ER/PR) and HER-2/neu. The HER-2/neu oncogene is closely related to the human epidermal growth factor. Grading the tumor indicates its differentiation, or how closely the cells resemble normal tissue. A well-differentiated tumor has a more favorable prognosis than a poorly differentiated lesion (Entrekin, 1992). ER/PR positive tumors are more likely to respond to hormonal manipulation, while ER/PR negative tumors have a less favorable prognosis (Donegan & Spratt, 2002). Overexpression of HER-2, which occurs in 20–25% of breast cancers, is associated with more aggressive tumor cells and a poorer prognosis (Yaziji et al., 2004).

The status of the axillary lymph nodes is critical in determining treatment options for women with invasive breast cancer. For those with early stage tumors less than 5 cm in size and no palpable axillary lymph nodes, the sentinel node biopsy provides necessary staging information without the associated morbidities of a full dissection, such as lymphedema, immobility of the upper extremity, and accompanying diminished quality of life. Dye is injected into the region surrounding the tumor and drains into the sentinel axillary node, which is the first node draining the breast, and this node is removed (Hsueh, Hansen, & Giuliano, 2000). If the sentinel node is positive, dissection of the Level I and II axillary lymph nodes is required. Additional tests are performed to detect metastases. These routinely include a complete blood count, liver function tests, and a chest X-ray. Brain imaging, a bone scan, and abdominal CT, MRI, or ultrasound are not routine but may be warranted if metastases are suspected (National Comprehensive Cancer Network, 2004).

DIFFERENTIAL DIAGNOSES

A palpable breast mass can be caused by any of the benign conditions discussed previously. The most likely differential diagnosis for invasive lobular carcinoma is fibrocystic disease. The differential diagnoses for Paget's disease include eczema, psoriasis, contact dermatitis, and rarely, squamous cell carcinoma in situ arising in the skin (Bowen's disease). The differential diagnoses for inflammatory carcinoma include breast abscess, infection, and mastitis. The presence of any of these conditions in a woman who is not lactating is highly suspicious for malignancy.

PREVENTION

The selective estrogen receptor modulars (SERMs) tamoxifen (Nolvadex) and raloxifene (Evista) are used to prevent breast cancer in women who are at high risk for developing the disease (chemoprevention). Both medications are associated with hot flashes and thromboembolic events. Tamoxifen increases the risk of endometrial cancer, while raloxifene has the advantage of increasing bone density. There are currently more studies in which tamoxifen, rather than raloxifene, was used for chemoprevention (Kinsinger, Harris, Woolf, Sox, & Lohr, 2002). However, a large clinical trial of breast cancer prevention, the Study of Tamoxifen and Raloxifene (STAR), is underway to compare the two medications with results expected in 2005 (National Surgical Adjuvant Breast and Bowel Project, n.d.). Those women who are at very high risk for breast cancer may elect to undergo prophylactic mastectomy. The benefits of risk reduction and decreased anxiety about the possibility of developing cancer must be weighed with the risks of the surgery itself. Although it is uncommon, women must be advised that breast cancer can develop in the chest wall after prophylactic mastectomy (Dowdy, Stefanek, & Hartmann, 2004).

MANAGEMENT

Suspected or diagnosed breast cancer requires collaborative care with breast cancer specialists, such as a surgeon or medical oncologist. The primary treatment strategies for breast cancer are surgery, chemotherapy, radiation, and hormonal manipulation. A combination of these modalities is often used. Breast-conserving surgery, lumpectomy or partial mastectomy, removes the cancer but not the breast itself. In addition to removal of breast tissue alone (total or simple mastectomy), mastectomy may include removal of the breast and Level I and II lymph nodes (modified radical mastectomy). Radical mastectomy, which includes removal of the breast, pectoralis major and minor muscles, and Level I–III lymph nodes, is no longer performed, as there are severe morbidities and no survival advantage over less radical surgery. Breast-conserving surgery may be performed instead of mastectomy depending on the disease stage. Studies comparing surgical treatment outcomes in women for 20 years after the procedures indicate that breast-conserving surgeries do not increase the future risk of death from recurrent disease when compared to mastectomy (Fisher et al., 2002; Veronesi et al., 2002). When mastectomy is performed, breast reconstruction is an option. Chemotherapy may be administered after surgery (adjuvant therapy) or preoperatively (neoadjuvant therapy) to decrease the size of a large tumor prior to surgery. Radiation therapy may also be used postoperatively following breast-sparing surgery to treat the breast. Radiation is also useful for treatment of locally advanced disease of the chest wall or breast, palliation for bone pain from bone metastases, or to strengthen a region that contains bony disease that is at risk for pathologic fracture. The SERM tamoxifen and the aromatase inhibitors are the hormonal therapies used in breast cancer treatment when ER/PR receptors are positive. The optimal duration of tamoxifen therapy is still under investigation, but more than five years is not recommended (National Cancer Institute, 2004). The aromatase inhibitors, letrozole (Femara), exemestane (Aromasin), and anastrazole (Arimidex), are currently second-line therapy for women who have previously taken tamoxifen. Both letrozole and exemestane improve disease-free survival (Coombes et al., 2004; Goss et al., 2003). The aromatase inhibitors are also used as treatment for women who develop metastatic disease and have previously taken tamoxifen. Due to the increased risk of developing osteoporosis, the use of the aromatase inhibitors is not recommended prior to menopause (Donegan & Spratt, 2002).

Ductal Carcinoma in Situ   Until recently, DCIS was treated with mastectomy, but this can be more radical surgery than is necessary for a carcinoma that may not progress to invasive carcinoma (Harris et al., 2000). Current options for DCIS treatment include breast-conserving surgery, with or without radiation, and total mastectomy. Tamoxifen therapy after surgery will be recommended in the ER/PR positive individual. The treatment options depend on the extent of disease (National Cancer Institute [NCI], 2004; National Comprehensive Cancer Network, 2004).

Lobular Carcinoma in Situ   The optimal management of LCIS is controversial. Treatment options include careful observation, chemoprevention with tamoxifen, and bilateral prophylactic mastectomy for those at high risk for breast cancer (NCI, 2004; National Comprehensive Cancer Network, 2004). The effectiveness of chemoprevention with raloxifene for women with LCIS is being evaluated in the STAR trial (National Surgical Adjuvant Breast and Bowel Project, n.d.).

Invasive Breast Cancer   Treatment of invasive carcinoma is dependent on the size and grade of the tumor, the involvement of lymph nodes, the presence of metastases, whether the cancer is being diagnosed for the first time or is recurrent, and the results of ER/PR and HER-2 testing. A combination of surgery, chemotherapy, radiation, and hormonal manipulation may be used. Other treatment options include ovarian ablation with gonadotropin-releasing hormone (GnRH) agonists or oopherectomy and use of trastuzumab for HER-2 positive breast cancer with metastases. When the cancer has metastasized, the goal of treatment is control or palliative, rather than curative (NCI, 2004; National Comprehensive Cancer Network, 2004).

Paget's Disease   If no underlying tumor is present, initial conservative treatment with steroidal cream often results in transient improvement in presenting symptoms. If complete resolution of the nipple changes does not occur in one to two weeks, referral to a surgeon for nipple biopsy is recommended. In the past, surgical treatment of Paget's disease of the nipple involved total mastectomy. Currently, breast-conserving surgery with complete excision of the nipple and areola to clear margins, followed by radiation, is recommended. If the margins are positive, mastectomy should be considered (Harris et al., 2000).

Inflammatory Carcinoma   Women with signs and symptoms of inflammatory breast carcinoma may initially be treated with antibiotics. If a 10–14 day course of antibiotic coverage does not result in resolution of symptoms, or if the cutaneous findings are highly suspicious, surgical referral for skin biopsy is indicated (Harris et al., 2000). Treatment of inflammatory carcinoma involves multiple modalities including surgery, chemotherapy, radiation, and hormonal manipulation (NCI, 2004).

EMERGING EVIDENCE THAT MAY CHANGE PRACTICE

Recommendations regarding breast cancer screening, diagnostic techniques, and management are constantly evolving. A search of the National Cancer Institute Web site in October 2004 identified over 250 ongoing clinical trials related to breast cancer. These trials will inevitably change clinical practice related to breast cancer, and providers must keep abreast of new developments. In addition, women at high risk for, or who have breast cancer, should be made aware of the option to participate in clinical trials.

SPECIAL CONSIDERATIONS

Pregnant Women   One in 200 pregnant or lactating women has breast cancer, and 1–2% of all malignancies are diagnosed in pregnant women (Cady et al., 1998). Ultrasound is usually preferable to mammography in pregnant and lactating women, and surgical biopsy is not delayed until birth or weaning because prompt diagnosis is necessary. Management of breast cancer during pregnancy must take into account the benefits and risks for both the mother and the fetus, and can involve making complex decisions.

REFERENCES

Ader, D. N., & Browne, M. W. (1997). Prevalence and impact of cyclic mastalgia in a United States clinic-based sample. *American Journal of Obstetrics and Gynecology, 177,* 126–132.

Ader, D. N., South-Paul, J., Adera, T., & Deuster, P. A. (2001). Cyclical mastalgia: Prevalence and associated health and behavioral factors. *Journal of Psychosomatic Obstetrics and Gynecology, 22,* 71–76.

American Cancer Society. (2004). *Cancer facts & figures 2004.* Atlanta, GA: Author.

American Joint Committee on Cancer. (2002). *AJCC cancer screening manual* (6th ed.). New York: Springer.

Barbosa-Cesnik, C., Schwartz, K., & Foxman, B. (2003). Lactation mastitis. *Journal of the American Medical Association, 289,* 1609–1612.

Barros, A. C., Mottola, J., Ruiz, C. A., Borges, M. N., & Pinotti, J. A. (1999). Reassurance in the treatment of mastalgia. *The Breast Journal, 5,* 162–165.

Beral, V., Bull, D., Doll, R., Peto, R., Reeves, G., & Collaborative Group on Hormonal Factors in Breast Cancer. (2002). Breast cancer and abortion: Collaborative reanalysis of data from 53 epidemiological studies, including 83,000 women with breast cancer from 16 countries. *Lancet, 363,* 1007–1016.

Cady, B., Steele, G. D., Morrow, M., Gardner B., Smith B. L., Lee, N. C., et al. (1998). Evaluation of common breast problems: Guidance for primary care providers. *CA: A Cancer Journal for Clinicians, 48,* 46–63.

Colak, T., Ipek, T., Kanik, A., Ogetman, Z., & Aydin, S. (2003). Efficacy of topical nonsteroidal antiinflammatory drugs in mastalgia treatment. *Journal of the American College of Surgeons, 196,* 525–530.

Collaborative Group on Hormonal Factors in Breast Cancer. (1996). Breast cancer and hormonal contraceptives: Collaborative reanalysis of individual data on 53,297 women with breast cancer and 100,239 women without breast cancer from 54 epidemiological studies. *Lancet, 347,* 1713–1727.

Collaborative Group on Hormonal Factors in Breast Cancer. (1997). Breast cancer and hormone replacement therapy: Collaborative reanalysis of data from 51 epidemiological studies of 52,705 women with breast cancer and 108,411 women without breast cancer. *Lancet, 350,* 1047–1059.

Collaborative Group on Hormonal Factors in Breast Cancer. (2002a). Alcohol, tobacco and breast cancer—collaborative reanalysis of individual data from 53 epidemiological studies, including 58,515 women with breast cancer and 95,067 women without the disease. *British Journal of Cancer, 87,* 1234–1245.

Collaborative Group on Hormonal Factors in Breast Cancer. (2002b). Breast cancer and breastfeeding: Collaborative reanalysis of individual data from 47 epidemiological studies in 30 countries, including 50,302 women with breast cancer and 96,973 women without the disease. *Lancet, 360,* 187–195.

Coombes, R. C., Hall, E., Gibson, L. J., Paridaens, R., Jassem, J., Delozier, T., et al. (2004). A randomized trial of exemestane after two to three years of tamoxifen therapy in postmenopausal women with primary breast cancer. *New England Journal of Medicine, 350,* 1081–1092.

Davies, E. L., Cochrane, R. A., Stansfield, K., Sweetland, H. M., & Mansel, R. E. (1999). Is there a role for surgery in the treatment of mastalgia? *The Breast, 8,* 285–288.

Dietz, J. R., Crowe, J. P., Grundfest, S., Arrigain, S., & Kim, J. A. (2002). Directed duct excision by using mammary ductoscopy in patients with pathologic nipple discharge. *Surgery, 132,* 582–588.

Donegan, W., & Spratt, J. (Eds.). (2002). *Cancer of the breast* (5th ed.). St. Louis, MO: Saunders.

Dowdy, S. C., Stefanek, M., & Hartmann, L. C. (2004). Surgical risk reduction: Prophylactic salpingo-oopherectomy and prophylactic mastectomy. *American Journal of Obstetrics and Gynecology, 191,* 1113–1123.

Entrekin, N. (1992). Breast cancer. In J. Clark & R. McGee (Eds.), *Core curriculum for oncology nursing* (2nd ed., p. 415). Philadelphia: Saunders.

Falkenberry, S. S. (2002). Nipple discharge. *Obstetrics and Gynecology Clinics of North America, 29,* 21–29.

Fiorica, J. V., Schorr, S. J., & Sickles, E. A. (1998, March). Benign breast disorders: First rule out cancer. *Contemporary OB/GYN,* 154–172.

Fisher, B., Anderson, S., Bryant, J., Margolese, R. G., Deutsch, M., Fisher E. R., et al. (2002). Twenty-year follow-up of a randomized trial comparing total mastectomy, lumpectomy, and lumpectomy plus irradiation for the treatment of invasive breast cancer. *New England Journal of Medicine, 347,* 1233–1242.

Garbe, E., Levesque, L., & Suissa, S. (2004). Variability of breast cancer risk in observational studies of hormone replacement therapy: A meta-regression analysis. *Maturitas, 47,* 175–183.

Goss, P., Ingle, J., Martino, S., Robert, N. J., Muss, H. B., Piccart, M. J., et al. (2003). A randomized trial of letrozole in postmenopausal women after five years of tamoxifen therapy for early-stage breast cancer. *New England Journal of Medicine, 349,* 1793–1802.

Gumm, R., Cunnick, G. H., & Mokbel, K. (2004). Evidence for the management of mastalgia. *Current Medical Research and Opinion, 20,* 681–684.

Hadi, M. S. (2000). Sports brassiere: Is it a solution for mastalgia? *The Breast Journal, 6,* 407–409.

Harris, J. R., Lippman, M. E., Morrow, M., & Hellman, S. (Eds.) (2000). *Diseases of the breast* (2nd ed.). Philadelphia: Lippincott-Raven.

Holmes, M. D., & Willett, W. C. (2004). Does diet affect breast cancer risk? *Breast Cancer Research, 6,* 170–178.

Hsueh, E., Hansen, N., & Giuliano, A. (2000). Intraoperative lymphatic mapping and sentinel lymph node dissection in breast cancer. *CA: A Cancer Journal for Clinicians, 50,* 279–288.

Ingram, D. M., Hickling, C., West, L., Mahe, L. J., & Dunbar, P. M. (2002). A double-blind randomized controlled trial of isoflavones in the treatment of cyclical mastalgia. *Breast, 11,* 170–174.

Jones, D. P. (2004). Cultural views of the female breast. *The Association of Black Nursing Faculty Journal, 15,* 15–21.

Kerlikowske, K., Smith-Bindman, R., Ljung, B., & Grady, D. (2003). Evaluation of abnormal mammography results and palpable breast abnormalities. *Annals of Internal Medicine, 139,* 274–284.

Khan, H. N., Rampaul, R., & Blamey, R. W. (2004). Local anaesthetic and steroid combined injection therapy in the management of non-cyclical mastalgia. *The Breast, 13,* 129–132.

Kinsinger, L. S., Harris, R., Woolf, S. H., Sox, H. C., & Lohr, K. N. (2002). Chemoprevention of breast cancer: A summary of the evidence for the U.S. Preventive Services Task Force. *Annals of Internal Medicine, 137,* 59–69.

Lanng, C., Eriksen, B. Ø., & Hoffman, J. (2004). Lipoma of the breast: A diagnostic dilemma. *The Breast, 13,* 408–411.

Lester, J. (2000). Breast tenderness/nipple discharge/swelling/lumps. In D. Camp-Sorrell & R. A. Hawkins (Eds.), *Clinical manual for the oncology advanced practice nurse* (pp. 921–925). Pittsburgh, PA: Oncology Nursing Press.

Marchant, D. J. (2002). Benign breast disease. *Obstetrics and Gynecology Clinics of North America, 29,* 1–20.

Millet, A. V., & Dirbas, F. M. (2002). Clinical management of breast pain: A review. *Obstetrical and Gynecological Survey, 57,* 451–461.

National Cancer Institute. (2004). *Breast cancer (PDQ®): Treatment. Health professional version.* Retrieved October 10, 2004, from http://www.cancer.gov/cancertopics/pdq/treatment/breast/Health-Professional.

National Comprehensive Cancer Network. (2004). *Breast cancer. Clinical practice guidelines in oncology—v.1.2004.* Retrieved October 10, 2004, from http://www.nccn.org/professionals/physician_gls/PDF/breast.pdf.

National Surgical Adjuvant Breast and Bowel Project. (n.d.). *Study of tamoxifen and raloxifene.* Retrieved October 8, 2004, from http://www.nsabp.pitt.edu/star/index.html.

Osuch, J. R. (2002). Breast health and disease over a lifetime. *Clinical Obstetrics and Gynecology, 45,* 1140–1161.

Rossouw, J. E., Anderson, G. L., Prentice, R. L., LaCroix, A. Z., Jackson, R. D., Beresford, S. A. A., et al. (2002). Risks and benefits of estrogen plus progestin in healthy postmenopausal women: Principal results from the Women's Health Initiative randomized controlled trial. *Journal of the American Medical Association, 288,* 321–333.

Sauter, E. R., Schlatter, L., Lininger, J., & Hewett, J. E. (2004). The association of bloody nipple discharge with breast pathology. *Surgery, 136,* 780–785.

Simmons, R., Adamovich, T., Brennan, M., Christos, P., Schultz, M., Eisen, C., et al. (2003). Nonsurgical evaluation of pathologic nipple discharge. *Annals of Surgical Oncology, 10,* 113–116.

Smith, B. L., & Souba, W. W. (1995). Breast disease. Algorithm and explanation: Assessment and management of breast complaints. *Scientific American Surgery, VIII,* 1–16.

Smith, M., & Kent, K. (2002). Breast concerns and lifestyles of women. *Clinical Obstetrics and Gynecology, 45*, 1129–1139.

Smith, R. L., Pruthi, S., & Fitzpatrick, L. A. (2004). Evaluation and management of breast pain. *Mayo Clinic Proceedings, 79*, 353–372.

Speroff, L., & Fritz, M. (2005). *Clinical gynecologic endocrinology and infertility* (7th ed.). Baltimore: Lippincott Williams & Wilkins.

Tavaf-Motamen, H., Ader, D. N., Browne, M. W., & Shriver, C. D. (1998). Clinical evaluation of mastalgia. *Archives of Surgery, 133*, 211–213.

Veronesi, U., Cascinelli, N., Mariani, L., Greco, M., Saccozzi, R., Alberto, L., et al. (2002). Twenty-year follow-up of a randomized study comparing breast-conserving surgery with radical mastectomy for early breast cancer. *New England Journal of Medicine, 347*, 1227–1232.

Westhoff, C. L. (1999). Breast cancer risk: Perception versus reality. *Contraception, 59*(Suppl. 1), 25S–28S.

Winer, E., Morrow, M., Osborne, C. K., & Harris, J. R. (2001). Malignant tumors of the breast. In V. DeVita, S. Hellman, & S. Rosenberg (Eds.), *Cancer principles and practice of oncology* (6th ed., pp. 1683–1684). Philadelphia: Lippincott Williams & Wilkins.

Yaziji, H., Goldstein, L. C., Barry, T. S., Werling, R., Hwang, H., Ellis, G. K., et al. (2004). HER-2 testing in breast cancer using parallel tissue-based methods. *Journal of the American Medical Association, 291*, 1972–1977.

Young, I. (1998). Breasted experience. In R. Weitz (Ed.), *The politics of women's bodies: Sexuality, appearance, and behavior* (pp. 125–136). Oxford, England: Oxford University Press.

Chapter 14

FEMALE SEXUAL DYSFUNCTION

SUSAN CHASSON

We live in a society where men, women, and children are constantly bombarded with messages about the importance of sexuality. Unfortunately these messages create a limited view of sexuality, usually emphasizing physical desirability to a partner and a person's ability to achieve orgasm. When society has a limited view of sexuality, there is the potential for using a limited approach to solving sexual problems. With the advent of sildenafil (Viagra) many clinicians have expressed concerns that the treatment of sexual dysfunction is becoming too medicalized. The greatest concern is that researchers are spending the majority of their time looking for a magic pill that will cure female sexual dysfunction and are not looking at the complex and multiple factors that may be causes of sexual dysfunction.

When examining sexuality and sexual dysfunction, it is important to look at a broad definition of sexuality. Poorman (1988) gives us a definition of sexuality that goes beyond basic sexual function, allowing us to examine sexuality in a more holistic and comprehensive manner by stating:

> Sexuality is interwoven with every aspect of human existence, and in its broadest sense, sexuality is defined as a desire for contact, warmth, tenderness, or love (Aletkey, 1980). Humans express and live their sexuality in their daily lives. Sexuality is not limited to an act of seduction or intercourse but encompasses every area in our lives: the way we relate to others, our friends, our family, and our work. It is evident in what we believe, how we behave, and the way we look. (p. 1)

Using a broader definition of sexuality allows the clinician to look at sexual problems in the context of both the patient as an individual and as a member of a larger society.

Evaluating and treating sexual dysfunction is a challenging area of women's health care. Composed of a complex combination of physical, psychological, and cultural components, our sexuality is shaped from conception by influences as diverse as genetics, religion, family, and the media (Morley & Kaiser, 2003). To provide care to women with sexual problems, the clinician must begin her or his practice with a correct understanding of female genital anatomy and physiology. Many health care providers are unaware that the clitoris is a wishbone shaped structure measuring between nine and eleven centimeters in length, because most medical textbooks describe what is actually the glans of the clitoris as the entire structure (Berman & Berman, 2001). The clinician must also be comfortable talking about sexual issues in a nonjudgmental fashion when dealing with the sexual problems of a patient.

CLASSIFICATION OF SEXUAL DYSFUNCTION

There are various approaches to classifying sexual dysfunction. This chapter will follow the structure developed by the American Foundation of Urologic Disease in the *Report on the International Consensus Development Conference on Female Sexual Dysfunction Definitions and Classifications* (International Consensus), which can be found in Box 14–1 (Basson et al., 2000). In 1998 a group of 19 experts in the field of female sexuality met to develop a new classification system for female sexual dysfunction. The purpose of the new classification was to combine the approach of the *DSM-IV: Diagnostic and Statistical Manual of Mental Disorders* (American Psychiatric Association, 1994), which looks mainly at psychological causes of sexual dysfunction, with organic causes of sexual dysfunction (Basson et al., 2000).

This classification of sexual dysfunction identifies problems within the three phases of sexual response—desire, arousal, and orgasm—and also includes the sexual pain disor-

---

BOX 14–1 CLASSIFICATION OF FEMALE SEXUAL DYSFUNCTION

 I. Sexual desire disorders:
  a. Hypoactive sexual desire disorder
  b. Sexual aversion disorder
 II. Sexual arousal disorder
 III. Orgasmic disorder
 IV. Sexual pain disorders:
  a. Dyspareunia
  b. Vaginismus
  c. Other sexual pain disorders

Source: Reprinted with permission from Basson, R., Berman, J., Burnett, A., Derogatis, L., Ferguson, D., Fourcroy, J., et al. (2000). Report of the International Consensus Development Conference on female sexual dysfunction: Definitions and classifications. *Journal of Urology, 163,* 888–893.

ders. The classification does not distinguish between dysfunction caused by psychological or physical problems, instead recognizing that most sexual problems are the result of many factors. An important part of both the classification system and the evaluation of sexual problems is determining whether or not the patient perceives the sexual dysfunction as a problem (Basson et al., 2000). For example, a woman who is unable to achieve orgasm but is satisfied by the sexual relationship with her partner is not considered to have sexual dysfunction. The development of the classification system has been met with some criticism, including conflicts of interest caused by major funding of the participants by the pharmaceutical industry, and lack of ability to define and measure personal distress (Shaw, 2001; Sugrue & Whipple, 2001); however, it gives the clinician a basis for looking at the problem of sexual dysfunction.

SCOPE OF THE PROBLEM

Many women have concerns about sexual issues. In one survey about sexual concerns, 43% of women acknowledged one or more problems with six different aspects of sexual response. Of the 1486 women, 27–32% reported a lack of interest in sex, 22–28% were unable to achieve orgasm, 17–27% reported sex was not pleasurable, 18–27% described trouble lubricating, 6–16% were anxious about performance, and 8–21% experienced pain during sex (ranges reflect variations among age groups) (Laumann, Paik, & Rosen, 1999). In another study of 1480 women seeking annual gynecologic care from a military hospital, 98.8% of the women surveyed reported one or more sexual concerns (Nusbaum, Gamble, & Heiman, 2000). These included lack of interest in sex, orgasm difficulty, lubrication, dyspareunia, body image, and other issues, including sexually transmitted diseases and sexual abuse (Nusbaum et al.).

There are several studies that recognize the prevalence of sexual problems among women, but critical information is missing from these surveys. There is no attempt in most of the studies to determine whether the problems identified are related to the patient or related to a problem with the patient's relationship with her partner (Bancroft, 2002). Although acknowledging difficulties with sexual response does not give a patient a diagnosis of sexual dysfunction, these surveys do indicate that sexual concerns are common.

ETIOLOGY

Developmental, health-related, partner, and relationship factors, as well as sociocultural influences may all contribute to female sexual dysfunction (see Chapter 8). Physical and psychological etiologies are possible, and an individual woman may have multiple causes of sexual dysfunction. Women with sexual concerns may also be experiencing normal variations of sexuality, and this must be considered in the assessment.

GENERAL ASSESSMENT FOR SEXUAL CONCERNS

This section describes the general assessment of any woman presenting with sexual concerns. Screening for sexual concerns is discussed in Chapter 8. Additional assessments specific to the different types of sexual dysfunction are detailed later in this chapter. The purpose of the assessment is to help identify all of the possible psychological or physical sources for the problem. When assessing the patient for sexual dysfunction, it is necessary to determine whether or not the problems are partner specific. Relationship stressors need to be evaluated to determine the source of sexual dysfunction. For example, if a patient is in an abusive relationship, changing the time and location of sexual relations will probably not increase sexual desire.

HISTORY

When evaluating the patient with a sexual problem, reviewing normal sexual response may be all that is needed to reassure the patient that what she is experiencing is normal. The clinician may also need to evaluate the patient's understanding of normal sexual anatomy and function. One technique is to use a diagram to discuss genital anatomy and physiology. Many women do not understand normal sexual response. For example, many people do not realize that the majority of women cannot achieve orgasm without direct or indirect stimulation of the clitoris. Women who cannot achieve orgasm through intercourse often believe they have a problem. Discussing and describing sexual anatomy may give the patient enough information to allow her to understand and improve her sexual response.

Assessment of the patient with sexual concerns requires a comprehensive health history that includes physical, psychological, and social history questions. Investigation of physical concerns should include surgeries, chronic illnesses, medications, and allergies. Surgeries that could impact vascular or neurologic function of the genital tract might indicate a need for further investigation. Chronic illnesses that involve neurologic, endocrine, or vascular problems (e.g., thyroid disease, diabetes, hypertension) are particularly of interest because of their potential impact on sexual function (MacLaren, 1995). A review of medications is important because several drugs are known to cause or exacerbate sexual problems (Box 14–2). Screening the patient for latex allergies should be a standard part of any gynecologic examination, because latex products used both for contraception and during pelvic examinations may be a source of sexually related pain.

A social history should include prior or present history of physical, emotional, or sexual abuse. It is important to inquire about the use of recreational drugs, alcohol, and cigarettes, because these habits may also be a factor in sexual dysfunction. Screen the woman for risk factors associated with sexual activity, including multiple sexual partners and use of contraception. Sexually transmitted infections may be a source of sexual pain, and oral contraceptives may cause decreased desire in some women. The cultural and religious beliefs of the patient should be considered when evaluating and recommending treatment

BOX 14-2   MEDICATIONS THAT CAN CAUSE OR EXACERBATE FEMALE SEXUAL DYSFUNCTION

Anorectics

Anticholinergics

Anticonvulsants

Antidepressants

Antiestrogens

Antihistamines

Antihypertensives

Antipsychotics

Antiulcer drugs

Barbiturates

Benzodiazepines

Gonadotropin-releasing hormone (GnRH) agonists

Narcotics

Oral contraceptives

Sources: Berman & Berman, 2001; Brassil & Keller, 2002; Fogel, 2004; Phillips, 2000.

for sexual dysfunction. For example, if a patient is unable to achieve orgasm through intercourse, encouraging self-stimulation may not be an option if that practice conflicts with religious or cultural beliefs.

A psychological history should examine issues such as life stressors, coping mechanisms, and body image. Women should also be assessed for signs and symptoms of major depression and other mental health problems, such as post-traumatic stress disorder and obsessive compulsive disorder that affect sexual function. In addition to asking general questions about the patient's physical, mental, and social health, Maurice (1999) suggests the clinician use a framework of questions about seven topic areas to identify the specific sexual problem. These topics include duration of problem, circumstances, description, patient's sex response cycle, partner's sex response cycle, patient and partner's reaction, and motivation for treatment.

PHYSICAL EXAMINATION

The physical examination should specifically look for potential health problems that could affect sexual function such as undiagnosed diabetes or hypertension. Height, weight, and vital signs should be recorded. Neurologic and vascular systems should be examined. The genital examination should include inspection and palpation of both external and internal genital structures (see Chapter 6 for examination techniques).

DIAGNOSTIC TESTING

Laboratory tests should be considered when there is a clinical indication. Cultures to determine the presence of a vaginal infection are indicated in a patient experiencing pain with intercourse. Other tests to consider include: thyroid studies for problems with decreased desire; hemoglobin A1C and lipid profile to determine a vascular source of sexual dysfunction; measurement of sex hormone-binding globulin (SHBG), free and total testosterone levels to look at problems caused by androgen deficiencies; and follicle-stimulating hormone (FSH) and estradiol levels to examine ovarian function (Clayton, 2003).

DIFFERENTIAL DIAGNOSES

The clinician should begin by categorizing the type of sexual dysfunction into one or more of the classifications developed by the International Consensus and found in Box 14–1 (Basson et al., 2000). Using the information obtained in the history and physical examination, the clinician should then determine whether the source of the dysfunction is psychological or physical. The rest of this chapter will look at specific assessment and management for each type of sexual dysfunction.

FURTHER ASSESSMENT AND MANAGEMENT OF SPECIFIC TYPES OF SEXUAL DYSFUNCTION

HYPOACTIVE SEXUAL DESIRE DISORDER

Hypoactive sexual desire disorder is defined as the "persistent or recurrent deficiency (or absence) of sexual fantasies/thoughts, and/or desire for or receptivity to sexual activity, which causes personal distress" (Basson et al., 2000, p. 890). In 2000, Dr. Rosemary Basson proposed a new model for female sexual response based on a changed perspective of female sexual dysfunction and desire disorders. Instead of the traditional model of arousal, desire, orgasm, and resolution, Basson (2000) describes many women as moving from a state of sexual neutrality to a state where they become motivated to seek stimuli that will cause sexual arousal. Further discussion and a diagram of Basson's model can be found in Chapter 8.

Basson (2000) believes that many women are motivated to initiate sexual activity by things other than a desire for sexual gratification. These motivating factors for sexual relations may include "emotional closeness, increased commitment, bonding, and tolerance of imperfections in the relationship" (Basson, p. 53). If a woman achieves these nonsexual goals, she will view her sexual experience as positive whether or not she personally experiences sexual gratification. Therefore, when assessing a woman for desire disorder, it is important to look at what motivates the patient's desire for sexual relations.

Assessment of Hypoactive Sexual Desire Disorder   Assessment of sexual desire disorder should start with determining the duration of the problem. Has the patient always felt this way, or is this a change in her level of desire? It is important to look for any negative factors, either psychological or physical, that may affect desire. Are there conflicts about other issues in the patient's relationship with her partner? Is the patient experiencing pain with intercourse? Other social factors that may impact desire include financial stress, small children that continue to require care at night, or work schedules that make it difficult for couples to find the time or energy to plan for sexual intimacy.

Frequency of sexual relations is another important factor to evaluate. Many couples report a decrease in frequency of sexual relations with time (Laumann, Gagnon, Michael, & Michaels, 1994). Instead of experiencing a lack of sexual desire caused by a physical or psychological source, the problem may be linked to a difference in expectations between the patient and her partner. In one study, married couples reported the following frequencies of sexual activity—not at all, 1.3%; a few times a year, 12.8%; a few times a month, 42.5%; two to three times a week, 36.1%; and four or more times a week, 7.3% (Laumann et al., 1994). These statistics give the clinician a baseline for looking at decrease in desire as it relates to frequency of sexual activity.

It is also important to inquire about whether or not change in desire has resulted in a change in sexual frequency. Does the woman continue to have sexual relations even when the encounters are unwanted? A woman who believes she does not have a choice about frequency of sexual relations may first need to deal with issues of power and control in the relationship before determining if there is a physical basis for her problem.

Using Basson's model (2000), if the patient does not initiate sexual relations, it is necessary to find out if she is willing to participate in and able to enjoy sexual relations if sexual intercourse is initiated by her partner. This patient may simply need to be told that her pattern of response is normal for many women. With the patient, explore any changes that may have altered her satisfaction with her sexual relationship. Does the woman experience orgasm with sexual relations? Although many anorgasmic women report satisfying sexual relationships, over time the lack of physical pleasure may decrease motivation for sexual relations.

Investigate the timing of sexual relations, and what occurs after intercourse. Although most men find sexual intercourse sedating, many women have increased mental arousal after sexual relations. In this situation, a woman may be more concerned about the loss of sleep than achieving the feelings of closeness that may result from sexual relations.

Do the negatives that result from sexual relations outweigh the positive rewards? If a woman's need for intimacy is not being met during the sexual encounter, because of either lack of time or fatigue, then she may lose her motivation for future sexual encounters. Although the hormonal changes associated with menopause can affect desire, a woman's inability to achieve pregnancy—a previous motivating factor for sexual relations—may act as a factor in decreasing desire for sexual relations after menopause or tubal ligation.

Do associated physical symptoms indicate that a patient's lack of desire is the result of underlying illness? Fatigue may be related to thyroid dysfunction or sleep disorders. Does the patient have chronic medical problems, such as arthritis or back pain, that make sexual relations painful or uncomfortable? Desire disorders are also associated with thyroid disease, epilepsy, and renal disease. Screen the patient for medications (Box 14–2) or surgeries that could alter desire by changing hormone levels, particularly oral contraceptives, GnRH agonists, antiestrogens, and hysterectomy or oophorectomy.

Menopause may be a time of decreased desire, and the reasons for this change may go beyond alterations in hormone levels. Decreased desire may be the result of insomnia, hot flashes, increased vaginal dryness, or decreased vaginal elasticity that results in pain (Weismiller, 2002). Recently androgen deficiency has been targeted as a source of decreased desire in perimenopausal and menopausal women. Studies show that androgen deficiency may be associated with problems with arousal, genital sensation, libido, and orgasm (Berman & Goldstein, 2001).

Androgens are produced both by the ovaries and the adrenal glands. The ovaries produce testosterone and androstenedione, and the adrenal glands produce dehydroepiandrosterone (DHEA) and dehydroepiandrosterone-sulfate (DHEAS). Androstenedione, DHEA, and DHEAS levels decrease 25 to 50% between the ages of 30 and 50 years (Knochenhauer & Azziz, 2001). Despite the 20–30% decrease in testosterone during menopause, a corresponding decrease in SHBG causes the levels of bioavailable, free testosterone to rise or remain the same (Lobo, 2003). Androgen levels can vary significantly from one woman to another, and the two main factors that can decrease androgen levels are oophorectomy and oral estrogen therapy. Oophorectomy can result in a 50% loss of testosterone production and oral estrogen therapy can increase SHBG, causing a relative decrease in free testosterone levels. In addition to drug-related and ovarian failure androgen deficiency, hypopituitarism, and adrenal insufficiency can also cause abnormal levels of androgens (Bachmann et al., 2002). For menopausal women with symptoms of androgen deficiency that cannot be explained by other conditions, laboratory testing that demonstrates abnormal androgen levels can diagnose idiopathic androgen insufficiency (Bachmann et al.).

There are problems with testing for androgen levels. Serum testosterone testing was initially designed for men, who have much higher blood levels of testosterone. Recent studies indicate two methods that will give an accurate representation of testosterone levels in women. Free testosterone calculated from the law of mass action, which requires the measurement of total testosterone and SHBG, and free testosterone measured by equilibrium dialysis, give the most accurate levels of bioavailable testosterone (Miller et al., 2004). Although normal levels of total testosterone range from 4–60 pg/ml, and free testosterone levels range from 0.6–6.8 pg/ml, some clinicians believe androgen therapy should be considered in women whose total testosterone levels are less than 20 pg/ml or whose free testosterone levels are less than 0.9 pg/dl (Berman & Goldstein, 2001). Androgen therapy has become a popular treatment for women's sexual dysfunction (Rako, 1996). It is important for the clinician to have a specific diagnosis prior to treating a patient with androgens (Bachmann et al.). Informed consent should include discussing with the patient the potential risks of "acne, weight gain, excess facial and body hair, permanent lowering of the voice, emotional changes, and adverse lipid changes" (Bachmann et al., p. 664).

Management of Hypoactive Sexual Desire Disorder   Treatment for hypoactive sexual desire disorder depends upon the type of problem identified. Patients with undiagnosed or untreated physical or mental health problems require interventions to remedy the underlying illness. Consider changing medications that may be affecting sexual desire (Box 14–2). If decreased desire is related to pain with intercourse, the source of the pain should be diagnosed and treated. If sexual dysfunction already exists, be aware of how medical interventions may cause the sexual problems to increase in severity. For example, decreased libido has been documented as a symptom in 70% to 80% of patients with depression (Clayton, 2002). At the same time, selective serotonin reuptake inhibitors (SSRIs) have a 36–43% rate of sexual dysfunction reported with their use (Clayton).

Women should be educated about normal alterations in desire that result from life changes such as those resulting from pregnancy, lactation, and menopause. Individual or couple counseling may help patients whose decreased desire is the result of life stressors or relationship problems. Some strategies for the primary care provider include encouraging couples to communicate about their sexual needs and differences, having couples vary the time of day or location for sexual activities, and making sure couples set aside planned time for intimacy (Phillips, 2000).

Women who have sexual side effects from the SSRIs may be helped by buproprion SR (Wellbutrin), given in doses of 300 to 400 mg a day (Clayton, 2002). Adding 30–60 mg of buspirone (Buspar) per day may also be used and has been shown to be twice as effective as a placebo in relieving sexual side effects of SSRIs. Switching the patient to an antidepressant with minimal sexual side effects, such as mirtrazapine, nefazadone, or trazadone, is another option (Clayton; Phillips & Slaughter, 2000).

For the woman experiencing physiologic changes related to menopause, estrogen therapy may eliminate hot flashes, insomnia that creates fatigue, and mood changes that result in decreased desire. Vaginal estrogen preparations may be used to decrease pain resulting from atrophic vaginitis. There is a Food and Drug Administration (FDA)-approved oral preparation of methyltestosterone in combination with estradiol (Estratest) for the woman with documented androgen deficiency. Proponents of androgen supplements often recommend obtaining topical preparations of methyltestosterone or testosterone proprionate from a compounding pharmacy (Berman & Goldstein, 2001). It is important to remember that the known adverse affects from androgen supplementation include decrease of high-density lipoprotein (HDL) cholesterol, hirsutism, deepening of the voice, liver damage, hair loss, and enlargement of the clitoris. There are also no prospective randomized controlled trials of androgen therapy to support the efficacy and safety of long-term androgen supplementation in menopausal women (Modelska & Cummings, 2003).

SEXUAL AVERSION DISORDER

Sexual aversion disorder is defined as "the persistent or recurrent phobic aversion to and avoidance of sexual contact with a sexual partner that causes personal distress" (Basson et al., 2000, p. 890). Sexual aversion or phobia is often associated with physical, sexual, or emotional abuse as a child or an adult. Theories about the development of sexual aversion include association of sexual stimuli with pain or physical trauma, and association of sexual relations with helplessness and loss of control (Bartoi, Kinder, & Tomianovic, 2000).

Assessment of Sexual Aversion Disorder Women with sexual aversion should be asked about prior history of abuse. Some women who display signs and symptoms of previous sexual trauma may not be able to remember any abuse. This lack of memory may be related to the age at which the abuse occurred, or to psychological protective mechanisms (Penner & Penner, 1993). Women with sexual aversion should be screened for depression, anxiety, and substance abuse, as these problems are often associated with child and adult sexual abuse and assault (Bartoi et al., 2000). Other problems associated with a history of sexual abuse are eating disorders such as anorexia nervosa or bulimia, and chronic pelvic pain. Although sexual aversion is often associated with trauma, it may also be the result of fear of harming the patient's sexual partner or fear of performance anxiety (Morley & Kaiser, 2003).

Management of Sexual Aversion Disorder Treatment should attempt to determine the underlying cause for the aversion. Therapy should be directed at resolving issues of abuse or trauma. Women with sexual aversion may respond to behavioral therapy that uses desensitization to teach a patient to become comfortable, first with her own body, and then with increased sexual intimacy with a partner (Finch, 2001). It is important that women with sexual aversion disorder are referred to an appropriate mental health provider for counseling to deal with the underlying issues of trauma or abuse.

SEXUAL AROUSAL DISORDER

Sexual arousal disorder is defined as "the persistent or recurrent inability to attain or maintain sufficient sexual excitement, causing personal distress, which may be expressed as a lack of subjective excitement, or genital (lubrication/swelling), or other somatic responses" (Basson et al., 2000, p. 890). Arousal disorders may be caused by medications, hormonal changes, physiological, or psychological problems (Brassil & Keller, 2002). Women should be asked whether they are experiencing vaginal lubrication or feelings of genital engorgement. It is also important to determine whether or not the woman is having adequate stimulation to achieve arousal prior to her partner attempting intercourse.

Assessment of Sexual Arousal Disorder Patients with difficulties in achieving arousal should be examined for physiological problems causing vascular or neurologic changes to the body. Diabetes, hypertension, and coronary artery disease can affect genital vasculature. The patient should also be questioned about exercise or physical activities such as bicycle riding or gymnastics, which can result in nerve trauma (Brassil & Keller, 2002). Medications associated with arousal problems include anticholinergics, antihistamines, monoamine oxidase (MAO) inhibitors, SSRIs, tricyclic antidepressants, and antihypertensives. Smoking and alcohol use can also affect a woman's ability to achieve sexual arousal.

Management of Sexual Arousal Disorder   If arousal problems are the result of inadequate stimulation of the clitoris, instructing the patient in the use of artificial lubricants and clitoral stimulation may allow for adequate arousal to achieve orgasm. Treatments for medical conditions associated with arousal disorder are usually based on trying to restore blood flow to the genital tissues. Vaginal lubricants may help increase stimulation. A warm bath may also cause vasodilation. For menopausal women with atrophic vaginitis, localized estrogen therapy may be beneficial. The FDA has also approved a device called the Eros-CTD (clitoral therapy device). This device fits over the clitoris and increases blood flow to the area by creating gentle suction (Berman & Berman, 2001).

Herbal preparations used for treating problems with sexual arousal include yohimbe and ginko biloba. Both appear to help women with orgasm problems related to antidepressant use (Rowland & Tai, 2003). There are no clinical research data to support the use of ginseng for sexual dysfunction (Rowland & Tai). Avimil and Zestra are two over-the-counter (OTC) products advertised for sexual dysfunction (Rowland & Tai). Currently there are no published clinical trials using Avimil (Kellogg-Spadt, 2003). Zestra, a topical massage oil, was tested in a sample size of 20 women and found to improve multiple aspects of sexual dysfunction (Ferguson et al., 2003). Clinicians should be cautious about recommending OTC preparations, because most contain multiple ingredients that may place a patient at risk for potential adverse reactions.

Although not approved for use in women, sildenafil (Viagra) has been tested in clinical trials. The outcomes of these trials have produced mixed results (Caruso, Intelisano, Lupo, & Agnello, 2002; Kaplan et al., 1999; Modelska & Cummings, 2003). There is some indication that sildenafil may be useful in treating arousal disorders in woman being treated with SSRIs, but these studies did not use placebo-controlled trials (Modelska & Cummings, 2003). Sildenafil should not be used in women with cardiovascular disease.

Future therapies being examined for arousal disorder include alprostadil, tibolone, and testosterone. Application of 1 gm of 0.2% alprostadil, a prostaglandin E_1, compounded into a topical gel, has been demonstrated to increased clitoral blood flow when applied topically (Becher, Bechara, & Casabe, 2001). Another medication being investigated is tibolone (Livial). Tibolone is a synthetic steroid given orally that has estrogenic, androgenic, and progestagenic properties. Tibolone has been used in Europe for many years to treat menopausal women, but it has not been approved by the FDA for use in the United States. In one small, randomized, double-blind trial, tibolone improved vaginal blood flow and vaginal lubrication (Modelska & Cummings, 2002).

Testosterone preparations designed for women are also being tested for alleviating sexual arousal disorder. Some clinicians are presently using off-label 1% testosterone gel (AndroGel), or they are prescribing compounded testosterone cream for arousal disorders (Berman & Berman, 2001). Achieving proper dosing for women can be difficult, because testosterone gel is packaged in a dose for male replacement. It is important to remember that testosterone is category X and contraindicated in pregnancy.

ORGASMIC DISORDER

Orgasmic disorder is "the recurrent difficulty, delay, or absence of attaining orgasm following sufficient sexual stimulation and arousal, which results in personal distress" (Basson et al., 2000, p. 890). In one study, only 29% of women reported always having an orgasm with their partner, compared to 75% of men. Yet 46.6% of men and 40.5% of women reported being extremely physically satisfied with their relationship (Laumann et al., 1994).

Assessment of Orgasmic Disorder   Assessment of orgasmic disorder begins with determining the duration and extent of the problem. Has the patient ever experienced an orgasm? Is the patient able to reach orgasm through self-stimulation, or has the patient experienced orgasm with a different partner? For a woman who has never experienced an orgasm either by self or partner stimulation, determine if she has experienced an orgasm while sleeping. Inability to achieve orgasm is usually related to lack of sufficient stimulation, or involuntary inhibition of the orgasmic reflex (Phillips, 2000). Inhibition of the orgasmic reflex may be psychological, or may be a response to genital pain. Neurologic and vascular problems can create problems achieving orgasm. Medications can also alter orgasmic function (Box 14–2).

Management of Orgasmic Disorder   There is no specific method for a woman to achieve orgasm. Laumann and colleagues (1994) describe orgasm as "a complex response to socially contextualized physical and mental stimuli and that, in any specific individual, there will be a variety of sources of effective stimulation, both physically and mentally" (p. 113). For the woman who has never experienced orgasm, the clinician should begin by using a diagram to demonstrate genital anatomy to the patient. It is important to explain to the patient that most women can achieve orgasm only through direct or indirect stimulation of the clitoris. Patients should be asked to try self exploration of their genital area to determine what type of touching achieves the best response. Practicing Kegel exercises allows the woman to control her muscular tension, which may decrease inhibition of her orgasmic response. For some women, the use of a vibrator will produce the required stimulation to achieve orgasm (Phillips, 2000). *Becoming Orgasmic* (Heiman & Lopiccolo, 1988) is an excellent self-help guide available for women who need more coaching to achieve orgasm. Patients who are uncomfortable with self stimulation may be able to instruct their partners to provide direct clitoral stimulation either manually or with a vibrator to achieve orgasm.

SEXUAL PAIN DISORDERS

Sexual pain disorders are described as three separate entities:

- Dyspareunia is the recurrent or persistent genital pain associated with sexual intercourse.
- Vaginismus is the recurrent or persistent involuntary spasm of the musculature of the outer third of the vagina that interferes with vaginal penetration and causes personal distress.
- Noncoital sexual pain disorder is the recurrent or persistent genital pain induced by noncoital sexual stimulation. (Basson et al., 2000, p. 890)

Assessment of Dyspareunia   In the evaluation of sexual pain, it is important to determine when the patient first experienced pain and the location of the pain. Patients who report persistent pain at the vaginal introitus, or inability to achieve penetration secondary to pain, should be evaluated for vulvar vestibulitis. Many of these women will describe experiencing pain while attempting to insert tampons prior to their first intercourse. To evaluate a patient for vulvar vestibulitis gently palpate the area anterior to the hymen with a cotton swab. The patient will often describe a sharp or burning sensation when touched with the swab. Pain is most often elicited at the region of six o'clock in the vestibule or fossa navicularis.

The etiology of vulvar vestibulitis is unknown. Several theories have been proposed including urinary excretion of oxalates, chronic candida, and human papillomavirus. Biopsies of the area usually demonstrate chronic inflammation (Gerber, Bongiovanni, Ledger, & Witkin, 2002). The clinician should rule out the presence of vaginal infections or dermatologic disorders before making the diagnosis of vulvar vestibulitis. Dermatologic disorders that may cause pain with intercourse include lichen sclerosces, lichen planus, lichen simplex chronicus, contact dermatitis, and psoriasis (Metts, 1999). A biopsy should be performed to diagnose any chronic skin conditions (see Chapter 22).

The patient with burning or pain after intercourse should be evaluated for vaginal infections, such as candida, group ß streptococcus, human papillomavirus, herpes simplex virus, trichomoniasis, and bacterial vaginosis (Heim, 2001). If the woman is using a latex barrier method for contraception, it is important to consider a latex allergy as the source of the pain.

Although fairly rare, some patients are sensitive to human semen. A woman with semen hypersensitivity can demonstrate localized symptoms of edema and burning after intercourse or systemic symptoms of hives, uticaria of the hands and face, cough, and dyspnea (DeCuyper, Bogaerts, Vanderkerchhove, & Gunst, 1996; Yocum, Jones, & Yunginger, 1996). If the clinician suspects a patient has a seminal fluid allergy, and use of latex condoms does not alleviate symptoms, the patient should also be assessed for a concurrent latex allergy.

Women who are perimenopausal or lactating should be evaluated for atrophic vaginitis. Medications that can also cause vaginal atrophy include antiestrogens, such as tamoxifen (Nolvadex), raloxifen (Evista), and leuprolide acetate (Lupron Depot). Women with atrophic vaginitis may have excessive dryness and burning after intercourse. Physical examination may demonstrate an alteration of the vaginal pH from the normal 4.7 to a pH between 6 and 7, mucosal color change, and decreased vaginal discharge (Wisniewski & Wilkinson, 1991).

Deep pelvic pain or pain with thrusting may be caused by endometriosis, pelvic adhesions, or adnexal pain (Heim, 2001). Trying to duplicate the pain during pelvic examination may give an indication of the source of the pain. Trauma related to episiotomy or obstetric lacerations may also be a source of sexual pain with pressure during intercourse placed on the perineum or the outer third of the vagina causing pain. Signorello, Harlow, Chekos, and Repke (2001) found that 26.7% of women who had a third or fourth-degree laceration with childbirth had pain with intercourse six months after giving birth.

Management of Dyspareunia   Treatment of dyspareunia will depend on the etiology of the pain. Women with signs and symptoms of vulvar vestibulitis may initially be treated conservatively with discontinuation of irritants to the vulvar area, such as excessive bathing, tight clothing, and sanitary pads (Edwards, 2003). Topical xylocaine 2% jelly or 5% ointment can be applied 20 minutes before intercourse. Some physical therapists are now receiving special training in pelvic floor rehabilitation. Techniques used by these therapists to decrease pelvic pain include using biofeedback to teach the patient to control her pelvic musculature, and myofascial massage to release painful trigger points in the pelvic area. In one retrospective study of patients receiving physical therapy for vulvar vestibulitis, 51.5% percent of patients reported a great improvement, or complete resolution of pain (Bergeron et al., 2002).

Some patients achieve pain relief with amitriptyline in doses up to 150 mg per day, or gabapentin (Neurontin) in doses up to 3600 mg per day (Edwards, 2003). For many women, surgical removal or laser treatment of the vestibule appears to have the best success for long-term pain relief. In a study of 111 women with primary and secondary vulvar vestibulitis, 80% of women with primary vestibulitis and 85% of women with secondary vestibulitis reported a satisfactory response to surgery (Bornstein, Maman, & Abramovici, 2001).

Vaginal infections should be treated with appropriate antibiotic or antifungal medication. Skin diseases of the genital area can usually be treated with short-term topical corticosteroids such as 2.5% hydrocortisone ointment or 0.1% triamcinolone (Metts, 1999). Atrophic vaginitis in the postpartum patient can be treated with short-term topical estrogen. In one small study, 11 women with postpartum atrophic vaginitis, treated with 2 gm twice a week of conjugated estrogen vaginal cream, experienced a resolution of symptoms within 28 days (Wisniewski & Wilkinson, 1991).

There are a variety of estrogen preparations for local administration available to menopausal women with atrophic vaginitis. Women who dislike the discharge associated with vaginal estrogen creams often prefer using the estradiol tablet (Vagifem) that is placed in the vagina, or the estradiol ring (Estring) that can be left in the vagina for three months. It is important to remember that women being treated with oral and transdermal estrogen therapy for menopausal symptoms may not be getting sufficient estrogen levels to treat atrophic vaginitis.

Treatment for pelvic pain with intercourse will depend on the source of the pain. Many patients report periodic sharp pain when their partner thrusts during intercourse. This pain is often the result of the penis against an ovary. Teaching the patient to shift the position of her hips to change the angle of the uterus and ovaries should eliminate this type of pelvic pain. Women with pelvic infections or endometriosis should receive appropriate treatment to remedy these problems. Physical therapy that teaches the patient to relax her pelvic muscles may also be beneficial in reducing pelvic pain.

Assessment of Vaginismus   Women with vaginismus are often not able to complete a pelvic examination. Involuntary contractions of the vaginal muscles prevent insertion of a speculum or the examiner's fingers. If the patient's partner is able to insert his penis into the vagina during sexual relations, he may describe intercourse as painful because of constriction of the penis by the muscles of the vagina. Patients with vaginismus may give a history of sexual abuse, or a history of pain or trauma resulting from medical procedures such as catheterization. Patients with dyspareunia may also develop vaginismus in response to repeated painful stimuli.

Management of Vaginismus   The treatment for vaginismus is progressive muscle relaxation. Kegel exercises can teach a patient to control her vaginal muscles. Referral to a physical therapist can provide the patient with the opportunity to use biofeedback to learn to control the vaginal muscles. The biofeedback machines use electrodes placed externally to the vagina to measure muscle tone. The patient then learns to consciously contract and relax the vaginal muscles and receives positive reinforcement when she practices the technique correctly. Once the patient successfully controls voluntary contraction and relaxation of the muscles, a series of dilators are used inside of the vagina until the woman can accommodate an object the size of a penis.

REFERRAL TO A THERAPIST SPECIALIZING IN SEXUAL DYSFUNCTION

The clinician who sees women with sexual dysfunction should be aware of counseling resources in his or her community. Problems that should be referred to a therapist are long-standing dysfunction, multiple dysfunctions, current or past abuse, a psychological disorder or acute psychological event, dysfunction with an unknown etiology, or a dysfunction with no response to therapy (Phillips, 2000). The American Association of Sex Educators, Counselors, and Therapists (AASECT) is a national organization that provides certification for sex counselors and sex therapists. Sex therapists are mental health professionals with specialized training in psychotherapy for sexual problems. The AASECT Web site (http://www.aasect.org) can help clinicians locate a certified sex therapist in their community.

REFERENCES

American Psychiatric Association. (1994). *DSM-IV: Diagnostic and Statistical Manual of Mental Disorders* (4th ed.). Washington, DC: Author.

Bachmann, G., Bancroft, J., Braunstein, G., Burger, H., Davis, S., Dennerstein, L., et al. (2002). Female androgen insufficiency: The Princeton consensus statement on definition, classification, and assessment. *Fertility and Sterility, 77,* 660–665.

Bancroft, J. (2002). The medicalization of female sexual dysfunction: The need for caution. *Archives of Sexual Behavior, 31,* 451–455.

Bartoi, M. G., Kinder, B. N., & Tomianovic, D. (2000). Interaction effects of emotional status and sexual abuse as an adult. *Journal of Sex and Marital Therapy, 26,* 1–25.

Basson, R. (2000). The female sexual response: A different model. *Journal of Sex and Marital Therapy, 26,* 51–65.

Basson, R., Berman, J., Burnett, A., Derogatis, L., Ferguson, D., Fourcroy, J., et al. (2000). Report of the International Consensus Development Conference on female sexual dysfunction: Definitions and classifications. *Journal of Urology, 163,* 888–893.

Becher, E. F., Bechara, A., & Casabe, A. (2001). Clitoral hemodynamic changes after a topical application of alprostadil. *Journal of Sex and Marital Therapy, 27,* 406–410.

Bergeron, S., Brown, C., Lord, M. J., Oala, M., Binik, Y. M., & Khalife, S. (2002). Physical therapy for vulvar vestibulitis syndrome: A retrospective study. *Journal of Sex and Marital Therapy, 28,* 183–192.

Berman, J., & Berman, L. (2001). *For women only: A revolutionary guide for overcoming sexual dysfunction and reclaiming your life.* New York: Henry Holt.

Berman, J., & Goldstein, I. (2001). Female sexual dysfunction. *Urologic Clinics of North America, 28,* 405–416.

Bornstein, J., Maman, M., & Abramovici, H. (2001). "Primary" versus "secondary" vulvar vestibulitis: One disease, two variants. *American Journal of Obstetrics and Gynecology, 148,* 28–31.

Brassil, D. F., & Keller, M. (2002). Female sexual dysfunction: Definitions, causes, and treatment. *Urologic Nursing, 22,* 237–284.

Caruso, S., Intelisano, G., Lupo, L., & Agnello, C. (2002). Premenopausal women affected by sexual arousal disorder treated with sildenafil: A double blind, cross-over, placebo-controlled study. *British Journal of Obstetrics and Gynecology, 108,* 623–628.

Clayton, A. H. (2002). Female sexual dysfunction related to depression and antidepressant medications. *Current Women's Health Reports, 2,* 182–187.

Clayton, A. H. (2003). Sexual function and dysfunction in women. *Psychiatric Clinics of North America, 26,* 673–682.

DeCuyper, C., Bogaerts, Y., Vanderkerchhove, F., & Gunst, J. (1996). Intravaginal desensitization and successful pregnancy in a woman with seminal fluid allergy. *Journal of Allergy and Clinical Immunology, 97,* 1428.

Edwards, L. (2003). New concepts in vulvodynia. *American Journal of Obstetrics and Gynecology, 189* (Suppl. 3), S24–S30.

Ferguson, D. M., Steidle, C. P., Singh, G. S., Alexander, J. S., Weihmiller, M. K., & Crosby, M. G. (2003). Randomized, placebo-controlled, double blind, crossover design trial of the efficacy and safety of Zestra for Women in women with and without female arousal disorder. *Journal of Sex and Marital Therapy, 29,* 33–44.

Finch, S. (2001). Sexual aversion disorder treated with behavioural desensitization. *Canadian Journal of Psychiatry, 46,* 563–563.

Fogel, C. I. (2004). Women and sexuality. In E. Q. Youngkin & M. S. Davis (Eds.), *Women's health: A primary care clinical guide* (3rd ed., pp. 109–129). Upper Saddle River, NJ: Pearson Prentice Hall.

Gerber, S., Bongiovanni, A. M., Ledger, W. J., & Witkin, S. S. (2002). Defective regulation of the proinflammatory immune response in women with vulvar vestibulitis syndrome. *American Journal of Obstetrics and Gynecology, 186,* 696–700.

Heim, L. J. (2001). Evaluation and differential diagnosis of dyspareunia. *American Family Physician, 63,* 1535–1544.

Heiman, J. R., & Lopiccolo, J. (1988). *Becoming orgasmic.* New York: Simon & Schuster.

Kaplan, S. A., Reis, R. B., Kohn, I. J., Ikeguchi, E. F., Laor, E., Te, A. E., et al. (1999). Safety and efficacy of sildenafil in postmenopausal women with sexual dysfunction. *Urology, 53,* 481–486.

Kellogg-Spadt, S. (2003). Sex Rx: When it comes to botanical prosexual preparations, clinicians and consumers beware! *Nurse Practitioners in Women's Health, 2*(11), 15–16.

Knochenhauer, E., & Azziz, R. (2001). Ovarian hormones and adrenal androgens during a woman's lifespan. *Journal of the American Academy of Dermatology, 45*(Suppl. 3), 105–115.

Laumann, E. O., Gagnon, J. H., Michael, R. T., & Michaels, S. (1994). *The social organization of sexuality: Sexual practices in the United States.* Chicago: University of Chicago Press.

Laumann, E. O., Paik, A., & Rosen, R. C. (1999). Sexual dysfunction in the United States: Prevalence and predictors. *Journal of the American Medical Association, 281*, 537–544.

Lobo, R. A. (2003). The physiology of androgens after menopause: What constitutes androgen deficiency? Menopause and sexuality: The impact of hormones [Special edition]. *Patient Care for the Nurse Practitioner, 4*–10.

MacLaren, A. (1995). Comprehensive sexual health assessment. *Journal of Nurse-Midwifery, 40*, 104–119.

Maurice, W. L. (1999). *Sexual medicine in primary care.* St. Louis, MO: Mosby.

Metts, J. F. (1999). Vulvodynia and vulvar vestibulitis: Challenges in diagnosis and management. *American Family Physician, 59*, 1547–1556.

Miller, K. K., Rosner, W., Lee, H., Hier, J., Sesmilo, G., Schoenfeld, D., et al. (2004). Measurement of free testosterone in normal women and women with androgen deficiency: Comparison of methods. *Journal of Endocrinology and Metabolism, 89*, 525–533.

Modelska, K., & Cummings, S. (2002). Tibolone for postmenopausal women: Systemic review of randomized trials. *Journal of Clinical Endocrinology and Metabolism, 87*, 16–23.

Modelska, K., & Cummings, S. (2003). Female sexual dysfunction in postmenopausal women: Systematic review of placebo-controlled trials. *American Journal of Obstetrics and Gynecology, 188*, 286–293.

Morley, J. E., & Kaiser, F. E. (2003). Female sexuality. *Medical Clinics of North America, 87*, 1077–1090.

Nusbaum, M. R., Gamble, G., & Heiman, J. (2000). The high prevalence of sexual concerns among women seeking routine gynecological care. *Journal of Family Practice, 49*, 229–232.

Penner, C. L., & Penner, J. J. (1993). *Restoring the pleasure.* Dallas: Word.

Phillips, N. A. (2000). Female sexual dysfunction: Evaluation and treatment. *American Family Physician, 62*, 127–136, 141–142.

Phillips, R. L., & Slaughter, J. S. (2000). Depression and sexual desire. *American Family Physician, 62*, 782–786.

Poorman, S. G. (1988). *Human sexuality and the nursing process.* Norwalk, CT: Appleton & Lange.

Rako, S. (1996). *The hormone of desire: The truth about testosterone, sexuality, and menopause.* New York: Three Rivers Press.

Rowland, D. L., & Tai, W. (2003). A review of plant-derived and herbal approaches to the treatment of sexual dysfunctions. *Journal of Sex and Marital Therapy, 28*, 185–205.

Shaw, J. (2001). Another procrustean bed for female sexual functioning. *Journal of Sex and Marital Therapy, 27*, 211–214.

Signorello, L. B., Harlow, B. L., Chekos, A. K., & Repke, J. T. (2001). Postpartum sexual functioning and its relationship to perineal trauma: A retrospective cohort study of primiparous women. *American Journal of Obstetrics and Gynecology, 184*, 881–890.

Sugrue, D. P., & Whipple, B. (2001). The consensus-based classification of female sexual dysfunction: Barriers to universal acceptance. *Journal of Sex and Marital Therapy, 27*, 221–226.

Weismiller, D. G. (2002). The perimenopause and menopause experience: An overview. *Clinics in Family Practice, 4*, 1–12.

Wisniewski, P. M., & Wilkinson, E. J. (1991). Postpartum vaginal atrophy. *American Journal of Obstetrics and Gynecology, 165*, 1249–1254.

Yocum, M. W., Jones, R. T., & Yunginger, J. W. (1996). Concurrent sensitization to natural rubber latex and human seminal fluid. *Journal of Allergy and Clinical Immunology, 98*, 1135–1136.

Chapter 15

UNINTENDED PREGNANCY

KATHERINE SIMMONDS
FRANCES E. LIKIS

Nearly half of all pregnancies in the United States are unintended, and for many women the discovery that they are pregnant is a time of personal crisis that requires complex decision making. Clinicians who provide gynecologic health care frequently encounter these women in the clinical setting and are often responsible for providing them with diagnoses, counseling, and other needed services or referrals. These responsibilities necessitate an understanding of unintended pregnancy, the conflicts that clinicians may experience when caring for women experiencing unintended pregnancies, and the appropriate assessment and management when providing this care.

SCOPE OF THE PROBLEM

An estimated 49% of pregnancies in the United States are unintended, and unintended pregnancies occur among women of all ages and socioeconomic groups (Brown & Eisenberg, 1995; Henshaw, 1998). The only age group in which the unintended pregnancy rate is less than 40% is women ages 30 to 34 years (Henshaw, 1998). Unintended pregnancies occur more frequently among women who are unmarried, living in poverty, or are at either end of their reproductive years (Brown & Eisenberg). According to the rates of unintended pregnancy in 1994 (the most recent year for which comprehensive data are available), it is estimated that the average woman can anticipate having 1.42 unintended pregnancies by the age of 45 years (Henshaw).

Approximately 47% of unintended pregnancies end in abortion, 40% result in live births, and 13% end in miscarriage (Henshaw, 1998). It is estimated that 1.31 million abortions took place in the United States in 2000 (Finer & Henshaw, 2003). Placing the infant for adoption is another alternative to parenting for the woman who chooses to carry an unintended pregnancy to term. Comprehensive adoption statistics have not been collected in the United States for over 10 years; thus current information about how frequently adoption is the outcome of unintended pregnancy is limited (National Adoption Information Clearinghouse, 2003). Estimates from the 1995 National Survey of Family Growth indicate that less than 1% of infants born to never-married women under 45 years of age were relinquished for adoption between 1989 and 1995 (Chandra, Abma, Maza, & Bachrach, 1999).

Consequences of the decision to continue an unintended pregnancy and to parent the child include potentially adverse effects for both women and their children. Unintended pregnancy is associated with later entry into prenatal care, a lower number of total prenatal visits, tobacco and alcohol use during pregnancy, low birth weight, infant mortality, child abuse, and insufficient resources for child development (Brown & Eisenberg, 1995). Unintended pregnancy precludes the opportunity to receive preconception care that may improve pregnancy outcomes. Women with unintended pregnancies are also at greater risk for physical abuse and depression. Couples experiencing unintended pregnancy are more likely to end their relationships, and they may forfeit their educational and professional aspirations (Brown & Eisenberg). Historically, unintended pregnancies have been subdivided into two categories: mistimed and unwanted. Pregnancies are defined as "mistimed" if the woman wanted to have a child or another child in the future, but not now. Pregnancies are considered "unwanted" if the woman never wanted to have a child or additional children. Negative effects of unintended pregnancy appear stronger among women with unwanted, rather than mistimed, pregnancies (Brown & Eisenberg).

ETIOLOGY

The most obvious reason why unintended pregnancies occur is inconsistent or incorrect use of contraceptives. Contraceptive nonuse and misuse results from numerous causes, including lack of knowledge; barriers to access; and complex personal, interpersonal, socioeconomic, and cultural factors (Brown & Eisenberg, 1995). Even perfect contraceptive use does not guarantee avoiding pregnancy because inherent method failures are possible. A recent study of over 10,000 women who had abortions found that 54% were using a contraceptive method in the month they conceived (Jones, Darroch, & Henshaw, 2002a). According to the Alan Guttmacher Institute (2000), "The typical American woman spends roughly three decades—or about 75% of her reproductive life—trying to avoid unintended pregnancy" (p. 10). Preventing pregnancy is an often underestimated undertaking that requires prolonged and concerted effort. The scale of this task, the obstacles to perfect contraceptive use, and the unavoidable failures of contraceptive methods provide insight into why unintended pregnancies are common.

CONFLICTS IN CARING FOR WOMEN WITH UNINTENDED PREGNANCIES

Clinicians may experience complex personal responses when providing care to women with unintended pregnancies. Reactions may range from complete acceptance to deep disturbance about a woman's situation or chosen course of action, with myriad possible emotions between these extremes. No matter what personal feelings are stirred by these clinical encounters, clinicians have professional responsibilities when providing patient care. Values clarification is a process that can help clinicians to explore the intersection of their personal beliefs and professional responsibilities, so that ultimately patients' rights are upheld (Simmonds & Likis, in press).

PROFESSIONAL RESPONSIBILITIES

Clinicians have professional responsibilities to uphold patient rights and autonomy, and to treat patients with respect and compassion. These responsibilities are codified by several professional organizations, including the American Academy of Physician Assistants (2004), the American College of Nurse-Midwives (1997), the American College of Obstetricians and Gynecologists (ACOG) (2004), and the National Organization of Nurse Practitioner Faculties and the American Association of Colleges of Nursing (2002). These documents (Box 15–1) provide an ethical and legal mandate for clinicians to ensure patient access to comprehensive reproductive health services, including pregnancy options counseling. Applying these principles in the clinical setting means that women must be given the opportunity to express their concerns, desires, and need for additional information in a supportive environment. Creating such conditions can be challenging.

BOX 15–1   STATEMENTS OF PROFESSIONAL ORGANIZATIONS

American Academy of Physician Assistants (2004):

Reproductive Decision Making: Patients have a right to access the full range of reproductive health care services, including fertility treatments, contraception, sterilization, and abortion. Physician assistants (PAs) have an ethical obligation to provide balanced and unbiased clinical information about reproductive health care.

When the PA's personal values conflict with providing full disclosure or providing certain services such as sterilization or abortion, the PA need not become involved in that aspect of the patient's care. By referring the patient to a qualified provider, the PA fulfills their ethical obligation to ensure the patient access to all legal options.

American College of Nurse-Midwives (1997):

Certified nurse-midwives (CNMs) and certified midwives (CMs) believe that every individual has the right to safe, satisfying health care with respect for human dignity and cultural variations. We support each person's right to self-determination, to complete information, and to active participation in all aspects of care. We acknowledge that the cultural, religious and ethnic diversity of CNMs and CMs and their clients allow for a variety of personal and professional choices.

(continues)

BOX 15–1 continued

Therefore, the ACNM holds the following positions:

- That every woman has the right to make reproductive choices;
- That every woman has the right to access to factual, unbiased information about reproductive choices, in order to make an informed decision; and
- That women with limited means should have access to financial resources for their reproductive choices.

American College of Obstetricians and Gynecologists (ACOG, 2004):

A pregnant woman should be fully informed in a balanced manner about all options, including raising the child herself, placing the child for adoption, and abortion. The information conveyed should be appropriate to the duration of the pregnancy. The professional should make every effort to avoid introducing personal bias.

ACOG supports access to care for all individuals, irrespective of financial status, and supports the availability of all reproductive options. ACOG opposes unnecessary regulations that limit or delay access to care.

National Organization of Nurse Practitioner Faculties and American Association of Colleges of Nursing (2002):

Upon graduation/entry into practice, Women's Health Nurse Practitioners should be able to:

i) facilitate access to reproductive health care services and provide referrals in an unbiased, timely, and sensitive manner;
ii) support a woman's right to make her own decisions regarding her health and reproductive choices within the context of her belief system;
iii) demonstrate effective communication skills in addressing sensitive topics related to sexuality, risk-taking behaviors, and abuse.

Opinions about what patients "should" do may subtly or overtly influence the therapeutic relationship, particularly for providers who are not fully aware of the boundaries between their personal beliefs and professional responsibilities. Though a woman may make a decision that is different from what a clinician wishes or believes is best, upholding patient autonomy is paramount (Simmonds & Likis, in press).

VALUES CLARIFICATION

Because unintended pregnancy and its outcomes—including such possibilities as adolescent pregnancy, single parenthood, and abortion—are socially and politically controversial, it is important for those who provide care to women of reproductive age to clarify their own values regarding these issues. Ideally, this self-assessment should take place before having a clinical encounter with a woman faced with an unintended pregnancy. In addition, because personal beliefs and professional work environments are dynamic, engaging in a process of values clarification throughout their careers benefits clinicians and the women they care for (Simmonds & Likis, in press).

Several resources have been developed to assist health care clinicians to clarify their personal beliefs about pregnancy options, and to help them examine the intersection of these beliefs with their responsibilities as professionals. These include books, articles, and exercises that may be used individually or in groups (Table 15–1). Given the heightened controversy surrounding abortion in the United States, many of these resources focus largely or exclusively on that option. Though this may be warranted, exploring beliefs about women's decisions to parent or place a child for adoption are equally important. Unexamined personal beliefs about these options can also inadvertently affect clinical encounters. For example, a clinician may have strong personal feelings about a teenager who reports she has decided to parent a child, or about a woman who has no hesitation about placing her infant for adoption. During the values clarification process, attention to all pregnancy options is worthwhile.

The ultimate goal of values clarification is to ensure that women with unintended pregnancies receive care that is free from bias, without judgment, and nondirective. By engaging in a process of values clarification, clinicians can identify situations in which they experience conflict between their personal beliefs and professional responsibilities, as well as situations where such tensions are not present. Areas of perceived conflict warrant further examination.

If after in-depth exploration clinicians determine that conflicts between their personal beliefs and professional responsibilities are irreconcilable, they must acknowledge this conflict. It is their professional obligation to make a feasible plan to ensure that women who come into their care will not be denied their right to comprehensive, respectful pregnancy options counseling. This may require that the clinician refer patients to a colleague or to a different setting entirely. Alternative plans should not create undue hardship for women, such as necessitating long travel distances or paying out of their own pockets for services rendered, nor should they result in significant delays in delivery of care. Familiarity with the practices of the referral site is also essential. If women are referred to another facility for options counseling, they must be assured that the counseling offered in that site will include factual information about all of the available options and be nondirective. Clinicians who identify a high level of personal conflict in providing comprehensive pregnancy options counseling are advised not to choose to work in settings where it is a frequent job responsibility (Higginbotham, 2002).

ASSESSMENT

A pregnancy test should be performed for diagnosis or when warranted to confirm previous testing. Estimate gestational age, preferably by ascertaining the woman's last menstrual

TABLE 15-1   Resources for Values Clarification

Title	Type of Resource	Where to Obtain
Abortion and Options Counseling: A Comprehensive Reference	Book	The Hope Clinic For Women, Ltd. 1602 21st Street Granite City, IL 62040 (800) 844-3130 www.hopeclinic.org
Caring for the Woman with an Unintended Pregnancy	CD-ROM	The Reproductive Options Education Consortium for Nursing c/o MGH Institute of Health Professions 36 First Avenue Charlestown, MA 02129 (617) 726-8007 www.roeconsortium.org
"Options Counseling: Techniques for Caring for Women with Unintended Pregnancies"	Article	Singer, J. (2004). Options counseling: Techniques for caring for women with unintended pregnancies. *Journal of Midwifery and Women's Health, 49*, 235–242. See Appendix A of the article for values clarification exercises.
Educating about Abortion, 2nd edition	Workbook	The Center for Family Life Education Planned Parenthood of Greater Northern New Jersey 196 Speedwell Avenue Morristown, NJ 07960 (973) 539-9580 Ext. 120
The Issue of Abortion in America: An Exploration of a Social Controversy	CD-ROM	Routledge 10650 Toebben Drive Independence, KY 41051 (800) 634-7064 (800) 248-4724 www.routledge.com

Obtaining Abortion Training: A Values Clarification Guide	Workbook	National Abortion Federation 1755 Massachusetts Avenue NW, Suite 600 Washington, DC 20036 (202) 667-5881 www.prochoice.org
"Induced Abortion: An Ethical Conundrum for Counselors"	Article	Millner, V. S., & Hanks, R. B. (2002). Induced abortion: An ethical conundrum for counselors. *Journal of Counseling & Development, 80*, 57–63.
Values Clarification Workshop	Workshop outline including exercises	The Access Project: www.theaccessproject.org/getting_started/ValuesClarificationWS.html

period (LMP). Bimanual examination for uterine size or ultrasound may be warranted to determine gestational age if the LMP is unknown. Assessment of pregnancy intention is more complex and is discussed in the next section.

MANAGEMENT

PREVENTION

Ideally all pregnancies would be wanted and planned. Toward this goal, the *Healthy People 2010* objectives include increasing the percentage of pregnancies that are intended to 70% (US Department of Health and Human Services, 2000). The primary way to prevent unintended pregnancy is for couples to use contraception with every act of intercourse during which they do not want to get pregnant. Improving contraception education and counseling, eliminating practice routines that impede obtaining timely services (e.g., long waits for appointments for contraceptive services, the requirements for a pelvic examination prior to prescribing hormonal contraception, etc.), and removing financial barriers to contraceptive access are important strategies to reduce unintended pregnancy (Moos, 2003).

Because perfect contraceptive use is unrealistic, emergency contraception (EC) has emerged as an important method for the prevention of unintended pregnancy. EC has the potential to prevent half of the unintended pregnancies in the United States, and EC is estimated to have prevented 51,000 abortions in 2000 (Finer & Henshaw, 2003; Trussell, Stewart, Guest, & Hatcher, 1992). More information about EC can be found in Chapter 9.

PREGNANCY OPTIONS COUNSELING

Options counseling provides women faced with an unintended pregnancy with an opportunity to explore whether they will carry the pregnancy and parent, carry the pregnancy and place the infant for adoption, or have an abortion. Although pregnancy options counseling is sometimes referred to as abortion counseling, the two are distinct. Options counseling is for a woman who knows she is pregnant and needs to clarify her thoughts and feelings about her alternatives. Abortion counseling is provided when a woman has made the decision to terminate a pregnancy (Baker, 1995). Clinicians counseling women with unintended pregnancies need to understand the options available as well as the fundamental principles of pregnancy options counseling to provide adequate quality care.

It is essential for the clinician who is providing pregnancy options counseling to be nondirective in her approach, and to withhold personal judgment about the woman's situation and decision. Equally important is ensuring patient confidentiality. Fear that parents, a partner, or others will find out about an unintended pregnancy may prevent some women from seeking counseling.

Other essentials of providing pregnancy options counseling include establishing rapport, using neutral language, and asking open-ended questions. It is important to remember that options counseling is a form of crisis intervention that usually takes place during one clinician–patient interaction. As such, it is short term, addresses an immediate problem, and involves a major life crisis needing a time-limited decision (Baker, 1995).

Though every patient encounter is unique—necessitating variations in approach—the following four general steps are suggested for clinicians when providing pregnancy options counseling (Simmonds & Likis, in press).

Explore How the Woman Feels About the Pregnancy and Her Options   Asking, "How do you feel about being pregnant?" is a neutral, open-ended question that may be used to begin the counseling session, and encourages the woman to share her emotions without being directed as to what her answer should be. Avoid questions or statements that make assumptions about feelings, such as "Are you happy about the pregnancy?" or, "Congratulations!" The questions "Do you know what your choices are?" or "What are your thoughts about becoming a parent, adoption, and abortion?" help the clinician ascertain the woman's level of understanding of the available options and her feelings about each choice. Listing the risks and benefits, or pros and cons, of each option may help the woman to assess her situation and make an informed decision.

Help the Woman to Identify Support Systems and Assess Risks   Asking the woman who she has told that she is pregnant, how these people have responded, and their significance to her allows for a greater understanding of her situation. This will help the provider identify women who may be isolated and in need of additional support. Assessing for risk of interpersonal violence should also be a standard component of pregnancy options counseling. Women experiencing an unintended pregnancy are at higher risk for intimate partner violence (Saltzman, Johnson, Gilbert, & Goodwin, 2003). Asking adolescents about their parents' potential reaction to the pregnancy can help identify situations where child abuse is present or possible.

Another important topic to address is the potential for coercion regarding the decision about the pregnancy. Coercion from partners, parents, or other significant relationships may be an issue with regard to any of the options. Women may feel pressured to continue pregnancies, place children for adoption, or have abortions against their will.

Encouraging the woman to talk with those she feels will be supportive of her decision, and helping her to explore what it would be like to tell someone who may not be supportive, can be valuable aspects of the counseling session, particularly in the case of adolescents. Arrange for additional follow-up for patients who report they are unable to tell anyone about the pregnancy. This may include referral to a professional counselor.

Help the Woman to Reach a Decision or Discuss a Timetable for Decision Making   Women may present for pregnancy options counseling, having just found out they are pregnant or already having been aware for some time. Some may need time to accept their situation or to discuss it with others, or both. Some may not want to discuss the matter with a clinician at all. Together with the woman, determine whether to proceed immediately with complete pregnancy options counseling, or to postpone it until a later time. In either case, be sure that she is aware of the current estimated gestational age of the pregnancy, and that her decision is time sensitive when establishing a follow-up plan. Some women may benefit from other resources to further explore their options on their own (Table 15–2).

TABLE 15–2 Patient Resources for Exploring Pregnancy Options

Title	Type	How to Obtain	Description
www.pregnancyoptions.info	Web site	Online only	Contains online resources including exercises for the woman who is undecided about what to do about a pregnancy, as well as information on all three options.
Pregnant? Need Help? Pregnancy Options Workbook	Workbook	Online: www.ferre.org/workbook Order print copies from: Ferre Institute 124 Front Street Binghamton, NY 13905 (607) 724-4308	Comprehensive workbook of information and exercises for women exploring pregnancy options. Includes all three options and addresses topics such as decision making, getting support, male partners, fetal development, and spiritual and religious concerns.
Unsure About Your Pregnancy? A Guide to Making the Right Decision for You	Brochure	Online: www.prochoice.org (click on "Your Choices") Order print copies from: The National Abortion Federation 1755 Massachusetts Avenue NW, Suite 600 Washington, DC 20036 (202) 667-5881	Provides exercises for pregnant women who are undecided about their pregnancy. The Web site also provides links to information about all three options.

If the woman is ready to make a decision, assess whether or not she needs any additional information, or if she would like to discuss any of the options further. For some women, resources that allow a better understanding or visualization of fetal development can be helpful during this stage of the decision-making process, whereas for others they may not. Accurate patient education resources on fetal development should be made available for those who express interest.

Refer or Provide the Woman with Appropriate Services   Depending on what a woman chooses to do, she may be able to receive the services she needs within that setting, or she may be referred elsewhere. Knowing what resources are available for pregnant women—whether they choose to continue a pregnancy, place a child for adoption, or terminate a pregnancy—is essential. The National Adoption Information Clearinghouse and the National Abortion Federation (Box 15–2) both offer information about the services available in

---

BOX 15–2   REPRODUCTIVE OPTIONS, LEGISLATION, AND POLICIES RESOURCES

The Alan Guttmacher Institute

www.agi-usa.org
Research and analysis for individual states
http://www.guttmacher.org/statecenter

The Kaiser Family Foundation

www.kff.org
Specifics regarding state policies and legislation
State Health Facts On-line
http://www.statehealthfacts.kff.org (click on Women's Health)

The National Abortion Federation

www.prochoice.org

The National Abortion Rights Action League

www.naral.org
Specifics regarding state legislation
The National Abortion Rights Action League State-by-State Guide to Legislative Bills
http://mail.naral.org/longdoc.nsf

The National Adoption Information Clearinghouse

http://naic.acf.hhs.gov

specific geographic areas. However, it is also important to consult colleagues and others in the community about the reputation and practices of any agency or clinic prior to referring patients there. Finally, when providing referrals, be sure that women understand how to access them.

OPTIONS FOR WOMEN EXPERIENCING UNINTENDED PREGNANCIES

Continuing the Pregnancy Parenting is a long-term commitment that carries immense responsibility. Optimally those who choose to parent would have the time and ability to care for a child; adequate financial resources; and support from spouses or partners, family members, and friends. Clinicians can provide pregnant women with information about state and local programs that provide social and financial support to pregnant women and their children. Such information may prove critical to their decision. Women who decide to continue a pregnancy should begin prenatal care, either in the setting where options counseling occurred, if those services are provided, or by referral to a prenatal care provider.

Adoption Arrangements for adoption vary according to state law. Children may be placed for adoption through public or private agencies, independently using an adoption lawyer or facilitator, or directly between the birth and adoptive parents. Adoptions may be closed or open. Parents in a confidential or closed adoption do not know each other or have contact, but the adoptive parents are given relevant information about the birth parents such as medical histories. Open adoption is a wide continuum that may span from birth parents reading about families and selecting one, to an ongoing relationship between the families (National Adoption Information Clearinghouse, 2003).

Abortion Options for pregnancy termination in the United States (as of this writing) include surgical, medical, and labor induction methods. The decision about which method is employed in an individual situation depends on several factors, including the gestational age of the pregnancy, preference of the patient, and provider training and availability. Clinicians need to be familiar with which abortion options are available for women in their care to provide accurate counseling and referrals. In addition, nurse practitioners, nurse-midwives, and physician assistants can legally provide medical or surgical abortion in some states. The specific laws and regulations that determine whether abortion provision lies within the scope of practice of these different clinician groups vary from state to state (Kruse, 2000).

Surgical abortion is currently the most common method of pregnancy termination in the United States, with medical abortion the next most common (Elam-Evans et al., 2003; Finer & Henshaw, 2003). Less than 1% of abortions are performed by labor induction, and because of their high rates of morbidity and mortality, hysterotomy and hysterectomy have fallen out of favor as techniques for abortion in this country and are rarely used (Haskell, Easterling, & Lichtenberg, 1999). The most recent data on the timing of abortions indicate that 87% are performed prior to 13 weeks gestation, and only 1.4% are performed at or after 21 weeks (Elam-Evans et al., 2003).

Surgical abortion may be performed as early as a pregnancy is detected, though to ensure that the pregnancy has been terminated some providers prefer to postpone the procedure until a gestational sac can be visualized by ultrasound or directly during postprocedure tissue examination (generally between four and six weeks). Research has demonstrated that surgical abortion prior to six weeks is safe and effective, particularly if protocols that guard against missed ectopic or continuing pregnancies are followed (Edwards & Carson, 1997). Upper limits beyond which surgical abortion may be performed are based on legal, rather than medical restrictions, and vary from state to state. See Box 15–2 for resources to locate information on state laws.

All surgical abortion methods involve removing the products of conception (POCs) by vacuum aspiration, which is performed by introducing a cannula attached to a source of suction through the cervical os into the uterine cavity. Suction can be generated by either manual or electric pumps (MVA or EVA). MVA is generally used only for pregnancy terminations earlier than 13 weeks gestation (McInerney, Baird, Hyman, & Huber, 2001). The decision to use MVA or EVA depends on provider preference and training as well as equipment availability.

In early pregnancy terminations, evacuation of the uterus takes only a few minutes, and may be accomplished through the use of suction alone. Some providers choose to curette the walls of the uterus after suctioning (referred to as dilation and curettage or D & C) to ensure that the procedure is complete. However, this technique has been associated with an increased risk of uterine perforation, and has not been shown to decrease the risk of retained products of conception or continuing pregnancy (Edwards, Darney, & Paul, 1999).

When performing surgical terminations after the first trimester, forceps are often used as an adjunct to suction to remove the POC. This technique is termed dilation and evacuation (D & E). Generally, with advancing gestational age the abortion procedure takes longer and requires more advanced training on the part of the provider. Research has shown D & E to be both safer and less physically and emotionally stressful for patients than labor induction (Blumenthal, Castleman, & Jain, 1999; Henshaw, 1999). In a small, randomized, controlled trial comparing D & E and labor induction, 62% of potential participants declined study enrollment primarily because of their preference for D & E (Grimes, Smith, & Witham, 2004). However, the decision to employ labor induction instead of D & E is often made because of the lack of providers skilled in this technique (Haskell et al., 1999). Dilation and extraction (D & X) is an advanced surgical technique that involves reduction of the fetal skull prior to removal. D & X is rare in the United States, and would not likely be the method used in instances of unintended pregnancy termination; therefore, further discussion is beyond the scope of this chapter.

Dilation of the cervix is usually necessary to remove the POC except in very early surgical abortions (Edwards et al., 1999; Haskell et al., 1999). The degree of dilation required depends on the gestational age of the pregnancy. It may be accomplished either by inserting dilating rods of increasing diameter into the cervical os immediately before inserting the cannula, or by placing osmotic dilators into the cervix several hours to a day before the procedure. In general, osmotic dilators are used in later pregnancy terminations, though provider training and experience may also guide this decision. Oral or vaginal pharmacologic agents, such as misoprostol, are also used in some settings to promote cervical ripening and subsequent dilation.

In the United States, women are offered several options for pain relief during and following surgical abortion (Maltzer, Maltzer, Wiebe, Halvorson-Boyd, & Boyd, 1999). In most settings, a paracervical block is routinely administered with a local anesthetic, such as lidocaine, prior to cervical dilation. In addition, many providers offer patients the options of additional intravenous (IV) sedation or oral pain medications, as well as non-pharmacologic interventions, for pain and anxiety relief. General anesthesia is offered in some settings, but is usually recommended for use only in limited, special circumstances because it significantly increases the risks associated with the procedure.

Postoperative recovery after a surgical abortion is usually rapid. The vast majority of procedures are performed in outpatient settings, and women return home after a brief period of stabilization (Edwards et al., 1999; Finer & Henshaw, 2003). Women may resume regular activity as soon as they feel ready, though they are usually advised to avoid lifting heavy objects, engaging in vigorous exercise, or having intercourse for one to two weeks following the procedure. Evidence to support these recommendations is limited (McIntosh, Stewart, & Teplin, 1999). Typically women are advised to return to the facility where the abortion was provided or to their primary care provider for a routine exam in two to three weeks to ensure a complete and uncomplicated recovery, emotional well-being, and to initiate or follow up on a newly established contraceptive method. There is also little evidence to support this practice, which is costly for women and the health care system. Alternative approaches for follow-up care have been suggested, including better patient education regarding self-monitoring for postabortion complications, and improved delivery of contraceptive services at the time of the abortion (Grossman, Ellertson, Grimes, & Walker, 2004).

Medical abortion is a relatively new method for pregnancy termination in the United States. There are currently two prominent methods available: mifepristone and methotrexate, both of which are given in combination with misoprostol. These methods are currently used only for early terminations (up to 63 days); however, studies are underway to evaluate their effectiveness for later terminations. Efficacy rates vary depending on the type of medication used, gestational age of the pregnancy, and the specific protocol employed. In their meta-analysis of different regimens, Kahn et al. (2000) found an overall efficacy of 94–96% for both mifepristone–misoprostol and methotrexate–misoprosotol regimens when used for gestations of 49 days or less. Efficacy was found to decrease with advancing gestational age, though some regimens were able to achieve comparably high rates of success. Mifepristone is the most common form of medical abortion in the United States. After this drug was approved by the Food and Drug Administration (FDA) in 2000, an estimated 200,000 women used it during the first three years it was commercially available in this country

(Danco Laboratories, 2004). During the prior decade, the most common medical method used to terminate pregnancies was methotrexate, which had emerged as a nonsurgical method for managing ectopic pregnancies, but it was not labeled for either of these uses. Methotrexate is still in use in some settings, but mifepristone has become a more prominent method of medical abortion in the United States because of greater efficacy and advantages with other clinical features. Methotrexate does maintain certain advantages including lower cost, as well as the ability to be used in cases when ectopic pregnancy cannot be ruled out (Creinin & Aubeny, 1999).

Mifepristone works by binding to progesterone receptors more effectively than progesterone itself. As a result, the endometrium sloughs and the cervix softens, both of which promote expulsion of pregnancy tissue. By adding misoprostol (a prostaglandin), the efficacy of this regimen increases (National Abortion Federation, 2001).

Specific protocols for the use of mifepristone vary from site to site (National Abortion Federation, 2001). These alternative but evidence-based options often differ from the FDA-approved protocol with regard to medication doses, their administration and timing, use of ultrasound, gestational limits, and required follow-up visits. Currently in most settings in the United States, patients are given mifepristone (200–600 mg) on site following verification of gestational age via clinical exam or ultrasound. One to three days later, the woman administers misoprostol vaginally or orally at home. For more than 50% of women, bleeding and passage of the pregnancy ensue within four to five hours after misoprostol administration, but may take up to 24 hours or longer (Spitz, Bardin, Benton, & Robbins, 1998). A follow-up visit is required several days to weeks later to ensure that the pregnancy has been successfully terminated.

Medical abortion with methotrexate is similar to mifepristone with respect to the manner of service delivery, but has several distinguishing clinical features. Most obviously, methotrexate is administered via intramuscular injection rather than orally, which may lead some women to have a preference for mifepristone. However, the most important clinical difference may lie in the timing of bleeding and expulsion of the pregnancy tissue, which can take up to several weeks following administration of misoprostol. For many women this unpredictability renders methotrexate far less desirable than mifepristone (National Abortion Federation, 2001). In considering a mifepristone–misoprostol (or methotrexate–misoprostol) abortion, helping women to understand that a medical abortion is a process that may take several days or longer to complete is important. In cases of failed medical abortion, surgical evacuation of the pregnancy is required because misoprostol is a known teratogen and a pregnancy should not continue after its use (National Abortion Federation). Women may prefer medical abortion because of its less invasive nature and perceptions that it is more private and patient controlled (Harvey, Beckman, Castle, & Coyteaux, 1995).

Labor induction is a method of abortion that involves administering medications such as prostaglandins, oxytocin, or hypertonic saline to stimulate uterine contractions that eventually lead to the expulsion of a fetus (Blumenthal et al., 1999). As previously discussed, this method has been found to be generally less safe and more difficult for patients than D & E, and thus has become less common in the United States. Because this method is used primarily for pregnancy terminations after 20 weeks' gestation, and often for pregnancies that were desired, in-depth discussion of this method is beyond the scope of this chapter.

Risks associated with early pregnancy termination, including death, are relatively low when procedures are carried out under modern medical conditions. Legality is an important prerequisite for such conditions to be manifest. In places where abortion is illegal, associated mortality rates remain high. The World Health Organization (2004) estimates that 68,000 women die around the world each year as a result of unsafe abortion, rendering it one of the leading causes of maternal mortality. However, in the United States abortion mortality rates have decreased considerably since the 1970s, largely as a result of advances in technique and elimination of many legal restrictions (Henshaw, 1999). The current mortality rate for legal, reported abortions in the United States is 0.6 per 100,000 (Elam-Evans et al., 2003). For first trimester terminations, this risk is 11 times less than carrying a pregnancy to term. Risk of death increases with advancing gestational age, and after 20 weeks abortion and childbearing are statistically equivalent in this regard (Henshaw, 1999).

Serious and minor complications following legal abortion are also infrequent. Haskell et al. (1999) listed the following possible complications:

- Hematometra requiring additional uterine evacuation (under 0.2%)
- Infection (0.1–2.0%)
- Cervical tear (0.6–1.2%)
- Uterine perforation (0.4%)
- Missed or incomplete abortion (0.3–2.0%)
- Hemorrhage requiring transfusion (0.02–0.3%)

In general, these conditions are treatable and rarely lead to long-term sequelae or death. Of particular import to many women is the fact that there is no evidence that first trimester abortion with vacuum aspiration leads to difficulties with childbearing in the future. Data regarding the impact on fertility of abortions performed via other methods, such as later in pregnancy, or multiple times are less well studied and less clear (Hogue, Boardman, Stotland, & Peipert, 1999). Assisting women to seek services as early as possible from abortion providers who are experienced and helping them to prevent repeat unintended pregnancies are important strategies for clinicians to help women reduce potential risks in this regard.

SPECIAL CONSIDERATIONS

ADOLESCENTS

The rate of unintended pregnancy is highest among 15- to 19-year-old women (Henshaw, 1998). Adolescent mothers are less likely to complete high school, are more likely to be single parents, and may have increased complications during pregnancy. Children of adolescent mothers have higher rates of low birth weight and related health problems, are more likely to be abused or neglected, and frequently have poor school performance (National Campaign to Prevent Teen Pregnancy, 2004).

Abortion is common among adolescents. A study of over 10,000 women who had abortions in 2000–2001 found that nearly one in five (19%) of the terminations were performed in women aged 15 to 19 years (Jones, Darroch, & Henshaw, 2002b). The majority of these abortions were among 18- and 19-year-old women. Less than 1% of the abortions during this period occurred among those less than 15 years old (Jones et al., 2002b).

Clinicians who work with young women need to be familiar with current laws regarding adolescent rights to confidential reproductive health services. These rights are currently an area of great controversy in the United States, as reflected by legislative battles at both the federal and state levels. Though state laws vary, at the present time there is no state with laws that prohibit minors from receiving family planning services without parental consent (Lieberman & Feierman, 1999). However, in Texas and Utah there are prohibitions on the use of state funds to provide contraceptive services to minors without parental consent. This results in minors in those states being unable to receive confidential services from state-funded health care providers. In all states but Connecticut and Maine and the District of Columbia, adolescents choosing to terminate an unwanted pregnancy must have the consent of a parent, a guardian, or a judge (Boonstra & Nash, 2000). Where legislative conditions allow, reassuring adolescent patients that all counseling and follow-up related to pregnancy will be kept confidential is an important aspect of providing pregnancy options counseling to this population. Before delivering services, it is also essential to inform adolescents about clinical situations when parents or guardians may or must be informed. A full discussion of the reproductive health rights of adolescents is beyond the scope of this chapter, and readers are referred to the references cited and to the resource listing (Box 15–2) regarding laws specifically pertaining to adolescents in their practice location.

INFLUENCES OF CULTURE

It is important for clinicians providing pregnancy options counseling not to make assumptions about what option a woman will choose based on generalizations about her marital status, previous childbearing, educational level, religious affiliation, or ethnicity. Although most women who have abortions are single, one out of six who terminate a pregnancy are married. The majority of women who have an abortion have some college education (57%) and have had one or more previous births (61%) (Jones et al., 2002b). Nearly 80% of women who have an abortion report a religious affiliation. Many of these women—27% are Catholic, and 13% are "born-again" or evangelical—identify themselves with religions that typically prohibit abortion (Jones et al.). Although rates of unintended pregnancy and abortion are higher among African-American and Latina women than Caucasian women in the United States (Jones et al.), when providing pregnancy options counseling, it is imperative to treat women as individuals and to provide them with the same quality and type of care regardless of their racial or ethnic backgrounds.

REFERENCES

Alan Guttmacher Institute. (2000). *Fulfilling the promise: Public policy and U.S. family planning clinics.* New York: Author.

American Academy of Physician Assistants. (2004). *Guidelines for ethical conduct for the physician assistant profession.* Alexandria, VA: Author.

American College of Nurse-Midwives. (1997). *Reproductive choices* [Position statement]. Washington, DC: Author.

American College of Obstetricians and Gynecologists. (2004). *Abortion policy* [Policy statement]. Washington, DC: Author.

Baker, A. (1995). *Abortion and options counseling: A comprehensive reference.* Granite City, IL: Hope Clinic for Women.

Blumenthal, P. D., Castleman, L. D., & Jain, J. K. (1999). Abortion by labor induction. In M. Paul, S. Lichtenberg, L. Borgatta, D. Grimes, & P. Stubblefield (Eds.), *A clinician's guide to medical and surgical abortion* (pp. 139–154). New York: Churchill Livingstone.

Boonstra, H., & Nash, E. (2000). Minors and the right to consent to health care. *The Guttmacher Report on Public Policy, 3*(4).

Brown, S. S., & Eisenberg, L. (Eds.). (1995). *The best intentions: Unintended pregnancy and the well-being of children and families.* Washington, DC: National Academy Press.

Chandra, A., Abma, J., Maza, P., & Bachrach, C. (1999). *Adoption, adoption seeking, and relinquishment for adoption in the United States. Advance data from vital and health statistics* (No. 306). Hyattsville, MD: National Center for Health Statistics.

Creinin, M. D., & Aubeny, E. (1999). Medical abortion in early pregnancy. In M. Paul, S. Lichtenberg, L. Borgatta, D. Grimes, & P. Stubblefield (Eds.), *A clinician's guide to medical and surgical abortion* (pp. 91–106). New York: Churchill Livingstone.

Danco Laboratories. (2004) *Using mifeprex: What every woman should know.* Retrieved September 21, 2004, from http://www.earlyoptionpill.com/may_ what. php3.

Edwards, J., & Carson, S. A. (1997). New technologies permit safe abortion at less than six weeks' gestation and provide timely detection of ectopic gestation.

American Journal of Obstetrics and Gynecology, 176, 1101–1106.

Edwards, J., Darney, P. D., & Paul, M. (1999). Surgical abortion in the first trimester. In M. Paul, S. Lichtenberg, L. Borgatta, D. Grimes, & P. Stubblefield (Eds.), *A clinician's guide to medical and surgical abortion* (pp. 107–122). New York: Churchill Livingstone.

Elam-Evans, L. D., Strauss, L. T., Herndon, J., Parker, W. Y., Bowens, S. V., Zane, S., et al. (2003). Abortion surveillance—United States, 2000. *Morbidity and Mortality Weekly Report Surveillance Summaries, 52*(SS12), 1–32.

Finer, L. B., & Henshaw, S. K. (2003). Abortion incidence and services in the United States in 2000. *Perspectives on Sexual and Reproductive Health, 35,* 6–15.

Grimes, D. A., Smith, M. S., & Witham, A. D. (2004). Mifepristone and misoprostol versus dilation and evacuation for midtrimester abortion: A pilot randomised, controlled trial. *British Journal of Obstetrics and Gynaecology, 111,* 148–153.

Grossman, D., Ellertson, C., Grimes, D. A., & Walker, D. (2004). Routine follow-up visits after first trimester induced abortion. *Obstetrics and Gynecology, 103,* 738–745.

Harvey, S. M., Beckman, L. I., Castle, M. A., & Coyteaux, F. (1995). Knowledge and perceptions of medical abortion among potential users. *Family Planning Perspectives, 27*(5), 203–207.

Haskell, W. M., Easterling, T. R., & Lichtenberg, E. S. (1999). Surgical abortion after the first trimester. In M. Paul, S. Lichtenberg, L. Borgatta, D. Grimes, & P. Stubblefield (Eds.), *A clinician's guide to medical and surgical abortion* (pp. 123–138). New York: Churchill Livingstone.

Henshaw, S. K. (1998). Unintended pregnancy in the United States. *Family Planning Perspectives, 30,* 24–29, 46.

Henshaw, S. K. (1999). Unintended pregnancy and abortion: A public health perspective. In M. Paul, S. Lichtenberg, L. Borgatta, D. Grimes, & P. Stubblefield (Eds.), *A clinician's guide to medical and surgical abortion* (pp. 11–22). New York: Churchill Livingstone.

Higginbotham, E. (2002). When your beliefs run counter to care. *RN, 65*(11), 69–72.

Hogue, C. J., Boardman, L. A., Stotland, N. A., & Peipert, J. F. (1999). Answering questions about long-term outcomes. In M. Paul, S. Lichtenberg, L. Borgatta, D. Grimes, & P. Stubblefield (Eds.), *A clinician's guide to medical and surgical abortion* (pp. 217–228). New York: Churchill Livingstone.

Jones, R. K., Darroch, J. E., & Henshaw, S. K. (2002a). Contraceptive use among US women having abortions in 2000–2001. *Perspectives on Sexual and Reproductive Health, 34,* 294–303.

Jones, R. K., Darroch, J. E., & Henshaw, S. K. (2002b). Patterns in the socioeconomic characteristics of women obtaining abortions in 2000–2001. *Perspectives on Sexual and Reproductive Health, 34,* 226–235.

Kahn, J. G., Becker, B. J., MacIsaac, L., Amory, J. K., Neuhaus, J., Olkin, I., et al. (2000). The efficacy of medical abortion: A meta-analysis. *Contraception, 61,* 29–40.

Kruse, B. (2000). Advanced practice clinicians and medical abortion: Increasing access to care. *Journal of the American Women's Medical Association, 55*(suppl. 3), 167–168.

Lieberman, D., & Feierman, J. (1999). Legal issues in the reproductive health care of adolescents. *Journal of the American Medical Women's Association, 54,* 109–114.

Maltzer, D. S., Maltzer, M. C., Wiebe, E. R., Halvorson-Boyd, G., & Boyd, C. (1999). Pain management. In M. Paul, S. Lichtenberg, L. Borgatta, D. Grimes, & P. Stubblefield (Eds.), *A clinician's guide to medical and surgical abortion* (pp. 73–90). New York: Churchill Livingstone.

McInerney, T., Baird, T. L., Hyman, A. G., & Huber, A. B. (2001). *A guide to providing abortion care.* Chapel Hill, NC: IPAS.

McIntosh, K. M., Stewart, G. K., & Teplin, D. (1999). Routine aftercare and contraception. In M. Paul, S. Lichtenberg, L. Borgatta, D. Grimes, & P. Stubblefield (Eds.), *A clinician's guide to medical and surgical abortion* (pp. 185–196). New York: Churchill Livingstone.

Moos, M-K. (2003). Unintended pregnancies: A call for nursing action. *MCN: The American Journal of Maternal/Child Nursing, 28,* 24–30.

National Abortion Federation. (2001). *Early options: A provider's guide to medical abortion.* Washington, DC: Author.

National Adoption Information Clearinghouse. (2003). Retrieved September 1, 2004, from http://naic.acf.hhs.gov.

National Campaign to Prevent Teen Pregnancy. (2004). *Teen pregnancy—so what?* Retrieved September 1, 2004, from http://www.teenpregnancy.org/whycare/sowhat.asp.

National Organization of Nurse Practitioner Faculties and American Association of Colleges of Nursing. (2002). *Nurse practitioner primary care competencies in specialty areas: Adult, family, gerontological, pediatric, and women's health.* Rockville, MD: Department of Health and Human Services.

Saltzman, L. E., Johnson, C. H., Gilbert, B. C., & Goodwin, M. M. (2003). Physical abuse around the time of pregnancy: An examination of prevalence and risk factors in 16 states. *Maternal and Child Health Journal, 7,* 31–43.

Simmonds, K. E., & Likis, F. E. (in press). Providing options counseling for women with unintended pregnancies. *Journal of Obstetric, Gynecologic, and Neonatal Nursing.*

Spitz, I. M., Bardin, C. W., Benton, L., & Robbins, A. (1998). Early pregnancy termination with mifepristone and misoprostol in the United States. *New England Journal of Medicine, 338,* 1241–1247.

Trussell, J., Stewart, F., Guest, F., & Hatcher, R. A. (1992). Emergency contraceptive pills: A simple proposal to reduce unintended pregnancies. *Family Planning Perspectives, 24,* 269–273.

US Department of Health and Human Services. (2000). *Healthy People 2010* (2nd ed.). Washington, DC: US Government Printing Office.

World Health Organization (2004) *Unsafe abortion: Global and regional estimates of incidence of unsafe abortion and associated mortality in 2000* (4th ed.). Geneva, Switzerland: Author.

16

INFERTILITY

ELLEN OLSHANSKY

The inability to become a mother or a father is a profound and extremely difficult challenge for a significant portion of the population. Infertility is a condition that generates a variety of meanings among those experiencing it, including those who care for people with infertility, family members and friends of people with infertility, and the society in which infertility occurs. People who are unable to conceive and bear a child often suffer immensely from this inability. Others choose infertility and specifically seek it out through surgical means, such as tubal ligation or vasectomy. Thus, there is both unwanted infertility and wanted infertility. Unwanted infertility is estimated to occur in 15% to 20% of couples in the United States (Carcio, 1998a). Unwanted infertility is often unrecognized as a serious problem because it is not a life-threatening illness. For those experiencing it, however, infertility often has a significant impact and is viewed as a major life crisis (Olshansky, 1996a).

We live in a pronatalist society, which adds to the emotionally charged nature of infertility. Definitions of femininity are socially constructed and interlaced with the ability to give birth. Many women internalize these societal expectations, seeing themselves as failures if they are unable to conceive (Olshansky, 1992).

Infertility is distressing to many who experience it, and social issues influence the experience. There is often a feeling of injustice when a woman is not able to conceive. A common response is "Why me?" There are those who do not understand the "drivenness" felt by women with infertility. There are also particular issues related to secondary infertility and to miscarriage. There is often even the inability to stop treatment within our technological context, as new treatments continue to be discovered. There are also ethical issues related to infertility treatment, including who receives treatment.

Historically, infertility has been viewed as a woman's problem. This view is changing as a result of enhanced abilities to diagnose infertility that have led to the recognition that both male and female factors cause infertility. Nevertheless, matters of reproduction, childbearing, and childrearing continue to be viewed primarily as women's issues. Many women have grown up rehearsing to be mothers, believing that their femininity and identity are interrelated with childbearing. Finding they are unable to conceive can be both shocking and devastating. Some women may be able to deconstruct such ideas through involvement in organizations and groups that support greater choices of lifestyles for women. Yet even women who may not feel that it is their duty to bear children may continue to profoundly desire children.

Infertility has also raised some issues and opportunities that were generally ignored before the advent of technological approaches to treat this condition. For example, people of childbearing age who are treated with cancer drugs and radiation may now preserve their fertility through the freezing of sperm or eggs. Other technological advances have led to ethical dilemmas, including issues of who has the right to a frozen embryo, who is the real parent, and who is considered eligible for certain treatments.

This chapter provides an overview of the pathophysiology of infertility, including the various causes of infertility, the diagnostic procedures related to infertility, and the treatments for infertility. The chapter also includes a discussion about the various options available beyond trying to conceive, including adoption and child-free living. Ethical issues are discussed, and a section on the sociocultural and psychological issues related to infertility is presented. Finally, suggestions are made for ways that health care providers can assist those experiencing infertility to have a better quality of life during and after the infertility experience.

DEFINING INFERTILITY

The medical definition of infertility is failure to conceive after one year of unprotected (without contraception) sexual intercourse. Some clinicians extend the definition to include the inability to carry the resulting embryo or fetus to a live birth (Benasutti, 2003). For women over 35 years of age, this medical definition is sometimes revised to six months instead of one year because the remaining time to conceive is limited (Domar, 2002). The assumption that 35 years old is a significant age in regard to infertility may be wrong, as maternal age cannot be looked at separately from the context of the relationship between the woman and her partner, social conditions, and physical problems in the male (Hanson, 2003). Advanced maternal age is occurring more frequently as a result of both the social change toward greater acceptability of older parents and the technological advances that have been made (Bickstein, 2003).

Male fertility takes a much different trajectory than female fertility. The sperm count of men usually does not decrease significantly until about 55 years of age. Even with that decrease, men are usually able to father children throughout their lives. Despite men's longer potential reproductive capability, male infertility represents only approximately 35% of all infertility problems (Speroff & Fritz, 2005).

From a personal perspective however, an individual often constructs his or her own definition of infertility, which is influenced by the social context in which he or she lives. For example, a couple who has been trying to conceive for three months and has many friends who have recently become pregnant with no apparent difficulty may begin to see themselves as infertile even though they are not considered infertile according to the medical definition. The couple may become very anxious and seek health care, but are turned away because they do not fit the medical definition of infertility. Meanwhile, their anxiety may increase, which could have a detrimental effect on their ability to conceive (Domar, 2002).

Conversely, a 40-year-old nulligravida may go for a routine gynecologic examination and her health care provider may warn her that she should consider conceiving very soon because her childbearing years are almost over. There may be an assumption that this woman—and all women, for that matter—choose to be mothers. For this particular woman, her life goals may not include parenting. Although it was correct to provide her with information about childbearing, it would have been more appropriate to ask her, in a nonjudgmental manner, about her goals related to childbearing with the recognition that not all women choose to become mothers.

OVERVIEW OF ANATOMY AND PHYSIOLOGY RELATED TO INFERTILITY

An understanding of the anatomy and physiology of the female and male reproductive systems as well as the processes of conception and implantation is crucial to understanding the etiology of infertility. Women's reproductive anatomy and physiology are discussed in Chapter 5; therefore, the discussion in this chapter is limited to an overview of men's reproductive anatomy and physiology, conception, and implantation.

ANATOMY AND PHYSIOLOGY OF THE MALE REPRODUCTIVE SYSTEM

The anatomic components of the male reproductive system include the penis, urethra, seminal vesicles, prostate gland, vas deferens, epididymis, and testes (testicles). See Figure 16–1 and Table 16–1. Mature sperm are generated approximately every 90 days. Sperm production relies on a functioning hypothalamic-pituitary-testicular axis that has many similarities to the hypothalamic-pituitary-ovarian axis in women. The pituitary produces follicle-stimulating hormone (FSH) and luteinizing hormone (LH) in response to secretion of gonadotropin-releasing hormone (GnRH) by the hypothalamus. FSH and LH initiate testicular production of sperm and testosterone, which are also required for spermatogenesis. Sperm mature in the epididymis and then travel out of the vas deferens during ejaculation.

CONCEPTION AND IMPLANTATION

The processes of conception (also known as fertilization) and implantation involve several steps. Sperm must be produced as described previously. The sperm must be deposited in

TABLE 16–1 Functions of the Male Reproductive Anatomy

Penis	External organ through which semen and urine are expelled
Urethra	Tube that carries semen and urine through the penis; its external opening is at the tip of the penis
Seminal vesicles	Two internal saclike structures that secrete fructose and other substances into the seminal fluid to promote viability of the semen
Prostate gland	Internal gland that secretes substances into the seminal fluid to nourish and increase the motility of the sperm
Vas deferens	Bilateral tubes through which sperm are propelled from each epididymis to the urethra for ejaculation
Epididymis	Stores sperm while they mature and connects the testicles to the vas deferens; each testicle has an adjacent epididymis
Testes	Produce testosterone and immature sperm; suspended externally in the scrotum
Bulbourethral gland	Two internal glands that produce an alkaline mucoid secretion that coats and lubricates the urethra

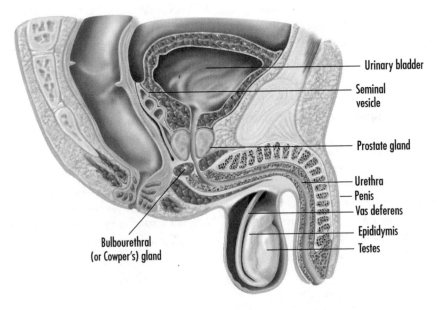

Urinary bladder

Seminal vesicle

Prostate gland

Urethra
Penis
Vas deferens

Epididymis
Testes

Bulbourethral (or Cowper's) gland

FIGURE 16–1 Mid-Sagittal View of the Male Reproductive System

the vagina and then transported through the vagina, cervix, and fallopian tubes. In the fallopian tubes the sperm are transformed by a process called capacitation, which changes the surface characteristics of sperm. Capacitation is essential to the sperm's ability to fertilize an egg and enables the sperm to undergo acrosome reaction, to bind to the zona pellucida, and to acquire hypermotility, all of which help to increase the sperm's ability to penetrate the ovum. The ovaries must produce a mature ovum (oocyte), which requires integrated functioning along the hypothalamic-pituitary-ovarian axis. The ovum is transported from the ovary into the fallopian tube where it is fertilized by the sperm. The fertilized ovum then travels down the fallopian tube into the uterus. Implantation is the process by which the fertilized ovum attaches to the uterine wall and penetrates the uterine epithelium and the maternal circulatory system. Implantation can occur only if there is destruction of the zona pellucida, which is the surface of the fertilized ovum.

PATHOPHYSIOLOGY AND ETIOLOGIES OF INFERTILITY

There are many causes of infertility, with about 55% of the causes attributable to female factors, 35% attributable to male factors, and 10% for which the cause remains unexplained (Speroff & Fritz, 2005). When presenting or discussing the pathophysiology of infertility, attention should be given to avoiding the use of terms that reflect negatively upon women. For example, cervical mucus that is not receptive to sperm is commonly referred to as "hostile cervical mucus," and a cervix that prematurely dilates is commonly called an "incompetent cervix." Although some may view such adjectives as innocuous, this terminology actually reflects negatively upon women, connoting blame on the woman's part for the infertility.

FEMALE ETIOLOGIES

The majority of female infertility is caused by ovulatory dysfunction and tubal and pelvic problems. Unexplained infertility, and combined or interactional infertility, which are discussed separately, account for most other cases of infertility among women. Ovulatory dysfunction may be the total lack of ovulation or the occurrence of irregular ovulation. Anovulation is usually, but not always, evidenced by irregular menstrual bleeding patterns or amenorrhea. There are numerous causes of ovulatory dysfunction, which can result from any interruption of the hypothalamic-pituitary-ovarian axis. Etiologies of ovarian dysfunction include polycystic ovarian syndrome, physiologic anovulation at either end of the reproductive spectrum, hyperprolactinemia, thyroid disorders, eating disorders, medications, and possibly stress. Further information about etiologies of anovulation can be found in Chapters 20 and 21.

A short duration of the luteal phase can also cause female infertility and is considered a subtle form of ovulatory dysfunction. A short luteal phase is also commonly referred to as luteal phase deficiency or defect, because it is associated with abnormally low levels of progesterone production by the corpus luteum. However, use of the latter terminology is discouraged because it may reflect negatively upon women as previously explained. The luteal phase is considered short when less than 13 days elapse between the midcycle LH surge and the onset of menses (Speroff & Fritz, 2005). This can lead not only to infertility, but also to recurrent miscarriage.

Tubal problems are usually related to blockages within the tubes, making it difficult or impossible for the sperm and ovum to meet. These blockages may be anatomic, but more frequently occur as a result of sexually transmitted infections (STIs) that have progressed to pelvic inflammatory disease (PID, see Chapter 18). These STIs may have been asymptomatic and thus gone unrecognized and untreated resulting in tubal scarring; however, tubal scarring may result even when STIs are treated. Tubal problems can also result from previous ectopic pregnancy or tubal surgery.

Other pelvic problems to consider when assessing for causes of infertility include endometriosis, uterine factors, and congenital anomalies. Endometriosis is a condition in which menstrual tissue grows in areas outside of the uterus rather than being sloughed off with each menstrual period. Endometriosis may or may not cause pain, and paradoxically, pain may not correlate with the extent of the disease process. For example, slight pain may correlate with severe endometriosis. This disease process can be elusive (see Chapter 22 for further information about endometriosis). Potential uterine causes of infertility include leiomyomatas, intrauterine adhesions, endometrial polyps, and chronic endometritis. The exact impact of these factors on fertility is not known, and they are not a common cause of infertility. Congenital anomalies of the reproductive tract, such as a bicornuate uterus or septate uterus, are also associated with infertility.

MALE ETIOLOGIES

Male factor infertility may be caused by anatomic or structural problems, abnormalities in sperm production or function, and sexual, hormonal, and genetic conditions. A structural cause of male infertility is undescended testes (cryptorchidism) after the age of two years. The testes are normally descended and are therefore external to the body, but if undescended they are exposed to higher temperatures that cause damage to the sperm. Hypospadias is a congenital anomaly that results in the urethral outlet being located on the shaft of the penis rather than at the end. This type of structural problem may make it difficult to deposit semen in the woman's vagina. Untreated or recurrent STIs in the male may result in scarring and blockage of the reproductive tract. Finally, a varicocele or varicose vein in the scrotum may affect male fertility. It is theorized that this causes an elevation in scrotal temperature and thus affects spermatogenesis.

Men who contract mumps later in life, particularly after adolescence, may become infertile, because the illness can result in a condition known as orchitis or testicular inflammation. However, because the condition is usually unilateral, sterility rarely results.

Infection, particularly in the prostate gland, can cause a decreased sperm count. Decreased blood flow to the testes, which can occur as a result of testicular torsion, can also lead to a decreased sperm count. Environmental factors can also negatively affect sperm production, though more research is needed in this area. There are also certain temporary causes of sperm abnormalities, such as being exposed to high temperatures due to illness accompanied by a high fever, or the use of hot tubs or saunas. In these instances, the decreased sperm count and/or motility will likely be improved after a three-month period of removing this exposure.

Other causes of male infertility are attributed to sexual difficulties, in particular erectile dysfunction. Hormonal problems, such as decreased testosterone production, can interfere with spermatogenesis. Genetic problems, such as Klinefelter's syndrome, can cause azoospermia (absence of sperm). Despite the many known etiologies, male factor infertility is often idiopathic.

COMBINED CAUSES

Combined or interactional causes of infertility include the inability of sperm to survive in the woman's cervical mucus because of the presence of antisperm antibodies. These antibodies can be present in the male or female, and their presence causes the sperm to agglutinate or clump, which decreases their motility. Testing for antisperm antibodies is no longer performed routinely because of advances in infertility treatments; therefore, this condition may go undetected. Other interactional causes of infertility include simultaneous female and male causes of infertility that together increase the risk for infertility and sexual difficulties. Emotional problems in one or both partners may or may not contribute to infertility, and these may also occur as a result of infertility.

UNEXPLAINED INFERTILITY

Unexplained infertility refers to situations in which no specific cause for the infertility can be found. Unexplained infertility is a diagnosis of exclusion, meaning that all other possible causes for the infertility have been ruled out. Interestingly, before the increased use of various technological means to diagnosis infertility problems, the rate of unexplained infertility was much higher. As scientific advances have increased the ability to diagnose an increasing number of causes of infertility, fewer people are diagnosed with unexplained infertility.

ASSESSMENT OF INFERTILITY

Evaluation of infertility begins with a thorough history and physical examination. Clinicians who provide gynecologic care often perform limited assessment of male partners (for example, obtaining relevant history and ordering semen analysis) and then refer men to another provider if additional evaluation is needed. Diagnostic tests for infertility are most useful and cost-effective if they proceed sequentially in a logical order.

HISTORY

Initially, it is essential that the clinician obtain an accurate and detailed history from the patient and her partner. This includes general medical, family, social, emotional, occupational, recreational, and lifestyle histories. The clinician should identify the duration of infertility and any previous evaluation or treatment. A detailed gynecologic history, with particular attention to the menstrual and obstetric histories as well as any previous surgeries or procedures (see Chapter 6), is crucial to the infertility evaluation. The frequency of coitus, any sexual difficulties, and history of STIs in either partner are also important to collect. When asking about previous pregnancies, clarify whether the woman and her partner have ever become pregnant together or with other partners. During the review of systems, ask the woman specifically about nipple discharge, hirsutism, pelvic pain, and symptoms of thyroid disorders. Ideally, the woman and her partner would each be interviewed separately and then together to encourage the most complete evaluation. This may be a stressful time for the individuals or couple because an initial infertility assessment also acknowledges the problem of infertility (Devine, 2003).

PHYSICAL EXAMINATION

A complete physical examination, including a pelvic examination, should be performed. During the general examination it is particularly important to note weight and body mass index (BMI); the presence of acne, hirsutism, or alopecia that could indicate a hyperandrogenic disorder; thyroid abnormalities, such as enlargement, nodule, or tenderness; and nipple discharge or visual changes that could indicate a pituitary mass. The pelvic examination should focus on identifying any abnormalities of the internal genitalia, such as enlargement, tenderness, and masses, as well as evidence of gynecologic infections and/or STIs. If infection is suspected, microscopic examination of vaginal secretions and chlamydia and gonorrhea testing should be performed (see Chapter 6). The male should also have a complete physical examination, with attention to the reproductive organs to rule out structural problems.

DIAGNOSTIC TESTING AND PROCEDURES

The basic and simple diagnostic procedures that should be done with an initial evaluation include ovulation detection and semen analysis. More specific tests that may be warranted include laboratory testing, postcoital testing, hysterosalpingogram, endometrial biopsy, laparoscopy, and sperm penetration assay. The couple's history should guide the clinician's decisions as to which testing is needed. Evaluation generally proceeds from less to more invasive tests. If a woman is ovulatory, it is preferable to organize the infertility evaluation according to the menstrual cycle. This way, many of the tests can be performed within the same month.

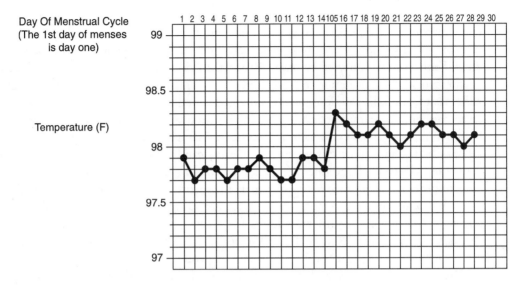

FIGURE 16–2   Sample Basal Body Temperature Chart

Ovulation Detection   Women can detect ovulation by monitoring and recording their basal body temperature (BBT) each day upon awakening. A BBT thermometer is different from a fever thermometer in that the BBT thermometer is calibrated in tenths of degrees, allowing for the detection of smaller changes in temperature. The BBT should be measured before eating or drinking and is most accurate if taken before rising from bed. If a woman ovulates, there will be a biphasic cycle that is indicated by temperature recordings consistently lower than 98°F during the follicular phase and consistently higher than 98°F during the luteal phase. There will be fluctuations within each of the phases, but plotting the temperatures on a graph makes a biphasic pattern clearly evident. Usually there is a slight drop in temperature just prior to ovulation, and a surge in temperature with ovulation (Figure 16–2). Recording the BBT is helpful because it provides useful data for assessment. The BBT should be recorded for at least three months because one menstrual cycle does not provide enough information. It is best to have a record of at least three menstrual cycles to assess whether or not there is a pattern in the cycles. Basal body temperature charting is a noninvasive test that is controlled by the woman.

Although keeping a record of one's BBT provides useful information, a more recent method of ovulation detection is available in the form of over-the-counter urine tests for LH. Women can do these tests in their home. The presence of a surge in LH (which is noted as a color change on the test strip) in the first morning urine indicates that ovulation will likely occur in 24 to 48 hours (Carcio, 1998b). Urine LH testing may become cost prohibitive if used for an extended period of time.

Semen Analysis Most male factor infertility is detected with semen analysis. It is important that semen analysis be performed early in the infertility evaluation so that male factor infertility can be diagnosed before the woman undergoes extensive, invasive diagnostic procedures. Semen can be collected by masturbation with ejaculation into a sterile container or by intercourse with ejaculation into a special collection condom if a man is uncomfortable with masturbation. Instructions include a defined period of abstinence of between two and seven days prior to sample collection. No more than one hour should elapse between collection and microscopic examination of the semen sample. The sample should be kept at room or body temperature during transport (American Urological Association [AUA] and American Society for Reproductive Medicine [ASRM], 2001). The semen analysis provides information about the volume of semen, the sperm count, motility, and morphology. There is not universal agreement on the reference ranges for semen analysis. A normal semen specimen is 1.5–5.0 ml in volume, has a concentration of more than 20 million sperm per ml, and includes more than 50% motile sperm. Cutoffs for normal morphology are greater than 14%, 30%, or 50% of sperm, depending on the criteria used (AUA and ASRM). A complete male evaluation usually includes an initial semen analysis and, if abnormalities are detected, two to three additional semen analyses to see if any patterns exist, as well as an endocrine evaluation (Boyle, Vlahos, & Jarow, 2004).

Laboratory Testing Various infertility tests are performed on blood samples. Initial evaluation usually includes measurement of thyroid stimulating hormone (TSH) and prolactin levels, as patients may have asymptomatic thyroid disease or hyperprolactinemia. An elevated prolactin level in the absence of lactation requires imaging of the sella turcica to rule out a pituitary mass. If BBT charting or LH urine testing does not demonstrate a biphasic curve, measuring serum progesterone levels midway during the luteal phase can be helpful in detecting whether or not a woman is ovulating. Serial progesterone tests to detect short luteal phase are not recommended (Speroff & Fritz, 2005). Additional laboratory tests, such as FSH, LH, and testosterone may be indicated if the woman is amenorrheic, or has signs and symptoms of a hyperandrogenic disorder (see Chapters 20 and 21).

Some clinicians perform assessments of "ovarian reserve" prior to infertility treatment as a predictor of the likelihood of success, particularly among women who are aged 35 years or older. One method is to obtain a serum FSH level on cycle day 3. Another protocol is the clomiphene citrate challenge, with measurement of serum FSH and estradiol levels on day 3, administration of clomiphene citrate from days 5–9, and another serum FSH level on day 10 (Speroff & Fritz, 2005). These tests are not typically part of the initial evaluation, but are mentioned because they are a frequent topic in the lay literature.

Postcoital Test A postcoital test (PCT) is done to evaluate the interaction of the sperm and cervical mucus around the time of ovulation. After the couple has sexual intercourse, a sample of the woman's cervical mucus is obtained by the health care provider for microscopic examination. Normally live, motile sperm will be seen. If there are problems, such as the cervical mucus being too acidic, or the man having an abnormally low sperm count, one might see predominantly immotile sperm or no sperm at all. With the advent of other assessment tools, the PCT is done much less frequently than a decade ago. Some advocate that this test is still a useful tool in infertility evaluation, but others recommend the PCT be performed only when it will influence the treatment strategy (Practice Committee of the ASRM, 2004a).

Hysterosalpingogram   A hysterosalpingogram (HSG) is a procedure in which a radio-opaque dye is injected through the woman's cervix into her uterus. During the HSG, the transport of the dye is observed by radiologic imaging. This procedure is performed after menstruation but before ovulation to avoid pushing away an ovum after ovulation, or pushing menstrual tissue back toward the ovaries. In a normal HSG, the dye travels unobstructed through the uterus and into the fallopian tubes. This test indicates whether the fallopian tubes are patent or if there is a structural abnormality in the uterus or tubes. An added benefit of having an HSG with oil-based dye is that the oil-based dye can cause dislodgement of tiny mucus plugs or peritoneal adhesions, which may be therapeutic in opening up areas of the fallopian tubes and enabling fertilization (Carcio, 1998b).

Endometrial Biopsy   Endometrial biopsy (EMB) of the uterine lining is used in infertility assessment because it allows evaluation of endometrial development. This procedure is done at approximately the midpoint of the luteal phase when there is a chance that conception has occurred. Endometrial biopsy can interfere with implantation, however, and therefore the woman may choose to use barrier contraception during the cycle in which the procedure is scheduled or a very sensitive pregnancy test may be performed immediately prior to the biopsy. During the procedure, an endometrial sampling device is inserted through the cervix into the uterus to obtain endometrial cells for laboratory evaluation. After the biopsy is performed, the cells are microscopically examined to assess the phase of the menstrual cycle. The day of the woman's menstrual cycle is compared with the phase of the endometrial tissue to determine if the two are consistent. This test had been considered the gold standard for the diagnosis of short luteal phase for many years, but recent research has found it is not a valid diagnostic tool. Speroff and Fritz (2005) recommend calculation of the length of the luteal phase, using BBT charting or urine LH testing, as the best method for diagnosis of short luteal phase in clinical practice.

Laparoscopy   The outside surfaces of the uterus, tubes, and ovaries can be observed via a laparoscope, which is inserted into the abdomen through the umbilicus. The pelvic organs are examined for any abnormalities, including structural alterations, endometriosis, or pelvic adhesions. Laparoscopy can be used not only for diagnosis of endometriosis and pelvic adhesions, but also for treatment. In addition, hysteroscopy may be performed simultaneously to evaluate the uterine cavity.

Sperm Penetration Assay Sometimes the cause of infertility is the inability of the sperm to penetrate the ovum. In the sperm penetration assay, sperm are exposed to hamster eggs to determine their ability to penetrate, because there is a correlation between the ability of sperm to penetrate human eggs and hamster eggs. This test is mentioned because it highlights the fact that sperm problems are sometimes better understood in interaction with the ova. This test, however, is done less frequently as more sophisticated tests have been developed.

DIFFERENTIAL DIAGNOSIS

The differential diagnosis of infertility includes the etiologies detailed previously. It is important to recognize that several causes may exist simultaneously.

PREVENTION OF INFERTILITY

The focus in infertility has traditionally been diagnosis and treatment, but there has recently been attention to prevention. Young women can be taught to prevent STIs, or if they have symptoms or suspect they may have been exposed to infection, to seek care early to prevent PID and subsequent infertility. Paradoxically, certain contraceptive methods may protect future fertility by decreasing the risk of PID, ectopic pregnancies, and endometriosis (see Chapter 9). There may be environmental factors that should be avoided, but more definitive study is needed.

MANAGEMENT OF INFERTILITY

Treatments for infertility are usually specific to the cause. Sometimes treatments are general because a specific cause of infertility is not able to be diagnosed (unexplained infertility). Approaches to treatment in these instances raise complex issues about risks and benefits.

PATIENT EDUCATION

Education about when a woman is fertile during the menstrual cycle and coital timing can be extremely beneficial for some patients. The infertility evaluation is also an opportune time to suggest health promotion behaviors. Behaviors that may specifically improve fertility include achieving a BMI of 20–25 if the woman is underweight or overweight, stopping smoking, and reducing alcohol and caffeine consumption (Speroff & Fritz, 2005).

OVULATION INDUCTION

If there is evidence of anovulation or infrequent ovulation, medication to induce ovulation may be prescribed. Because ovulation induction medications are so widely used and are frequently called "fertility drugs," there is a misconception by the general public that these medications improve general fertility. These drugs specifically help with ovulation and are not warranted in women who ovulate but want to otherwise improve their fertility. Taking these medications in such a situation is actually contraindicated, as they have antiestrogenic effects that may adversely affect the cervical mucus and may actually interfere with fertility. Despite this, ovulation induction medications are used in the treatment of women with unexplained infertility who are ovulatory.

The first choice of medication for ovulation induction is usually clomiphene citrate (Clomid, Serophene), which works by binding estrogen receptors in the pituitary gland, thereby blocking those receptors from detecting circulating estrogen. As a result, the hypothalamus increases its secretion of GnRH, which stimulates the pituitary to secrete FSH and LH. These hormones stimulate and initiate an ovulatory menstrual cycle.

Clomiphene citrate (Clomid) is taken orally once a day for five consecutive days. The initial dose is usually 50 mg. The medication is typically started on the third to fifth day after menses begins spontaneously or is induced with progestin. Ovulation usually occurs 14 days after the first dose. The dose can be increased in increments of 50 mg if the woman does not respond to the lower dose (ovulation does not occur); however, most pregnancies occur as a result of dosages of 50 to 100 mg (Practice Committee of the ASRM, 2004b). Clomiphene citrate can be administered in doses as high as 250 mg, but other approaches should be considered if continued increases in the dose are unsuccessful. If ovulation does occur at a specific dose, the woman should remain on that dose each month because an increased dose provides no advantage. The addition of metformin to clomiphene citrate may be beneficial in women with polycystic ovary syndrome (see Chapter 21).

Side effects of clomiphene citrate include hot flashes, headaches, ovarian enlargement, multiple gestation, and less frequently, nausea and visual disturbances. Multiple gestations are a frequent concern among women taking ovulation induction medications. In pregnancies that occur among women taking clomiphene citrate, 8% are multiple gestations and the vast majority of these are twins. Appropriate monitoring of women using clomiphene citrate includes ovulation detection with BBT charting, urine LH testing, or serum progesterone levels to determine effectiveness of the treatment. Close follow-up for ovarian enlargement is also warranted, although monthly pelvic or ultrasound examinations are no longer routinely required. Treatment is limited to six ovulatory cycles (Practice Committee of the ASRM, 2004b).

More potent ovulation induction with injectable exogenous gonadotropins can be tried for women who do not respond to clomiphene citrate. Recombinant or purified FSH (Follistim, Gonal-F) or human menopausal gonadotropins containing FSH and LH (Pergonal, Repronex) are most commonly used. These medications work by directly stimulating development of the ovarian follicles and are used in conjunction with human chorionic gonadotropin (hCG), which is administered once maturation of the follicle occurs. Exogenous gonadotropins increase the risk of ovarian hyperstimulation and resulting multiple gestations more than clomiphene citrate. GnRH agonists are now used with the exogenous gonadotropins to try to limit these effects (Griesinger, Felberbau,

Schultze-Mosgau, & Diedrich, 2004). The complex protocols and potential serious side effects of exogenous gonadotropins require careful treatment and extensive monitoring that is best performed by clinicians who are experienced in their use.

Women undergoing ovulation induction therapy must be informed about the medication, including its mechanism of action and potential side effects and risks. Exogenous gonadotropins can be very expensive, which is a consideration for many people. Some research suggests there may be a link between a woman's use of ovulation-inducing medication and later development of ovarian cancer. A recent meta-analysis found no increase in ovarian cancer among women with infertility who were treated when compared to those who were not (Kashyap, Moher, Fung, & Rosenwaks, 2004). However, judicious use of ovulation induction medications remains prudent.

TREATMENT OF SHORT LUTEAL PHASE

There is an association between hyperprolactinemia and a short luteal phase. Treatment to normalize the prolactin level may lengthen the luteal phase. In the absence of this identifiable cause, treatment of short luteal phase can be ambiguous. One theory of treatment is that the follicular phase of the menstrual cycle should be enhanced with ovulation induction methods because short luteal phase is a form of ovulatory dysfunction. Clomiphene citrate or other ovulation induction medications may be used. Another theory is that the luteal phase of the menstrual cycle should be enhanced by administering progesterone, thus increasing the secretory endometrium. Progesterone is administered rectally or vaginally, beginning three days after midcycle and continuing until menstruation. The usual dose is 12.5 to 25 mg every 12 hours. Sometimes women experience local irritation of the vagina and external genitalia and therefore choose to use the injectable form of progesterone in oil instead. If the woman conceives, she continues progesterone therapy throughout the first trimester. There is no evidence to support one strategy as more beneficial than the other (progesterone administration versus ovulation induction medications) (Speroff & Fritz, 2005).

TREATMENT FOR MALE FACTOR INFERTILITY

Treatment for male factor infertility depends upon the specific problem. For example, certain hormonal problems respond to medical therapy, and surgical repair of a varicocele can be beneficial. However, many causes of male factor infertility are not amenable to treatment. Pregnancy can still be achieved with artificial insemination, intrauterine insemination (IUI), or intracytoplasmic sperm injection (the latter is discussed in the section on assisted reproductive technologies).

Insemination procedures begin with the man masturbating to collect the semen, which is then processed in a laboratory to remove the seminal plasma, creating a more highly concentrated specimen of motile sperm. For artificial insemination, the clinician then places the semen into the woman's cervix. With IUI, the semen is placed directly into her uterus, bypassing the cervix. This is particularly warranted if there is a problem with the cervical mucus. Artificial and intrauterine insemination must be performed in a precisely timed manner based on the woman's menstrual cycle. These procedures can lead to increased stress for the couple. The man may feel greater pressure to perform by producing the semen, and the woman may feel more anxious about having intercourse at "appropriate" times and abstaining at "inappropriate" times. Intrauterine insemination is often used with ovulation induction even if no male factors are identified. This is done to increase the success of the ovulation induction by enhancing the precision and accuracy of timing.

OPTIONS FOR WOMEN AND MEN WITH INFERTILITY

Technological advances have led to an increasing array of procedures for becoming pregnant, including the possibility of collaborative reproduction. Women and men may also choose adoption or child-free living. These options are presented in this section, and their psychological and ethical considerations are the focus of the next section.

ASSISTED REPRODUCTIVE TECHNOLOGIES

In vitro fertilization (IVF) is the most widely used assisted reproductive technology (ART) procedure. The ovaries are hyperstimulated with medication and then several mature ova are surgically retrieved, placed in a laboratory dish, and then mixed with sperm. Fertilization takes place in vitro and, after fertilization, one or more embryos are transferred directly into the woman's uterus for implantation. IVF bypasses the fallopian tubes and is thus commonly attempted in women who have tubal blockage, either because of structural problems or secondary to pelvic infection or scar tissue. It is also used when infertility is unexplained.

Gamete intrafallopian transfer (GIFT) is another form of ART, but in this case fertilization occurs in vivo rather than in vitro. The egg and sperm are both placed directly into the fallopian tube via laparoscopy so that fertilization can occur. The woman must have at least one patent fallopian tube for GIFT to be successful. Women and men who are Catholic may choose this method over IVF because the Catholic church condones GIFT, but not IVF.

Zygote intrafallopian transfer (ZIFT) is a process in which the ovaries are hyperstimulated and the ova are surgically retrieved. They are fertilized in vitro, as with IVF. The zygotes are placed in the fallopian tube laparoscopically the day after fertilization.

Intracytoplasmic sperm injection (ICSI) is a newer technique in which the egg is directly injected with one sperm. This procedure is used when the man has a low sperm count or other instances of male factor infertility. Intracytoplasmic sperm injection is used in conjunction with IVF or ZIFT.

COLLABORATIVE REPRODUCTION

Collaborative, or third-party, reproduction refers to the involvement of a person who will not be raising the child, such as a sperm or egg donor or surrogate mother. One person may donate sperm or eggs (genetic parent) and/or carry the pregnancy (gestational mother) for another person or couple who will raise the child (rearing parents). Collaborative reproduction may involve artificial or intrauterine insemination, or ARTs. Collaborative reproduction may be chosen when infertility treatment or ARTs have been unsuccessful or are not possible because of individual factors. Women who are situationally infertile, or those who are unable to conceive by virtue of not having a male partner, may also seek donor insemination. These women may be single or may be lesbians. Insemination is a very viable option for them.

Use of donor sperm is the most common type of collaborative reproduction, but women may also become pregnant with donor eggs. For example, a known or anonymous woman donates her eggs to an individual or couple. The eggs are fertilized in vitro with sperm, most likely from the man of the couple with infertility (rearing father), and then transferred to the woman with infertility for gestation. In this instance, the egg donor is the genetic mother and the woman who becomes pregnant is the gestational and rearing mother. Surrogate mothers can be genetic and gestational mothers if they carry a fetus who is conceived from their own egg, or solely gestational mothers if they carry a fetus conceived from another couple's egg and sperm, such as from a woman who can conceive but not carry a pregnancy.

ADOPTION

For those who are able to separate pregnancy from parenting, adoption is often an ideal option. Couples who choose to adopt usually go through a home study by an adoption agency prior to being approved for adoption. Other couples go through private attorneys to find a woman who is willing to give her child up for adoption. International adoption has become increasingly popular as more people go to other countries, such as China or Russia, to adopt children. Although adoption is often an excellent option for individuals or couples seeking parenthood, this is not always the case in all cultures. In India, infertility is referred to as "adoption gone awry," and people seek solutions in secret, thus making adoption an unacceptable option because it is difficult to keep that secret (Bharadwaj, 2003).

CHILD-FREE LIVING

Some individuals or couples eventually come to a decision to live their lives without children. The term "child-free" connotes that this has now become a choice rather than something occurring against their will. People without children may be referred to as "childless," but this term indicates a loss or absence. Granted, this situation was initially "childlessness" for those who hoped to conceive, but through the process of reconciling their loss, these people are able to come to a conclusion of their own volition to remain childfree.

EVIDENCE FOR BEST PRACTICES RELATED TO INFERTILITY CARE

Practices that offer ARTs are urged to follow the guidelines developed by the American Society for Reproductive Medicine and the Society for Assisted Reproductive Technology (2003). The guidelines address minimum requirements for all personnel, the specialized training and experience required for personnel, minimum standards to follow for each technological procedure, ethical and experimental procedures, recordkeeping, and informed consent. These guidelines are updated periodically and are considered the standard for the delivery of ART. The ASRM (2004) has several additional reports that are helpful for other clinical aspects of infertility care.

SPECIAL CONSIDERATIONS

This section presents some of the controversial issues related to infertility and its treatment. Infertility can have psychosocial effects on the individuals and couples involved as well as their larger families. The new technologies used to both diagnose and treat infertility create many ethical issues. The psychosocial and ethical issues are the focus of this section.

PSYCHOLOGICAL, FAMILY, RELATIONSHIP, AND SOCIAL ISSUES

Extensive research suggests that many psychological issues are related to infertility, whether the psychological problems are causes or consequences of infertility. Historically, women were viewed as psychogenically infertile, a very negative term that implied that those women who were unable to conceive were psychologically unstable, had unresolved relationship issues with their mothers, or were hysterical or neurotic. Psychoanalytic theory in the 1950s and 1960s predominated in regard to explaining infertility as a woman's problem to the exclusion of any involvement by men. A few decades later, the scientific literature developed an increasing focus on psychological problems in both women and men that occurred as a consequence of infertility rather than as a cause, mitigating the negative labels on women. A better understanding was developed about the difficulties and stresses that both women and men experienced as a result of their inability to conceive or bear a child. Recently, scientific literature has taken a more complex view, indicating that there are both psychological causes and consequences of infertility for women and men.

In general, infertility is profoundly distressing for those experiencing it, whether this is a cause or a consequence. Olshansky (1996a) generated a theory of identity as infertile to reflect the experience of infertility becoming so central to one's definition of self that a person begins to take on an identity as an infertile person. Other identities are pushed to the periphery as the identity as infertile becomes central.

Recent research suggests that psychological problems, such as depression and anxiety, may contribute to the development of infertility, though much further study is needed. Domar (2002) found that using a mind–body approach to elicit a relaxation response helps some women conceive.

There are often complicated psychological issues surrounding a decision or inability to make a decision to stop infertility treatment. This is particularly true with the advances in reproductive technology that make new options continually available. New treatments raise hopes and make it difficult to stop treatment for fear that there will be a feeling of not having done everything possible to conceive, which could then make it difficult to resolve infertility later.

Infertility is directly intertwined with family issues because it represents the inability to expand a family. Some people even view it as an inability to have a family, implying that two people in a couple are not a family by virtue of not having children and further emphasizing a societal bent toward pronatalism. Family gatherings can be extremely difficult for persons dealing with infertility because they may confront directly their inability to conceive, especially if young children are present. Family issues may extend to others, such as the parents of people with infertility who are experiencing the loss related to not being grandparents. Family members may pressure couples with infertility with comments such as, "Why are they taking so long to have a baby?"

As stated earlier, women and men experience infertility within a socially pronatalist context. As a result they are often viewed as abnormal or as not fulfilling their responsibilities to continue the human race. Women, by virtue of the general social approach to and view of women's roles, may experience feeling even more "aberrant" than do men.

Social issues may vary in different societies and in different socioeconomic groups. For example, a recent study in South Africa found that although infertility is a large problem, the resources for treatment are limited (Stewart-Smythe & van Iddekinge, 2003). Tubal problems are the most frequently diagnosed cause of infertility in South Africa, and the best treatment is IVF. This is an expensive technique, however, and as such is less available and accessible in the public sector of South Africa. Inhorn (2003) corroborated this problem in her case study of infertility in Egypt, where she found that even though reproductive technologies are available, many structural and cultural constraints prevent access to such technologies. She further states that more attention should be paid to preventable infertility problems, specifically infections that lead to PID.

ETHICAL ISSUES

Many of the ethical issues related to infertility occur as a result of the increasing use of technology; however, it is important to note that ethical issues existed prior to and may be independent of advances in infertility treatment. Access to infertility treatment has always been an issue, but it has been particularly compounded by technology. The expense of infertility treatment raises the question of whether these therapies will be limited to those with the financial means to afford them. The ability to conceive with technology but without a partner leads to questions regarding whether single women, single men, lesbian couples, or gay men will be treated.

Other ethical issues concern who the parents are in situations where extra embryos have been frozen and the couple subsequently divorces, or when a surrogate mother decides she no longer wants to relinquish the infant. In fact, the larger issue is how "real parent" is defined. There are the genetic mother, the surrogate mother, the gestational mother, the adoptive or rearing mother, and the birth mother to be considered. Egg donation is one example of a treatment that raises many ethical, as well as legal issues (Robertson, 1995).

Another ethical dilemma can occur when several embryos are transferred into the woman's uterus and multiple embryos survive. The fact that there are multiple embryos may create a high risk for all of them and the woman may choose to selectively abort one or more. This creates complex ethical as well as emotional issues. Some infertility clinics limit the number of embryos they transfer to eliminate the possibility of this situation, but other clinics take the attitude that if more embryos are transferred, the chance of a successful pregnancy increases.

Ethical concerns have also arisen about the ability to perform pre-implantation testing with ARTs. After in vitro fertilization, a cell is removed from the embryo for genetic testing. This allows couples with known inherited disorders to select nonaffected embryos for transfer, but leads to questions about genetic engineering. The sex of the embryo can also be determined, which is useful for sex-linked disorders, but is controversial when sex selection is purely for parental preference.

These are just a few of the many ethical issues in infertility care and treatment. There are no simple answers to these conflicts, but they warrant consideration both from a societal perspective and on the level of caring for individual patients. The ASRM (2004) has several reports that address ethical issues in infertility.

INFERTILITY AND CANCER

Progress in medicine has provided much better prognoses for many people with a diagnosis of cancer. As a result, people who survive cancer may be at reproductive age and may want to conceive. Conversely, some concern is raised about the possibility that infertility and its treatment may increase the risk for or development of cancer, though recent research has not confirmed this fear (Venn, Healy, & McLachlan, 2003). Infertility may occur as a result of treatments for cancer, and a recent body of scientific work is now focused on preserving fertility in people after a diagnosis of cancer. Fossa (2004) presented a review of males treated for testicular cancer and the consequences for treating infertility that indicates infertility is a problem in 10% to 15% of males who survive testicular cancer.

INFERTILITY AND WOMEN IN THE LATER YEARS OF CHILDBEARING

With the increased use of technology to treat infertility, more options have been developed for women at the end of their childbearing years. Thus, women in their mid-forties to even early fifties may conceive and carry a pregnancy to term. Although this creates more options for women, this situation also creates more complex decisions for women and their families. There are certain known genetic risks to the fetus, such as Down syndrome, when women are pregnant at later ages. At the same time, there may be advantages to women and their children in parenting at older ages. More research is needed in this area.

PATIENT COUNSELING

It is crucial for providers to recognize that treatment for infertility involves more than physical treatment. Olshansky (1996b) noted four important aspects of care that should be included in a counseling approach to persons with infertility. These aspects include the following:

1. Assist patients in confronting and analyzing the choices available to them by providing complete and accurate information while empowering them to make decisions that only they can make.
2. Assist patients in focusing on and reclaiming the successful parts of their lives by helping them to see positive aspects of themselves rather than defining themselves based on their infertility.
3. Assist patients in moving on with their lives by helping them to stop treatment when appropriate and seek other options.
4. Assist patients in developing and maintaining healthy interpersonal relationships by emphasizing the importance of relationships to good mental health.

Incorporating these aspects into clinical care can improve patients' quality of life both during and after infertility treatment.

REFERENCES

American Society for Reproductive Medicine. (2004). 2004 compendium of ASRM practice committee and ethics committee reports. *Fertility and Sterility, 82*(Suppl. 1).

American Society for Reproductive Medicine and Society for Assisted Reproductive Technology. (2003). Revised minimum standards for practices offering assisted reproductive technologies. *Fertility and Sterility, 80,* 1556–1559.

American Urological Association and American Society for Reproductive Medicine. (2001). *Report on the optimal evaluation of the infertile male.* Retrieved October 23, 2004, from http://www.asrm.org/Media/Practice/infertilemale.pdf.

Benasutti, R. D. (2003). Infertility: Experiences and meanings. *Journal of Couple and Relationship Therapy, 2*(4), 51–71.

Bharadwaj, A. (2003). Why adoption is not an option in India: The visibility of infertility, the secrecy of donor insemination, and other cultural complexities. *Social Science and Medicine, 56*(9), 1867–1880.

Bickstein, I. (2003). Motherhood at or beyond the edge of reproductive age. *International Journal of Fertility and Women's Medicine, 48*(1), 17–24.

Boyle, K. A., Vlahos, N., & Jarow, J. P. (2004). Assisted reproductive technology in the new millennium: Part I. *Urology, 63*(1), 2–6.

Carcio, H. A. (1998a). Causes of infertility. In H. A. Carcio (Ed.), *Management of the infertile woman* (pp. 25–48). Philadelphia: Lippincott.

Carcio, H. A. (1998b). The investigation. In H. A. Carcio (Ed.), *Management of the infertile woman* (pp. 111–166). Philadelphia: Lippincott.

Devine, K. (2003). Caring for the infertile woman. *MCN: The American Journal of Maternal-Child Nursing, 28*(2), 100–105.

Domar, A. D. (2002). *Conquering infertility.* New York: Viking Press.

Fossa, S. D. (2004). Long-term sequelae after cancer therapy: Survivorship after treatment for testicular cancer. *Acta Oncologica, 43*(2), 134–141.

Griesinger, G., Felberbau, R. W., Schultze-Mosgau, A., & Diedrich, K. (2004). Gonadotropin-releasing hormone antagonists for assisted reproductive techniques: Are there clinical differences between agents? *Drugs, 64*(6), 563–575.

Hanson, B. (2003). Questioning the construction of maternal age as a fertility problem. *Health Care for Women International, 24*(3), 166–176.

Inhorn, M. C. (2003). Global infertility and the globalization of new reproductive technologies: Illustrations from Egypt. *Social Science and Medicine, 56*(9), 1837–1851.

Kashyap, S., Moher, D., Fung, M. F., & Rosenwaks, Z. (2004). Assisted reproductive technology and the incidence of ovarian cancer: A meta-analysis. *Obstetrics & Gynecology, 103,* 785–794.

Olshansky, E. F. (1992). Redefining the concepts of success and failure in infertility treatment. *AACOG's Clinical Issues in Women's Health and Perinatal Nursing, 3*(2), 343–347.

Olshansky, E. (1996a). Theoretical issues in building a grounded theory: Application of a program of research on infertility. *Qualitative Health Research, 6*(3), 394–405.

Olshansky, E. (1996b). A counseling approach with persons experiencing infertility: Implications for advanced practice nursing. *Advanced Practice Nursing Quarterly, 2*(3), 42–47.

Practice Committee of the American Society for Reproductive Medicine. (2004a). Optimal evaluation of the infertile female. *Fertility and Sterility, 82*(Suppl. 1), S169–S172.

Practice Committee of the American Society for Reproductive Medicine. (2004b). Use of clomiphene citrate in women. *Fertility and Sterility, 82*(Suppl. 1), S90–S96.

Robertson, J. A. (1995). Legal issues in human egg donation and gestational surrogacy. *Seminars in Reproductive Endocrinology, 13*(3), 210–218.

Speroff, L., & Fritz, M. (2005). *Clinical gynecologic endocrinology and infertility* (7th ed.). Baltimore: Lippincott Williams & Wilkins.

Stewart-Smythe, G. W., & van Iddekinge, B. (2003). Lessons learned from infertility investigations in the public sector. *South African Medical Journal, 93*(2), 141–143.

Venn, A., Healy, D., & McLachlan, R. (2003). Cancer risks associated with the diagnosis of infertility. *Best Practice and Research in Clinical Obstetrics and Gynecology, 17*(2), 343–367.

Chapter 17

GYNECOLOGIC INFECTIONS

CATHERINE INGRAM FOGEL

Gynecologic infections, often associated with vaginal discharge, itching of the vulva and vagina, and vaginal or vulvar pain, are among the most frequent reasons a woman seeks help from a health care provider. Different women perceive discharge and itching in unique ways. One woman may be extremely uncomfortable, another may feel only minor distress, a third may be very anxious, and a fourth may be mildly concerned. Women's reactions depend on many factors, including their previous experiences or knowledge; societal, religious, and cultural beliefs; and the number and severity of symptoms.

VAGINAL SECRETIONS

NORMAL CHARACTERISTICS

Vaginal secretions are a normal, regularly occurring experience for women during their reproductive years. The numerous variations in the amount and characteristics of vaginal secretions are determined by physiology, emotions, and pathology. Women who have adequate endogenous or exogenous estrogen will have vaginal secretions. The major source of vaginal secretions is the cervical mucosa. Small amounts are secreted by the Bartholin's, sebaceous, sweat, and apocrine glands of the vulva. Vaginal lubrication, which is pushed through the semipermanent vaginal membrane as a result of increased vasocongestion in the sponge-like tissues surrounding the vagina, occurs during sexual excitement (Ayres, 2004).

Normal vaginal secretions are clear to cloudy in appearance and may turn yellow after drying. The discharge is slightly slimy, nonirritating, and has a mild unoffensive odor. The alkaline, shiny mucoid substance secreted by the cervix, on the other hand, is more abundant than vaginal secretions and is less viscous at ovulation. Normal vaginal secretions are acidic, with a pH range of 3.8 to 4.2. Doderlein's bacilli are customarily seen in the vaginal secretions of women during their reproductive years. The amount of vaginal discharge a woman experiences is not, in itself, an indication of infection.

LIFE CYCLE CHANGES

The female newborn may have a mucous discharge for 1 to 10 days following birth as a result of in utero stimulation of the uterus and vagina by maternal estrogen. A similar mucoid discharge may be seen a few years before and after menarche as a result of increased estrogen production by the maturing ovaries. Pregnancy often substantially increases mucus production, with a resulting profuse discharge, particularly during the last few weeks. A similar discharge may occur in a woman taking combined oral contraceptives (Hatcher et al., 1998).

Before menarche and following menopause, when estrogen levels are low, vaginal secretions are minimal. The vaginal epithelium is inactive and thin, the cells contain very little glycogen, Doderlein's bacilli are absent, and the vaginal pH is between 6 and 7. Such inactive mucosa is particularly susceptible to infection, whereas the estrogen-stimulated vaginal mucosa during the reproductive years is less susceptible.

Vaginal secretions normally vary throughout the menstrual cycle. During the immediate postmenstrual phase, when the estrogen level is low, the mucosa is thin and relatively inactive with little cervical cell secretion present. Vaginal cells proliferate and exfoliate rapidly as estrogen production increases. At the same time, the cervical cells secrete more and more mucus. Maximal estrogen production occurs at ovulation and causes a profuse watery discharge, primarily from the cervix. Secretions then decrease until just prior to menstruation.

VAGINITIS AND VAGINOSIS

Vaginitis is an inflammation of the vagina characterized by an increased vaginal discharge containing numerous white blood cells. In contrast, vaginosis is not associated with white blood cells. Vaginitis occurs when the vaginal environment is altered, either by a microorganism (Table 17–1) or by a disturbance that allows the pathogens found normally in the vagina to proliferate. Factors that can disturb the vaginal environment include douches, vaginal medications, antibiotics, hormones, contraceptive preparations (oral and topical), stress, sexual intercourse, and changes in sexual partners (Schaffer, 2003).

Vulvovaginitis or inflammation of the vulva and vagina may be caused by vaginal infection or copious amounts of leukorrhea, an increased amount of vaginal and cervical discharge consisting of epithelial cells and cervical mucus that can cause maceration of tissues. In addition, chemical irritants, allergens, and foreign bodies may produce inflammatory reactions. Bacterial vaginosis (BV), vulvovaginal candidiasis (VVC), and trichonomiasis are the most common causes of abnormal vaginal discharge (see Chapter 18 for a discussion of trichomoniasis).

TABLE 17-1 Vaginal Discharge

	Normal Discharge	Bacterial Vaginosis	Vulvovaginal Candidiasis
Vaginal pH	3.8–4.2	>4.5	<4.5 (usually)
Wet Prep	Normal flora	With saline solution: positive for clue cells, decreased lactobacilli	With potassium hydroxide: pseudohyphae with yeast buds
Discharge	White/clear Thin/mucoid	Thin, homogenous, grayish-white, adherent	Thick or thin; white, curd-like; "cottage cheeselike," adherent
Amine odor (KOH "whiff" test)	Normal body odor	Present (fishy)	None/yeasty, musty odor
Vulvar pruritis	No	Mild if present at all	Yes, swelling, excoriation, redness
Genital ulceration	No	No	Skin cracks with severe cases
Pelvic pain	No	No	No
Dysuria	No	Occasionally	Severe cases
Dyspareunia	No	Occasionally	Occasionally
Main patient concern	No	May be asymptomatic discharge, bad odor, possibly worse after intercourse; may report suprapubic pain	Itching/burning discharge
Risk of PID	No	Yes	No

Sources: CDC, 2002; Scharbo-DeHaan & Anderson, 2003.

PREVENTION MEASURES

Clinicians can do much to alleviate the discomfort associated with abnormal vaginal discharge by teaching preventive measures, providing information to assist in recognizing symptoms, and suggesting self-care activities to prevent and treat vaginitis. Preventive measures are important for all types of vaginal infections, particularly for women with recurrent episodes of vaginitis. General health promotion, including adequate rest, reduction of life stressors, and a healthy diet low in refined sugars, may help to decrease the likelihood of infection. Good personal hygiene is essential for preventing vaginal infections. The perineal area needs to be washed often to remove perspiration and smegma accumulations, then patted dry rather than rubbed. Towels, washcloths, sponges, douching equipment, vaginal diaphragms, cervical caps, and underwear should be clean and never shared. Bathtubs should be washed after each use.

Critical to prevention efforts is teaching women the proper way to wipe after voiding and defecation. One should always wipe from front to back (never the reverse) to avoid introducing bacteria into the vagina or urethra. Sprays, powders, soaps, and deodorants that are perfumed or irritating in any way should not be used. Any chemicals that irritate the skin or vaginal mucosa, or that alter the vaginal environment, should be avoided. Clothing that is too tight, does not allow free air flow to the perineum, or traps moisture should be avoided. Underwear and pantyhose should always have a cotton crotch. Women should not douche because douching can strip the vagina of its normal flora, introduce bacteria, and aggravate inflammation. The only exception to this is when medication is needed.

Women should be encouraged to change tampons, sanitary pads, and panty liners frequently. Women should be counseled not to wear tampons to bed and not to use them when flow is scanty because they may adhere to the vaginal wall or cervix and cause trauma when removed. In addition, women should avoid perfumed sanitary products because they can be an allergen or chemical irritant.

BACTERIAL VAGINOSIS

Bacterial vaginosis, formerly called nonspecific vaginitis, hemophilus vaginitis, or gardnerella, makes up 30–50% of all cases of vaginitis (Star & Deal, 2004) and is the most common vaginal infection in childbearing women (Calzolari, Masciangelo, Milite, & Vertaramo, 2000). African-American and Hispanic women have a much greater risk of having BV than do Caucasian and Asian women (Star & Deal). Bacterial vaginosis is a clinical syndrome in which normal hydrogen peroxide-producing *Lactobacilli* are replaced with high concentrations of anaerobic (e.g., *Prevotella*, *Peptostreptococcus*, *Eubacterium*, and *Mobiluncus* sp.), and facultative anaerobic (i.e., *Gardnerella vaginalis* and *Mycoplasma hominis*) bacteria. With the proliferation of anaerobes, the level of vaginal amines is raised and the normal acidic pH of the vagina is altered. Epithelial cells slough, and numerous bacteria attach to their surfaces (clue cells). When the amines are volatilized, the characteristic fishy odor of BV occurs. The cause of the microbial alteration is not completely understood, but BV is not considered a sexually transmitted infection (STI). What is known is that BV is associated with new or multiple sex partners, lesbian partnerships, douching, and a lack of vaginal lactobacilli (Fethers, Marks, Mindel, & Estcourt, 2000; McCaffrey, Varney, Evans, & Taylor-Robinson, 1999; Star & Deal). Women who have never been sexually active are rarely affected.

Bacterial vaginosis may cause serious infection in some women, including pelvic inflammatory disease (PID) and postoperative infections, such as posthysterectomy vaginal cuff infection, postabortion endometritis, and postcesarean wound infection (Centers for Disease Control and Prevention [CDC], 2002). Studies suggest that BV also increases a woman's risk of acquiring STIs, including human immunodeficiency virus (HIV), and of transmitting HIV infection (Koumans, Markowitz, & Hogan, 2002; Taha, Hoover, & Dallabetta, 1998). Additionally, failure to treat BV infection prior to insertion of an intrauterine device (IUD) is associated with increased incidence of PID in the first month after insertion (Hawkins, Roberto-Nichols, & Stanley-Haney, 2004).

As many as 50% of women with BV are asymptomatic. The most common symptom is a malodorous discharge. The "fishy odor" may be noticed by the woman or her partner after heterosexual intercourse because semen releases the vaginal amines. When present, the BV discharge is usually increased, thin, white or gray, and milky in appearance. Some women also may experience mild irritation, vulvar pruritus, postcoital spotting, irregular bleeding episodes, vaginal burning after intercourse, and urinary discomfort.

ASSESSMENT

A careful history may help distinguish BV from other vaginal infections if the woman is symptomatic. Reports of fishy odor and increased thin vaginal discharge are most significant. Reports of increased odor after intercourse are also suggestive of BV. Previous occurrences of similar symptoms, diagnoses, and treatments should be investigated because women may experience repeat episodes associated with antibiotic use, douching, or life stresses.

A speculum examination is done to inspect the vaginal walls and cervix. A microscopic examination of vaginal secretions is always performed with both normal saline and 10% potassium hydroxide (KOH). The presence of clue cells (vaginal epithelial cells coated with bacteria that obscure cell borders) in the saline smear is highly diagnostic because the phenomenon is specific to BV (Figure 17–1). KOH is used to test for amine odor. A fishy odor will be released when KOH is added to vaginal secretions on a slide or on the lip of the withdrawn speculum (whiff test). Vaginal secretions should also be tested for pH. Nitrazine paper is sensitive enough to detect a pH of 4.5 or greater. The smear should be taken from the lateral walls of the vagina, not the cervix, for an accurate pH. In

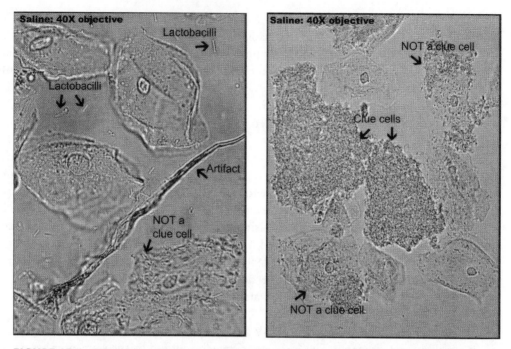

FIGURE 17-1 Wet Mount Findings with Bacterial Vaginosis. No bacterial vaginosis (left)—presence of normal epithelial cells and *Lactobacilli*. Bacterial vaginosis (right)—clue cells and absence of *Lactobacilli*. *Source:* Used with permission from Washington State Department of Health STD/TB Program, Seattle STD/HIV Prevention Training Center, and Cindy Fennell, MS, MT, ASCP.

asymptomatic women, BV can be reliably diagnosed by gram stain as well. Diagnosis is based on the presence of three out of four of the following Amsel criteria:

1. White, thin adherent discharge
2. pH > 4.5
3. Positive whiff test
4. Clue cells on wet mount (> 20% clue cells).

DIFFERENTIAL DIAGNOSIS

The differential diagnoses for BV are trichomoniasis, vulvovaginal candidiasis, presence of a foreign body, chemical vaginitis, contact vaginitis, chlamydia, gonorrhea, genital herpes, and normal physiologic discharge (Hawkins et al., 2004).

MANAGEMENT

Treatment guidelines can be found in Table 17–2. Vaginal metronidazole should not be given to women with a known allergy to oral metronidazole (CDC, 2002). Clindamycin cream is preferred in case of allergy or intolerance to metronidazole. Treatment of sexual partners is not recommended as sexual transmission of BV has not been proven (CDC). Alternative therapies for BV can be found in Table 17–3.

TABLE 17-2 Bacterial Vaginosis and Vulvovaginal Candidiasis Treatment

Vaginal Infection	Recommended Regimens	Alternative Regimens
Bacterial vaginosis	Metronidazole 500 mg orally twice a day x 7 days Metronidazole gel 0.75%, one full applicator (5g) intravaginally, daily x 5 days Clindamycin cream 2%, one full applicator (5g) intravaginally, at bedtime x 7 days	Metronidazole 2 g orally in a single dose Clindamycin 300 mg orally twice a day x 7 days Clindamycin ovules 100 g intravaginally once at bedtime x 3 days
	Pregnant Women Metronidazole 250 mg orally three times a day x 7 days Clindamycin 300 mg orally twice a day x 7 days	**Pregnant Women** None
Uncomplicated vulvovaginal candidiasis	**Intravaginal Medications** Butoconazole 2% cream 5 g intravaginally x 3 days* Butoconazole 2% cream 5 g (sustained release) single intravaginal application Clotrimazole 1% cream 5 g intravaginally x 7–14 days* Clotrimazole 100 mg vaginal tablet x 7 days Clotrimazole 100 mg vaginal tablet, 2 tablets x 3 days Clotrimazole 500 mg vaginal tablet, 1 tablet in single application Miconazole 2% cream 5 g intravaginally x 7 days* Miconazole 100 mg vaginal suppository, 1 for 7 days* Miconazole 200 mg vaginal suppository, 1 for 3 days* Nystatin 100,000-unit vaginal tablet, 1 x 14 days Tioconazole 6.5% ointment 5 g intravaginally in a single application* Terconazole 0.4% cream 5 g intravaginally x 7 days Terconazole 0.8% cream 5 g intravaginally x 3 days Terconazole 80 mg vaginal suppository, 1 x 3 days **Oral Agent** Fluconazole 150 mg oral tablet, 1 tablet single dose	

(continues)

TABLE 17–2   Bacterial Vaginosis and Vulvovaginal Candidiasis Treatment continued

Vaginal Infection	Recommended Regimens	Alternative Regimens
Complicated vulvovaginal candidiasis (VVC)	**Recurrent VVC Initial Therapy** Longer duration, 7–14 days of topical therapy or 150 mg dose of fluconazole repeated 3 days later **Recurrent VVC Maintenance Therapy** Clotrimazole 500 mg vaginal suppository weekly Ketoconazole 100 mg daily Fluconazole 100–150 mg dose weekly Itraconazole 400 mg once monthly or 100 mg daily **Severe VVC** 7–14 days of topical azole Fluconazole 150 mg in 2 sequential doses, 2nd dose 72 hours after initial dose **Non-albicans VVC** Nonfluconazole azole drug x 7–14 days **Recurrent non-albicans VVC** 600 mg boric acid in gelatin capsule vaginally each day x 14 days Maintenance regimen: 100,000 units nystatin vaginal suppository daily **Pregnancy** Topical azole therapy, applied for 7 days **HIV Infection** Should not differ from that of seronegative women	

*Over-the-counter (OTC) preparations.
Source: CDC, 2002.

TABLE 17-3   Alternative Therapies for Vaginitis

Intervention	Dosage	Administration	Use
Gentian violet	Few drops in water, 0.25% to 2%	Douche or local application	Vulvovaginal candidiasis
Vinegar (white)	1 tablespoon per pint of water	Douche every 5–7 days or twice a day for 2 days	Vulvovaginal candidiasis or trichomoniasis
	1–2 tablespoons per quart of water	Douche 1–2 times/week	Bacterial vaginosis
Acidophilus culture	2 tablespoons per pint of water	Douche twice a day	Vulvovaginal candidiasis
Vitamin C	500 mg two to four times daily	Orally	Vulvovaginal candidiasis
Acidophilus tablet	40 million–1 billion units (1 tab) daily	Orally	Vulvovaginal candidiasis
Yogurt	1 application to labia or in vagina	Hourly as needed	Vulvovaginal candidiasis
Goldenseal	1 teaspoon in 3 cups warm water, strain and cool	Douche	Bacterial vaginosis
Garlic clove	1 peeled clove wrapped in cloth dipped in olive oil	Overnight in vagina, change daily	Bacterial vaginosis
Boric acid powder	600 mg in gelatin capsule	Every day in vagina x 14 days	Bacterial vaginosis
Sassafras bark	Steep in warm water Compress	Wash affected area	Vulvovaginal candidiasis
Cold milk, cottage cheese, yogurt	Compress or insert in vagina	Apply to affected area	Pruritis

Sources: Balch & Balch, 1997; Hudson, 1999; Low Dog, 2004; Shaley, Battino, Weiner, Colodner, & Keness, 1996.

SPECIAL CONSIDERATIONS

Pregnant Women   Bacterial vaginosis is associated with miscarriage, chorioamnionitis, premature rupture of fetal membranes, preterm labor and delivery, postpartum or postabortion endometritis, and postpartum complications in the infant (CDC, 2002; Koumans et al., 2002). A test for BV may be done early in the second trimester for symptomatic pregnant women who are at risk for preterm labor and whenever high-risk women report increased vaginal discharge or symptoms of preterm labor. Current evidence is conflicting regarding whether treatment of asymptomatic pregnant women who are at low risk for preterm delivery reduces adverse outcomes of pregnancy; therefore, universal testing of all pregnant women regardless of risk status for BV is not recommended (CDC). Treatment guidelines can be found in Table 17–2. Clindamycin vaginal cream is not recommended in pregnancy because research has shown an increased number of premature births and neonatal infections in women who were treated with this medication (CDC).

Talking with the Patient   The importance of completing the course of medication and of not consuming alcohol while taking metronidazole (and for 48 hours after completing the treatment) must be emphasized. Women should be informed that metronidazole can cause nausea, vomiting, and cramps even if alcohol is not consumed. In addition, women should be counseled to avoid intercourse until symptoms cease, and to then use condoms until they complete their treatment. Women should be instructed to refrain from douching, both in general and during treatment. Clinicians should also emphasize general hygiene measures including wearing cotton underwear and loose clothing, not wearing underwear while sleeping, wiping from front to back after urination, and not using feminine deodorants or hygiene sprays.

VULVOVAGINAL CANDIDIASIS

Vulvovaginal candidiasis or yeast infection accounts for 20% to 25% of all vaginal infections and is the second most common type of vaginal infection in the United States. It is estimated that three-fourths of all women will have at least one episode of VVC in their lifetimes, and 40% to 45% will have two or more episodes (CDC, 2002; Klebanoff et al., 2001). It is difficult to determine the actual incidence of VVC as it is not a reportable condition and the recent availability of over-the-counter (OTC) treatments prevents many cases from being seen by health care providers (Scharbo-DeHaan & Anderson, 2003). Most (80% to 90%) women who have VVC will have uncomplicated VVC (Table 17–4).

The most common cause of VVC is *Candida albicans.* It is estimated that 80–95% of yeast infections in women are caused by this organism. However, in the past 10 years, the incidence of non-albicans infections has risen steadily. Non-albicans species include *Candida tropicalis, Candida glabrata, Candida parapsilosis,* and *Candida krusei* (Hawkins et al., 2004). Women with recurrent infections—defined as four or more clinically proven infections in one year (CDC, 2002)—often are infected with a higher percentage of non-albicans species than are women who are experiencing their first infection or who have few recurrences.

TABLE 17-4   Classification of Vulvovaginal Candidiasis (VVC)

Uncomplicated VVC	Complicated VVC	Recurrent VVC
Sporadic or infrequent VVC	Recurrent VVC	4 or more episodes in symptomatic VVC in 1 year
Mild to moderate VVC	Severe VVC	
Likely to be *C. albicans*	Non-albicans candidiasis	Predisposing factors: diabetes, immunosuppression, corticosteroid use, commercial perineal hygiene or vaginal douche products use, greater number of lifetime sexual partners
Nonimmunocompromised women	Women with uncontrolled diabetes, debilitation, immunosuppression, or who are pregnant	

Sources: CDC, 2002; Scharbo-DeHaan & Anderson, 2003; Sinclair, 2004.

Numerous factors have been identified as predisposing a woman to yeast infections including the following:

- Repeated courses of systemic or topical antibiotic therapy, particularly broad-spectrum antibiotics such as ampicillin, tetracycline, cephalosporins, and metronidazole
- Diabetes, especially when uncontrolled
- Pregnancy
- Obesity
- Diets high in refined sugars or artificial sweeteners
- Use of corticosteroids and exogenous hormones
- Immunosuppressed states, including HIV seropositivity
- Local allergic or hypersensitivity reactions

Clinical observations and research have suggested that tight fitting clothing and underwear or pantyhose made of nonabsorbent materials create an environment in which vaginal fungus can grow.

The most common symptom of yeast infections is vulvar and possibly vaginal pruritis (Table 17–1). The itching may be mild or intense, interfere with rest and activities, and occur during or after intercourse. Some women report a feeling of dryness. Others may experience painful urination as the urine flows over the vulva; this usually occurs in women who have excoriation resulting from scratching. Most often the discharge is thick, white, lumpy, and cottage cheeselike. Often the discharge is found in patches on the vaginal walls, cervix, and labia. The vulva is commonly red and swollen as are the labial folds, vagina, and cervix. Although there is not a characteristic odor with yeast infections, sometimes a yeasty or musty smell occurs. Although vaginal candidiasis infections are common in healthy women, those seen in women with HIV infection are often more severe and persistent. Genital candidiasis lesions may be painful, coalescing ulcerations necessitating continuous, prophylactic therapy.

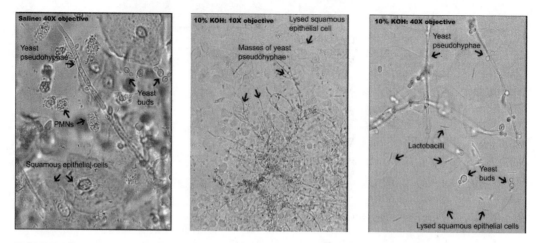

FIGURE 17–2   Wet Mount Findings with Vulvovaginal Candidiasis. PMNs = polymorphonuclear leukocytes/white blood cells. *Source:* Used with permission from Washington State Department of Health STD/TB Program, Seattle STD/HIV Prevention Training Center, and Cindy Fennell, MS, MT, ASCP.

ASSESSMENT

In addition to obtaining a careful record of the woman's symptoms (their onset and course), the patient history is a valuable screening tool for identifying predisposing risk factors. Physical examination should include a thorough inspection of the vulva and vagina. A speculum examination, saline and KOH wet smears, and vaginal pH are performed. Vaginal pH is normal with a yeast infection. If the pH is >4.5, one should suspect trichomoniasis or BV. The characteristic pseudohyphae may be seen on a wet smear done with normal saline; however, they may be confused with other cells and artifacts. Pseudohyphae are best seen on the KOH wet smear (Figure 17–2). Fasting plasma glucose and oral glucose tolerance (measurement two hours after 75 g of oral glucose) testing should be considered for women with recurrent infections. Testing for chlamydia, gonorrhea, and HIV should be done if the patient history indicates risk factors for STIs (see Chapter 18). Cultures for yeast should be obtained in recurrent or resistant cases to confirm the diagnosis and identify unusual species, and with suspected candidiasis when the KOH prep is negative (CDC, 2002).

DIFFERENTIAL DIAGNOSIS

The differential diagnosis for VVC includes BV, trichomoniasis, chemical vaginitis, contact vaginitis, chlamydia, gonorrhea, genital herpes, and normal physiologic discharge. Clinicians should also consider candidiasis secondary to diabetes, pregnancy, HIV seropositivity, and non-albicans species such as *Candida glabrata* or *Candida tropicalis* (Hawkins et al., 2004).

MANAGEMENT

A number of antifungal preparations are available for the treatment of VVC (Table 17–1), and no single brand is significantly more effective than another. Women must be counseled that the creams and suppositories recommended for treatment of VVC are oil based and may weaken latex condoms and diaphragms. Many of the effective topical azole drugs (e.g., Monistat and Gyne-Lotrimin) are available OTC. Self-treatment with OTC medications should be used only by women who have been previously diagnosed with VVC and who are experiencing the same symptoms. Any woman whose symptoms persist or who has a recurrence of symptoms within two months of treatment should seek medical care (CDC, 2002). Unnecessary or inappropriate use of OTC preparations is common and can lead to delays in treating other causes of vulvovaginitis. If vaginal discharge is extremely thick and copious, vaginal debridement with a cotton swab followed by application of vaginal medication may be useful. Alternative therapies for VVC can be found in Table 17–3. Women who have extensive irritation, swelling, and discomfort of the labia and vulva may find sitz baths helpful in decreasing inflammation and increasing comfort. Adding Aveeno powder to the bath may also increase the woman's comfort.

SPECIAL CONSIDERATIONS

Pregnant Women Pregnant women who suspect they have candidiasis should be counseled not to self-treat their infection and to contact their health care provider. Oral medication for VVC is not recommended in pregnancy. Only topical azole therapies, applied for seven days, are recommended for use among pregnant women (CDC, 2002).

Talking with the Patient Bathing daily with lots of water and minimal soap may help prevent recurrent infections. Additional measures to minimize the moist environment of the vagina and thus prevent recurrences include: not wearing underwear to bed, wearing loose-fitting slacks and jeans, and wearing cotton-crotched underwear or pantyhose. Completing the full course of treatment prescribed is essential to removing the pathogen, and women are instructed to continue medication even during menstruation. Women should be counseled not to use tampons as they will absorb the medication. If possible, intercourse should be avoided during treatment; if this is not feasible, the woman's partner should use a condom to prevent the introduction of more organisms. Women should be counseled to avoid feminine hygiene sprays, deodorants, scented tampons or pads, perfumed or colored toilet paper, and fabric softeners—all of which may cause irritation and allergies. Vitamin C, oral acidophilous, or live culture yogurt taken to increase vaginal acidity may also be helpful (Hawkins et al., 2004).

TOXIC SHOCK SYNDROME

Toxic shock syndrome (TSS) is sepsis caused by a *Staphylococcus aureus* infection that originates in the reproductive tract, most often during menses associated with tampon use that is usually within five days of symptom onset (Shannon, 2004; Sinclair, 2004). Toxic shock syndrome is rarely associated with diaphragm use, contraceptive sponge use, or postabortion or postpartum endometritis. Because the occurrence of TSS is unknown (Brown, 2004), in cases involving menstruation 99% are associated with tampon use. Symptoms include a temperature greater than 102°F (38.8°C), headache, erythematous rash with desquamation two to three weeks later, myalgia, nausea, vomiting, profuse watery discharge, dizziness, syncope, and hypotension that develops into shock (CDC, 1980; Shannon).

ASSESSMENT

In addition to a careful history of the woman's symptoms, their onset, and course, the history is a valuable screening tool for identifying predisposing risk factors such as menses with tampon use (usually within five days of onset of symptoms), history of TSS, and history of recent surgery, wound, or nasal packing (Shannon, 2004). Upon physical examination, dermatologic findings may differ depending on the stage of the illness. Early signs may include generalized erythematous and macular rash; generalized, nonpitting edema; and erythema of palms and soles. After the acute phase, findings may include generalized maculopapular rash and desquamation of fingers, palms, toes, and soles. Pelvic examination may reveal vaginal erythema or ulcerations, blood, or a tampon in the vaginal vault. The diagnosis of TSS is made on the basis of clinical manifestations meeting the 1980 CDC case definition (Table 17–5). Although there are no specific laboratory tests to con-

TABLE 17–5   CDC Case Definition for Toxic Shock Syndrome

CDC criteria used for diagnosing toxic shock syndrome

1. Fever: temperature >38.9°C (102°F)
2. Rash: diffuse macular erythroderma
3. Desquamation: 1–2 weeks after the onset of the initial rash, especially involving the palms and soles
4. Hypotension: systolic blood pressure <90 mm Hg for adults or <5th percentile by age for children, or orthostatic syncope
5. Involvement of three or more of the following symptoms:
   - Gastrointestinal system: vomiting or diarrhea at onset of symptoms
   - Musculoskeletal system: severe myalgia or creatinine kinase >2 times normal level
   - Mucous membranes: vaginal, oropharyngeal, conjunctival hyperemia
   - Renal system: serum blood urea nitrogen (BUN) or creatinine ≥2 times normal levels or 5 white blood cells per high-powered field on microscopic urinalysis in the absence of a urinary tract infection
   - Hepatic system: bilirubin or transaminase >2 times normal levels
   - Hematologic system: platelets <100,000/mmm3
   - CNS system: disorientation or altered consciousness without focal neurologic signs when a fever and neurologic signs are absent
6. Negative results for the following tests (if obtained):
   - Culture of blood, throat, cerebrospinal fluid
   - Serology for Rocky Mountain spotted fever, leptospirosis, or measles

Source: CDC, 1980.

firm a diagnosis, various studies will provide information on the patient's status and possible invading organism. Clinicians should obtain a complete blood count (CBC) with differential, bacterial culture of the cervix and vagina, serum chemistry panel, and serum antibody testing for TSS toxin-1 (Brown, 2004; Shannon; Sinclair, 2004).

DIFFERENTIAL DIAGNOSIS

Differential diagnosis should include Rocky Mountain Spotted Fever, leptospirosis, measles, and shock from another origin (Brown, 2004; Sinclair, 2004).

MANAGEMENT

All women with a suspected case of TSS should be referred to a physician. Hospitalization is often necessary. After hospitalization, close monitoring is required for symptom resolution. All menstruating women and others at risk for TSS should be educated about the signs and symptoms of TSS and ways to prevent its occurrence, such as using low-absorbency tampons, changing tampons frequently, and removing barrier contraception within 24 hours. Women who have had TSS should be instructed not to use barrier methods of birth control or tampons.

BARTHOLIN'S CYST OR ABSCESS

The Bartholin's glands are two mucous-secreting, nonpalpable glandular structures with duct openings within the posterolateral vulvar vestibule that provide minimal lubrication. Occlusion of a duct with mucus retention results in a nontender mass approximately 1 to 4 cm (and up to 10 cm) in size. Occlusion occurs from congenital stenosis or atresia, thickened mucus at the outlet, mechanical trauma, or neoplasm (suspected when cyst formation occurs in women older than the age of 40 years). Abscess formation occurs when the cystic fluid becomes infected. Originally it was thought that gonorrhea was the primary cause of Bartholin's abscess; however, further research has documented a number of causative organisms including *E. coli*, *Bacteroides*, *Proteus*, and *Peptostreptococcus* (Star & Appelmans, 2004).

Most women with a Bartholin's cyst are asymptomatic. An abscess usually develops rapidly over a two- to three-day period and may spontaneously rupture within 72 hours. Symptoms include varying amounts of pain or tenderness, difficulty sitting or walking, and dyspareunia. Extensive inflammation may cause systemic symptoms.

ASSESSMENT

A Bartholin's cyst may be an incidental finding during a routine pelvic examination. The cyst appears as a visible round or oval mass causing a crescent-shaped vestibular entrance. It is nontender but tense, and there is palpable swelling that is usually unilateral and without erythema or inflammation. A Bartholin's abscess is a very tender, edematous fluctuant mass with erythema of the overlying skin. Labial edema and distortion are observed on the affected area. Size of the area affected is rarely greater than 5 cm. An area of softening or "pointing" suggests an impending rupture. Cultures of purulent abscess fluid and of the cervix for *N. gonorrhoeae* and *C. trachomatis* should be obtained to rule out an STI. A CBC should be obtained when extensive inflammation exists (Sinclair, 2004).

DIFFERENTIAL DIAGNOSIS

Differential diagnoses include cyst versus abscess, neoplasm, STI, or sebaceous cyst.

MANAGEMENT

Small asymptomatic cysts do not require treatment. Treatment is indicated when there is rapid cyst enlargement; increased pain, pressure, or introital obstruction; hemorrhage into the cyst cavity; and abscess formation. The aim of treatment for a cyst or abscess is to create a fistulous tract from the dilated duct to the vestibule by incision and drainage (I&D) or marsupialization (Star & Appelmans, 2004). Referral for I&D should be made if the provider is not experienced with the procedure. Referral is indicated for marsupialization, recurrent cyst or abscess formation, or for women over 40 years of age to rule out neoplasm. Broad-spectrum antibiotics (Cephalexin 500 mg orally four times a day for 7–14 days, or Amoxicillin 500 mg/clavulanic acid 125 mg, 1 tablet orally twice a day for 7–14 days) may provide initial symptomatic relief, prevent additional soft-tissue involvement, and delay ripening or pointing of the abscess. Star and Appelmans note that an acute abscess treated only with sitz bath may spontaneously rupture within 72 hours but often recurs.

REFERENCES

Ayres, T. (2004). Sexual dysfunction. In W. Star, L. Lommel, & M. Shannon (Eds.), *Women's primary health care* (2nd ed., 12-132–12-134). San Francisco: UCSF Nursing Press.

Balch, J. F., & Balch, P. A. (1997). *Prescription for prevention* (2nd ed.). Garden City Park, NY: Avery.

Brown, K. (2004). *Management guidelines for women's health nurse practitioners* (2nd ed.). Philadelphia: F. A. Davis.

Calzolari, E., Masciangelo, R., Milite, V., & Vertaramo, R. (2000). Bacterial vaginosis and contraceptive methods. *International Journal of Gynecology and Obstetrics, 70,* 341–346.

Centers for Disease Control and Prevention. (1980). Toxic-shock syndrome—United States. *Morbidity and Mortality Weekly Report, 29,* 227–229.

Centers for Disease Control and Prevention. (2002). Sexually transmitted diseases treatment guidelines 2002. *Morbidity and Mortality Weekly Report, 51*(RR-6), 1–80.

Fethers, K., Marks, C., Mindel, A., & Estcourt, C. S. (2000). Sexually transmitted infections and risk behaviors in women who have sex with women. *Sexually Transmitted Infections, 76,* 345–349.

Hatcher, R. A., Trussell, J., Stewart, F., Cates, W., Stewart, G. K., Guest, F., et al. (1998). *Contraceptive technology* (17th ed.). New York: Ardent Media.

Hawkins, J. W., Roberto-Nichols, D. M., & Stanley-Haney, J. L. (2004). *Guidelines for nurse practitioners in gynecologic settings* (8th ed.). New York: Springer.

Hudson, T. (1999). *Women's encyclopedia of natural medicine.* Los Angeles: Keats.

Klebanoff, M. A., Carey, J. C., Hauth, J. C., Hillier, S. L., Nugent, R. P., Thom, E. A., et al. (2001). Failure of metronidazole to prevent preterm delivery among pregnant women with asymptomatic *tri-*

chomonas vaginalis infection. *New England Journal of Medicine, 345,* 487–493.

Koumans, E. H., Markowitz, L. E., & Hogan, V. (2002). Indications for therapy and treatment recommendations for bacterial vaginosis in nonpregnant and pregnant women: A synthesis of data. *Clinical Infectious Diseases, 35,* S152–S172.

Low Dog, T. (2004). *Women's health in complementary and alternative medicine.* St. Louis, MO: Elsevier.

McCaffrey, M., Varney, P., Evans, B., & Taylor-Robinson, D. (1999). Bacterial vaginosis in lesbians: Evidence for lack of sexual transmission. *International Journal of STD & AIDS, 10,* 305–308.

Schaffer, S. D. (2003). Vaginitis and sexually transmitted diseases. In E. Q. Youngkin & M. S. Davis (Eds.), *Women's health: A primary care clinical guide* (3rd ed., pp. 261–290). Upper Saddle River, NJ: Pearson Prentice Hall.

Scharbo-DeHaan, M., & Anderson, D. G. (2003). The CDC 2002 guidelines for the treatment of sexually transmitted diseases: Implications for women's health care. *Journal of Midwifery & Women's Health, 48,* 96–104.

Shaley, E., Battino, S., Weiner, E., Colodner, R., & Keness, Y. (1996). Ingestion of yogurt containing *Lactobacillus acidosis* compared with pasteurized yogurt as prophylaxis for recurrent candidal vaginitis and bacterial vaginosis. *Archives of Family Medicine, 5,* 593–596.

Shannon, M. (2004). Toxic shock syndrome. In W. Star, L. Lommel, & M. Shannon (Eds.), *Women's primary health care* (2nd ed., pp. 12–147 to 12–150). San Francisco: UCSF Nursing Press.

Sinclair, C. (2004). *A midwife's handbook.* St. Louis, MO: Saunders.

Star, W. L., & Appelmans, C. L. (2004). Large lesions of the vulva. In W. Star, L. Lommel, & M. Shannon (Eds.), *Women's primary health care* (2nd ed., pp. 12–211–12–215). San Francisco: UCSF Nursing Press.

Taha, T. E., Hoover, D. R., & Dallabetta, G. A. (1998). Bacterial vaginosis and disturbances of vaginal flora: Association with increased acquisition of HIV. *AIDS, 12,* 1699–1706.

Chapter 18

SEXUALLY TRANSMITTED INFECTIONS

CATHERINE INGRAM FOGEL

Healthy sexual relations and reproductive experiences should be free of infection (Hatcher et al., 2004). Unfortunately, sexual activity can result in sexually transmitted infections (STIs). STIs are a "hidden epidemic of tremendous health and economic consequences in the United States" and represent a "growing threat to the Nation's health" (Institute of Medicine, 1997, p. 28). Despite more than 20 years of the US Surgeon General targeting STIs as a priority for prevention and control efforts (Public Health Service, 1979), these infections continue to be among the most common health problems in the United States today. STIs affect approximately 15 million Americans every year (Cates, Alexander, & Cates, 1998). At the current rate at least one in four—and possibly as many as one in two—Americans will contract an STI during their lifetime (Gonen, 1999). In some regions of the United States, notably the Southeast, rates exceed those of some developing countries. STIs are a direct cause of tremendous human suffering, place heavy demands on health care services, and cost up to $8.4 billion dollars a year to treat (Cates et al.).

An STI is not any one specific disease; rather, the term includes more than 25 infectious organisms that are transmitted through sexual activity and dozens of clinical syndromes that they cause (Schmid, 2001). Common STIs are found in Table 18–1. These terms have replaced the older designation, venereal disease, which primarily described gonorrhea and syphilis. STIs may be caused by a wide spectrum of bacteria, viruses, protozoa, and ectoparasites (organisms that live on the outside of the body such as a louse). Historically, many STIs were considered to be symptomatic illnesses usually afflicting men; however, women and children have more severe symptoms and sequelae from these infections than men.

Preventing, identifying, and managing STIs are essential components of women's health care. Clinicians can assume an essential role in promoting women's reproductive and sexual health by counseling women about the risks of STIs and human immunodeficiency

TABLE 18–1 Common Sexually Transmitted Infections

Infection	Causative Organism
Chancroid	*Haemophilus ducreyi*
Chlamydia	*Chlamydia trachomatis*
Genital herpes	Herpes simplex virus
Genital warts	Human papillomavirus (HPV)
Gonorrhea	*Neisseria gonorrhoeae*
Hepatitis	Hepatitis B virus (HBV), Hepatitis C virus (HCV)
HIV infection and acquired immunodeficiency syndrome (AIDS)	Human immunodeficiency virus (HIV)
Molluscum contagiosum	Molluscum contagiosum virus
Pubic lice	*Phthirus pubis*
Syphilis	*Treponema pallidum*
Trichomoniasis	*Trichomonas vaginalis*

virus (HIV), encouraging sexual and other risk-reduction measures, incorporating education regarding HIV and STI prevention in their practice, and by being familiar with assessment and management strategies. In doing so, clinicians can assist women in avoiding STIs and in living better with the sequelae and chronic infections of STIs.

This chapter begins with an overview of STI transmission, screening, and detection. Topics that need to be addressed when talking with a woman diagnosed with an STI are presented. The remaining sections address specific STIs, including human papillomavirus, genital herpes simplex virus infection, chancroid, pediculosis, trichomoniasis, chlamydia, gonorrhea, pelvic inflammatory disease (PID), syphilis, hepatitis B virus (HBV), and HIV infection.

TRANSMISSION OF STIs

The chance of contracting, transmitting, or suffering complications from HIV and STIs depends on multiple biologic, behavioral, social, and relationship risk factors (Table 18–2). Microbiologic, hormonal, and immunologic factors influence individual susceptibility and transmission potential for STIs. These factors are partially influenced by a woman's sexual practices, substance use, and other health behaviors. Health behaviors, in turn, are influenced by socioeconomic factors and other social influences.

BIOLOGIC FACTORS

Women are biologically more likely to become infected with STIs than men. For example, the risk of a woman contracting gonorrhea from a single act of intercourse is 60% to 90% while the risk for a man is 20% to 30%. Further, men are two to three times more

TABLE 18-2   Risk Factors for STIs And HIV

Individuals who are at increased risk for STIs and HIV include:

- Those who are or were recently sexually active, especially persons with multiple sexual partners
- Those who use alcohol or illicit drugs
- Gay or bisexual men who have sex with other men
- Persons with a previous history of a documented STI/HIV infection and/or a previous history in their sexual contacts
- Persons involved in the exchange of sex for drugs or money
- Persons living in areas where the prevalence of HIV infection and STIs is high
- Health care workers, particularly those who experience a needle stick or are exposed to contaminated body fluids
- Victims of abuse
- Persons with tattoos/pierced body parts
- Those practicing anal sex
- Individuals at the initiation of sexual activity

Sources: CDC, 2002a; Institute of Medicine, 1997; Schmid, 2001.

likely to transmit HIV to women than the reverse. The vagina has a larger amount of genital mucous membranes exposed and is an environment more conducive for infections than the penis (Cates et al., 1998). Further, risk for trauma is greater during vaginal intercourse for women than for men (Kurth, 1998). The cervix, particularly the squamocolumnar junction or transformation zone and the endocervical columnar epithelial cells, are most susceptible to HIV; however, the virus can invade the vaginal epithelium as well (Futterman, 2001).

More than 50% of bacterial STIs and 90% of viral STIs are asymptomatic in women and thus likely to be undetected. Additionally, when or if symptoms develop, they are often confused with those of other diseases not transmitted sexually. The frequency of asymptomatic and unrecognized infections results in delayed diagnosis and treatment, chronic untreated infections, and complications. Further, it is more difficult to diagnose STIs in a woman because the anatomy of her genital tract makes clinical examination more difficult. For example, to diagnose gonorrhea in men all that is needed is a urethral swab and Gram stain; yet in women, a speculum examination and specific cervical culture are necessary. Lesions that occur inside the vagina and on the cervix are not readily visible, and the normal vaginal environment (warm, moist, enriched medium) is ideal for infection.

Some infections occur more commonly in young persons, whose lack of immunity and biologic susceptibility are contributing factors. Age and gender influence an individual's risk for an STI. Specifically, young women (ages 20–24 years) and female adolescents (ages 10–19 years) are more susceptible than their male counterparts. Eighty percent of all adolescent girls are sexually active by the age of 18 years with the end result being many young women at risk for STIs (Alan Guttmacher Institute, 1999). The earlier a woman begins to have sexual intercourse, the longer her period of sexual activity is, the greater her number of partners, and the less apt she is to use barrier contraception (Schmid, 2001). Compared to older women prior to menopause, female adolescents and young women are more susceptible to cervical infections, such as chlamydial infections, gonorrhea, and HIV because of the ectropion of the immature cervix and resulting larger exposed surface area of cells unprotected by cervical mucus. The cells eventually recede into the inner cervix as women age. Postmenopausal women also are at increased risk because of thin vaginal and cervical mucosa. Further, women who are pregnant have higher rates of cervical ectropion (Cunningham et al., 2002). Both younger and postmenopausal women are at greater risk for acquiring HIV because of a thinner vaginal epithelium and resulting increased friability, thus providing direct access to the bloodstream (Kurth, 1998).

Other biologic factors that may increase risk for acquiring, transmitting, or developing complications of certain STIs include vaginal douching, risky sexual practices, use of hormonal contraceptives, and bacterial vaginosis. Risk for contracting the infections that can lead to PID may be increased with vaginal douching, and risk for PID may also increase with greater frequency of douching (Centers for Disease Control and Prevention [CDC], 2002a). Certain sexual practices such as anal intercourse, sex during menses, and insertive vaginal sex without sufficient lubrication (dry sex) may predispose a woman to acquiring an STI. This may be because the bleeding and tissue trauma that can result from these practices facilitates invasion by pathogens. The role of oral contraceptives in the acquisition and transmission of STIs is not fully understood. Several studies have found oral contraceptives to be associated with a decreased risk (10% to 70%) of developing PID (Dickey, 2000). Cervical ectopy is positively associated with use of oral contraceptives and with chlamydial infections. A meta-analysis of studies on the effects of oral contraceptives on HIV susceptibility reported that the use of oral contraceptives may be associated with a small increased risk of HIV infection (Wang & Celum, 2001). Normal vaginal flora may confer nonspecific immunity, and recent data suggest that women with bacterial vaginosis are at increased risk for HIV seroconversion (Wang & Celum).

SOCIAL FACTORS

Preventing the spread of STIs and HIV is difficult without addressing community and individual issues that have a tremendous influence on prevention, transmission, and treatment of these infections. Societal factors such as poverty, lack of education, social inequity, and inadequate access to health care indirectly increase the prevalence of STIs and HIV in at-risk populations.

Persons with the highest rates of many STIs are often those with the least access to health care, and health insurance coverage influences if and where a woman obtains STI services and preventive services. Further, even if a woman of lower socioeconomic status perceives herself to be at risk for an STI, she may not practice protective behaviors if survival is an overarching concern, or if there are other risks that appear to be more threatening or imminent (Mays & Cochran, 1988). The need to secure shelter, food, clothing, money, and safety for herself and her children may override any concerns about preventive health and thus prevent her from changing risky behaviors (Nyamanthi & Lewis, 1991; Stevens et al., 1995).

SOCIAL INTERACTIONS AND RELATIONSHIPS

STIs are the only illnesses whose spread is directly caused by the human urge to share sexual intimacy and reproduce. Sexual behavior within the context of relationships is a critical risk factor for preventing and acquiring STIs, because intimate human contact is the common vehicle of transmission. The gender-power imbalance and cultural proscriptions often associated with sexual relationships make it difficult for women to protect themselves from infection (Miller, Exner, Williams, & Ehrhardt, 2000; Mize, Robinson, Bockting, & Scheltma, 2002). Women may have less say than men over when and under what circumstances intercourse occurs. Young women are particularly at risk as they may have sex with older men, and because of the difference in power within the relationship. These young women may lack the negotiating skills, self-efficacy, and self-confidence needed to successfully negotiate for safer sex practices. Lifestyles of premarital, intermarital, and extramarital sexual activity are common for many women; yet because of the secrecy and cultural proscriptions surrounding such activities, women often engage in them without preparation, leading to risk for themselves and their partners.

Women may be dependent upon an abusive male partner or a partner who places a woman at risk by his own risky behaviors (Kurth, 1998). The risk of acquiring STIs or HIV infection is high among women who are physically and sexually abused. Past and current experiences with violence, particularly sexual abuse, erode women's sense of self-efficacy to exercise control over sexual behaviors, engender feelings of anxiety and depression, and increase the likelihood of risky sexual behaviors (Maman, 2000). Additionally, fear of physical harm and loss of economic support hamper women's efforts to enact protective practices. Further, past and current abuse is strongly associated with substance abuse, which also increases the risk of contracting an STI.

Risk of acquiring an STI is determined not only by the woman's actions but by her partner's as well. Although prevention counseling customarily includes recommending that women identify any partner who is at high risk and the nature of their sexual practices, this advice may be unrealistic or culturally inappropriate in many relationships because of drugs and medical factors. Women who engage in sexual activities only with other women may also be at risk for infection. Many women who identify themselves as lesbians have had intercourse with a man by choice, by force, or by necessity. Their female partners may also have had intercourse with a man. In addition, some lesbians may use drugs and share needles, may have received blood transfusions, or may be artificially inseminated.

SOCIETAL NORMS

Relationships and sexual behavior are regulated by cultural norms that influence sexual expression in interpersonal relationships. Women are still socialized to please their partners and to place men's needs and desires first and may find it difficult to insist on safer sex behaviors. Traditional cultural values associated with passivity and subordination may diminish the ability of many women to adequately protect themselves.

Power imbalances in relationships are the product of and contribute to the maintenance of traditional gender roles that identify men as the initiators and decision makers of sexual activities and women as passive gatekeepers (Miller et al., 2000). As long as traditional gender norms define the roles in sexual relationships as men having the dominant role in sexual decision making, negotiating condom use by women will remain difficult. Additionally, cultural norms define talking about condoms as implying a lack of trust that runs counter to the traditional gender norm expectations for women (Maman, 2000). Women often do not request condom use because of a need to establish and maintain intimacy with partners. Research has demonstrated that women at risk for HIV place significant importance on and investment in their heterosexual relationships, and that these dynamics impact on the women's risk taking and risk management (MacRae & Aalto, 2000). Urging women to insist on condom use may be unrealistic, because traditional gender roles do not encourage women to talk about sex, initiate sexual practices, or control intimate encounters.

SUBSTANCE USE

The use of alcohol and drugs is associated with increased risk of HIV and STIs. For example, in many areas crack use has paralleled trends in syphilis, gonorrhea, chancroid, and HIV infection. There are several possible reasons for this association, including social factors such as poverty and lack of educational or economic opportunities, and individual factors such as taking risks and low self-efficacy. In addition to the risk from needle sharing, use of drugs and alcohol may contribute to risk of HIV infection by undermining cognitive and social skills, thus making it more difficult to engage in HIV-protective actions (Harris & Kavanagh, 1995). Further, depression and other psychological problems or a history of sexual abuse are associated with substance abuse and thus contribute to risky behaviors. Being high and unable to clean drug paraphernalia can be a pervasive barrier to protective practice. Further, drug use may take place in settings where persons participate in sexual activities while using drugs. Cocaine abusers have demonstrated higher levels of sexual risk behaviors than other addict populations (McCoy, McCoy, & Lai, 1998). Finally, women who use drugs may be at higher risk because they may exchange sex for drugs or money, and may have higher numbers of sexual partners and encounters (Dolcini, Coates, Catania, Kegeles, & Hauck, 1995).

Past and current physical, emotional, and sexual abuse characterize the lives of many, if not most, women using drugs (Kearney, 2001; McFarlane, Parker, & Cross, 2001). For women who have experienced violence, use of alcohol and drugs can become a coping mechanism by which they self-medicate to relieve feelings of anxiety, guilt, fear, and anger stemming from the violence (Grella, Anglin, & Annon, 1996). Women's drug use is strongly linked to relationship inequities and the ability of some men to mandate women's sexual behavior. Sexual degradation of women is described as an intimate part of crack cocaine use (Henderson, 1997).

STI SCREENING AND DETECTION

Prompt diagnosis and treatment are predicated on the assumption that any person who believes he or she may have contracted an STI, has symptoms of an STI, has had sexual relations with someone who has symptoms of an STI, or has a partner who has been diagnosed with an STI will seek care. To obtain prompt diagnosis and treatment, patients must know how to recognize the major signs and symptoms of all STIs and must obtain health care if they experience symptoms or have sexual contact with someone who has an STI. Clinicians have the responsibility of educating their patients regarding the signs and symptoms of STIs. This may be done when a woman comes in for her annual health examination, seeks contraception, obtains preconceptual care, or comes to her clinician for prenatal care. Clinicians also must ensure that patients know where and how to obtain care if they suspect they might have contracted an STI. Many local health departments have clinics specifically designed to treat STIs, and often free treatment can be obtained at local emergency departments.

SCREENING

All women who are sexually active should be screened regularly through history, physical examination, and laboratory studies. To identify those at risk, specific questions should be asked during the collection of a health history (Tables 18–3 and 18–4). Risk assessment depends on a woman's willingness to self-identify risk factors that may be seen as socially unacceptable or stigmatizing. It is possible that women may not reveal such risk factors directly to health care providers, but will do so if asked to fill out a questionnaire using questions similar to those given in the Sexual Risk History (Table 18–3). Current recommendations (CDC, 2001b; CDC, 2002a) are that all women 25 years of age and younger should be screened at least yearly for STIs. After the age of 25 years, the timing of screening is dependent on risk factors present and whether or not the woman is pregnant. All pregnant women must be screened for gonorrhea, syphilis, chlamydia, and HBV. In addition, all pregnant women should be counseled regarding the need to be tested for HIV infection. Any woman who has been diagnosed with an STI should be screened for other STIs, because many of these infections (e.g., chlamydia, gonorrhea, syphilis, hepatitis B) can be asymptomatic.

ASSESSMENT

The diagnosis of an STI is based on the integration of relevant history, physical, and laboratory data. A history that is accurate, comprehensive, and specific is essential for accurate diagnosis. Generally the history should be taken first, with the woman dressed. Information should be collected in a nonjudgmental manner, avoiding assumptions of sexual preference. All partners should be referred to as partners and not by gender. It is helpful to

TABLE 18–3 Sexual Risk History

Risk Screening

- Are you sexually active? Have you had sex/intercourse with anyone in the past six months/year?
- If no, ask, "Have you had intercourse in the past?"
- If yes, ask,

  "Have your partners been men, women, or both?"
  - With how many different people: _____ 1 _____ 2–3 _____ 4–10 _____ >10
  - How many different people are you having sex with right now?
  - Does your partner have any other partners that you know of?
  - Have you ever had sex with someone who had been in jail?
  - Have you ever had sex with someone who has had a blood transfusion or hemophilia?
  - Have you ever had sex with someone whom you were afraid put you at risk for HIV/STI?
    - Someone who had a positive AIDS test?
    - Someone you think might have AIDS?
    - Someone who uses drugs? IV drugs? Cocaine?
    - A partner(s) who might have had sex with a prostitute or with both men and women?
    - Have you ever been told that you had an STI?
      - _____ Never
      - _____ Chlamydia
      - _____ Gonorrhea
      - _____ Trichomoniasis
      - _____ Syphilis
      - _____ Other (list): _____
- Have you ever been told that you had a pelvic infection or PID?
- Many women have sex when they have drunk too much alcohol or have been using drugs. Has this happened to you?
  - What kinds of drugs do you use?
    - _____ Opioids: types _____ Route of administration _____ Frequency _____
    - _____ Stimulants: types _____ Route of administration _____ Frequency _____
    - _____ Crack cocaine? Frequency _____ Have you had sex in a crack house?
    - _____ Alcohol: types: _____ Frequency _____
- Have you ever blacked out from alcohol or drugs, especially during sex?
- Have you ever traded sex for drugs, money, food, housing, or anything else?
- Do you ever have sex when you are high?

TABLE 18–3   continued

Risk Screening

- Can you tell me the kinds of sex that you have? This will help determine what your risks are.

  Yes/No

mouth on penis or vulva	protected _____	unprotected _____
penis in vagina	protected _____	unprotected _____
penis in the rectum	protected _____	unprotected _____
mouth on anus	protected _____	unprotected _____

For every sexually active woman, ask:

- Are you worried about catching a sexually transmitted infection or HIV (the AIDS virus)?
- Do you do anything to prevent catching an infection?
- Have you had sex without a condom?
- When did you start using condoms?
- Have you performed oral sex on a man or woman without a barrier (dental dam, Saran wrap, condom)?

Sources: Brown, 2004; Carcio, 1999; Fogel, 1995; Fogel & Lauver, 1990; Kurth, 1998; MacLauren, 1995; Starr, Lommel, & Shannon, 2004.

TABLE 18–4   Menstrual/Gynecologic History Questions to Assess Risk of STIs

Do you experience now or have you ever experienced:

- Frequent vaginal infections
- Unusual vaginal discharge/odor
- Vaginal itching/burning/sores/warts
- Sexually transmitted infections (ask about individual diseases)
- Abdominal pain
- Pelvic inflammatory disease/infection of the uterus, tubes, ovaries
- Rape
- Physical, emotional, sexual abuse
- Abnormal Pap smear
- Pain/bleeding with intercourse
- Severe menstrual cramps occurring at end of period
- Ectopic pregnancy

begin with open-ended questions that often elicit information that might otherwise be missed. These can be followed with symptom-specific questions and relevant history. Specific areas to address include the reason why the woman has sought care and any symptoms she has noticed; a sexual history, including a description of the date and type of sexual activity; number of partners; whether or not she has had contact with someone who recently had an STI; and potential sites of infection (mouth, cervix, urethra, rectum). Pertinent medical history includes anything that will influence the management plan, such as history of drug allergies, previously diagnosed chronic illnesses, and general health status. A menstrual history, including the date of the woman's last menstrual period, must always be obtained so that pregnancy may be ruled out because certain medications used to treat STIs are contraindicated in pregnancy. When indicated, an HIV-oriented systems review should be conducted. Any positive answers regarding symptoms should be followed up to elicit information about onset, duration, and specific characteristics, such as color, amount, and consistency of discharge.

Before the actual physical examination is performed, the clinician should discuss the examination with the woman so that she is prepared. The physical examination begins with careful visualization of the external genitalia, including the perineum. Erythema, edema, distortions, lesions, or trauma from scratching, sexual activity, sports activity, or injury are noted. Palpation can locate areas of tenderness. During the speculum examination, the vagina and cervix are inspected for edema, thinning, lesions, abnormal coloration, trauma, discharge, and bleeding. Thorough palpation of inguinal area and pelvic organs, milking of the urethra for discharge, and assessment of vaginal secretion odors are essential. Lesions should be evaluated and cervical specimens obtained when appropriate. Appropriate laboratory studies will be suggested, in part, by the history and physical examination results. Additional laboratory studies may be done because women are often infected with more than one STI simultaneously and because many are asymptomatic. These include Pap tests, wet mounts, chlamydia and gonorrhea testing, Venereal Disease Research Laboratory (VDRL) or rapid plasma reagent (RPR) testing for syphilis, and a hepatitis B panel. When an STI is diagnosed, testing for other STIs is essential. Cultures for herpes simplex virus (HSV) should be obtained when indicated by history or physical examination. The woman should be offered HIV testing (see the section on HIV testing later in this chapter). When indicated, a complete blood count, sedimentation rate, urinalysis, or urine culture and sensitivity should be obtained. Further, if history or physical examination indicate, a pregnancy test should be performed.

REPORTING

Accurate identification and timely reporting of STIs are integral components of successful infection control efforts. Health care providers are required to report certain STIs to the state public health officials. All states require that gonorrhea, syphilis, and acquired immune deficiency syndrome (AIDS) be reported to public health officials. Chlamydial infection is reportable in most states. The requirements for reporting other STIs differ from state to state. Additionally, individuals with STIs should be asked to identify and notify all partners who might have been exposed. Health care providers are legally responsible for reporting all cases of those infections identified as reportable and should know the requirements of the state in which they practice. The patient must be informed when a case will be reported and told why. Failure to inform the patient the case will be reported is a serious breech of professional ethics. Confidentiality is a crucial issue for many patients. When an STI is reportable, women need to be told they may be contacted by a health department representative. They should be assured the information reported to and collected by health authorities is maintained in strictest confidence. Reports are protected by statute from subpoena in most jurisdictions. Every effort, within the limits of one's public health responsibilities, should be made to reassure patients.

TALKING WITH THE PATIENT

Patient counseling is essential (Tables 18–5 and 18–6). The woman with an STI will need support in seeking care at the earliest possible stage of symptoms. Counseling women about STIs is essential for the following reasons:

- Preventing new infections or reinfection
- Increasing compliance with treatment and follow-up
- Providing support during treatment
- Assisting patients in discussions with their partners

TABLE 18–5   Patient Information

The only certain way to prevent STIs is to avoid sexual contact with others. If you choose to be sexually active, there are things you can do to decrease your risk of developing an STI:

- Have sex with only one person who doesn't have sex with anyone else and who has no infections.
- Always use a condom and use it correctly.
- Use clean needles if you inject any drugs.
- Prevent and control other STIs to decease your susceptibility to HIV infection and to reduce your infectiousness if you are HIV positive.
- Wait to have sex for as long as possible. The younger you are when you have sex for the first time, the more likely you are to catch an STI. The risk of acquiring an STI also increases with the number of partners you have over a lifetime.

Anyone who is sexually active should do the following:

- Always use protection unless you are having sex with only one person who doesn't have sex with anyone else and who has no infections.
- Have regular checkups for STIs even if you have no symptoms and especially when having sex with a new partner.
- Learn the common symptoms of STIs. Seek health care immediately if any suspicious symptoms develop, even if they are mild.
- Avoid having sex during menstruation. Women with HIV are probably more infectious, and women without HIV are probably more susceptible to becoming infected during that time.
- Avoid anal intercourse, but if practiced, use a condom.
- Avoid douching. It removes some of the normal protective bacteria in the vagina and increases the risk of getting some STIs.

Anyone diagnosed as having an STI should do the following:

- Be treated to reduce the risk of transmitting an STI to another person.
- Notify all recent sex partners and urge them to get a checkup as soon as possible to decrease the risk of catching the infection again from them.
- Follow the health care provider's recommendations and complete the full course of medication prescribed. Have a follow-up test if necessary.
- Avoid all sexual activity while being treated.

TABLE 18–6 Sexual Risk Practices

Safest	Low Risk	Possibly Risky (Possible exposure)	High Risk (Unsafe)
Behavior	Behavior	Behavior	Behavior
• Abstinence	• Wet kissing	• Cunnilingus	• Unprotected anal intercourse
• Self-masturbation	• Vaginal intercourse with condom	• Fellatio	• Unprotected vaginal intercourse
• Monogamous (both partners and no high risk activities)	• Anal intercourse with condom	• Mutual masturbation with skin breaks	• Oral–anal contact
• Hugging*, massage*, touching*	• Fellatio interruptus	• Vaginal intercourse after anal contact without new condom	• Fisting
• Dry kissing	• Urine contact with intact skin	Prevention	• Multiple sexual partners
• Mutual masturbation	Prevention	• Dental dam or female condom with cunnilingus	• Sharing sex toys, douche equipment
• Drug abstinence	• Avoid exposure to potentially infected body fluids	• Use condom with fellatio	• Sharing needles
Prevention	• Consistently use condom & spermicide	• Use latex gloves	Prevention
• Avoid high risk behaviors	• Avoid anal intercourse		• Avoid exposure to potentially infected body fluids
			• Consistently use condom & spermicide
			• Avoid anal penetration
			• If having anal penetration, use condom with intercourse, latex glove with hand penetration
			• Avoid oral-anal contact
			• Do not share sex toys, needles, douching equipment
			• If sharing needles, clean with bleach before and after use

Note: *assumes no breaks in skin.

Sources: Adapted from Fogel, 1995; Star, 2004.

Women must be made aware of the serious potential consequences of STIs and the behaviors that increase their likelihood of infection.

The health care provider must make sure that the woman understands what infection she has, how it is transmitted, and why it must be treated. Women should be given a brief description of the infection in language they can understand. This description should include modes of transmission, incubation period, symptoms, infectious period, and potential complications. Effective treatment of STIs necessitates a careful, thorough explanation of the treatment regimen and follow-up procedures. Comprehensive and precise instructions about medications must be provided, both verbally and in writing. Side effects, benefits, and risks of medications should be discussed. Unpleasant side effects or early relief of symptoms may discourage women from completing their medication course. Patients should be strongly urged to continue their medication until it is finished, regardless of whether their symptoms diminish or disappear in a few days. Comfort measures that decrease symptoms such as pain, itching, or nausea should be suggested. Providing written information is a useful strategy because this is a time of high anxiety for many women, and they may not be able to hear or remember what they were told. A number of booklets on STIs are available, or the clinician may wish to develop literature specific to the practice setting and patient population.

In general, women will be advised to refrain from intercourse until all treatment is finished and repeat testing, if appropriate, is done. After the infection is cured, women should be urged to continue using condoms to prevent recurring infections, especially if they have had one episode of PID or continue to have intercourse with new partners. Women may wish to avoid having sex with partners who have many other sexual partners. All women who have contracted an STI should be taught safer sex practices if this has not been done already. Follow-up appointments should be made as needed.

Addressing the psychosocial component of STIs is essential. Remember that a woman may be afraid or embarrassed to tell her partner and ask him or her to seek treatment, or she may be concerned about confidentiality. The effect of a diagnosis of an STI on a committed relationship for the woman (who is now faced with the necessity of dealing with uncertain monogamy) can be significant. In other instances the woman may be afraid that telling her partner may place her in danger of escalating abuse. This potential consequence must be discussed with each patient.

For most STIs, sexual partners should be examined; thus the woman is asked to identify and notify all partners who might have been exposed (partner notification). Often, she will find this difficult to do. Empathizing with the woman's feelings and suggesting specific ways of talking with partners will help decrease her anxiety and assist in efforts to control infection. For example, the clinician might suggest that the woman say, "I care about you and I'm concerned about you. That's why I'm calling to tell you that I have a sexually transmitted infection. My clinician is _____ and she will be happy to talk with you if you would like" (Fogel, 1995). Offering literature and role-playing situations with the woman may also be of assistance. It is often helpful to remind the woman that, although this is an embarrassing situation, most persons would rather know than not know they have been exposed. Health professionals who take time to counsel their patients on how to talk with their partners can improve compliance and case finding. In situations when patient referral may not be effective or possible, health departments should be prepared to assist the woman—either through contact referral or provider referral. Contact referral is the process by which a woman agrees to notify her partners by a certain time. If her partners do not obtain medical evaluation and treatment within the given time period, then clinician referral is implemented. Clinician referral is the process by which partners named by identified patients are notified and counseled by health department providers (CDC, 2002a).

HUMAN PAPILLOMAVIRUS

Human papillomavirus (HPV) infection, previously named genital or venereal warts, is an STI that was first described in the year AD 25, and is now the most prevalent viral STI in the United States (Schaffer, 2003; Wiley et al., 2002). The exact incidence of HPV infections is not known, because health care providers are not required to report these infections. However, it is estimated that as many as one million new HPV infections occur yearly (CDC, 1995). It is likely that at least 60% of sexually active adolescents and young adults will harbor subclinical infections.

HPV is part of the papovirus family. This double-stranded DNA virus has over 70 known serotypes, of which more than 30 can infect the genital tract, including the external genitalia, vagina, urethra, and anus (Gall, 2001). Most HPV infections are asymptomatic, subclinical, or unrecognized. The incubation period is at least one to six months and may be as long as 30 years (Hawkins, Roberto-Nichols & Stanley-Haney, 2004). Although the period of communicability is unknown, approximately 50% of those who have a partner with genital warts will also develop them. In addition to the general risk factors for STIs noted earlier, cigarette smoking has been found to be a risk factor for HPV.

HPV lesions in women are most frequently seen in the posterior part of the introitus; however, lesions also are found on the buttocks, vulva, vagina, anus, and cervix. Typically the lesions present as small (2–3 mm in length, 10–15 mm in height), soft, papillary swellings occurring singularly or in clusters on the genital and anal–rectal region. Warts are usually flesh colored or slightly darker on Caucasian women, black on African-American women, and brownish on Asian women. Infections of long duration may appear as a cauliflower-like mass. In moist areas such as the vaginal introitus, the lesions may appear to have multiple, fine, fingerlike projections. Vaginal lesions are often multiple. Flat-topped papules, 1 to 4 mm in diameter, are seen most often on the cervix. Often these lesions are visualized only under magnification. Women with visible genital warts can be infected with multiple HPV strains, and cervical or vaginal lesions are present in up to 70% of women with vulvar lesions. Usually painless, the lesions may also be uncomfortable, particularly when very large, inflamed, or ulcerated. Chronic vaginal discharge, pruritis, or dyspareunia also can occur.

Visible genital lesions are usually caused by HPV types 6, 11, 42, 43, and 44 and are low risk for invasive cancer. Other types (e.g., 31, 33, 35, 51, and 52) have been strongly associated with cervical dysplasia, and HPV types 16, 18, 45, and 56 are associated with invasive cancer (Gall, 2001). Cervical infection with oncogenic types of HPV is associated with up to 95% of all cervical squamous cell carcinomas and nearly all preinvasive cervical neoplasms (Schaffer, 2003). Further, women with HPV infection of the cervix are 10 times more likely to develop invasive cervical cancer compared to women without HPV (Gall; IOM, 1997). HIV infection may increase the risk that HPV infection will progress to cervical, vaginal, vulvar, and anal cancers.

ASSESSMENT

A woman with HPV lesions may have symptoms such as a profuse, irritating vaginal discharge, itching, dyspareunia, or postcoital bleeding. She may also report "bumps" on her vulva or labia. History of known exposure is important because of the potentially long latency period and the possibility of subclinical infections in men. However, the lack of a history of known exposure cannot be used to exclude a diagnosis of HPV infection.

Physical inspection of the vulva, perineum, anus, vagina, and cervix is essential whenever HPV lesions are suspected or seen. Speculum examination of the vagina may block some lesions; thus it is important to rotate the speculum blades until all areas are visualized. When lesions are visible, the characteristic appearance previously described is considered diagnostic. However, in many instances, cervical lesions are not visible and some vaginal or vulvar lesions also may be unobservable to the naked eye. Gloves should be changed between vaginal and rectal examinations to prevent the potential spread of vulvar or vaginal lesions to the anus. Diagnosis is made by careful, thorough clinical examination of visible genital warts or by biopsy of cervical lesions and (rarely) of lesions at other sites if the diagnosis is not clear.

It is imperative that women with vulvar HPV or who have partners with HPV have cervical cancer screening. Pap tests of the cervical transformation zone are a screening technique and not diagnostic, as the sample can miss a lesion. Thus a negative Pap test does not indicate absence of disease. To identify cervical HPV infection, a cervical swab is taken of the transformation zone for laboratory identification of HPV DNA. It is important that any grossly visible suspicious cervical lesion be biopsied regardless of Pap test findings. Further, the severity of any cervical lesion identified on Pap test is best determined by colposcopy and biopsy. Vinegar solution has been used in the past to highlight early or flat cervical lesions, but a positive reaction to vinegar may also be obtained with any inflammatory reaction, after sexual intercourse, and with vaginal trauma.

DIFFERENTIAL DIAGNOSES

HPV lesions must be differentiated from molluscum contagiosum, condylomata lata, and carcinoma. Molluscum contagiosum lesions are half-domed, smooth, flesh-colored to pearly white papules with depressed centers. Condylomata lata are a form of secondary syphilis and generally are flatter and wider than genital warts. Cancers to be ruled out are squamous cell carcinoma, carcinoma in situ, and malignant melanoma. An extensive list of other differential diagnoses for vulvar lesions can be found in Chapter 22.

MANAGEMENT

The primary goals of treatment of visible genital warts (also known as condylomata acuminata or condyloma) are removal or reduction of warts and relief of signs and symptoms—not the eradication of HPV (CDC, 2002a). Often treatment can induce wart-free periods. If left untreated, genital warts may resolve, remain unchanged, or increase in size and number (CDC). Treatment of genital warts is often very difficult. The patient often must make multiple office visits, and frequently many different treatment modalities will be used. Eradication of the virus is not considered conclusive even after there is no visible evidence of wart tissue because of the high incidence of recurrence.

Treatment of genital warts should be guided by preference of the woman, available resources, and experience of the clinician. None of the treatments are superior, and no one treatment is ideal for all warts (CDC, 2002a). Available treatments are outlined in Table 18–7. Any concurrent vaginal infections or STIs should also be treated.

Women who have cervical warts must be evaluated for dysplasia before treatment is started and should be referred to an expert in the field of gynecologic dysplasia. Biannual Pap tests should be done for the first two years after treatment and annually thereafter on women who have been treated for HPV infections (CDC, 2002a). When the cervix is treated, a Pap test should be done in four to six months. An annual Pap test can be performed after two negative Pap smears at 6-month intervals (CDC).

Women who are experiencing discomfort associated with genital warts may find that bathing with an oatmeal solution and drying the area with a hair dyer on a lower setting will

TABLE 18–7   Treatment of Genital Warts

Patient-Applied Regimens	Provider-Administered Regimens	Alternative Regimens
Podofilox 0.5% solution gel	Cryotherapy with liquid nitrogen or cryoprobe	Intralesional interferon
Imiquimod 5% cream	Podophyllin resin 10%–25% in compound tincture of benzoin	Laser surgery
	Trichloroacetic acid (TCA) or bichloroacetic acid (BCA) 80–90%	
	Surgical removal	

Source: CDC, 2002a.

provide some relief. Keeping the area clean and dry will also decrease the growth of warts. Cotton underwear and loose fitting clothes that decrease friction and irritation also may decrease discomfort. Women should be advised to maintain a healthy lifestyle to aid the immune system. Women can also be counseled regarding diet, rest, stress reduction, and exercise. All women who smoke should be counseled in smoking-cessation techniques.

EMERGING EVIDENCE

Recent research findings suggest that a vaccine against HPV 16, the primary cause of cervical cancer, will reach the market in the next few years. A clinical trial involving 1500 young women who were negative for HPV 16 demonstrated the vaccine appeared to be 100% effective in preventing HPV 16 infection and low-grade cervical cytologic abnormalities attributable to HPV 16 (Koutsky et al., 2002).

TALKING WITH THE PATIENT

Counseling messages for women with HPV can be found in Table 18–8. The partners of women with HPV should be evaluated and treated if lesions are present. Condoms should be used until both partners are lesion free and up to nine months after the appearance of lesions, as subclinical condylomata may be infectious. All sexually active women with multiple partners or a history of HPV should be encouraged to use latex condoms during intercourse to decrease acquisition or transmission of condylomata. The link between cervical cancer and the need for close follow-up should be discussed. Semiannual or annual health examinations are recommended to assess disease recurrence and screening for cervical cancer. Women should understand the advisability of treatment before becoming

---

TABLE 18–8   Counseling Messages for Women with Human Papilloma Virus

Based on a new understanding of the life history of the human papillomavirus, the CDC recommends that the following key counseling points be conveyed to all persons with HPV:

- HPV is a viral infection that is common in sexually active persons and is almost always transmitted through sexual activity.
- Sexual partners are usually infected when a woman is diagnosed, even though they may be asymptomatic, because the incubation period is variable.
- Genital warts are usually benign. The types of HPV that cause genital warts are usually not the ones associated with cervical cancer. Recurrence of genital warts within the first several months after treatment is common and usually indicates recurrence rather than reinfection.
- The likelihood of transmission and duration of infectivity after treatment is unknown. Although information on prevention is lacking, the use of latex condoms is associated with a lower rate of cervical cancer.
- The value of telling future partners about a past diagnosis of HPV is unclear, because genital HPV is very common and the duration of infectivity is not known. Nevertheless, candid discussions about other STIs are encouraged.

Source: CDC, 2002a.

pregnant. Women with HPV infection may radically alter their sexual practices both from fear of transmission to or from a partner, and from genital discomfort associated with treatment, which may have a negative impact on their sexual relationships. Unless the partner accepts and understands the necessary precautions, it may be difficult for the woman to follow the treatment regimen. The clinician can offer to discuss feelings that the woman may have and, when indicated, joint counseling can be suggested.

GENITAL HERPES SIMPLEX VIRUS INFECTION

Unknown until the middle of the twentieth century, genital HSV infection is now one of the most common STIs in the United States, especially for women, who contract it far more often than men. Although HSV infection is not a reportable infection, it is estimated that approximately one half million cases are diagnosed annually and that 55 million Americans are infected with genital herpes. Prevalence is higher in women with multiple sex partners. The greatest numbers of new cases occur in individuals between 15 and 34 years of age (CDC, 2002a).

Genital herpes is a recurrent, incurable viral infection characterized by painful vesicular eruption of the skin and mucosa of the genitals. Two serotypes of HSV have been identified: herpes simplex virus I (HSV-1) and herpes simplex virus II (HSV-2). HSV-2 is usually transmitted sexually and HSV-1, nonsexually. Although HSV-1 is more commonly associated with gingivostomatitis and oral ulcers (fever blisters), and HSV-2 with genital lesions, both types are not exclusively associated with the respective sites.

An initial or primary genital herpes infection characteristically has both systemic and local symptoms and lasts about three weeks. Women generally have a more severe clinical course than do men. Flu-like symptoms with fever, malaise, and myalgia first appear about a week after exposure, peak within four days, and subside over the next week. Multiple genital lesions develop at the site of infection, usually the vulva. Other common sites are the perianal area, vagina, and cervix. The lesions begin as small painful blisters or vesicles that become "unroofed," leaving ulcerated lesions. Individuals with primary herpes often develop bilateral, tender, inguinal lymphadenopathy; vulvar edema; vaginal discharge; and severe dysuria.

Ulcerative lesions last 4 to 15 days before crusting over. New lesions may develop up to the 10th day during the course of the infection. Cervicitis is also common with initial HSV-2 infections. The cervix may appear normal or be friable, reddened, ulcerated, or necrotic. A heavy, watery to purulent vaginal discharge is common. Extragenital lesions may be present because of autoinoculation. Urinary retention and dysuria may occur secondary to autonomic involvement of the sacral nerve root.

Women experiencing recurrent episodes of HSV infections commonly will have only local symptoms that are usually less severe than those associated with the initial infection. Systemic symptoms are usually absent, although the characteristic prodromal genital tingling is common. Recurrent lesions are unilateral, less severe, and usually last 7 to 10 days without prolonged viral shedding. Lesions begin as vesicles and progress rapidly to ulcers. Very few women with recurrent disease have cervicitis.

ASSESSMENT

A history of exposure to a person with HSV infection is important, although infection from an asymptomatic individual is possible. A history of viral symptoms, such as malaise, headache, fever, or myalgia, is suggestive of HSV infections. Local symptoms such as vulvar pain, dysuria, itching or burning at the site of infection, and painful genital lesions that heal spontaneously also are very suggestive of HSV infections. The clinician should also ask about prior history of a primary infection, prodromal symptoms, vaginal discharge, dysuria, and dyspareunia.

During the physical examination, the clinician should assess for inguinal and generalized lymphadenopathy and elevated temperature. The entire vulvar, perineal, vaginal, and cervical areas should be carefully inspected for vesicles or ulcerated or crusted areas. A speculum examination may be very difficult for the patient because of the extreme tenderness often associated with herpes infections.

Although a diagnosis of HSV infection may be suspected from the history and physical examination, it is only confirmed by laboratory studies. Screening of asymptomatic women is not recommended. Isolation of HSV in cell culture is the preferred virologic test in women who have genital ulcers or other mucocutaneous lesions. Viral culture has a sensitivity of 70% to 80% (CDC, 2002a; Schaffer, 2003). Culture yield is best if the specimen is taken during the vesicular stage of the disease because the sensitivity of a culture declines rapidly as lesions begin to heal. In a primary infection, viral shedding is prolonged and the HSV is more easily isolated.

Type-specific serologic tests are useful in confirming a clinical diagnosis because false negative HSV cultures are common, especially with healing lesions or recurrent infection. The POCkit-HSV-2 assay is a point-of-care test that provides results for HSV-2 antibodies from capillary blood or serum during a clinic visit (CDC, 2002a). Sensitivity varies from 80% to 90% and false negative results can occur, especially in early stages of infection. Specificity of the assay is greater than 96%, and false positive results may occur in patients with a low likelihood of HSV infection.

DIFFERENTIAL DIAGNOSES

Differential diagnoses include syphilis, chancroid, lymphogranuloma venereum, granuloma inguinale, as well as non-STI vulvar lesions (see Chapter 22).

MANAGEMENT

Genital herpes is a chronic and recurring disease for which there is no known cure. Systemic antiviral drugs partially control the symptoms and signs of HSV infections when used for the primary or recurrent episodes, or when used as daily suppressive therapy.

TABLE 18–9   Treatment of Genital Herpes

Primary infection:

Acyclovir 400 mg orally three times a day for 7–10 days

Acyclovir 200 mg orally five times a day for 7–10 days

Famciclovir 250 mg orally three times a day for 7–10 days

Valacyclovir 1 g orally twice a day for 7–10 days

Recurrent infection:

Acyclovir 400 mg orally three times a day for 5 days

Acyclovir 200 mg orally five times a day for 5 days

Acyclovir 800 mg orally twice a day for 5 days

Famciclovir 125 mg orally twice a day for 5 days

Valacyclovir 500 mg orally twice a day for 5 days

Valacyclovir 1 g (1000 mg) orally once a day for 5 days

Suppressive therapy:

Acyclovir 400 mg orally BID

Famciclovir 250 mg orally BID

Valacyclovir 500 mg orally once a day

Valacyclovir 1 g (1000 mg) orally once a day

Source: CDC, 2002a.

However, these drugs do not cure the infection, nor do they alter subsequent risk, frequency, or recurrences after discontinuation. Three antiviral medications provide clinical benefits for genital herpes: acyclovir, valacyclovir, and famciclovir (CDC, 2002a). Treatment recommendations are given in Table 18–9. Safety and efficacy have been clearly demonstrated in persons taking acyclovir daily for up to three years.

Cleaning lesions twice a day with saline will help prevent secondary infection. Coexisting bacterial infections must be treated with appropriate antibiotics. Oral analgesics, such as aspirin or ibuprofen, may be used to relieve pain and systemic symptoms associated with initial infections. Any topical agents should be used with caution, because the mucous membranes affected by herpes are very sensitive. Ointments containing cortisone should be avoided. Women should be informed that occlusive ointments may prolong the course of infections.

Complementary measures that may increase comfort for women when lesions are active include warm sitz baths with baking soda; keeping lesions warm and dry by using a hair dryer set on cool or patting dry the area with a soft towel; wearing cotton underwear and loose clothing; applying cold milk or witch hazel compresses followed by aloe vera gel or Burrow's solution (Domeboro) to lesions four times a day for 30 minutes; oatmeal baths; applying cool, wet, black tea bags to lesions; and applying compresses with an infusion of cloves or peppermint oil and clove oil to lesions (Sinclair, 2004; Star, Lommel, & Shannon, 2004).

A diet rich in Vitamins C, B-complex, zinc, and calcium is thought to help prevent recurrences. Daily use of kelp powder (2 capsules) and sunflower seed oil (1 tbsp) also have been recommended to decrease recurrences. The amino acid L-lysine has been used in doses of 750 to 1000 mg daily while lesions are active and 500 mg during asymptomatic periods. It is thought that L-lysine has an inhibitory effect on the multiplication of HSV (Fogel, 1995). Minimizing the following foods that contain L-arginine may help as well: coffee, grains, chicken, chocolate, corn, dairy products, meat, peanut butter, nuts, and seeds. Avoiding citrus foods may also be helpful (Balch & Balch, 1997; Page, 2000; Sinclair, 2004)

A number of herbal remedies may also help with the discomforts of herpes infections. Liquid Burdock (15 to 60 g/L) can be applied as a compress or taken orally at a dose of 6 to 25 drops of tincture three times a day (Griffith, 2000; Nissim, 1996; Page; Stapleton & Tiran, 2000). Calendula comes in an ointment or infused oil that can be applied locally, as a tea that can be used to make a sitz bath, or as a tincture that is diluted with one to three parts water and applied to lesions with a cotton swab three times a day (Cummings & Ullman, 1997; Griffith; Nissim; Page; Sinclair; Singingtree, 1993; Stapleton & Tiran). Echinacea extract has antiviral properties, stimulates the body's immune system, and is useful in treating herpes infections. It may be taken orally or applied locally to reduce inflammation and pain. It should be used at the first indication of a herpes outbreak (Balch & Balch; Griffith; Page). Nissim suggests 25 drops of echinacea tincture be taken with a little water every two hours for six to eight hours, and then continuing four times a day for the length of the outbreak. Goldenseal may be taken by capsule, tea, or extract, or applied locally to decrease inflammation and pain (Balch & Balch; Griffith; Page). Myrrh can be applied locally as a diluted tincture or as a compress to decrease pain and inflammation. When applied to the lesions, diluted tincture of myrrh has a drying effect, though it stings (Balch & Balch; Page; Stapleton & Tiran). Tea tree oil stimulates the immune system and can be applied locally or added to bath water (Page; Sinclair; Stapleton & Tiran).

TALKING WITH THE PATIENT

Women should be advised that viral shedding and thus transmission to a partner is most likely with active lesions, but can occur even when they are asymptomatic. Women should refrain from sexual contact from the onset of prodrome until the complete healing of lesions. Women should be taught how to examine themselves for herpetic lesions using a mirror and good light source to look, and a wet cloth or finger covered with a finger cot to rub lightly over the labia. The clinician should ensure that patients understand that when lesions are active, sharing intimate articles (e.g., washcloths, wet towels) that come into contact with the lesions should be avoided. Women should be taught that stress, menstruation, trauma, febrile illnesses, chronic illness, and ultraviolet light have all been found to trigger genital herpes. A common misconception that may cause anxiety for women is that HSV causes cancer. This myth should be dispelled because the role of HSV-2 in cervical cancer is (at most) that of a cofactor rather than a primary etiologic agent (CDC, 2002a).

CHANCROID

Chancroid is a bacterial infection of the genitourinary tract caused by the gram-negative bacteria, *Haemophilus ducreyi*. The acute localized infection of chancroid is found more often in Asia, Africa, and South America, but also occurs in discrete outbreaks in the United States. The infection also is endemic in some areas. For example, sex workers appear to have a high incidence of chancroid in areas such as Los Angeles, Boston, Dallas, New York City, and parts of Georgia and Florida. About 10% of persons in the United States who have chancroid are coinfected with HSV or syphilis. Chancroid is a genital ulcer; thus it is a cofactor for HIV infection. The major way chancroid is acquired is through sexual contact and trauma. Infection through autoinoculation of fingers or other sites occasionally occurs. The incubation period, though not well established, is usually four to seven days but may be as long as three weeks.

Typically the woman presents with a history of a painful macule on the external genitalia that rapidly changes to a pustule and then to an ulcerated lesion. The patient may develop enlarged unilateral or bilateral inguinal nodes know as buboe. After one to two weeks, the skin overlying the lymph node becomes erythematous, the center necroses, and the node becomes ulcerated.

ASSESSMENT

A probable diagnosis of chancroid can be made when painful genital ulcers are present and there is no evidence of syphilis or HSV infection. Definitive diagnosis of chancroid is difficult because the organism can only be identified by culture on a special media that is not used routinely. A cotton or calcium alginate swab is used to obtain the specimen from the ulcer base after gentle removal of necrotic exudate with saline. Culture sensitivity is no higher than 80% and is usually lower (CDC, 2002a). Testing for gonorrhea, chlamydia, and syphilis should be performed. HIV testing should be done at the time of diagnosis and repeated in three months.

DIFFERENTIAL DIAGNOSES

Differential diagnoses include syphilis, herpes simplex, lymphogranuloma venereum, folliculitis, metastatic genital cancer (cervical, vagina, vulvar), and other vulvar lesions (see Chapter 22).

MANAGEMENT

The recommended treatments for chancroid are azithromycin, 1 gram orally in a single dose; ceftriaxone, 250 mg IM in a single dose; ciprofloxacin, 500 mg orally twice a day for three days; or erythromycin base, 500 mg orally four times a day for seven days (CDC, 2002a). Women with HIV may require retreatment after single dose therapy.

Patients should be reexamined three to seven days after beginning therapy. If treatment is successful, there should be symptomatic improvement within three days of starting therapy. Note that it may take more than two weeks for complete healing of the ulcers. All sexual partners who have had sexual contact within 10 days preceding the onset of symptoms with a person diagnosed with chancroid should be evaluated regardless of whether symptoms are present.

PEDICULOSIS

Pediculosis is a parasitic infection caused by the following three species of lice:

- *Pediculosis humanus capitus* (head louse infecting the scalp)
- *Pediculosis humanus corporus* (body or clothing louse infecting the trunk)
- *Phtirus pubis* (pubic lice or "crabs")

Phtirus pubis inhabit the genital area but may also be found in other hair-bearing areas of the body, including the axillae, chest, thighs, eyelashes, and head. A woman is infected through contact with infected clothing or bedding, and by sexual transmission.

ASSESSMENT

A patient usually presents with pruritus, caused by the lice ingesting saliva, and then depositing digestive juices and feces into the skin. Women may report seeing the lice or known exposure to a household member or sexual partner with head, body, or pubic lice. A history of shared clothing, bathing equipment, or bedding may also be given. Diagnosis is made by direct examination of the egg cases (nits) in the involved area. These are usually visible to the naked eye but a hand lens and light can be helpful. Black dots (excreta) may be visible on the surrounding skin and underclothing, and crusts or scabs in the pubic area may also be seen.

DIFFERENTIAL DIAGNOSES

Differential diagnosis includes anogenital eczema and pruritis, seborrheic dermatitis, pruritis vulvae, folliculitis, tinea cruris, and scabies. Other concomitant STIs should be ruled out.

MANAGEMENT

Pediculosis pubis is treated with permethrin 1% cream (Nix) rinse, or pyrethrins with piperonyl butoxice (RID, Clear, A-200, Pronto). These medications are applied to the affected areas and washed off after 10 minutes. Lindane 1% can also be used and is applied for four minutes to the affected area and then thoroughly washed off (Shannon, 2004). Patients should be told to wash in hot water and dry thoroughly on the hot cycle all clothing, bed linen, and towels to destroy lice and nits.

TRICHOMONIASIS

Trichomoniasis is caused by *Trichomonas vaginalis*, an anaerobic one-celled protozoan with characteristic flagellae. The organism lives in the vagina, urethra, Bartholin's, and Skene's glands in women, and in the urethra and prostate gland in men. Trichomoniasis causes up to 20% of vaginitis and occurs in approximately three million women annually in the United States (Gorroll, 2001). It is transmitted during vaginal-penile intercourse and over 70% of exposed partners become infected (Benenson, 1995). It is infrequently transmitted by wet, warm fomites, but intravaginal inoculation is still necessary (Nissim, 1996). Trichomoniasis is believed to facilitate HIV transmission.

Although trichomoniasis may be asymptomatic in nearly half of women with the infection, women commonly experience a characteristically yellow to greenish, frothy, mucopurulent, copious, malodorous discharge. However, Wheeler (2002) notes that clinicians are notoriously unable to make a diagnosis only on the appearance of the discharge. Inflammation of the vulva, vagina, or both may be present and the woman may have irritation and pruritis. Dysuria and dyspareunia are often present. Typically, the discharge worsens during and after menstruation.

ASSESSMENT

In addition to the history of current symptoms, a careful sexual history including last intercourse and last sexual contract should be obtained. Any history of similar symptoms in the past and treatment used should be noted. The clinician should determine whether or not the woman's partners were treated and if she has had subsequent relations with new partners. Additional important information includes last menstrual period, method of birth control (if any), and other medications.

The external genitalia should be observed for excoriation, erythema, edema, ulceration, and lesions. On speculum examination, note the quantity, color, consistency, and any odor of the vaginal discharge. Often the cervix and vaginal walls will demonstrate the characteristic "strawberry spots" or tiny petechiae, and the cervix may bleed on contact. In severe infections, the vaginal walls, cervix, and occasionally the vulva may be acutely inflamed. The pH of vaginal discharge is elevated. Diagnosis is usually made by wet prep visualization of the typical one-celled flagellate trichomonads (Figure 18–1). However, this method has a sensitivity of only approximately 60% to 70% (CDC, 2002a). Microscopic examination of the wet mount may also reveal increased numbers of white blood cells. Culture is the most sensitive, specific method of diagnosis, but it is expensive and not widely available. Pap smear results frequently include reports of trichomonads; however, the sensitivity of the method is low (65%) and is not acceptable for diagnosing trichomoniasis in asymptomatic women.

DIFFERENTIAL DIAGNOSES

Differential diagnoses for trichomoniasis include other conditions that cause vaginal discharge, such as vulvovaginal candidiasis, bacterial vaginosis, chlamydia, and gonorrhea.

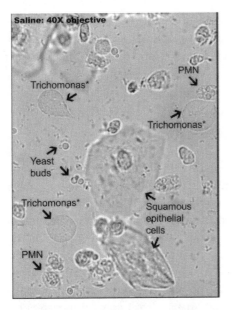

FIGURE 18-1   Wet Mount Findings with Trichomoniasis. PMNs = polymorphonuclear leukocytes/white blood cells. Trichomonads must be motile for conclusive diagnosis. *Source:* Used with permission from Washington State Department of Health STD/TB Program, Seattle STD/HIV Prevention Training Center, and Cindy Fennell, MS, MT, ASCP.

MANAGEMENT

The recommended treatment is 2 g metronidazole orally in a single dose (CDC, 2002a; Forna & Gulmezoglu, 2002). Metronidazole (Flagyl) is an antiprotozoal and antibacterial agent. When oral metronidazole is taken, the patient is advised not to drink alcoholic beverages, or she will experience severe abdominal distress, nausea, vomiting, and headache. Although the male partner is usually asymptomatic, it is recommended that he receive treatment also, because he often harbors the trichomonads in the urethra or prostate. Garlic has been suggested as an effective agent against trichomonas infection. A goldenseal douche is reputed to act as an antibiotic and to stimulate the immune system (Griffith, 2000; Sinclair, 2004)

CHLAMYDIA

Chlamydia is the most common bacterial STI in American women with almost 800,000 cases reported to the CDC in 2001 (CDC, 2002b). Up to 80% of these infections are silent (Faro, 2001), and the symptoms, when present, are nonspecific. The causative organism is *Chlamydia trachomatis*. Risk factors include multiple partners and nonuse of barrier methods of contraception. Chlamydia is more common among adolescents than older women. Sexually active women younger than 20 years of age are two to three times more likely to become infected with chlamydia than women between 20 and 29 years. Women over the age of 30 years have the lowest rate of infection. Lower socioeconomic status may be a risk factor, especially with respect to treatment-seeking behaviors. Acute salpingitis or PID is the most serious complication of chlamydial infections (see the section on PID in this chapter). Additionally, chlamydial infection of the cervix causes inflammation resulting in microscopic cervical ulcerations, and thus may increase the risk of acquiring HIV infection.

ASSESSMENT

In addition to obtaining information regarding the presence of risk factors, the clinician should inquire about the presence of any symptoms. Although chlamydia is usually asymptomatic, some women may experience spotting or postcoital bleeding, mucoid or purulent cervical discharge, urinary frequency, or dysuria. Bleeding results from inflammation and erosion of the cervical columnar epithelium. Women on oral contraceptives may also experience breakthrough bleeding. Occasionally women report lower abdominal pain and dyspareunia.

Physical examination findings of guarding, referred pain, or rebound upon abdominal examination should raise suspicion for PID. Cervical friability may be detected with the speculum examination. Discharge, if present, is characteristically mucopurulent. During the bimanual examination, a woman may report pain with cervical movement, and the examiner may detect adnexal fullness and uterine tenderness. These findings are also suggestive of PID.

The CDC has expanded recommendations for chlamydia screening among asymptomatic women. All sexually active women ages 25 years and under should be screened for chlamydia at least annually, even if no symptoms are reported (CDC, 2002b). Women over 25 years old with risk factors (history of previous STI, inconsistent or incorrect condom use, new or multiple partners) should also be screened. A sexual risk history should always be assessed and may indicate more frequent screening for some women. Culture, once considered the gold standard for identification of chlamydia, is time consuming, expensive, and infrequently used today (Faro, 2001). Recommended screening procedures for chlamydial infection (in order of preference) are: nucleic acid amplification test (NAAT) of an endocervical sample (if a pelvic examination is acceptable) or a urine sample (if a pelvic examination is not acceptable) (CDC). Endocervical NAAT is preferred because it provides the highest sensitivity of any screening test. Women with a positive urine test should have a pelvic examination to identify complications, such as PID.

There is a high prevalence of reinfection in women who have had chlamydial infections in the preceding several months, usually from reinfection by an untreated partner (CDC, 2002a). Clinicians should advise all women, especially adolescents, with a chlamydial infection to be rescreened three to four months after treatment, because reinfection rates are high and the risk of complications increases with reinfection.

DIFFERENTIAL DIAGNOSES

Differential diagnoses include gonorrhea, trichomoniasis, PID, appendicitis, and cystitis.

TABLE 18-10   Treatment of Chlamydial Infections

Recommended regimens:

Azithromycin 1 g orally once

Doxycycline 100 mg orally twice a day for 7 days

Alternative regimens:

Erythromycin base 500 mg orally four times a day for 7 days

Erythromycin ethylsuccinate 800 mg orally four times a day for 7 days

Ofloxacin 300 mg orally twice a day for 7 days

Levofloxacin 500 mg orally for 7 days

Source: CDC, 2002a.

MANAGEMENT

Recommendations for treatment of urethral, cervical, and rectal chlamydial infections are found in Table 18–10. Azithromycin is often prescribed when compliance may be a problem because only one dose is needed; however, expense is a concern with this medication. A test of cure is not necessary for women who complete treatment with doxcycline or azithromycin unless symptoms persist or reinfection is a possibility. A test of cure may be considered if the woman is treated with erythromycin.

GONORRHEA

Gonorrhea is probably the oldest communicable disease in the United States. An estimated one million American men and women contract gonorrhea each year. Age is likely the most important risk factor associated with gonorrhea. The majority of those contracting gonorrhea are less than 20 years old. In a single act of unprotected sex with a partner who has gonorrhea, a teenage woman has a 50% change of contracting the infection.

Gonorrhea is caused by the aerobic, gram-negative diplococci *Neisseria gonorrhoeae.* Gonorrhea is almost exclusively transmitted by sexual activity, primarily through genital-to-genital contact; however, it is also spread by oral-to-genital and anal-to-genital contact. Sites of infection in females are the cervix, urethra, oropharynx, Skene's glands, and Bartholin's glands. Although the gonorrhea organism has been recovered from inanimate objects artificially inoculated with the bacteria, there is no evidence that natural transmission occurs this way (Schaffer, 2003). Other risk factors include early onset of sexual activity and multiple sexual partners. The incidence of drug-resistant cases of gonorrhea, in particular penicillinase-producing *N. gonorrhoeae,* is rising dramatically in the United States (CDC, 2002a; Star & Deal, 2004a).

The main complication of gonorrheal infections is PID. Women may also have a pelvic abscess or Bartholin's abscess. Disseminated gonococcal infections (DGI) are a rare (0.5% to 3%) complication of untreated gonorrhea. DGI occurs in two stages: the first stage is characterized by bacteremia with chills, fever, and skin lesions, and is followed by the second stage during which the patient experiences acute septic arthritis with characteristic effusions, most commonly of the wrists, knees, and ankles (Star & Deal, 2004a).

ASSESSMENT

Women are often asymptomatic (up to 80%). When symptoms are present, they are often less specific than the symptoms in men. Women may report dyspareunia, leukorrhea or a change in vaginal discharge, unilateral labial pain and swelling, or lower abdominal discomfort. Later in the infection's course, women give a history of purulent, irritating vaginal discharge, or rectal pain and discharge. Menstrual irregularities may be the presenting symptom with longer, more painful menses. Women may also give a history of chronic or acute lower abdominal pain. Generally women report symptoms worsening postmenstrually. Unilateral labial pain and swelling may indicate Bartholin's gland infection (see Chapter 17), and periurethral pain and swelling may indicate inflamed Skene's glands. Infrequently, dysuria, vague abdominal pain, or low backache prompt women to seek care. Later symptoms may include fever (possibly high), nausea, vomiting, joint pain and swelling, or upper abdominal pain (liver involvement).

Women may develop a gonococcal rectal infection following anal intercourse and report symptoms of profuse purulent anal discharge, rectal pain, and blood in the stool. Rectal itching, fullness, pressure, and pain are also common symptoms. Women with gonococcal pharyngitis may appear to have viral pharyngitis, as some individuals will have a red, swollen uvula and pustule vesicles on the soft palate and tonsils similar to streptococcal infections. A diffuse vaginitis with vulvitis is the most common form of gonococcal infection in prepubertal girls. There may be few signs of infection in this age group, or there may be vaginal discharge, dysuria, and swollen, reddened labia.

Physical examination is individualized based on a woman's presenting symptoms. Vital signs should be obtained and a general skin inspection conducted for signs of classic DGI lesions, which are painful necrotic pustules on an erythematous base, approximately 1 mm to 2 cm in diameter. The pharynx and oral cavity are inspected for erythema, edema, and lesions. Palpation for cervical lymphadenopathy should be performed. The abdomen should be palpated and masses, tenderness, and rebound tenderness noted. During the speculum examination, the vaginal walls are inspected for discharge and redness, and the cervix is inspected for mucopurulent discharge, ectopy, and friability. During the bimanual examination, the clinician observes for cervical motion tenderness, uterine tenderness, adnexal tenderness, and adnexal masses. These findings are associated with PID.

Cultures are considered the gold standard for diagnosis of gonorrhea, but require specific conditions for storage and transport (see Chapter 6). Cultures should be obtained from the endocervix, rectum, and when indicated, the pharynx. Thayer–Martin cultures are recommended to diagnose gonorrhea in women. NAAT or nucleic acid hybridization of an endocervical swab specimen may be used if viable organisms cannot be maintained for culture analysis (CDC, 2002b). Any woman suspected of having gonorrhea should have chlamydia and

TABLE 18–11   Treatment of Gonococcal Infections

Cefixime 400 mg orally once

Ceftriaxone 125 mg IM once

Ciprofloxacin 500 mg orally once

Ofloxacin 400 mg orally once

Levofloxacin 250 mg orally once

   Plus, if chlamydia is not ruled out

Azithromycin 1 g orally once or Doxycycline 100 mg orally twice a day for 7 days

Source: CDC, 2002a.

syphilis testing if these tests have not been performed in the past two months. All patients with gonorrhea should be offered confidential counseling and testing for HIV infection.

DIFFERENTIAL DIAGNOSES

Differential diagnoses include chlamydia, trichomoniasis, PID, appendicitis, and cystitis.

MANAGEMENT

Management of gonorrhea is straightforward, and the cure is usually rapid with appropriate antibiotic therapy (Table 18–11). Penicillin is no longer used to treat gonorrhea because of the high rate of penicillin-resistant strains of the organism. Single-dose efficacy is a major consideration in selecting an antibiotic regimen for women with gonorrhea. Another important consideration is the high percentage (45%) of women with coexisting chlamydial infections. The CDC (2002a) suggests concomitant treatment for chlamydia because coinfection is common. Gonorrhea is a highly communicable infection. Recent (past 30 days) sexual partners should be examined, tested, and treated with appropriate regimens. Most treatment failures result from reinfection.

Treatment failure in women with uncomplicated gonorrhea who are treated with any of the recommended regimens is rare (less than 5%); therefore, a follow-up test of cure is not essential. A more cost-effective approach is reexamination with testing one to two months after treatment. This approach will detect both treatment failures and reinfections.

PELVIC INFLAMMATORY DISEASE

Pelvic inflammatory disease is a spectrum of inflammatory disorders of the upper female genital tract including any combination of endometritis, salpingitis, tubo-ovarian abscess, and pelvic peritonitis (CDC, 2002a). Each year more than 1 million women in the United States will have an episode of symptomatic PID (Hatcher et al., 2004). Teenagers have the highest risk for PID because of their decreased immunity to infectious organisms and increased risk of gonorrhea and chlamydia (Star & Deal, 2004a).

Multiple organisms have been found to cause PID, and most cases are associated with more than one organism. In the past the most common causative agent was thought to be *N. gonorrhoeae*; however, *C. trachomatis* is now estimated to cause one-half of all cases of PID. In addition to gonorrhea and chlamydia, a wide variety of anaerobic and aerobic bacteria such as *Streptococcus, E. coli,* and *Gardnerella vaginalis* can cause PID (CDC, 2002a).

Most PID results from the ascending spread of microorganisms from the vagina and endocervix to the upper genital tract. This spread most frequently happens at the end of or just after menses following the reception of an infectious agent. During the menstrual period, several factors facilitate the development of an infection—the cervical os is slightly open, the cervical mucus barrier is absent, and menstrual blood is an excellent medium for growth. PID also may develop following an abortion, pelvic surgery, or childbirth. Young age at first intercourse, frequent sexual intercourse, multiple sex partners, and a history of STIs also increase a woman's risk for PID. In addition, cigarette smoking and douching may increase a woman's risk for acute PID. The CDC (2002a) states that women who use IUDs are probably at increased risk for PID that may not be STI related, and that most of this risk occurs in the first few weeks after IUD insertion.

Major medical complications are associated with PID. Short-term consequences include acute pelvic pain, tubo-ovarian abscess, tubal scarring, and adhesions. At least 25% of women experience long-term sequelae from PID, including chronic pelvic pain, dyspareunia, ectopic pregnancy as a result of partial tubal scarring and blockage, tubal infertility, increased need for reproductive tract surgery, and recurring PID (CDC, 2002a; Gonen, 1999).

PID may be caused by a wide variety of infectious agents and encompasses a wide variety of pathologic processes; therefore, the infection can be acute, subacute, or chronic, and has a wide range of symptoms. Diagnosis of PID is difficult because almost all of the most common signs and symptoms could accompany other urinary, gastrointestinal, or reproductive tract problems.

ASSESSMENT

History taking must be comprehensive (Fogel, 1995). A menstrual history is useful in establishing the relationship of the onset of pain to menses and in identifying any variations from normal in the cycle. Other relevant history includes recent pelvic surgery, abortion, childbirth, dilatation of the cervix, IUD insertion (within the last month), purulent vaginal discharge, irregular bleeding, and a longer, heavier menstrual period. A thorough sexual risk history should be obtained, including current or most recent sexual activity, number of partners, and method of contraception, and will assist in identifying possible increased risk for STI exposure. Intestinal and bladder symptoms are important to review (Star & Deal, 2004a). Women may report various symptoms ranging from minimal pelvic discomfort to dull, cramping, and intermittent pain, or severe, persistent, and incapacitating pain. Pelvic pain usually develops within 7–10 days of menses, remains constant, is bilateral, and is most severe in the lower quadrants. Pelvic discomfort is exacerbated by Valsalva maneuver, intercourse, or movement. The woman with acute PID also may have intermenstrual bleeding (Hawkins et al., 2004). Symptoms of STIs in a woman's partners also should be noted.

Vital signs are obtained and a complete physical examination performed. A fever of 102° F or above is characteristic. Physical examination reveals adnexal tenderness, abdominal tenderness, with or without rebound, and exquisite tenderness with cervical movement. Pelvic tenderness is usually bilateral. There may or may not be a palpable adnexal swelling or thickening. Fever and peritonitis are more characteristic of gonococcal PID than of PID caused by other organisms, which are more likely to be "silent" (Hawkins et al., 2004).

Subacute PID is far less dramatic, with a great variation in the severity and extent of symptoms. At times symptoms are so mild and vague that the woman ignores them. Symptoms that suggest subacute PID are chronic lower abdominal pain, dyspareunia, menstrual irregularities, urinary discomfort, low-grade fever, lower backache, and constipation. Abdominal examination usually reveals no rebound tenderness. Slight adnexal tenderness with cervical movement and cervical or urethral discharge (often purulent in nature) may be present.

There is no single laboratory test that can be used to detect upper genital tract infections. Endocervical testing for chlamydia and gonorrhea should be performed, but negative results do not rule out their presence in the upper genital tract. Other laboratory tests that are commonly performed include the wet mount, CBC, erythrocyte sedimentation rate (ESR), and C-reactive protein (CRP). Laboratory data are useful only when considered in conjunction with history and physical examination findings.

Clinical diagnosis of PID is imprecise; nevertheless, most diagnoses of PID are clinical because laparoscopy and biopsy are too expensive and invasive to be practical screening tools. The CDC established new minimum criteria for beginning treatment in 2002 (Table 18–12), because delay in diagnosis and treatment of PID is associated with severe sequelae. In addition, a diagnosis of PID should be considered in a woman with any pelvic tenderness or sign of lower genital tract inflammation.

DIFFERENTIAL DIAGNOSES

Symptoms of PID may mimic other disease processes such as ectopic pregnancy, endometriosis, ovarian cyst with torsion, pelvic adhesions, inflammatory bowel disease, or acute appendicitis.

MANAGEMENT

Perhaps the most important action a clinician can take is prevention counseling. Primary prevention would be education in avoiding STIs, whereas secondary prevention involves prompt treatment of lower genital tract infections to prevent ascension to the upper genital tract. Instructing women in self-protective behaviors such as practicing safer sex and using barrier methods is critical. Also important is the detection of asymptomatic gonorrheal and chlamydial infections through routine screening of women with risk factors. Partner notification when an STI is diagnosed is essential to prevent reinfection.

TABLE 18-12 Diagnosing PID

Empiric treatment of PID should be initiated for sexually active young women and others at risk for STIs if these minimum criteria are present and no other cause(s) for the illness can be found:

- Uterine/adnexal tenderness or
- Cervical motion tenderness

Additional criteria to support a diagnosis of PID include:

- Oral temperature > 101° F (> 38.3° C)
- Abnormal cervical or vaginal mucopurulent discharge
- Presence of white blood cells (WBCs) on saline microscopy of vaginal secretions
- Elevated erythrocyte sedimentation rate
- Elevated C-reactive protein
- Laboratory documentation of cervical infection with *N. gonorrheae* or *C. trachomatis*.

The most specific criteria for diagnosing PID include:

- Endometrial biopsy with histopathologic evidence of endometriosis
- Transvaginal sonography or magnetic resonance imaging techniques showing thickened, fluid-filled tubes with or without free pelvic fluid or tubo-ovarian complex
- Laparoscopic abnormalities consistent with PID

Source: CDC, 2002a.

In the past, the majority of women with PID were hospitalized so that bed rest and parenteral therapy could be started. Today approximately three-fourths of women with PID are not hospitalized (Ness & Brooks-Nelson, 2000). A randomized, controlled trial of 831 women with mild to moderate PID found no difference in short-term improvement and long-term reproductive outcomes (e.g., pregnancy rates, PID recurrence, chronic pelvic pain, and ectopic pregnancy) between those treated in inpatient and outpatient settings (Ness & Brooks-Nelson). The decision of whether or not to hospitalize should be based on each woman's individual circumstances. To guide clinicians' decisions regarding hospitalization, the CDC (2002a) has developed specific criteria for hospitalization including the need to rule out surgical emergencies (e.g., appendicitis); pregnancy; no clinical response to oral antimicrobial therapy; inability to follow or tolerate an outpatient oral regimen; severe illness, nausea and vomiting, or high fever; and tubo-ovarian abscess.

There are no current data to suggest that adolescents would benefit from hospitalization for treatment; however, there is some evidence that women over the age of 35 years are likely to have a more complicated course and thus may benefit from hospitalization (CDC, 2002a). Although treatment regimens vary with the infecting organism, a broad-spectrum antibiotic is generally used. Several antimicrobial regimens have proved to be effective, and no single therapeutic regimen of choice exists (Table 18–13). Minimal pelvic examinations should be done during the acute phase of the disease, and analgesics can be given for pain. During the recovery phase, the woman should restrict her activity and make every effort to get adequate rest and a nutritionally sound diet. Follow-up laboratory studies after treatment should include endocervical gonorrhea and chlamydia tests of cure.

TABLE 18–13   Treatment of Pelvic Inflammatory Disease

Parenteral Regimens	Oral Regimens
Parenteral Regimen A	*Oral Regimen A*
Cefotetan 2 g IV every 12 hours or	Ofloxacin 400 mg orally twice a day for 14 days
Cefoxitin 2 g IV every 6 hours	or
Plus Doxycycline 100 mg orally or IV every 12 hours	Levofloxacin 500 mg orally once daily for 14 days
	With or without Metronidazole 500 mg orally twice a day for 14 days
Parenteral Regimen B	
Clindamycin 900 mg IV every 8 hours	*Oral Regimen B*
Plus Gentamicin loading dose IV or IM (2 mg/kg of body weight) followed by a maintenance dose (1.5 mg/kg) every 8 hours. Single day dosing may be substituted.	Ceftriaxone 250 mg IM in a single dose or
	Cefoxitin 2 g IM in a single dose and Probenecid 1 g orally administered concurrently in a single dose or
Alternative Parenteral Regimen	Other parenteral third-generation cephalosporin (e.g., ceftizoxime or cefotaxime)
Ofloxacin 400 mg IV every 12 hours or Levofloxacin 500 mg IV once daily	Plus Doxycline 100 mg orally twice a day for 14 days
With or without Metronidazole 500 mg IV every 8 hours or Ampicillin/Sulbactam 3 g IV every 6 hours	With or without Metronidazole 500 mg orally twice a day for 14 days
Plus Doxycycline 100 mg orally or IV every 12 hours	

Source: CDC, 2002a.

Health education is central to effective management of PID. Clinicians should explain to women the nature of their infection and should encourage them to comply with all therapy and prevention recommendations, emphasizing the necessity of taking all medication, even if symptoms resolve. Any potential problems that would prevent a woman from completing a course of treatment, such as lack of money for prescriptions or lack of transportation to return to a clinic for follow-up appointments, should be identified and the importance of follow-up visits emphasized. The woman diagnosed with PID will need supportive care, because PID is so closely tied to sexuality, body image, and self-concept. Her feelings need to be discussed, and her partners included when appropriate.

SYPHILIS

Syphilis is one of the earliest described STIs and is a systemic disease. There are an estimated 40,000 cases of primary and secondary syphilis in the United States each year. During 1986–1990, an epidemic of syphilis occurred throughout the United States

(CDC, 1998). In 1991, syphilis rates began to decline and have continued to drop. The only area of the country that did not achieve the national health objectives for 2000 is the South, where rates remain substantially higher than the rest of the country. Syphilis rates are higher for heterosexual African-American and Hispanic women than they are for Caucasian women. Currently, approximately as many women as men have primary or secondary syphilis, which has also led to an increase in cases of congenital syphilis. In contrast to other bacterial STIs that affect mostly teens and adults under 34 years old, syphilis persists into the early 30s in both men and women. Additionally, as many as 15% of adolescents and adults with syphilis are HIV-positive.

Syphilis is caused by *Treponema pallidum*, a motile spirochete. The disease is characterized by periods of active symptoms and periods of asymptomatic latency. It can affect any tissue or organ in the body. Transmission is thought to be by entry in the subcutaneous tissue through microscopic abrasions that can occur during sexual intercourse. The infection can also be transmitted through kissing, biting, or oral-genital sex. A single sexual exposure to a person with active mucocutaneous syphilis carries up to a 50% risk of acquiring the disease (Jacobs, 2001).

Syphilis is a complex infection that can lead to serious systemic disease and even death when untreated. Infection manifests itself in distinct stages with different symptoms and clinical manifestations (Table 18–14). Primary syphilis is characterized by a primary lesion, or a chancre, which often begins as a painless papule at the site of inoculation and then erodes to form a nontender, shallow, indurated, clean ulcer several millimeters to a few centimeters in size. The chancre is loaded with spirochetes and is most commonly found on the genitalia though it may occur on the cervix, perianal area, or mouth. Secondary syphilis is characterized by a widespread, symmetrical maculopapular rash on the palms and soles and generalized lymphadenopathy. The woman may also experience fever, headache, and malaise. Condylomata lata (wartlike infectious lesions) may develop on the vulva, perineum, or anus. If the patient is untreated, she enters a latent phase that is asymptomatic for the majority of individuals. If left untreated, about one-third of patients will develop tertiary syphilis. Cardiovascular (chest pain, cough), dermatologic (multiple nodules or ulcers), skeletal (arthritis, myalgia, myositis), or neurologic (headache, irritability, impaired balance, memory loss, tremor) symptoms can develop in this stage. Neurologic complications are not limited to tertiary syphilis; rather, a variety of syndromes (e.g., meningitis, meningovascular syphilis, general paresis, and tabes dorsalis) may span all stages of the disease. In recent years, there has been evidence that the disease is shifting from these more traditional symptomatic forms of neurosphyilis to asymptomatic central nervous system involvement with subtler, less well-defined syndromes (Star & Deal, 2004b).

ASSESSMENT

Women with primary syphilis may be asymptomatic or they may report an anogenital lesion, typically raised, painless, and indurated. Seventy percent of women with secondary

TABLE 18–14   Stages of Syphilis

	Primary	Secondary	Early Latent	Late Latent	Tertiary
Time after exposure	9–90 days	6 weeks to 6 months	3–12 mo	>1 yr	Years
Duration	Weeks	Weeks	<2 yrs	>2 yrs	Variable
Infectious	Yes	Yes	No	No	Yes
Clinical symptoms	Chancre Painless lymphadenopathy	Skin lesions; papular rash of soles & palms; patchy alopecia; condylomata Symptoms of systemic illness (fever, malaise, anorexia, weight loss, headache, myalgias)			Symptomatic CNS disease Cardiovascular syphilis Skin lesions (gumma) Progressive bone destruction
Laboratory changes	Dark-field positive; serology often negative or rising titers VDRL & FTA-ABS	Dark-field positive; Peak antibody titers Seroconversion of FTA-ABS or MHA-TP positive CSF abnormal in up to 50% Proteinuria	CSF VDRL negative Falling VDRL titers	CSF VDRL negative Falling VDRL titers	CSF: VDRL positive or increased cells & protein, Serum treponemal positive; nontreponemal positive or negative VDRL remains positive indefinitely with declining titer

Sources: Hawkins, Roberto-Nichols, & Stanley-Haney, 2004; Star & Deal, 2004b.

syphilis will give a history of flu-like symptoms including sore throat, malaise, headache, fever, myalgias, arthralgias, hoarseness, and anorexia. These women may also report skin rashes on the trunk, extremities, palms, and soles that may be pruritic (Star & Deal, 2004b). Approximately 25% of patients will also report a persistent primary chancre. Some women will experience alopecia and have a "moth-eaten" look or lose the lateral one-third of an eyebrow. Occasionally women will have a history of low-grade fever. When syphilis is suspected, a comprehensive sexual risk history should be obtained.

The physical examination includes a general examination of the skin for alopecia and rash of feet, palms, and condylomata lata. Additionally, a pharyngeal examination and inspection for enlarged inguinal nodes should be conducted. The external genitalia are inspected for vulvar lesions and chancre at the point of inoculation. A speculum examination is done to inspect for lesions on the vaginal walls and cervix and for vaginal and cervical discharge. A bimanual examination is conducted to assess uterine size, shape, consistency, mobility, and tenderness, and to palpate for adnexal masses and tenderness. When history and clinical findings suggest the need, a neurologic examination should be done.

Darkfield examination and direct fluorescent antibody tests of lesion exudates or tissue provide definitive diagnosis of early syphilis. Diagnosis is dependent on serology during latency and late infection. Any test for antibodies may not be reactive in the presence of active infection, as it takes time for the body's immune system to develop antibodies to any antigens. A presumptive diagnosis is possible with the use of two serologic tests: nontreponemal and treponemal.

Nontreponemal antibody tests such as the VDRL and RPR are used as screening tests, and are relatively inexpensive, sensitive, moderately nonspecific, and fast. False positive results are not unusual with these tests, particularly when conditions such as acute infection, autoimmune disorders, malignancy, pregnancy, and drug addiction exist, and after immunization or vaccination. A high titer (> 1:16) usually indicates active disease. A four-fold drop in the titer indicates a response to treatment. Treatment of primary syphilis usually causes a progressive decline to a negative VDRL within two years. In secondary, latent, or tertiary syphilis, low titers persist in about 50% of cases after two years. Rising titer (four times) indicates relapse, reinfection, or treatment failure (Wallach, 1996).

The treponemal tests, fluorescent treponemal antibody absorbed (FTA-ABS) and microhemagglutination assays for antibody to *T. pallidum* (MHA-TP), are used to confirm positive results. Test results in patients with early primary or incubating syphilis may be negative. Seroconversion usually takes place six to eight weeks after exposure so testing should be repeated in one to two months when a suspicious genital lesion exists. Treponemal antibody tests frequently stay positive for life regardless of treatment or disease activity; therefore, treatment is monitored by the titers of the VDRL or RPR. Sequential serologic tests should be obtained by using the same method (VDRL or RPR), preferably by the same laboratory. Tests for concomitant STIs should be done, HIV testing offered and, if indicated, wet preps carried out.

TABLE 18–15   Treatment of Syphilis

Recommended	**Primary, secondary, and early latent syphilis:** Benzathine penicillin G 2.4 million units IM once **Late latent syphilis or latent syphilis of unknown duration:** Benzathine penicillin G 7.2 million units total, administered as three doses of 2.4 million units IM each at 1-week intervals
Alternatives if penicillin allergic*	**Primary, secondary, and early latent syphilis:** Doxycycline 100 mg orally twice a day for 14 days or Tetracycline 500 mg orally four times daily for 14 days **Late latent syphilis or latent syphilis of unknown duration:** Doxycycline 100 mg orally twice a day for 14 days or Tetracycline 500 mg orally four times daily for 14 days

*There are limited data to support these regimens; thus close follow-up is warranted.
Source: CDC, 2002a.

MANAGEMENT

Parenteral penicillin G is the preferred drug for treating patients with all stages of syphilis (Table 18–15). It is the only proven therapy that has been widely used for patients with neurosyphilis, congenital syphilis, or syphilis during pregnancy. Single dose therapy is used to treat primary, secondary, and early latent syphilis, although women who have had syphilis for longer than one year (late latent or tertiary stage) require weekly treatment for three weeks. Monthly follow-up is mandatory so that additional treatment may be given if needed. Clinicians should emphasize the necessity of long-term serologic testing even in the absence of symptoms.

HEPATITIS B

Hepatitis B virus (HBV) is a blood-borne pathogen transmitted by exposure to infectious blood or body fluids (e.g., semen, saliva). In 1998, an estimated 181,000 persons were infected with HBV in the United States, and an estimated 1.25 million people are chronically infected with HBV (CDC, 2002a). Overall prevalence of HBV infection differs among racial and ethnic populations and is highest among persons who have emigrated from areas with a high endemicity of HBV infections, such as Asia, the Pacific islands, Africa, and the Middle East (CDC, 2003). Hepatitis B chronic infection affects 5% of the world population.

Hepatitis B infection is caused by a large DNA virus and is associated with three antigens and their antibodies. Screening for active or chronic disease or disease immunity is

TABLE 18–16   Parameters of Hepatitis B Testing

HBsAg	Hepatitis B surface antigen
	Indicates patient has the infection and can transmit it to others
Anti-HBs	Hepatitis B surface antibody
	Indicates immunity resulting from vaccination or previous infection
Anti-HBc	Total hepatitis B core antibody
	Indicates previous or ongoing infection
IgM anti-HBc	IgM antibody to hepatitis B core antigen
	Indicates current infection or infection within the past six months

based on testing for these antigens and their antibodies (Table 18–16). HBV is approximately 100 times more infectious than HIV and 10 times more infectious than Hepatitis C virus (CDC, 2003). HBV infection is transmitted parenterally and through intimate contact. Hepatitis B surface antigen (HBsAg) has been found in blood, saliva, sweat, tears, vaginal secretions, and semen. Perinatal transmission does occur; however, the fetus is not at risk until it comes in contact with contaminated blood at birth. HBV has also been transmitted by artificial insemination.

Factors considered to place a woman at risk for HBV are those associated with STI risk in general (history of multiple sexual partners, multiple STIs, intravenous drug use), behaviors that are associated with blood contact (e.g., work or treatment in a dialysis unit), history of multiple blood transfusions, public safety workers exposed to blood in the workplace, health care workers, and persons born in a country with a high incidence of HBV infection. Although HBV can be transmitted via blood transfusion, the incidence of such infections has decreased significantly since the testing of blood for the presence of HBsAg became possible. Women who abuse drugs and share needles are at risk, as are women with a history of jail or prison experiences and a history of needlestick injury, tattoos, or body piercing.

HBV infection is a disease of the liver and is asymptomatic in up to one-third of persons with the infection. In both a child and an adult the course of the infection can be fulminating and the outcome fatal. Symptoms of HBV infection include arthralgias, arthritis, lassitude, anorexia, nausea, vomiting, headache, fever, and mild abdominal pain. Later the patient may have clay-colored stools, dark urine, increased abdominal pain, and jaundice. Between 6% and 10% of adults with HBV have a persistence of HBsAg and become chronically infected. Up to 25% of chronically infected individuals will die from primary hepatocellular carcinoma or cirrhosis of the liver.

ASSESSMENT

Components of the history to be obtained when hepatitis B is suspected include symptoms of the disease and risk factors outlined earlier. Women also should be asked about taste and smell peculiarities and intolerance of fatty foods and cigarettes. The clinician should ask about darkened urine and light-colored stools as well. Physical examination includes inspection of the skin for rashes, inspection of the skin and conjunctiva for jaundice, and palpation of the liver for enlargement and tenderness. Weight loss, fever, and general debilitation should be noted.

Interpretation of testing for hepatitis B is complex (Table 18–16). Women who have negative HBsAg, anti-HBc, and anti-HBs tests are susceptible to infection, and vaccination should be considered (see section on management). A woman with a positive anti-HBs test with negative HBsAg and anti-HBc tests has immunity from vaccination. A woman with a negative HBsAg test and positive anti-HBc and anti-HBs tests has immunity from previous infection that is now resolved. A woman with acute hepatitis B infection will have positive HBsAg, anti-HBc, and IgM anti-HBc tests and a negative anti-HBs test. A woman with chronic hepatitis B infection will have positive HBsAg and anti-HBc tests and negative IgM anti-HBc and anti-HBs tests. A woman with a positive anti-HBc test and negative HBsAg and anti-HBs tests should be referred for further evaluation, as this result has multiple interpretations. Women who have hepatitis B should be prepared for repeat testing as HBV serologic markers may also be used to monitor the progression of the disease. HIV testing should also be offered.

MANAGEMENT

All nonimmune women at high or moderate risk of hepatitis B should be informed of the existence of hepatitis B vaccine. Vaccination is recommended for all individuals who have had multiple sex partners within the past six months (CDC, 2002a). In addition, intravenous (IV) drug users, residents of correctional or long-term care facilities, persons seeking care for an STI, prostitutes, women whose partners are IV-drug users or bisexual, and women whose occupation exposes them to high risk should be vaccinated. Vaccination is not associated with serious side effects and does not carry a risk for contracting HIV. The vaccine is given as a series of three (some authorities recommend four) doses over a 6-month period with the first two doses given within one month of each other. In adults, the vaccine should be given in the deltoid muscle, never in the gluteus or quadriceps muscle. Women with a definite exposure to hepatitis B should be given hepatitis B immunoglobulin intramuscularly in a single dose as soon as possible within a seven-day period after exposure (CDC). There is no specific treatment for acute hepatitis B. Recovery is usually spontaneous in 3 to 16 weeks. Rest and a high-protein, low-fat diet are important. Education about preventing transmission of HBV to others is paramount. Women should be advised to increase their fluid intake, and to avoid medications metabolized in the liver, drugs, and alcohol. Women with chronic HBV should be referred to a specialist.

HUMAN IMMUNODEFICIENCY VIRUS

In the early summer of 1981, the occurrence of several rare illnesses such as *Pneumocystis carinii pneumonia, Mycobacterium,* and *M. intracellulare* infections, cryptosporidiosis, Kaposi's sarcoma, and non-Hodgkin's lymphoma in a cluster of gay and bisexual men represented a medical mystery that was solved by the identification of a single infectious agent that was destroying the immune system of infected persons—the human immunodeficiency virus (CDC, 1981). Although the earliest identified victims of the AIDS epidemic were typically homosexual men, symptoms of the syndrome were identified in a woman within two months of the earliest reports of the disease in men. Within the first year of the epidemic, female partners of hemophiliacs infected with HIV, female IV-drug abusers, and female partners in heterosexual relationships in poor countries, notably Haiti, were diagnosed with AIDS.

Deeply ingrained social and cultural forces that tend to devalue women, and particularly poor women of color, perpetuated the tendency for HIV and AIDS to be considered a "men's disease," and more specifically, a disease of homosexual men, that was underdiagnosed in women, However, the rapid spread of HIV among women is indisputable, with current estimates indicating that almost 17.6 million women worldwide are living with HIV and AIDS (CDC, 2002c; National Institute of Allergy and Infectious Diseases [NIAID], 2003).

The numbers of persons infected with HIV has increased rapidly since the virus was first identified almost two decades ago. Through the middle of 2001, 455,750 persons were reported to be living with HIV and AIDS in the United States (CDC, 2002c). AIDS is the fifth leading cause of death among women between the ages of 25 and 44 years, and the third leading cause of death in African-American women in this age group (CDC).

The growing number of women living with HIV and AIDS is a dominant feature of the AIDS epidemic (Anderson, 2001). Of persons with AIDS in 1992, 14% were women; by 1998, 20% of persons with AIDS were women (CDC, 2002c). Current CDC estimates are between 120,000 and 160,000 HIV-positive adult and adolescent women living in the United States (CDC, 2002c). Of the new infections among women in the United States, approximately 75% were infected through heterosexual sex and 25% through injection drug use (NIAID, 2003). Seventy-seven percent of all AIDS cases in the United States among women have occurred in African-American and Hispanic women, who compose less than a quarter of all women in the country (CDC, 2002d).

THE EFFECT OF HIV ON THE IMMUNE SYSTEM

The human immune system functions to protect the body from invasion by a variety of microbes and tumor cells. The immune system is composed of two arms: humoral immunity, involved with antibody production, and cellular immunity, effected largely through cytotoxic T-cells. Central components of the cellular arm of the immune system are macrophages and CD4+ T-cells. HIV is a retrovirus that specifically targets CD4+ T-cells, binding to the cell surface protein known as the CD4+ receptor. The virus affects the cells two ways. First, the absolute numbers of these cells are depleted; second, the function of the remaining cells is impaired, resulting in a gradual loss of immune function. Progressive depletion of CD4 cells in peripheral blood is the hallmark of advancing HIV disease (Greenblatt & Hessol, 2001).

Unimpeded, HIV can destroy up to one billion CD4 cells per day. In addition to its aggressive destruction, HIV is genetically highly variable, mutating with apparent ease.

HIV TRANSMISSION ISSUES SPECIFIC TO WOMEN

Women have several HIV transmission issues directly related to their age, anatomy, and to specific anatomic changes related to age. Several factors affect the relative ease with which women are infected with HIV during heterosexual vaginal intercourse. Of particular importance is the woman's age. Younger women have greater vaginally exposed cervical columnar epithelium, known to be a risk factor in the transmission of other STIs. Women taking oral contraceptives and pregnant women also have an increased exposure of columnar epithelium. This tissue is associated with endocervical inflammatory cells, and can bleed more easily during intercourse than does the stratified squamous epithelium found in the cervical os of older women.

The integrity of the tissues of the lower genital tract influence HIV transmission risk. Trauma during intercourse, STI-related inflammation or cervicitis, and an STI ulcer or chancre increase susceptibility to HIV infection. Postmenopausal women may be at a higher theoretic risk because of the thinning of vaginal tissues related to decreased estrogen, increasing their risk of trauma during intercourse (Stratton & Alexander, 1997). Any activity or condition that disrupts the tissues of the vagina may predispose a woman to infection with HIV. This includes the use of highly absorbent tampons, which are associated with vaginal desquamation with long-term use. Similarly, the disruption of tissues through receptive penile-anal intercourse provide a highly efficient means of HIV transmission (Stratton & Alexander).

HIV can be transmitted through receptive oral sex with ejaculation. Any condition that interrupts the integrity of oral tissues, including periodontal disease, increases the risk of HIV transmission in this manner.

Female to female sex poses a small risk of transmission, especially in sexual activities that may result in some level of vaginal trauma. Women who have sex with women may also have a history of sex with men. Assuming that a woman is of very low risk for HIV because she has an expressed sexual preference for women overlooks the fact that many lesbians have a history of sexual intercourse with men, or may have other risk factors for HIV infection.

ASSESSMENT

Pretest Counseling   HIV testing is a serious matter with a number of social, ethical, and psychological implications, in addition to the obvious health care related issues. A woman who chooses HIV testing is in need of both pre- and posttesting counseling and education, regardless of the test results. An overview of counseling is provided here, and the reader is referred to the CDC (2001a) guidelines on this topic for detailed information. State laws vary regarding disclosure of a positive diagnosis for HIV to persons other than the patient, such as spouses or sexual contacts. The clinician must inform the patient of these regulations prior to testing, so that she can be fully informed as to the social and legal implications of a positive test. For many women, partner notification may make her very vulnerable to abuse and violence in the event she is HIV positive. Informed consent must be obtained prior to HIV testing, and some states require written consent (CDC, 2002a). Informed consent must indicate that the individual understands that she is being tested for HIV and is doing so voluntarily. Testing for HIV is recommended and should be offered to all women seeking evaluation for and treatment of STIs (CDC). All women seeking HIV testing should also be tested for HBV.

Diagnostic Tests   HIV infection is usually diagnosed by tests for antibodies against HIV-1 and HIV-2. The enzyme-linked immunosorbent assay (ELISA) is the most commonly used test to detect HIV antibodies. Two tests on the same sample must be reactive for a person to be considered HIV antibody-positive. If the ELISA is reactive, then a more specific confirmatory test such as the Western Blot (WB) or an immunofluorescence assay (IFA) is conducted. Antibodies to HIV can be detected in 95% of persons within three months after exposure to the virus. Although a negative antibody test usually indicates that a person is not infected, these tests cannot detect a recent infection. A patient with a negative test who is at very high risk for contracting the virus should be retested at three to six months after the initial baseline test. A person with a specific exposure to HIV, such as in an occupational setting or via unprotected sexual contact with a person known to have HIV, should be tested serially. Testing should occur at the time of the exposure to determine the baseline serologic status, then at three- and six-month intervals until seroconversion is determined, or the person remains seronegative for one year.

Posttest Counseling   Regardless of the results, the posttest visit is very emotional for the patient. Test results should be disclosed immediately in the visit because the patient may be very anxious regarding the outcome. A patient who is seronegative for HIV should receive counseling and education regarding behavioral changes to reduce the risk of contracting HIV. The news that one is negative for HIV will be met with relief and immediate reduction of anxiety. However, it is crucial that patients who are tested for HIV based on risky behaviors be counseled carefully. The patient will also need to be counseled that she may want to be tested serially if she has engaged in very high-risk behaviors. This is to prevent the ongoing assumption that the woman is seronegative for HIV, when in fact she may have been tested between the time of infection and the development of antibodies. Hepatitis B vaccination is recommended for all women who are not immune to hepatitis B.

If the test is positive for HIV, the woman must be given time to react emotionally. She must assimilate a lot of information at the time of this visit. Allowing her to express her feelings prior to discussing issues related to partner notification, treatments, and other issues may allow her to take in the some of the important information that must be conveyed at this time.

Women with HIV must understand that although they may exhibit no signs or symptoms of HIV disease, they are still infectious, and will be for life. Basic information regarding minimizing transmission risk must be relayed to the patient at this time. A specific goal is to minimize the risk of transmission of the virus to others; therefore, the patient needs to understand immediately the implications of her HIV seropositivity in terms of transmission risk. Furthermore, the clinician must assess the need for further supportive services for the psychological and emotional needs of the newly diagnosed HIV positive patient.

A plan for treatment must be established. For many patients, this means referral to an infectious disease setting that can provide expert care for her infection. Unless the patient is clearly immunocompromised and in need of immediate treatment for opportunistic infection, there is likely to be an interval between diagnosis and treatment decisions. This time can be used by the woman to begin to adapt emotionally and psychologically to her diagnosis. She can make decisions about who must be told about her infection, and institute behaviors that are required of her to minimize the risk of transmitting the virus to others. Sensitive and nonjudgmental care at this time can assist the newly diagnosed HIV positive woman to make healthy adaptations to her diagnosis.

MANAGEMENT

Effective management and treatment of the patient with HIV involves the use of antiretroviral therapy (ART) to slow viral replication. The goal of ART is to decrease the peripheral blood levels of the virus to levels undetectable by current means of measurement. There are three categories of HIV ARTs:

1. Nucleoside reverse transcriptase inhibitors (NRTIs)
2. Nonnucleoside reverse transcriptase inhibitors (NNRTIs)
3. Protease inhibitors (PIs)

NRTIs and NNRTIs work by disrupting the work of reverse transcriptase, an enzyme that changes the virus's chemical genetic message into a form that can be easily inserted inside the nucleus of an infected cell. This process occurs early in the viral replication cycle. Reverse transcriptase inhibitors interrupt the duplication of genetic material necessary for the virus to replicate. PIs work inside infected cells late in the HIV replication process. After HIV has infected a cell, it continues relentlessly to replicate itself. However, the newly produced genetic material, in the form of long chains of proteins and enzymes, is functional only after these long chains have been cut into shorter pieces by the HIV enzyme protease. By inhibiting the function of protease, PIs reduce the number of new infectious copies of HIV. Combination therapy with multiple ARTs is currently recommended for most patients. Chemoprophylaxis for opportunistic infections may also be warranted. Basic health practices such as adequate sleep and rest, good nutrition, exercise, smoking cessation, and avoidance of stress should be recommended to persons with HIV.

Current guidelines by the Panel on Clinical Practices for Treatment of HIV Infection (1999) recommend that care of persons with HIV be supervised by an expert in infectious disease. Prompt referral should be initiated. Detailed treatment of HIV is beyond the scope of this chapter. The research and development of new therapies and the testing of different combinations of therapies can quickly change the state of the science. Clinicians are encouraged to use reliable sources (e.g., CDC, National Institutes of Health) available on the Internet for the most current recommendations and practices in HIV care. A list of reliable Web sites is found at the end of the references for this chapter.

Very few diseases in history have been associated with the high levels of stigmatization that may accompany an HIV diagnosis. Many persons with HIV choose to keep their diagnosis a secret from family, friends, and coworkers. Although this means they must hide clinic visits, medications, and HIV-related illnesses, they may feel this is preferable to experiencing the stigma that accompanies this diagnosis. Persons with HIV may face the dissolution of important relationships when and if the diagnosis becomes known. Clinicians can assist patients in identifying supportive persons who can be helpful as the patient adapts to the diagnosis and ART when initiated. However, the clinician must take care not to assume that the patient can tell anyone, and should respect the patient's decisions about disclosure of the diagnosis.

Clinicians can help patients reframe their understanding of HIV, particularly in terms of understanding it as a chronic disease that can be managed, rather than as a terminal illness. Many patients on learning of their HIV become seriously depressed, expect to die soon and with much pain. Intervening early with these patients may prepare them to live with the disease, rather than simply waiting to die. Furthermore, many persons with HIV are recognized as long-term nonprogressors who, although infected with HIV, do not progress to AIDS even years after infection. Researchers have found that there are psychological and behavioral factors that may play a role in the continuing viral suppression of nonprogressors. These factors include the following:

1. Viewing HIV as a manageable illness
2. Taking care of their physical health
3. Staying connected with others in supportive relationships
4. Taking care of their emotional and mental health
5. Nurturing their spiritual well-being (Barroso, 1999)

These means of adapting to the very serious diagnosis of HIV can assist the woman with HIV to regain a sense of control and hope. Clinicians stand in a unique position to understand the multiplicity of factors and issues that face persons with HIV. Awareness of these factors can enhance health care by improving both the physical and mental health of patients, as well as the long-term health outcomes for women with HIV.

SEXUALLY TRANSMITTED INFECTIONS DURING PREGNANCY

Perinatal outcomes can be affected by various STIs because pregnant women may transmit the infection to their fetus, newborn, or infant through vertical transmission (via the placenta, during vaginal birth, or after birth through breastfeeding) or horizontal transmission (close physical or household contact). Some STIs (like syphilis) cross the placenta and infect the fetus in utero. Other STIs (like gonorrhea, chlamydia, hepatitis B, and genital herpes) can be transmitted as the baby passes through the birth canal. HIV can cross the placenta during pregnancy, be transmitted during the birth process and, unlike most other

STIs, can infect the baby during breastfeeding. The harmful effects of STIs may include stillbirth, low birth weight (less than five pounds), conjunctivitis, pneumonia, neonatal sepsis, neurologic damage (such as brain damage or lack of coordination in body movements), blindness, deafness, acute hepatitis, meningitis, chronic liver disease, and cirrhosis. Some of these problems can be prevented if the woman is screened and treated for STIs during pregnancy. Other problems can be treated if the infection is found in the newborn. A pregnant woman with an STI may also have early onset of labor, premature rupture of the membranes, and uterine infection after delivery. STI treatment regimens may differ for pregnant women. Clinicians should consult the most current CDC treatment guidelines and selected chapter references for further information about STIs in pregnancy (Faro, 2001; Star et al., 2004).

CONCLUSION

STIs are among the most common health problems of women in the United States and the world. Women experience a disproportionate amount of the burden associated with these illnesses, including complications of infertility, perinatal infections, poor pregnancy outcomes, chronic pelvic pain, genital tract neoplasms, and potentially death. Additionally, these infections interfere with a woman's lifestyle and cause considerable distress, both emotional and physical. Clinicians can help to ameliorate the misery, morbidity, and mortality associated with STIs and other common infections through accurate, safe, sensitive, and supportive care. The reader should be aware that knowledge of STIs is constantly increasing and changing with new and improved prevention, diagnostic, and treatment modalities now being developed and reported. All clinicians have a responsibility to stay current with these developments through reviewing current journals, attending conferences, and being knowledgeable about recommendations and bulletins from the CDC. Furthermore, it is important that clinicians be aware of policies, recommendations, and guidelines of the state in which they practice, which also may change frequently.

REFERENCES

Alan Guttmacher Institute. (1999). *Facts in brief: Teen sex and pregnancy.* Retrieved November 11, 2004, from http://www.agi-usa.org/pubs/fb_teen_sex.html.

Anderson, J. R. (2001). *A guide to the clinical care of women with HIV.* Rockville, MD: U.S. Department of Health and Human Services, Health Resources and Service Administration, HIV/AIDS Bureau.

Balch, J. F., & Balch, P. A. (1997). *Prescription for prevention* (2nd ed.). Garden City Park, NY: Avery.

Barroso, J. (1999). Long-term nonprogressors with HIV disease. *Nursing Research, 48*(5), 242–249.

Benenson, A. S. (1995). *Control of communicable diseases manual* (16th ed.). Washington, DC: American Public Health Association.

Brown, K. (2004). *Management guidelines for nurse practitioners working with women* (2nd ed.). Philadelphia: F. A. Davis.

Carcio, H. (1999). *Advanced health assessment of women.* Philadelphia: Lippincott.

Cates, J., Alexander, L., & Cates, W. J. (1998). Prevention of sexually transmitted diseases in an era of managed care: The relevance for women. *Women's Health Issues, 8*(3), 169–186.

Centers for Disease Control and Prevention. (1981). Pneumocystis pneumonia—Los Angeles. *Mortality and Morbidity Weekly Review, 30,* 250–252.

Centers for Disease Control and Prevention. (1995). *Annual report 1994.* Atlanta, GA: U.S. Department of Health and Human Services.

Centers for Disease Control and Prevention (1998). Primary and secondary syphilis—United States, 1997. *Mortality and Morbidity Weekly Review, 47*(24), 493–497.

Centers for Disease Control and Prevention. (2001a). Revised guidelines for HIV counseling, testing, and referral. *Mortality and Morbidity Weekly Review, 50,* 1–58.

Centers for Disease Control and Prevention. (2001b). Special focus profiles: STDs in women and infants. In *Sexually transmitted disease surveillance 2000.* Atlanta, GA: U.S. Department of Health and Human Services.

Centers for Disease Control and Prevention. (2002a). Sexually transmitted diseases treatment guidelines 2002. *Mortality and Morbidity Weekly Review, 51*(RR-6), 1–80.

Centers for Disease Control and Prevention. (2002b). Screening tests to detect chlamydia trachomatis and neisseria gonorrhoeae infections—2002. *Mortality Morbidity Weekly Review, 51*(RR-15), 1–38.

Centers for Disease Control and Prevention. (2002c). *HIV/AIDS among US women: Minority and young women at continuing risk.* Retrieved November 11, 2004, from www.cdc.gov/hiv/pubs/facts/women.htm.

Centers for Disease Control and Prevention. (2002d). *Public health service task force recommendations for the use of antiretroviral drugs in pregnant women infected with HIV-1 for maternal health and for reducing perinatal HIV-1 transmission in the United States.* Retrieved November 11, 2004, from http://aidsinfo.nih.gov/guidelines/perinatal/PER_062304.html.

Centers for Disease Control and Prevention (2003). Prevention and control of infection with hepatitis viruses in correctional settings. *Mortality and Morbidity Weekly Review, 52*(RR-1), 1–3.

Cummings, S., & Ullman, D. (1997). *Everybody's guide to homeopathic medicines.* New York: Putman.

Cunningham, F. G., MacDonald, P. C., Gant, N. F., Leveno, K. J., Gilstrap, L. C., Hankins, et al. (2002). *Williams obstetrics* (21st ed.). Stamford, CT: Appleton & Lange.

Dickey, R. P. (2000). *Managing contraceptive pill patients* (10th ed.). Dallas, TX: Emis Medical.

Dolcini, M., Coates, T. J., Catania, J. A., Kegeles, S. M., & Hauck, W. W. (1995). Multiple sexual partners and their psychosocial correlates: The population-based AIDS in multiethnic neighborhoods (AMEN) study. *Health Psychologist, 14*(2), 22–31.

Faro, S. (2001). Chlamydia trachomatis. In S. Faro & D. E. Soper (Eds.), *Infectious diseases in women.* Philadelphia: W. B. Saunders.

Fogel, C. I. (1995). Sexually transmitted diseases. In C. I. Fogel & N. F. Woods (Eds.), *Women's health care.* Thousand Oaks, CA: Sage.

Fogel, C. I., & Lauver, D. (1990). *Sexual health promotion.* Philadelphia: Saunders.

Forna, F., & Gulmezoglu, A. M. (2002). Interventions for treating trichomoniasis in women (Cochrane Review). In *Cochrane Library, 4,* 2002. Oxford, UK: Update Software.

Futterman, D. (2001). Adolescents. In J. R. Anderson (Ed.), *A guide to the clinical care of women with HIV.* Rockville, MD: Womencare.

Gall, S. A. (2001). Human papillomavirus. In S. Faro & D. E. Soper (Eds.), *Infectious diseases in women.* Philadelphia: Saunders.

Gonen, V. (1999). Confronting STDs: A challenge for managed care. *Women's Health Issues, 9*(Suppl. 2), 36S–46S.

Gorroll, A. H. (2001). Approach to the patient with a vaginal discharge. In A. H. Gorroll & A. G. Mulley (Eds.), *Primary care medicine: Office evaluation and management of the adult patient.* Baltimore: Williams & Wilkins.

Greenblatt, R. M., & Hessol, N. A. (2001). Epidemiology and natural history of HIV infection in women. In J. R. Anderson (Ed.), *A guide to the clinical care of women with HIV.* Rockville, MD: Womencare.

Grella, C. E., Anglin, M. D., & Annon, J. J. (1996). HIV risk behaviors among women in methadone maintenance treatment. *Substance Abuse & Misuse, 31,* 277–301.

Griffith, H. W. (2000). *Healing herbs: The essential guide.* Tucson, AZ: Fisher Books.

Harris, R. M., & Kavanagh, K. H. (1995). Perception of AIDS risk and high-risk behaviors among women in methadone maintenance treatment. *Substance Abuse & Misuse, 31,* 277–301.

Hatcher, R. A., Trussell, J., Stewart, F., Nelson, A. L., Cates, W., Guest, F., et al. (2004). *Contraceptive technology* (18th ed.). New York: Ardent Media.

Hawkins, J. W., Roberto-Nichols, D. M., & Stanley-Haney, J. L. (2004). *Guidelines for nurse practitioners in gynecologic settings* (8th ed.). New York: Springer.

Henderson, D. (1997, November). *Transition to community for incarcerated addicted women.* Paper presented at the 49th Annual Meeting of the American Society of Criminology, San Diego, CA.

Institute of Medicine. (1997). *The hidden epidemic: Confronting sexually transmitted diseases.* Washington, DC: National Academy Press.

Jacobs, R. A. (2001). Infectious diseases: Spirochetal. In L. M. Tierney, S. J. McPhee, & M. A. Papadakis (Eds.), *Current medical diagnosis and treatment, 2001.* New York: Lange Medical Books/McGraw Hill.

Kearney, M. H. (2001). *Perinatal impact of alcohol, tobacco and other drugs* (2nd ed.). White Plains, NY: Educational Services, March of Dimes.

Koutsky, L. A., Ault, K. A., Wheeler, C. M., Brown, D. R., Barr, E., Alvarez, F. B., et al. (2002). A controlled trial of a human papillomavirus type 16 vaccine. *New England Journal of Medicine, 347*(21), 1645–1651.

Kurth, A. (1998). Promoting sexual health in the age of HIV/AIDS. *Journal of Nurse-Midwifery, 43*(3), 162–181.

MacLauren, A. (1995). Primary care for women: Comprehensive sexual health assessment. *Journal of Nurse-Midwifery, 40,* 104–119.

MacRae, R., & Aalto, E. (2000). Gendered power dynamics and HIV risk in drug-using sexual relationships. *AIDS Care, 12*(4), 505–514.

Maman, S. C. (2000). The intersections of HIV and violence: Directions for future research and interventions. *Social Science & Medicine, 50,* 459–478.

Mays, V. M., & Cochran, S. D. (1988). Issues in the perception of AIDS risk and risk reduction activities by black and Hispanic/Latina women. *American Psychology, 43,* 949–957.

McCoy, H. V., McCoy, C. B., & Lai, S. (1998). Effectiveness of HIV interventions among women drug users. *Women & Health, 271*(2), 49–66.

McFarlane, J., Parker, B., & Cross, B. (2001). *Abuse during pregnancy: A protocol for prevention and intervention* (2nd ed.). White Plains, NY: Educational Services, March of Dimes.

Miller, S., Exner, T. M., Williams, S. P., & Ehrhardt, A. A. (2000). A gender-specific intervention for at-risk women in the USA. *AIDS Care, 13*(3), 603–612.

Mize, S. J. S., Robinson, B. E., Bockting, W. O., & Scheltma, K. E. (2002). Meta-analysis of the effectiveness of HIV prevention interventions for women. *AIDS Care, 14*(2), 163–180.

National Institute of Allergy and Infectious Diseases. (2003). *HIV/AIDS Statistics.* Retrieved June 7, 2003, from www.niaid.nih.gov/factsheets/aidsstat.htm.

Ness, R., & Brooks-Nelson, D. (2000). Pelvic inflammatory disease. In M. B. Goldman & M. C. Hatch (Eds.), *Women and health.* San Diego, CA: Academic Press.

Nissim, R. (1996). *Natural healing in gynecology: A manual for women.* San Francisco: HarperCollins.

Nyamanthi, A. M., & Lewis, C. E. (1991). Coping of African American women at risk for AIDS. *Women's Health Issues, 1*(2), 53–62.

Page, L. (2000). *Healthy healing* (11th ed.). Carmel Valley, CA: Healthy Healing.

Panel on Clinical Practices for the Treatment of HIV Infection (1999). *Guidelines for the use of antiretroviral agents in HIV-infected adults and adolescents.* Washington, DC: U.S. Department of Health and Human Services and the Henry J. Kaiser Foundation.

Public Health Service. (1979). *Healthy people: The surgeon general's report on health promotion and disease prevention.* Washington, DC: GPO.

Schaffer, S. D. (2003). Vaginitis and sexually transmitted diseases. In E. Q. Youngkin & M. S. Davis (Eds.), *Women's health: A primary clinical guide* (3rd ed.). Upper Saddle River, NJ: Pearson Prentice Hall.

Schmid, G. P. (2001). Epidemiology of sexually transmitted infections. In S. Faro & D. E. Soper (Eds.), *Infectious diseases in women.* Philadelphia: Saunders.

Shannon, M. T. (2004). Pediculosis. In W. L. Star, L. L. Lommel, & M. T. Shannon (Eds.), *Women's primary health care* (2nd ed.). San Francisco: UCSF Nursing Press.

Sinclair, C. (2004). *A midwife's handbook.* St. Louis, MO: Saunders.

Singingtree, D. (1993). Herbal helps. *Midwifery Today, 26,* 16.

Stapleton, H., & Tiran, D. (2000). Herbal medicine. In D. Tiran & S. Mack (Eds.), *Complementary therapies for pregnancy and childbirth* (2nd ed.). Edinburgh, UK: Bailliere Tindall.

Star, W. (2004). Sexually transmitted diseases. In W. L. Star, L. L. Lommel, & M. T. Shannon (Eds.), *Women's primary health care* (2nd ed.). San Francisco: UCSF Nursing Press.

Star, W., & Deal, M. (2004a). Gonorrhea. In W. L. Star, L. L. Lommel, & M. T. Shannon (Eds.), *Women's primary health care* (2nd ed.). San Francisco: UCSF Nursing Press.

Star, W., & Deal, M. (2004b). Syphilis. In W. L. Star, L. L. Lommel, & M. T. Shannon (Eds.), *Women's primary health care* (2nd ed.). San Francisco: UCSF Nursing Press.

Star, W. L., Lommel, L., & Shannon, M. T. (2004). *Women's primary health care* (2nd ed.). San Francisco: UCSF Nursing Press.

Stevens, J., Zierlier, S., Cram, V., Dean, D., Mayer, K., & DeGroot, A. (1995). Risks for HIV infection in incarcerated women. *Journal of Women's Health, 4*(5), 569–577.

Stratton, P., & Alexander, N. (1997) Heterosexual spread of HIV infection. In D. Cotton & D. Watts (Eds.), *The medical management of AIDS in women.* New York: Wiley-Liss.

Wallach, J. (1996). *Interpretation of diagnostic tests.* Boston: Little, Brown.

Wang, C., & Celum, C. (2001). Prevention of HIV. In J. R. Anderson (Ed.), *A guide to the clinical care of women with HIV.* Rockville, MD: Womencare.

Wheeler, L. (2002). *Nurse-midwifery handbook: A practical guide to prenatal and postpartum care* (2nd ed.). Philadelphia: Lippincott Williams & Wilkins.

Wiley, D. J., Douglas, J., Beutener, K., Cox, T., Fife, K., Moscicki, et al. (2002). External genital warts: Diagnosis, treatment, and prevention. *Clinical Infectious Diseases, 35,* S210–S224.

INTERNET RESOURCES

http://aidsinfo.nih.gov

This site is dedicated to presenting the most up-to-date recommendations for HIV and AIDS management. The Panel on Clinical Practices for Treatment of HIV Infection posts its latest recommendations on this site, which is maintained by the HIV/AIDS Treatment Information Service.

www.cdc.gov

The Centers for Disease Control and Prevention maintains the site, which provides many STI and HIV/AIDS resources including the STD Treatment Guidelines.

www.engenderhealth.org

EngenderHealth's Web site has online minicourses about STIs and HIV/AIDS.

www.hopkins-aids.edu

This comprehensive site is maintained by the Johns Hopkins AIDS Service.

www.thebody.com

This site is also maintained by the HIV/AIDS Treatment Information Service. This site is highly informative, and is geared to the general public rather than specifically to health care providers, although its information is certainly useful to health care providers who are seeking simplified explanations or quick references. This site is typically very readable, and covers a wide variety of topics associated with HIV and AIDS.

| Chapter 19 | MENSTRUAL CYCLE PAIN AND DISCOMFORTS |

DIANA TAYLOR
KERRI DURNELL SCHUILING
BETH A. COLLINS SHARP

In the past decade, multidisciplinary efforts have increased women's power to institute changes in their health status through cross-disciplinary research that builds on the wisdom of early pioneers. Recently, an interdisciplinary group proposed a more precise classification—cyclic perimenstrual pain and discomfort (CPPD)—that encompasses a broader perspective about cyclic pelvic pain (CPP), cyclic moods, and physical discomforts (Association of Women's Health, Obstetric, and Neonatal Nurses [AWHONN], 2003). This original work provides scientific evidence about a widespread women's health problem overlooked by the majority of the health care community. The recognition of CPPD as an entity separate from previously identified medical or psychiatric diagnostic classifications is significant because it validates additional distressing symptoms as "real" and enables the development of effective treatment guidelines based on scientific evidence incorporating cross-disciplinary perspectives as well as personal evidence from women's own experiences.

HISTORICAL OVERVIEW

Most women, at some time during their childbearing years, experience CPP and other discomforts associated with the menstrual cycle (Collins Sharp, Taylor, Kelly-Thomas, Killeen, & Dawood, 2002). Historically, paternalistic views of menstrual related experiences prevailed and biomedical language predominated with little attention paid to alternative perspectives from other disciplines or, more importantly, from a woman's perspective.

In the mid-1980s, professional medical organizations in the United States and the United Kingdom met to define Premenstrual Syndrome (PMS), and the published proceedings established the medical basis for the presentation and clinical existence of PMS as a disease classification (Dawood, McGuire, & Demers, 1985; Halbreich, 1997). From that point forward, paternalistic labeling shifted to medical diagnosis. Recognized in the International Classification of Diseases Manual of the World Health Organization (WHO, 1992), the popular and quasi-medical term PMS describes the cyclical recurrence of symptoms that impair a woman's health, relationships, and occupational functioning. Although met with much controversy, the American Psychiatric Association (APA) has recognized the diagnostic term premenstrual dysphoric disorder (PMDD) in the third and fourth editions of its *Diagnostic and Statistical Manual* (APA, 1987, 1994). PMDD is a diagnostic label that applies to a much smaller number of menstruating women experiencing severe PMS with predominantly negative affect symptoms.

DEVELOPMENT OF EVIDENCE-BASED CLINICAL PRACTICE GUIDELINES

An interdisciplinary group of scientists and clinicians sponsored by AWHONN developed clinical practice guidelines (AWHONN, 2003) based on a broad range of clinical, empirical, and theoretical evidence (Collins Sharp et al., 2002). The goal was to provide a comprehensive description of a complex women's health problem that encompasses more than the individual concepts of dysmenorrhea, PMS, and PMDD. These guidelines recommend the term CPPD to differentiate normal cyclic changes associated with menstruation from the severe, debilitating menstrual and premenstrual symptom experiences that require professional or pharmacologic intervention. Perimenstrual refers to the period from about 7 to 10 days before menstrual flow begins until the first or second day of menstrual flow (Collins Sharp et al.; Woods, Most, & Dery, 1982a). Although the term CPPD references the negative end of the perimenstrual experience spectrum, it reflects the woman's experience, rather than her personal attributes or a medically imposed diagnosis, and is based on a range of rigorously reviewed empirical studies using both quantitative and qualitative methods. The AWHONN guidelines provide evidence-based clinical practice recommendations that are helpful to women's health professionals in accomplishing the following objectives:

- Screening for cyclic perimenstrual symptoms as routine in women's health care
- Conducting a targeted assessment to identify perimenstrual symptom patterns
- Implementing evidence-based therapeutic strategies applicable to cyclic perimenstrual symptoms (including PMS)
- Assisting women with self-care activities and referring them to other providers as appropriate (AWHONN, 2003)

The American College of Obstetricians and Gynecologists (ACOG) has also developed clinical management guidelines designed to aid practitioners in making decisions about appropriate PMS diagnosis and treatment (ACOG, 2000). The focus is on diagnosing and treating PMS—rather than on assessing a woman's symptom experience across the menstrual cycle—with the aim to assist her in developing symptom management or self-care strategies.

SCOPE AND PREVALENCE OF THE PROBLEM

The menstrual cycle is a normative process; however, about 10% of women experience severe recurring symptoms associated with their menstrual cycle. In well-designed studies of community-based, nonclinical samples, the prevalence of perimenstrual symptoms was 30% to 50%, with pain, fatigue, mood swings, and physical discomforts reported most commonly (Woods, Most, & Dery, 1982b). As the *Diagnostic and Statistical Manual-IV* (*DSM-IV)* definition of PMDD acknowledges, mild symptoms such as bloating and breast tenderness affect up to 70% of menstruating women; thus, these symptoms should not be considered "disordered" (APA, 1994). However, between 5% and 14% of women report perimenstrual symptoms so severe that they are disabling (Angst, Sellaro, Merikangas, & Endicott, 2001), and another 30% to 40% of women have perimenstrual symptoms that are bothersome enough that they seek professional advice (Woods, Lentz, et al., 1997; Woods, Taylor, Mitchell, & Lentz, 1992). A review of several recent studies suggests that between 4% and 7% of women qualify for a diagnosis of PMDD (Ross & Steiner, 2003). Based on these prevalence studies, an estimated 35 million women will experience mild to moderate PMS and 5–7 million will have severe PMS (Woods, Most, & Dery; Woods, Mitchell, Lentz, Taylor, & Lee, 1987). Table 19–1 provides a comparison of clinical labels and diagnostic classifications of the perimenstrual symptom experience.

Focusing on perimenstrual symptoms rather than a disease-oriented syndrome provides a model for understanding complex gender-specific conditions that include biologic, psychosocial, and cultural factors. This holistic model can be applied to other women's health problems such as stress-related conditions (heart disease, arthritis, and immune system disorders), psychiatric disorders, or normative menstrual cycle transitions (menarche, postpartum, and menopause).

TABLE 19–1   Perimenstrual Symptom Experience: Comparing Clinical Labels and Diagnostic Classifications

	Perimenstrual Symptom Experience		
Clinical Label and Diagnostic Classification	Cyclic Perimenstrual Pain and Discomforts (CPPD)	Premenstrual Syndrome (PMS)	
	Perimenstrual Symptoms–Primary Dysmenorrhea		Premenstrual Dysphoric Disorder (PMDD)
Intensity/Distress	Mild to Moderate	Moderate	Severe
Pattern	Few hours to 5 days	6–9 days	10–14 days

CLINICAL PRESENTATION

Research has identified several common patterns of perimenstrual symptoms (Collins Sharp et al., 2002; Moos, 1969; Taylor, 1986; Woods, Mitchell, & Lentz, 1999). In a factor and cluster analysis of data from a cross-sectional population-based sample, Woods, Mitchell, and Lentz identified four symptom clusters that accounted for much of the variance in women's experience of the premenstrual phase:

- *Turmoil*—Hostility, depression, anger, feeling out of control, tension, guilt feelings, tearfulness, anxiety, rapid mood changes, nervousness, irritability, desire to be alone, loneliness, and impatience
- *Fluid retention*—Weight gain, abdominal bloating or swelling, painful breasts, swelling of hands and feet, and skin disorders
- *Somatic symptoms*—Nausea, lowered desire to move, decreased food intake, abdominal pain, headaches, decreased sexual desire, and aches and pains
- *Arousal*—Bursts of energy or activity, increased sexual desire, impulsiveness, increased food intake, increased sense of well-being, and cravings for certain foods or tastes

Turmoil was the dominant symptom cluster in terms of explaining variance in premenstrual symptoms, and fluid retention was the most important cluster for distinguishing women with low-symptom severity from those with PMS or premenstrual magnification. Woods, Mitchell, and Lentz conclude that these symptom clusters are reliable indicators of premenstrual symptoms that are sensitive to cycle phase differences. Somatic symptoms and arousal symptoms were highly stable across the menstrual cycle, and these clusters were poorly correlated with each other. The researchers speculate that somatic and arousal symptoms might be independent of menstrual cycle phases.

Based on much of the research from Woods and associates, the AWHONN guidelines identify a composite diagnosis of three perimenstrual symptom clusters (Collins Sharp et al., 2002). For clinicians, considering symptom clusters is a more efficient and pragmatic approach to assessment and intervention. In addition to symptom clusters, the clinical presentation of CPPD or PMS includes symptom severity (mild to severe), symptom distress (degree of bother), and symptom pattern (by menstrual cycle phase).

CYCLIC PERIMENSTRUAL PAIN AND DISCOMFORT

Cyclic perimenstrual pain and discomfort addresses symptom clusters that occur both before and after the menstrual flow begins (Box 19–1). The primary feature of CPPD is a cluster of cyclic symptoms that includes pain, discomfort, and mood symptoms (Collins Sharp et al., 2002), and encompasses three nursing diagnoses, each representing a cluster of symptoms (AWHONN, 2003).

The recognition of CPPD as a diagnosis distinct from medical diagnoses relative to menstrual cycle pain and discomforts does not negate the importance of the biologic-based diagnoses and therapies. Instead, a more inclusive diagnosis encourages an integrated approach to assessment and treatment. This approach is woman centered and relies

> ## BOX 19-1   CPPD SYMPTOM CLUSTERS
>
> **Cyclic perimenstrual pain and discomforts (CPPD)** includes dysmenorrhea and pelvic pain as well as other perimenstrual physical and mood symptoms. It is distinguished by three major symptom clusters: cyclic pelvic pain, perimenstrual physical discomforts, and perimenstrual mood discomforts.
>
> Perimenstrual refers to the span of time from approximately 7–10 days before menstrual flow (premenstrual phase) begins through the first one to two days of menstrual flow (menstrual phase).
>
> **Cyclic Pelvic Pain (CPP)** is subjectively identified acute discomfort that occurs in the abdominal area circumscribed by the pelvis and that recurs in a pattern associated with the menstrual cycle. Other pain symptoms related to CPP are abdominal cramps, backache, nausea, vomiting, diarrhea, and change in bowel frequency.
>
> **Perimenstrual Physical Discomforts** are painful physical symptoms other than those commonly associated with CPP that escalate around the time of menstruation and subside after menses begins. Symptoms include fatigue, headaches, fluid retention, joint aches and pains, breast tenderness, leg/thigh discomforts, and change in energy and appetite.
>
> **Perimenstrual Mood Discomforts** are psychological symptoms that escalate around the time of menstruation and subside after menses begins. Symptoms include depression, irritability, tension, impatience, anxiety, anger, mood swings, hostility, change in sexual desire, guilt, feeling out of control, and tearfulness.
>
> *Source: AWHONN, 2003.*

on the woman as the expert "knower." Her description of symptoms, their severity, and affect on her life assists in the diagnosis and management of the problem. Using an integrated approach to assess, diagnose, and treat perimenstrual symptoms encourages the use of complementary and pharmacologic treatment modalities. An integrated approach also encourages women to participate in decision making and to take responsibility for those treatment regimens within their control such as nutrition and exercise.

CYCLIC PELVIC PAIN (PRIMARY DYSMENORRHEA)

Many women report experiencing CPP that significantly impacts their quality of life. This includes lost work or school time, expenses for self-care, over-the-counter (OTC) treatments, and visits to health care professionals (AWHONN, 2003). Between 30% and 60% of women of childbearing age will suffer from CPP, as previously defined by its medical diagnosis of primary dysmenorrhea (AWHONN; Smith, 1993). Dysmenorrhea is categorized as primary or secondary based on the presence of known etiology or pelvic pathology. As medically defined, primary dysmenorrhea is diagnosed by exclusion when painful menstruation occurs in the absence of pathology. Secondary dysmenorrhea involves an underlying pathology acting directly or indirectly on the pelvic anatomy to cause pain symptoms during menstrual flow. Another form of CPP is "mittelschmerz," a German term used to denote midcycle pain often associated with ovulation. This type of cyclic pelvic pain is far less common than dysmenorrhea.

Therefore, the term CPP more clearly specifies the woman's experience of menstrually related pain, and is defined as subjectively identified acute discomfort that occurs in the abdominal area circumscribed by the pelvis, and that recurs in a pattern associated with normative menstrual cycle processes (AWHONN, 2003). The incidence of CPP is as high as 80% for women in their teens and early twenties, with one-half of these women experiencing loss of time from school or work (Dawood, 1990). For 10% to 20% of women, CPP is so severe it is disabling (Harlow & Park, 1996; Smith, 1993). Young women in their teens and early twenties experience menstrual pain most often, with the onset occurring within three years of menarche (Sundell, Milsom, & Andersch, 1990).

PERIMENSTRUAL PHYSICAL AND MOOD SYMPTOMS

Perimenstrual symptoms are cyclic changes of mild intensity that are viewed as troublesome or problematic by women, but are usually not severe enough to interfere with a woman's ability to perform her typical roles (Woods, Mitchell, & Taylor, 1999). These symptoms express themselves as physical or mood discomforts. Symptoms usually escalate around the onset of the menses and subside shortly after menses begins; thus the term "perimenstrual." Factor and cluster analysis of perimenstrual symptoms in community-based populations have identified symptom clusters such as negative affect, fluid retention, pain and somatic symptoms, and behavioral changes (Woods, Mitchell, & Lentz, 1999). The most prevalent symptoms reported include cramps, mood swings, fatigue, swelling, irritability, tension, skin disorders, headache, depression, backache, breast tenderness, weight gain, anxiety, and crying (Woods, Most, & Dery, 1982c). These symptoms are either psychological or physical in nature, and some are not routinely considered in a medical model differential diagnosis of PMS or dysmenorrhea (AWHONN, 2003). Grouping the symptoms into clusters is important because it facilitates a better understanding of women's perimenstrual experiences and provides for a more accurate direction of therapeutic strategies.

OTHER MENSTRUAL DIAGNOSES

PREMENSTRUAL SYNDROME

The term PMS is used to indicate the cyclic recurrence of distressing physical, mood, and behavioral experiences that often affect interpersonal relationships, personal health, and a woman's ability to function (Woods, Mitchell, & Lentz, 1999) (Box 19–2). The hallmark of the syndrome has been defined as the repeated occurrence of behavioral, somatic, and mood symptoms severe enough to impair a woman's social and work-related functioning during the perimenstrual phase of the menstrual cycle (Mitchell, Woods, Lentz, & Taylor,

BOX 19-2   OTHER MENSTRUAL DIAGNOSES

Dysmenorrhea is difficult or painful menses. The medical literature differentiates primary and secondary dysmenorrhea. Primary dysmenorrhea is associated with multiple symptoms including: abdominal cramps, headache, backache, general body aches, continuous abdominal pain, and other somatic discomforts (Dawood & Ramos, 1990) and is more common than secondary dysmenorrhea. There is no evidence of organic pathophysiology in the uterus, fallopian tubes, or ovaries with primary dysmenorrhea (Kinch & Robinson, 1985). Secondary dysmenorrhea involves underlying pathology that causes pain during menses.

Premenstrual Syndrome (PMS) is a diagnostic term used to indicate cyclical recurrence of distressing physical, mood, and behavioral experiences that often affect interpersonal relationships and personal health and function (Woods, Mitchell, & Taylor, 1999). A PMS symptom pattern can be discerned by the absence of symptoms or low severity symptoms after menses (post-menses, defined as approximately days 6 through 10 of the cycle), followed by an escalation in symptoms premenses during the seven days preceding the next menses that subside again at the onset (or first few days) of menses.

Premenstrual Dysphoric Disorder (PMDD) is a diagnostic label now included in the *Diagnostic and Statistical Manual IV* of the American Psychiatric Association (1994) and replaces the earlier label of late luteal phase dysphoric disorder. This diagnosis applies to a subset of women suffering from severe PMS with an emphasis on mood symptoms.

Premenstrual Magnification (PMM) is a variant of the premenstrual syndrome pattern in which women experience moderately severe symptoms postmenses, and more severe symptoms premenses (Mitchell, Woods, & Lentz, 1991). This variant may represent an exacerbation of an ongoing mental health problem or physical disorder (Harrison, 1985). Women with conditions such as eating disorders, bipolar disorder, substance abuse disorder, major depression, anxiety, or personality disorders will experience symptoms of their disorder throughout the menstrual cycle, but the symptoms are more severe during the premenstrual phase.

1991). PMS has a distinct symptom pattern: no or low severity of symptoms after menses, followed by an escalation in symptom frequency and severity pre-menses, that subsides again at the onset (or first few days) of menses (Mitchell, Woods, & Lentz, 1994). Changes in other perceptions are also evident, such as emotional and physical feelings of stress, including anticipatory stress in advance of symptoms (Hamilton, Alagna, & Sharpe, 1985; Rubinow, Schmidt, & Roca, 1998a; Taylor, Woods, Lentz, Mitchell, & Lee, 1991; Woods, Lentz, Mitchell, Taylor, & Lee, 1992). Behavioral patterns, such as angry outbursts or low impulse control that precipitate interpersonal conflict, may also occur (Woods, Mitchell, & Lentz). Successful management of PMS begins with the assessment of symptom clusters, symptom severity patterns, and their degree of impact on a woman's functional status.

There is disagreement among clinicians about whether or not PMS is a distinct disease entity. Many argue that PMS is a culture-bound syndrome (Condon, 2004). This suggests that the experience of PMS is socially constructed and related in some way to society's beliefs about and attitudes toward the individuals experiencing the problem. Regardless of cause, the experience of PMS is very real and distressing for many women, and therefore assessment and effective treatment regimens are important for their overall health.

PREMENSTRUAL MAGNIFICATION

Premenstrual magnification (PMM) is another syndrome distinct from PMS (Box 19–2). This term refers to the exacerbation of somatic or mood symptoms in the late luteal or menstrual phase of the cycle (Harrison, 1985). Conditions that may worsen during the premenstrual or menstrual phase include depressive disorders, panic or anxiety disorders, migraines, seizure disorders, irritable bowel syndrome (IBS), asthma, chronic fatigue syndrome, and allergies (Mitchell, Woods, & Lentz, 1994). Premenstrual symptoms or CPPD may coexist with other conditions such as mood disorders, asthma, migraines, thyroid disorders, seizure disorders, or arthritis. This is considered a dual diagnosis. Women who have PMM of an illness or who feel sick before or during menstruation may also have some characteristics of CPPD or PMS.

PREMENSTRUAL DYSPHORIC DISORDER

PMDD is a separate diagnostic label that applies to a much smaller number of menstruating women and requires at least one affective symptom (Box 19–2). The APA first included the diagnostic term "late luteal phase dysphoric disorder" (LLPDD) in the third edition of its *Diagnostic and Statistical Manual (DSM-III)*, published in 1987 (APA, 1987). Although this term was listed in the research appendix, as a condition "requiring further study," it was given a diagnostic code, list of symptoms, and cutoff points, exactly like diagnostic labels in the main text of the *DSM-III* that were considered to be supported by scientific evidence. After an extensive literature review, an LLPDD subcommittee of the APA concluded in 1994 that very little research supported the existence of premenstrual mental illness (in contrast to PMS). Nevertheless, the term LLPDD was revised to PMDD and is included in the *DMS-IV* in the research appendix and also in the main text under Depressive Disorders (APA, 1994). There is no question that some women experience a more severe form of PMS, but the legitimization of PMDD or severe PMS as a psychiatric disorder troubles many feminist and medical scholars. In spite of the US Food and Drug Administration (FDA) approval of the antidepressant fluoxetine (Prozac/Sarafem) as a treatment for PMDD in 1999, a European drug regulator required the manufacturer (Lilly) to delete PMDD as an indicated disorder for fluoxetine treatment (Moynihan, 2004). The European Committee for Proprietary Medicinal Products found that "PMDD [was] not a well-established disease entity across Europe," was not listed in the International Classification of Diseases (ICD), and was listed only as a research diagnosis in the *DMS-IV* (Moynihan).

ETIOLOGY

BIOLOGIC

A strong body of knowledge supports a biologic etiology for cyclic menstrual pain or dysmenorrhea. Dawood and associates (1985) established that there is an increase or imbalance in the quantity of prostaglandins present in the menstrual fluid of women with dysmenorrhea. The excessive amounts of prostaglandins cause the uterus to contract abnormally and reduce uterine blood flow and oxygenation, giving rise to pain. However, almost any process that can affect the pelvic viscera and cause acute or intermittent recurring pain might be a source for cyclic perimenstrual pain, including urinary tract infection, endometriosis, pelvic inflammatory disease, uterine fibroids, interstitial cystitis, hernia, IBS, and pelvic relaxation (Dawood, 1990; Smith, 1993). Identifying the cause of perimenstrual cyclic pelvic pain can be difficult because the health care provider must distinguish dysmenorrhea from other pelvic pain that occurs in a cyclic manner outside the time of the menstrual flow (ACOG, 2004; Smith).

The etiologic mechanisms for cyclic perimenstrual physical and mood discomforts, PMS, or PMDD are even less clear. Although a number of biologic and neuroendocrine etiologies have been proposed, they have been mostly simple, direct, unsubstantiated pathophysiologic models such as hormonal imbalances, sodium retention, nutritional deficiencies, or abnormal hypothalamic-pituitary-adrenal axis function (Backstrom et al., 1983; Keye, 1989; O'Brien, 1987; Reid & Yen, 1981). A number of investigators have hypothesized the neuroregulatory effects of ovarian hormones on central serotonin systems in humans as inferred from (mostly animal) studies demonstrating the impact of gender, estrus cycle, or hormone manipulation (Rubinow, Schmidt, & Roca, 1998b). This menstrual cycle hormone-serotonin hypothesis is unconfirmed and is based primarily on indirect tests using selective serotonin reuptake inhibitor (SSRI) antidepressants (Freeman, 1997).

Integration of Biologic, Genetic, and Environmental Factors   More recent empirical and theory testing research points to an integrative etiology that links genetics, environmental stressors, and hormonal processes with individual vulnerabilities (Endicott, 2001; Halbreich, 1997, 1999; Kendler, Karkowski, Corey, & Neale, 1998; Rubinow & Schmidt, 1995; Schmidt, Nieman, Danaceau, Adams, & Rubinow, 1998; Taylor, Woods, Lentz, Mitchell, & Lee, 1991). Perimenstrual symptoms and syndromes may act as modulators of other disorders or they may be an abnormal response to normal biologic rhythms (e.g., the menstrual cycle, circadian rhythms, adrenocortical pulses) (Cahill, 1998; Lewis, Greenblatt, Rittenhouse, Veldhuis, & Jaffe, 1995; Reame et al., 1996; Reame, Marshall, & Kelch, 1992; Ross, Sellers, Gilbert-Evans, & Romach, 2004; Taylor et al.; Thys-Jacobs, 2000; Ussher, 2002). PMS is most likely a psychoneuroendocrine disorder whereby psychosocial variables become influential in lowering the individual's threshold to experience perimenstrual symptoms in response to normal or abnormal biologic changes of the menstrual cycle in the context of a multifaceted interaction between the central nervous system (CNS), hormones, and other modulators. A few well-designed studies have empirically tested the hypothesis that biologic and psychosocial variables interact to result in vulnerability to mood and behavioral changes across the menstrual cycle (Taylor et al.). The effect of stressors and stress response was not only direct, but operated through generalized distress mediated by poor health behaviors. Multiple well-crafted laboratory studies from the National Institutes of Mental Health Behavioral Endocrinology Branch have tested the putative roles of pituitary, ovarian, and adrenal steroids in the etiology of PMS, and results do not support a primary endocrine abnormality in PMS patients, but indicate that the understanding of these disorders lies in contextual factors rather than in hormonal excesses or deficiencies (Bloch, Schmidt, Su, Tobin, & Rubinow, 1998; Rubinow et al., 1998a; Schmidt et al., 1998).

In a study of 1312 menstruating twins, lifetime major depression, premenstrual tiredness, sadness, and irritability were retrospectively assessed twice over six years. Premenstrual depression and anxiety were moderately stable over time and the investigators estimate that the heritability of this stable component of premenstrual symptoms was 56%. Moreover, the results suggest that there is no close etiologic relationship between PMS and major depression. Although premenstrual symptoms and major depression were found to share genetic and environmental risk factors, 88% of the genetic variance for premenstrual symptoms, and 88% of the environmental variance were not shared with major depression (Kendler et al., 1998). PMDD may have a different pattern of heritability, as suggested by a recent report on the relationship between a polymorphism in the serotonin transporter gene and the severity of PMDD symptoms (Praschak-Rieder et al., 2002).

PSYCHOSOCIAL STRESSORS AND SOCIOCULTURAL FACTORS

A number of studies have suggested that the manifestation of PMS, particularly perimenstrual mood discomforts, may result from a combination of multiple stressors, a heightened stress response, few supports, and a vulnerable period of biologic reactivity. Stress perception and stressful experiences appear to influence the reporting of premenstrual symptoms, and biopsychosocial factors (altered stress hormones, low self-esteem, negative life changes, increased stress response) increase the severity of PMS (Gallant, 1991; Taylor et al., 1991; Woods et al., 1998). Women with PMS report more stressors and experience them as more distressing than women without PMS (Freeman, Sondheimer, & Rickels, 1988; Gise, Lebovits, Paddison, & Strain, 1990). Women with premenstrual symptoms may use relatively ineffective methods of coping with stress, such as avoidance or wishful thinking, rather than effective strategies such as problem-solving communication or direct action (Ross, 2004; Taylor, 1996a).

A history of sexual abuse, particularly in childhood, seems to be common among women seeking treatment for severe PMS. Among 42 women with severe PMS who agreed to be interviewed about their sexual abuse history, 95% reported at least one attempted or completed sexual abuse event, with 81% reporting rape with penetration (Golding, Taylor, Menard, & King, 2000).

Sociocultural factors appear to influence what symptoms women notice and what symptoms they consider to be problematic. Two of the largest cross-cultural studies suggest that the reported incidence of various premenstrual changes is high in many different countries and that a large number of women throughout the world report physical discomfort and mood changes associated with menstruation (Janiger, Riffenburgh, & Kersh, 1972; WHO, 1981). Perimenstrual symptom experiences appear to differ by geographic location, marital status, parity, education, and occupation (Futterman, Jones, Miccio-Fonseca, & Quigley, 1992; Huerta-Franco & Malacara, 1993; Woods, Dery, & Most, 1982). Some analyses of cross-cultural differences suggest that women in Western societies have been socialized to have negative expectations about menstruation. Mexican women who viewed a videotape describing the negative consequences of PMS later reported more severe premenstrual symptoms compared with women in a control group who watched a neutral video (Marvan, Diaz-Erosa, & Montesinos, 1998).

The onset of PMS or perimenstrual symptom severity seems to occur across the reproductive lifespan, although women who report experiencing the most severe symptoms tend to be in their late thirties. However, experiencing more severe symptoms at this time may be because they coincide with increasing stress in a woman's life (Lee & Rittenhouse, 1992; Taylor, 1996a, 1996b). The menopausal transition has also been associated with the onset of perimenstrual mood discomforts or PMS (Woods, Lentz, Mitchell, Heitkemper, & Shaver, 1997). One hypothesis suggests that as women age, brain receptors are not as resilient to hormonal fluctuations as they were in earlier years (Rubinow et al., 1998b). In general, studies reveal that older women report more symptoms premenstrually and younger women report more symptoms during menstruation. There is evidence that two-thirds of adolescent females have some degree of dysmenorrhea, with rates higher for adolescents than for adults (Freeman, Rickels, & Sondheimer, 1993; Sundell et al., 1990).

Young girls learn about symptoms from observing their mothers, sisters, and peers, including their expectations regarding menstrual experiences and the effects of menstruation on feelings and behavior (Woods, Mitchell, & Lentz, 1999). Mothers' experiences with premenstrual symptoms appear linked to daughters' subsequent symptom experiences and illness behavior. Indeed, exposure to a mother with premenstrual symptoms and teachings about negative effects of menstruation were associated with negative affect symptomatology during the premenses and menses for adult women (Taylor et al., 1991). Women who have perimenstrual symptoms may come to anticipate having them and perceive events around the time of menstruation as more stressful.

It is unlikely that any single general theory can explain the flare-up of premenstrual symptoms for all women. Although PMS and PMDD have been predominantly regarded as biologically based illnesses, there is strong evidence that variables such as life stress, stress response, history of sexual abuse, and cultural socialization are important determinants of perimenstrual symptoms. The prevailing view is that women with PMS are more sensitive to what are essentially normal hormonal shifts, and as a result develop symptoms that do not affect other menstruating women. Some of these physiologic changes may make more of a difference for some women who experience PMS than for others. For example, it may be that one woman is particularly sensitive to premenstrually induced low blood sugar, and another might be hypersensitive to changes in serotonin levels. Perhaps changes in the levels of gonadal steroids that are released by the pituitary gland trigger a change in some women's moods, or otherwise predispose them to mood instability. For some women, response to stress may be the key factor. Moreover, it may be that women with PMS have trouble coping with physiologic shifts as well as with other stressful aspects of their lives, which exacerbates the intensity of their premenstrual symptoms.

TRANSLATING RESEARCH INTO PRACTICE

Cyclic perimenstrual pain and discomfort represents a family of symptom clusters that require the clinician to balance several seemingly dichotomous views: normative versus pathologic, one dimensional versus multidimensional, acute versus chronic, and protocol versus individualized care. The goal for practice related to the menstrual cycle and perimenstrual experiences is to normalize these experiences for women, and to help women understand them in the context of their life transitions, personal characteristics, and environmental stressors.

A few of the assumptions that underpin the assessment and therapeutic strategies for women experiencing perimenstrual pain and discomforts include the following:

- Personal and social changes have health effects that are as important, if not more important, than the biologic changes of the menstrual cycle.
- Biologic changes should not be ignored, but rather viewed in the context of biobehavioral relationships, including, but not restricted to, the levels of hormones.
- Multiple factors both promote and prevent women from caring for their own health.

Clinicians can have a significant impact on the care of women with cyclic perimenstrual pain, discomforts, and PMS by using the evidence-based approach to assessing, diagnosing, and managing cyclic perimenstrual pain and discomfort as developed by AWHONN's science team (Collins Sharp et al., 2002) and the evidence-based clinical guideline (EBG) development group (AWHONN, 2003).

ASSESSMENT

The conventional medical approach to assessment and diagnosis focuses on ruling out pathology. Data for assessment and diagnosis are collected during the medical history, physical exam, laboratory assessments, and differential diagnoses. The challenge as women's health clinicians is to integrate the strengths of a feminist approach to clinical practice with biomedical knowledge and skills. A feminist model of intervention focuses on women-centered care, advocacy, health promotion, and self-care.

The goal for assessment is to understand each individual woman's perimenstrual experience and to help her define and manage distressing symptoms and their concomitant problems. Much of the assessment process can be assumed by the woman herself with the help of self-assessment tools (Taylor & Colino, 2002) and professional guidance (AWHONN, 2003). Prospective assessment of individual symptoms or symptom clusters is the recommended method and can be accomplished by the use of a calendar or symptom checklist kept for two to three consecutive cycles (Mitchell, 1991; Shaver & Woods, 1985).

Three professional societies have proposed diagnostic criteria for use in clinical assessment of perimenstrual symptoms. Each one emphasizes thorough symptom assessment. The AWHONN guidelines emphasize that assessment of difficulties related to the menstrual cycle require attention to the interaction of medical, psychological, sociocultural, and lifestyle factors. Figure 19–1 presents important questions for general screening and a focused health history (AWHONN, 2003).

In addition to a focused health history and physical examination, distinguishing perimenstrual symptoms and discomfort patterns across at least three menstrual cycle phases is optimal: premenstrual phase (up to 14 days prior to onset of menses), menstrual phase (days during menses), and the postmenstrual phase (after menses and before ovulation) (AWHONN 2003; Mitchell et al., 1991; Mitchell, 1991).

According to the ACOG, the key criteria for a diagnosis of PMS are as follows:

- Symptoms consistent with PMS
- Consistent occurrence of the symptoms only during the luteal phase of the menstrual cycle
- Negative impact of symptoms on some facet of the woman's life
- Exclusion of other diagnoses that may better explain the symptoms (ACOG, 2000)

For a diagnosis of PMDD, the APA requirements are the following:

- Five or more symptoms, including affective and physical symptoms, are present during the week before menses and are absent in the follicular phase
- One of the symptoms is irritability, depressed mood, anxiety, or affective lability
- The symptoms markedly interfere with occupational or social functioning
- The symptoms are not due to an exacerbation of another disorder
- The above criteria have been confirmed by prospective daily ratings over at least two menstrual cycles (APA, 1994)

However, recent evidence suggests there is not enough support to establish PMDD as a separate classification from severe PMS or CPPD (Moynihan, 2004).

Symptom Assessment Based on research and professional recommendations, CPPD and PMS are individualized experiences requiring a dynamic and personalized assessment and diagnosis, which includes self-monitoring of symptoms, rating symptom severity, and the identification of patient-specific symptom clusters and patterns. Screening should assess for pelvic pain at or around the time of menstruation, other related discomforts, and the

Focused Nursing Assessment

SCREENING QUESTIONS

- Do you ever have pelvic pain or cramps during or around the time of your period?
- Are you able to treat this pain so it doesn't bother you?
- Do you ever have other physical or mood discomforts during or around the time of your period?
- Are you able to treat these discomforts so they don't bother you?

FOCUSED HEALTH HISTORY

- **Investigation of presenting problem/chief complaint**
  - Identify the individual woman's pattern of CPPD. The cycle may be divided into three phases: premenstrual, early menstrual (days 1–3 or days of heavy flow) and late menstrual (day 4 and onward or days of lighter flow).
    - Pattern of severity of CPP across pre- and early menstrual phases
    - Rating of overall distress caused by CPP
    - Pattern of severity of other cyclic discomforts across pre- and early menstrual phases
    - Rating of overall distress caused by cyclic discomforts
    - Influences on the cyclic symptoms — e.g., work stress, diet or exercise
  - A symptom checklist and calendar are useful for collecting these data (Figure 19–2).
- **Medical history**
  - Medical problems
  - Depression, anxiety, eating disorders
  - Surgeries
- **Focused family history**
  - Maternal and sibling CPPD experience and beliefs
  - Family response to CPPD
  - Cultural remedies
- **Menstrual history**
  - Age at menarche
  - First day of last menstrual period
  - Description of usual cycle (length, flow, regularity)
  - Any changes in usual cycle
- **Present health status**
  - Health perception
  - Current medications, complementary therapies
  - Drug allergies

- **Identification of the individual woman's pattern of symptom management**
  - Interventions, including self-care strategies
  - Pattern of use across pre- and early menstrual phases
  - Rating of relief obtained from intervention
  - Rating of satisfaction with pain and symptom control
  - Rating of adherence (consistent use of treatment)
- **Sexual history**
  - Sexual orientation and current sexual activity
  - Number of partners
  - Satisfaction with current sexual practices
  - Protection from sexually transmitted infections
  - Contraception
  - Physical or sexual assault or abuse
  - Risk-taking behaviors (alcohol, drugs, age of partners)
- **Obstetric history**
  - Gravity, parity, abortions
  - Living children
  - Complications related to pregnancy and birth
- **Health behaviors/functional status**
  - Nutrition
  - Exercise
  - Sleep/rest
  - Self-perception/concept
  - Roles and relationships
  - Family, social and occupational stressors
  - Coping skills
    - Health promoting
    - Health damaging

FOCUSED PHYSICAL EXAMINATION

- Abdominal examination: inspection, auscultation, percussion, palpation
  - Assess rebound tenderness (peritoneal inflammation)
  - Iliopsoas and obturator muscle tests (appendicitis)
- Percussion for costovertebral angle tenderness and palpation for suprapubic tenderness (pyelonephritis, urinary tract infection)
- External examination: inspection, palpation
- Internal examination: inspection, palpation, assessment cervical motion and tenderness
- Laboratory evaluation as indicated by history and examination

Figure 19–1 Focused Health History & Physical Exam. *Source:* © 2003 by the Association of Women's Health, Obstetric, and Neonatal Nurses. All rights reserved.

effectiveness of currently used therapies. AWHONN (2003) suggests four screening questions (Figure 19–1), a focused health history and physical examination, and a CPPD symptom assessment (type, severity, pattern).

Symptom Monitoring   Symptom monitoring is essentially educating women in self-diagnosis. Getting in touch with symptoms includes simply listing and rating feelings, symptoms, and behavioral changes, as well as a focus on social and physical environmental factors. Careful symptom assessment through daily monitoring and use of a diary of daily experiences can be therapeutic (Taylor, 1996b). Women can see their own patterns of symptoms and the relationship between these symptoms and the circumstances of their lives as well as the menstrual cycle. Not only will daily monitoring of these factors help women determine the severity and pattern of their symptoms, but it will also provide the basis for making healthy changes all month long.

Although prospective assessment is the recommended method of assessing symptom severity, distress, and pattern, retrospective assessment can be an initial first step in determining symptom distress. Retrospective symptom severity reports are likely to overestimate severity and do not provide data about symptom patterns. Prospective ratings are critical to precise diagnosis and to rule out other chronic illnesses. Retrospective assessment can include the following questions:

- In your own words, describe the pain and discomforts that are the most severe and distressing to you.
- What is the pattern of pain and discomforts during a typical menstrual cycle? How many days before, during, or after your period do you notice symptoms? Do they occur around ovulation?
- Does anything in particular—such as work stress, dietary influences, or exercise— worsen or alleviate symptoms?

IDENTIFYING AND RATING SYMPTOM CLUSTER SEVERITY AND DISTRESS

Once a woman has identified her most distressing or bothersome discomforts by symptom cluster, she can then rate the severity and degree of distress prospectively over one to two menstrual cycles. Prospective assessment of cyclic pain and discomforts can be accomplished by the use of a calendar or symptom checklist. A menstrual or symptom calendar is useful for women who are able to describe their unique symptoms and symptom clusters, as well as to visualize symptom severity patterns. Women fill in their most distressing symptoms beginning on the first day of their last menstrual period, using the following 5-point rating scale:

0—No severity
1—Minimal severity
2—Mild severity
3—Moderate severity
4—Extreme severity

An example of a calendar method of symptom assessment can be found in Figure 19–2 (Taylor & Colino, 2002). Women who have difficulty describing their symptoms or who have many symptoms may find it easier to use a symptom-severity checklist to identify symptoms and symptom clusters (Mitchell et al., 1991; Mitchell, Woods, Lentz, Taylor, & Lee, 1992; Taylor & Colino).

DETERMINING SYMPTOM CLUSTER SEVERITY AND DISTRESS PATTERNS

It is important to clearly delineate symptoms, their patterns, and how they are related (or not) to the menstrual cycle because PMS and perimenstrual symptom clusters have no clearly defined cause. A number of investigators have found that many women who believed they had PMS were later found to have another problem, such as endometriosis, which worsened around the time of menstruation. In other instances, a woman's mood or behavior changes—which may have been heightened during the premenstrual phase—were attributed to PMS when, in fact, they were a result of external problems such as work-related stress, relationship difficulties, problems with children, on-the-job harassment, violence, and other legitimate sources of anxiety, fear, and frustration. Alternatively, when examining a completed chart, women discover that certain symptom clusters—pain and fatigue, for example—continue all month long but just worsen premenstrually. This exercise helps a woman to gain a sense of self-awareness and become more attuned to how her perimenstrual experiences manifest themselves as symptoms, feelings, or behaviors, as well as the degree to which they affect her life.

Once symptom clusters have been identified and tracked for one or two menstrual cycles, symptom patterns can be classified. There are three to four common classifications of cyclic pain and discomfort patterns:

- When women have a low severity of perimenstrual pain and discomforts, they experience few bothersome symptoms of low to mild severity in the menstrual or premenstrual phases, or they may have one or two symptoms that are rated as moderate to severe but last only for one or two days.
- The classic CPP (or in a medical model, dysmenorrhea) pattern includes multiple pain symptoms that are rated as moderate or severe for one day premenstrually and three to five menstrual days. Symptoms completely subside after menses but might also include cyclic headaches and physical discomforts such as bloating.
- The classic PMS pattern or cyclic perimenstrual mood and physical discomforts include symptoms that are rated as moderate to extremely severe for up to two weeks before the onset of menses, and symptoms that subsequently disappear or become much milder within one to four days of the onset of bleeding.
- With PMM, women have symptoms that are cyclic in the sense that they are present during the postmenstrual (follicular) and early premenstrual (luteal) phases, but often increase in severity during the premenstrual phase. Many women who have this pattern deserve careful evaluation to determine whether they are

CPPD Symptom Calendar

INSTRUCTIONS

Menstrual cycle day: Begin with the first day of menstrual flow and end with the last day of your menstrual cycle. If you are only experiencing symptoms during your menstrual flow (and not before), you may stop your calendar when your flow stops.

Month and date: Write the month and the corresponding date in the box under each menstrual cycle day.

Bleeding/menstrual flow: Record your menstrual flow or vaginal bleeding as heavy (H), moderate (M), light (L), spotting (S) or, if no bleeding, leave the box blank. Note the last day of your menstrual flow with an asterisk (*).

Symptoms: Rate these symptoms or behavior changes daily as mild (1), moderate (2), severe (3) or extreme (4) throughout the cycle.

Menstrual cycle day	1	2	3	4	5	6	7	8	9	10	11	12	13	14	15	16	17	18	19	20	21	22	23	24	25	26	27	28	29	30	31
Month/date																															
Bleeding/menstrual flow																															
Cyclic pelvic pain																															
• Abdominal cramps																															
• Nausea, vomiting																															
• Backache																															
• Change in bowel frequency																															
Physical discomforts																															
• Fatigue																															
• Headaches																															
• Fluid retention																															
• Joint aches and pain																															
• Breast tenderness																															
• Leg/thigh discomfort																															
• Change in energy and appetite																															
Mood discomforts																															
• Depression																															
• Irritability																															
• Tension																															
• Impatience																															
• Anxiety																															
• Anger																															
• Mood swings																															
• Hostility																															
• Change in sexual desire																															
• Guilt																															
• Feeling out of control																															
• Tearfulness																															

Note: From *Taking Back the Month: A Personalized Solution for Managing PMS and Enhancing Your Health* (p. 285), by D. Taylor and Stacey Colino, 2002, New York: Berkley Publishing. Copyright 2002 by Diana Taylor and Stacey Colino. Adapted with permission. This form may be duplicated for use in clinical practice only. Permission for use in any other form must be obtained from AWHONN.

Figure 19–2 Calendar Method for Perimenstrual Symptom Assessment

Source: © 2003 by the Association of Women's Health, Obstetric, and Neonatal Nurses. All rights reserved.

experiencing a premenstrual exacerbation of another disorder such as depression, anxiety, substance abuse, headaches, allergies, asthma, IBS, or chronic pelvic pain.

Laboratory Assessments   There are no specific tests for CPPD, PMS, or PMM, however, there are some laboratory tests that can be helpful in ruling out underlying problems. Simple blood tests can identify conditions such as anemia, thyroid disorders, diabetes, or hypoglycemia. Ovarian hormone testing is unnecessary unless premature menopause (before the age of 40 years) is suspected.

DIFFERENTIAL DIAGNOSES

The patterns and severity of symptoms are the best guide for sorting out whether a woman has cyclic or chronic perimenstrual pain, mild or severe perimenstrual physical or mood discomforts, PMM, severe PMS, or a dual diagnosis. Symptom-tracking charts and calendars along with menstrual and health history data will provide essential clues.

PMS and CPPD need to be distinguished from endocrine abnormalities and from conditions that are subject to PMM (discussed previously). Furthermore, the transition to menopause may be a vulnerable period when women experience the onset or a worsening of CPPD or PMS, especially mood disturbances and fatigue (Woods et al., 1997).

Although the underlying cause of this phenomenon is unknown, there is considerable evidence of many manifestations of PMM. Many medical and psychiatric conditions are exacerbated in the premenstrual or menstrual phase of the cycle, leading a woman to believe that she must be experiencing PMS. Thyroid disease is frequently overlooked because of the many symptoms associated with hypothyroid or hyperthyroid disease syndromes (Girdler, Pedersen, & Light, 1995). Mood disorders—primarily depression—are twice as common as anxiety disorders and both will exacerbate premenstrually (Rubinow & Schmidt, 1995; Yonkers & White, 1992). Other psychiatric disorders such as substance abuse and bulimia can be exacerbated during the luteal phase of the menstrual cycle. Many women with epilepsy experience changes in seizure frequency and severity with changes in reproductive cycles, including at puberty, over the menstrual cycle, with pregnancy, and at menopause.

Musculoskeletal pain syndromes, such as arthralgias, arthritis, and fibromyalgia, can cause symptoms that overlap with PMS (e.g., generalized pain, fatigue, sleep disturbances, or cognitive impairment) and may go undiagnosed in women with moderate to severe PMS (Shaver et al., 1997). Cyclic perimenstrual pain that is severe and begins at midcycle or worsens premenstrually may indicate an underlying gynecologic condition such as endometriosis, pelvic inflammatory disease, or chronic pelvic pain (see Chapters 18, 22, and 25). Clinical management guidelines for the diagnosis of chronic pelvic pain have been published recently by ACOG that differentiate pathophysiology between acute and chronic pelvic pain (ACOG, 2004). In addition, migraine-type headaches appear to increase during the premenstrual and menstrual phases. Menstrual migraines tend to occur one to three days before menstruation begins or during the first day or two of menstruation when hormone levels drop considerably.

All menstruating women report that gastrointestinal (GI) symptoms, such as stomach pain, nausea, and loose stools, are highest during menses and almost 50% of women with IBS report a perimenstrual increase in symptoms. Women with Crohn's Disease report more premenstrual and menstrual GI symptoms (diarrhea, abdominal pain, and constipation) than other women with bowel disease. Women with functional bowel disease (FBD)—that is not yet classified as a GI disorder—report more stomach pain, nausea, and diarrhea at menses than women without FBD.

Infections seem to increase or worsen during the premenstrual phase of the menstrual cycle. Vaginal infections, especially yeast infections, often occur right before or during menstruation and have been found to be related to alterations in the normal vaginal pH level. The incidence of urinary cystitis increases premenstrually and during menstruation for the same reasons. Viral infections, such as herpes, seem to flare up during this time. Some women report sinus congestion and symptoms of colds or other upper respiratory infection premenstrually, which disappear after the onset of their periods.

BEGINNING THE THERAPEUTIC PROCESS

SETTING GOALS

Sometimes the process of assessment is therapeutic in itself—raising self-awareness and validating women's symptom experience. Setting goals and outcome criteria formalizes the process while continuing an interactive process that includes and encourages the woman's participation.

The AWHONN EBG for CPPD (2003) outlines the possible expected therapeutic outcomes for CPPD that should be explicitly negotiated with each woman. For example, outcomes may include comfort level, type of treatment, pain and discomfort relief, role performance change, or economic costs. Setting goals should include both health-related outcomes and other outcomes, such as functional status and economic impact. In terms of functional status, the detrimental effects of inadequately treated cyclic perimenstrual pain range from missed life opportunities, such as work, school, or other activities, to increased costs for women seeking relief from pain (Dawood et al., 1985; Harlow, 1986; Harlow & Park, 1996; Smith, 1993).

The clinician—in collaboration with the woman—facilitates the therapeutic process which is dependent on the:

1. Desired patient outcome
2. Characteristics of the diagnosis
3. Research base associated with the intervention
4. Feasibility of successfully implementing the intervention
5. Acceptability of the intervention to the client
6. Capability of the clinician (Bulecheck & McCloskey, 1999)

THERAPEUTIC OPTIONS

Most women use OTC remedies to manage their pelvic pain. Drugs such as acetaminophen, naproxen, and ibuprofen have proven effective in managing pain (Jarrett, Heitkemper, & Shaver, 1995). Nonetheless, it appears that women—particularly adolescents—may not always use OTC medications effectively and would benefit from additional information on pain management and evidence-based self-care strategies (Campbell & McGrath, 1997).

Treatments for perimenstrual symptoms and PMS range from dangerous (ovarian radiation) to those treatments that obviously are ineffective (hiding in one's room). Until recently, the focus on singular (usually pharmacologic) therapy has dominated treatments for perimenstrual symptoms and PMS. Clinical research suggests that a combination of treatments is more satisfactory than a single treatment (Keye, 1988; Taylor, 1988, 1996b; Taylor & Woods, 1991). Moreover, outcomes from symptom-management programs suggest that when symptoms are comprehensively managed, people are more likely to remain in treatment and show improved outcomes. New models of symptom management that combine self-care, social support, medical therapies, and psychosocial strategies applied to specific conditions have shown promising results. In a clinical trial of multimodal symptom-management strategies for women experiencing severe PMS, Taylor (1999) found that women prefer to select multiple strategies for symptom management, that perimenstrual symptom severity will decline markedly within the first few months, and that this effect will be maintained over the long-term.

These strategies, although focused on perimenstrual symptom relief, are generally health promoting. Establishing healthy dietary and exercise habits along with managing personal and environmental stress during early adulthood may lead to lifelong healthy behaviors that result in chronic disease prevention in later adult life. Symptom management interventions can also be considered as complementary to pharmacologic therapy in women with a dual diagnosis or a depressive disorder that regularly worsens during a specific menstrual cycle phase.

AWHONN EVIDENCE-BASED CLINICAL PRACTICE GUIDELINES

CPPD SYMPTOM MANAGEMENT

Because the evidence-based clinical practice guidelines developed for CPPD form the basis for professional interventions as well as self-care remedies for CPP and perimenstrual mood and physical discomforts, the reader is referred to the AWHONN publication department (1-800-673-8499, toll free United States) or (800-245-0231, toll free Canada) or to the AWHONN online store to purchase the guidelines (www.awhonn.org). These guidelines provide the practicing clinician with a comprehensive care plan for assessing and managing menstrually related symptoms as well as a mechanism for integrating health-promoting strategies into patient care management.

Interventions within the guidelines have been organized into categories of clinician-sensitive and self-care therapeutics based on a model of symptom management. Each intervention has both specific recommendations along with referenced rationale statements. A pullout quick care guide serves as a clinically useful reference for the practicing clinician.

The following sections build on the AWHONN CPPD Management Guideline and add pharmacologic and emerging therapies for severe PMS. Table 19–2 presents an outline of the AWHONN model for CPPD management with an additional column for treatments for severe PMS.

CPPD symptom management begins with mutual goal setting, collaborative pain and discomfort assessment, and self-monitoring of symptoms and stressors as described in the previous sections. Symptom regulation is differentiated for CPP as well as for cyclic perimenstrual physical and mood discomforts. For example, symptom regulation for cyclic perimenstrual pain includes OTC and prescription medications such as prostaglandin inhibitors, analgesics, and oral contraceptives. Specific nutritional supplements, or nutraceuticals, have been shown to be effective for CPPD, and a growing body of evidence supports the use of dietary supplements prescribed at levels well above the US recommended daily allowance (RDA) for CPPD, particularly specific vitamins, minerals, and fatty acids (Stevinson & Ernst, 2001). The AWHONN guidelines recommend selected nutraceuticals based on Level I–II evidence. Topical cutaneous symptom regulation includes heat application, therapeutic massage, acupressure, and transcutaneous nerve stimulation, and is supported by Level I evidence.

Behavioral and cognitive strategies for symptom regulation of CPPD include body relaxation exercises for cyclic pain and physical discomforts, and mind relaxation strategies for perimenstrual mood discomforts. For example, in a study of perimenstrual symptom management (Level I evidence, see Chapter 3), Taylor (2000) tested a combination of behavioral and cognitive relaxation strategies and demonstrated that all women found mind–body relaxation strategies to be somewhat to very helpful in managing their perimenstrual symptoms as well as in managing their general stress response. Combining body relaxation strategies (e.g., breathing and muscle relaxation exercises) with cognitive stress reduction (e.g., meditation, guided imagery, prayer, or thought changing exercises) was critical for half of the women, especially during the premenstrual days when they felt unable to practice relaxation strategies because of uncontrollable worries, self-doubts, and critical self-talk. Learning proper breathing reduced symptoms of anxiety in this randomized clinical trial.

Based on the research by Taylor (2000), the CPPD guidelines include both personal and environmental modification strategies for perimenstrual symptom relief. Most stress reduction strategies focus on managing "inner" stress; however, a number of investigators have found that environmental stressors—"outside" stress such as interpersonal relationship stress and time pressures—were associated with increased perimenstrual symptom severity (Brown & Zimmer, 1986; Winter, Ashton, & Moore, 1991). Taylor (1999), in a clinical trial of the Perimenstrual Symptom Management program, found that learning to

TABLE 19–2   CPPD and PMS Interventions

CPPD and PMS Interventions: Interventions are organized within a conceptual framework of symptom management in the left column. Interventions for which there is an evidence base are identified under each symptom cluster. Specific details about implementation of the intervention are presented in this chapter, the AWHONN Evidence-based guideline (Collins Sharp et al., 2003) or Taylor and Colino (2002).

	Cyclic Pelvic Pain	Physical Discomforts	Mood Discomforts	Severe PMS
1. Fundamental symptom management				
• Collaborative symptom assessment & Self Monitoring	X Symptom cluster, severity, pattern assessment	X	X	X
• Mutual goal-setting	X	X	X	X
• Coping enhancement	X	X	X	X
2. Symptom-regulation				
a. Pharmacologic				
• Over-the-Counter Medication	X NSAIDs, Analgesics	X NSAIDs, Analgesics		
• Prescription Medication	X NSAIDs, Analgesics	X	X	X Antidepressants
• Hormones	X Oral contraceptives, Progesterone IUD	X Oral contraceptives		X Micronized progesterone (inconsistent evidence)
• Nutraceuticals	X Calcium, Magnesium, Essential fatty acids, Vitamin E, B1	X	X	X
b. Topical-Cutaneous				
• Heat Application	X	X		
• Therapeutic Massage	X	X	X	
• Acupressure	X	X		
• Transcutaneous Nerve Stimulation	X			
c. Behavioral-cognitive				
• Behavioral Relaxation	X Breathing, stretching, PMR	X	X Breathing, stretching, PMR, AT	
• Cognitive Relaxation			X Cognitive exercises, imagery, meditation, biofeedback	X
• Environmental Modification			X Time management, healthy communication, problem solving	X
3. Self-modification				
• Nutritional Counseling: General Dietary Modification	X Multivitamin-mineral supplement, low-fat and vegetarian diet, increase fluid premenstrually	X	X Decrease caffeine, alcohol, simple sugars, salt premenstrually, increase fluids, meal frequency	X
• Health Risk Reduction: Smoking Cessation	X			
• Exercise Promotion	X Aerobic exercise postmenstrually; premenstrual or menstrual activity modification	X	X	X
4. Referral and/or co-management				
• Acupuncture	X	X	X	
• Traditional Chinese Medicine	X	X	X	X
• Homeopathy		X	X	
• Botanical/Herbal Therapy			X	X Vitex, SAMe
• Chiropractic Therapy	X			
• Surgical Evaluation	X			
• Mental Health Evaluation			X	X
• Emerging Therapies			X	X Light therapy, SAM-e,

TABLE 19–3   Translating Research into Practice—Science-based PMS Self-Management

Putting the science back into self-care has been a significant extension of menstrual cycle research, resulting in consumer education about this research. Taylor and Colino (2002) have published one of the first science-based self-help books for women that describes step-by-step strategies for self-assessment and self-management of perimenstrual symptoms, PMS, and stress. This book can be used in combination with the ACOG or AWHONN guidelines in ways such as the following:

- Tracking symptoms and stress—Empowered self-diagnosis strategies
- The anti-PMS diet—How food increases and decreases stress and PMS
- Nutritional supplements for PMS and stress management
- Reducing body stress—Breathing, physical activity, and relaxation strategies
  - Behavioral relaxation strategies include breathing and stretching exercises that can be accomplished in a few minutes twice daily, along with how to choose between progressive muscle relaxation and autogenic training relaxation.
- Adding the mind to the body—Breaking the cycle of mental bad habits, dealing with thoughts that won't stop, changing thinking to change mood, retraining the mind, and thinking up better realities.
  - As body relaxation is effective for only 50% of women (Taylor, 1996b), cognitive relaxation strategies have been found to be helpful in relaxing the mind. For example, meditation, guided imagery, prayer, and biofeedback are ways to reduce mental stress. Instructions for thought stopping and reducing toxic self-talk have been found to be effective in reducing both mind and body tension.
- Managing stress from the "outside," such as making and taking time, learning to communicate effectively, developing an everyday talk therapy, and other effective ways to manage work, home, and relationship stress that increase perimenstrual negative moods and stress responses.
  - Managing time vs. letting time take over—Assessing time problems, managing time, and reclaiming time
  - Controlling relationship stress at home and work—Everyday talk therapy, revamping communication styles, developing a "can do" process for dealing with relationship stress, overcoming resistance from others, and starting a support group.
- Putting the pieces together—Developing a personalized prescription
- Solve new symptoms as they arise, such as common stress-related headaches, fatigue, insomnia, or menstrual pain and bloating.

manage time effectively across the menstrual cycle, along with learning effective communication and problem-solving strategies, ultimately reduced stress. By the end of the study, most women found these strategies helpful (70%) or very helpful (27%), and only 6% of the women did not use role redefinition or time-management strategies.

Based on these symptom management clinical trials, Taylor and Colino (2002) have published the first evidence-based, step-by-step guide for managing personal and environmental stress in a user-friendly format (Table 19–3). Mind-body relaxation strategies reduce internal symptoms and stress, and managing stress from the "outside" includes exercises such as making and taking time, learning to communicate effectively, developing and practicing everyday talk therapy, and other effective ways to manage work, home, and relationship stressors that increase perimenstrual negative moods and stress responses. These evidence-based self-care strategies expand the AWHONN guidelines.

The CPPD symptom management model includes strategies for both CPPD relief and general health promotion. Establishing healthy dietary and exercise habits along with personal and environmental stress management for perimenstrual symptoms has been found to lead to long-term health behaviors that are also related to chronic disease prevention (Taylor, 2000). This component of CPPD management is referred to as self-modification because the strategies are focused on overall personal and lifestyle modification. Nutritional counseling and exercise promotion include specific techniques for modifying diet and physical activity and are based on Level I (exercise modification, dietary modification, vitamin supplementation) and Level II (regular physical activity, aerobic exercise, reducing caffeine, smoking, and alcohol) evidence. Smoking cessation is also part of the symptom management plan (Level II evidence) because smoking can exacerbate painful menstrual cramps, and success with smoking cessation efforts may be improved by coordinating the effort with the time of the menstrual cycle phase (Perkins et al., 2000).

MANAGEMENT OF SEVERE PMS

EVIDENCE-BASED RECOMMENDATIONS

Some women experience severe PMS or have a dual diagnosis that includes noncyclic mood disorders, seasonal depression, or intense menstrual pain that may benefit from medication in combination with various aspects of a symptom-management program. Others may be so acutely sensitive to hormonal fluctuations that it may make sense to suppress the ovarian cycle for symptom relief.

Certain psychotropic medications, hormonal therapies, and diuretics have been found to be helpful in dealing with noncyclic moods, PMM, or severe mood and physical discomforts. Although the SSRI drugs appear to lessen the cyclic agitated–depressive symptoms, micronized progesterone has been found to act as an antianxiety agent, which means it may be better suited to the perimenstrual mood discomfort cluster of symptoms (tension, irritability, anger, feeling out of control, or mood swings). Women who are experiencing both CPPD and perimenopausal menstrual irregularities may be more responsive to micronized progesterone. If a woman is not sensitive to exogenous hormones and needs contraception, ovarian suppression using a combined contraceptive (in a pill, patch, or vaginal ring) may help decrease the mood, pain, and other physical symptoms that haven't been completely relieved by nonpharmacologic symptom-management strategies. General caveats for all the pharmacologic therapies include avoidance during pregnancy or pregnancy planning, and to try these medications for at least two or three menstrual cycles to gauge their effects on symptoms and to overcome any side effects.

PHARMACOLOGIC SYMPTOM MANAGEMENT

Antidepressants   For patients with severe PMS and for those who do not respond to fundamental symptom management, ACOG practice guidelines recommend SSRIs, particularly fluoxetine (Prozac) and sertraline (Zoloft) taken daily or intermittently during the premenstrual phase of the menstrual cycle (ACOG, 2000). Level I evidence supported by a meta-analysis and three placebo-controlled trials (Steiner, Korzekwa, Lamont, & Wilkins, 1997; Steiner et al., 1995, 2001) found SSRIs resulted in a 40–55% decrease in PMDD (especially negative mood symptoms) but had a high rate of side effects (especially at the 60 mg level of fluoxetine), even when used cyclically. Level II evidence suggests that SSRIs can be used for a shorter duration when combined with multimodal symptom-management strategies (Taylor, 2000).

Serotonergic-activating agents, including the SSRIs fluoxetine (Prozac), sertraline (Zoloft), paroxetine (Paxil), and citalopram (Celexa), have all been shown to mediate severe premenstrual symptoms. Recently, a relabeled form of fluoxetine was approved by the FDA for the treatment of PMDD or severe PMS under the brand name Sarafem. Notably, the European analog to the FDA has not approved these drugs for treatment of PMDD, claiming lack of evidence to establish PMDD as a treatable disorder (Moynihan, 2004).

The most common side effects of SSRIs are headaches, sleep disturbances, dizziness, weight gain, dry mouth, and decreased libido. Other, less often reported side effects include decreased appetite, weight loss, drowsiness, impaired concentration, altered taste, nausea, diarrhea, and nervousness. If these occur, they can usually be lessened with lower dosages of the medications. Notably, there is substantial evidence that SSRIs produce no increased risk of spontaneous abortion, major malformation, decreased birth weight, prematurity, or postnatal complications following in utero exposure, nor is there evidence that SSRIs are teratogenic.

Anxiolytic Drugs   The most commonly prescribed antianxiety medication for noncyclic anxiety or panic disorders is alprazolam (Xanax). Others include diazepam (Valium), lorazepam (Ativan), and buspirone (BuSpar). Research on the use of antianxiety medications has shown mixed results. In the only two randomized, crossover, placebo-controlled clinical trials of alprazolam for use during the premenstrual phase, women taking the drug experienced less anxiety, depression, and headaches (Freeman, Rickels, Sondheimer, & Polansky, 1995; Schmidt, Grover, & Rubinow, 1993). However, alprazolam has also been shown to stimulate increased appetite premenstrually, which could make it hard to control food cravings or binges. Furthermore, with alprazolam there is potential for addiction, tolerance, and bothersome sedation, and it is not recommended as a first-line treatment by the ACOG PMS Practice Guidelines (ACOG, 2000).

These medications are for short-term use only, and continued use should not exceed eight weeks without medical or psychiatric evaluation, because physical and psychological dependencies can occur quickly with these drugs. Physical tolerance develops quickly, and relying on pills supersedes the development of nonpharmacologic stress management. Side effects can include visual problems, mood swings, and joint stiffness. Other, less frequently reported side effects include drowsiness, headaches, dizziness, blurred vision, dry mouth, weakness, confusion, nausea, constipation, agitation, and depression. Oral contraceptives can increase the potency of antianxiety drugs, which can increase the risk of side effects. By contrast, alcohol, if consumed while taking an antianxiety drug, increases depression of the CNS.

HORMONAL THERAPY

SUPPLEMENTATION OR SUPPRESSION

A progesterone deficiency has not been proven as a causal mechanism for PMS, and results of research using progesterone as a treatment for PMS are inconsistent. A systematic review of 14 trials with progesterone and progestogens given orally, vaginally, or rectally did not support the use of progesterone therapy (Wyatt, Dimmock, Jones, Obhrai, & O'Brien, 2001). Although the US FDA has not approved progesterone therapy for PMS, micronized progesterone is an FDA-recognized hormone therapy for perimenopausal symptoms, especially when a woman is still menstruating and estrogen supplementation is contraindicated (Martorano, Ahlgrimm, & Colbert, 1998). Cyclic physical and mood discomforts that are experienced by women in the menopausal transition combined with menstrual irregularities have been successfully treated with 300 mg of micronized progesterone at bedtime or medroxyprogesterone (Provera) in a dose of 10 mg per day for 16 days of the menstrual cycle (Prior, 2002). Micronized progesterone appears to play a role in bone formation, whereas the synthetic progestins are implicated in bone loss (Prior et al., 2001). Micronized progesterone has been recognized as a treatment for PMS in the United Kingdom since the 1970s and few side effects have been reported beyond mild sedation or drowsiness, nor has it been linked with fetal abnormalities if it's used during pregnancy. Current contraindications to the use of oral progestins, such as medroxyprogesterone, include liver dysfunction, known or suspected cancer, genital bleeding of unknown cause, and blood clotting disorders.

A number of investigators have found that temporarily suppressing ovulation can reduce both cyclic perimenstrual pain as well as cyclic perimenstrual physical and mood discomforts in some women (Bjorn et al., 2002; Bjorn, Bixo, Nojd, Nyberg, & Backstrom, 2000; Freeman et al., 2001; Sanders, Graham, Bass, & Bancroft, 2001). There is Level III evidence that oral contraceptives will reduce perimenstrual negative mood symptom severity and variability (Oinonen & Mazmanian, 2002). However, in a controlled trial of a new oral contraceptive (Yasmin) with a new progestin, results indicated an insignificant decrease in mood symptoms (10% decrease in premenstrual mood symptoms and PMDD) and a 10–20% rate of side effects such as nausea, headaches, and depression that are similar to side effects reported for all oral contraceptives (Freeman et al., 2001). According to ACOG, oral contraceptives should be considered only if symptoms are primarily physical (ACOG, 2000).

There is limited and inconsistent evidence for hormonal ovulation suppression with gonadotropin-releasing hormone (GnRH) agonists or surgical oophorectomy. Although some women have benefited from these therapies, GnRH agonists are associated with significant side effects, and surgical oophorectomy is an irreversible therapeutic option.

Diuretics   Diuretics have commonly been prescribed for severe premenstrual bloating and fluid retention. However, no evidence exists that thiazide diuretics are of benefit, and they can actually make symptoms worse via potassium depletion, which results in stimulation of the autonomic nervous system. An aldosterone antagonist with antiandrogenic properties, spironolactone, is the only diuretic that has demonstrated evidence in reducing severe premenstrual bloating and headaches. According to ACOG, there is Level I evidence to support the use of spironolactone, although not all reports evaluating spironolactone have shown benefit (ACOG, 2000).

CO-MANAGEMENT AND REFERRAL

EMERGING THERAPIES

Several promising alternative or complementary therapies for perimenstrual pain and discomforts have come to light in recent years. These approaches are different from those used by conventional, Western medical practitioners, and although the science behind many of these nonmedicinal remedies is sparse, many of these treatments have some research to support their use. They are included because alternative or complementary treatments, such as herbal remedies, homeopathy, massage, and nutritional supplements, are popular among women who have perimenstrual discomforts.

Although the use of light therapy sprang from high-tech research interventions, many of the therapies included here, such as acupuncture, are based on centuries-old practices and ancient healing systems. Many of these techniques are based on Eastern philosophies that do not separate the body from the mind, or health from lifestyle. Instead, the Eastern view is of a woman's body as an integrated whole, with body and mind working in concert. The aim behind these disciplines is to create balance and harmony in the body, to produce subtle, positive effects over time, or to bolster the body's own healing abilities rather than relying on a potent drug that would intervene in a more aggressive way. Because of the complexity of these approaches, this section can only provide an overview of how they could help relieve various premenstrual symptoms. Note that to err on the side of caution, herbal or nutritional remedies are included in this section only if they are considered safe and have well-documented efficacy studies to support them.

ALTERNATIVE HEALING SYSTEMS: TRADITIONAL CHINESE MEDICINE AND HOMEOPATHY

In traditional Chinese medicine (TCM), both herbs and acupuncture are used separately or in combination to treat health conditions that result from disruptions to the flow of the body's vital energy (qi or chi), which represents an imbalance between the eternal opposites of yin and yang. The National Institutes of Health has found acupuncture, the ancient Chinese art of needle placement, to be helpful in the treatment of menstrual cramps, low back pain, joint pain, headaches, and severe PMS. Acupuncture treatment manipulates the vital energy sources of the body by introducing ultrathin needles into specific points along the "meridians," or energy pathways, of the body. Most TCM practitioners will also use a combination of acupuncture and herbs in the treatment of severe PMS.

Homeopathy is a holistic treatment system based on the principle that giving a person the right dose of a natural substance that might disturb the body in the wrong amounts can actually trigger healing. In a meta-analysis of 105 clinical trials of homeopathic treatments, researchers found that 75% of interpretable trials showed a positive result (Chapman, Angelica, Spitalny, & Strauss, 1994). More recently, a randomized, controlled double-blind clinical trial at The Hebrew University, Hadassah Medical School in Israel, found that 90% of the women experienced an improvement of more than 30% in their premenstrual symptoms after an oral dose of a homeopathic medication (Yakir et al., 2001). Although homeopathic remedies have no side effects and are available without a prescription, it is wise to consult a professional homeopath who can help choose the most appropriate treatments.

BOTANIC, HERBAL, AND ALTERNATIVE THERAPIES

Several herbs seem to have beneficial effects on PMS, as well as menstrual cramps. These include Vitex (chaste tree berry), cramp bark, and evening primrose oil, among others. All herbs are available without a prescription at pharmacies and health food stores. Not all herbs have enough clinical or research evidence to document their safety or efficacy. Only those herbs that have been recommended by the German Commission E (which was established more than 20 years ago and has reviewed all the available literature on more than 300 herbs) or by the late Varro Tyler, PhD, a professor of pharmacognosy at Purdue University and author of *The Honest Herbal* (Foster & Tyler, 2000), are included here. To learn about safe, therapeutic dosages, the reader may want to consult *The American Pharmaceutical Association Practical Guide to Natural Medicines* (Pierce, 1999) or the American Botanical Council's *ABC Guide to Herbal Medicines* (American Botanical Council, 2003).

Vitex agnus-castus (Chaste Tree Berry)   The only botanical treatment with Level I evidence is chaste tree berry. Native to the Mediterranean and central Asia, chaste tree (also called Vitex) is a shrub that produces dark brown to black fruit the size of a peppercorn. Preparations of the fruit as an extract or in powdered form have been approved by German health authorities for the treatment of menstrual irregularities, such as PMS and breast pain associated with a woman's menstrual period. It appears to have a dopamine like activity and effect on the pituitary gland, which helps to reinstate the normal balance between estrogen and progesterone during the luteal phase of the menstrual cycle. Clinical trials have shown that chaste tree berry extract keeps the overproduction of progesterone in check and effectively reduces breast pain associated with a woman's menses (Schellenberg, 2001). In the first placebo-controlled trial to clearly demonstrate the herb's effectiveness in treating PMS, German scientists found that women taking 20 mg of Vitex reported a 52% overall reduction in PMS symptoms compared with only 24% for those taking placebo (Berger, Schaffner, Schrader, Meier, & Brattstrom, 2000; Schellenberg). Reports of side effects were rare, with only 5% of the women experiencing mild symptoms, such as acne, skin rash, and bleeding between their periods. None of these symptoms caused women to drop out of the study.

Although chaste tree berry extracts do not contain hormones, they should not be used with birth control pills or other hormone replacement therapies without the guidance of a health care professional. Chaste tree berry extract also should not be used during pregnancy as it can stimulate premature lactation.

Evening Primrose Oil   The seed oil of the evening primrose, a weed that is native to North America, is high in the essential fatty acid gamma linolenic acid, which is a precursor to prostaglandin. Over 120 studies in 15 countries have reported on the potential use of evening primrose oil, and the studies of its use for PMS suggest that it helps to regulate hormones (American Botanical Council, 2003). Two well-controlled studies failed to show any beneficial effects for evening primrose oil, although because the trials were relatively small modest effects cannot be excluded. Although the results of research have been mixed, some researchers have found that consuming evening primrose oil supplements decreases premenstrual mood symptoms, breast pain, and fluid retention (Budeiri, Li Wan Po, & Dornan, 1996). Safety of the herb seems well-established but about 2% of those who take evening primrose oil may experience stomach discomfort, nausea, or headaches.

SAM-e   S-adenosylmethionine, or SAM-e, is neither a drug nor an herb. SAM-e is a molecule manufactured in the body from the amino acid methionine during metabolism and has been discovered to be related to metabolic disturbances found in patients with psychiatric and neurologic disorders. Available by prescription for years in Europe, SAM-e has been shown to be both safe and effective in treating depression and comparable to standard tricyclic antidepressants according to a 1994 meta-analysis (Bressa, 1994). A recent double-blind, placebo-controlled trial found no difference between the antidepressive efficacy of 1600 mg of Sam-e and 400 mg of imipramine, except that Sam-e was more easily tolerated (Delle Chiaie, Pancheri, & Scapicchio, 2002). Dr. Bottiglieri, a neuropharmacologist at Baylor University Medical Center Institute of Metabolic Disease in Dallas, Texas, has been studying SAM-e for more than 15 years and considers it to be safe and effective for mild to moderate depressive symptoms (Bottiglieri, 2002). It has also been found to be helpful in reducing joint pain associated with osteoarthritis and used as an alternative for people who have side effects from nonsteroidal anti-inflammatory drug (NSAID) agents. SAMe has been reported to cause mild and transient insomnia, nervousness, lack of appetite, constipation, headaches, heart palpitations, nausea, dry mouth, sweating, and dizziness.

Because SAM-e is converted into homocysteine in the body, a protein associated with heart disease, it is unclear whether rising levels of homocysteine secondary to SAM-e metabolism will increase the risk of heart disease. SAM-e must be taken with a daily multivitamin along with a diet high in fruits and vegetables. Three of the B vitamins (folic acid [B_3], B_6 and B_{12}) can lower the homocysteine levels that SAM-e elevates.

Unfortunately there is no way to find a standardized dose of SAM-e, and because raw SAM-e degrades quickly unless stored at proper temperatures, there is no guarantee that the pills available for sale have been properly handled. SAM-e is also very expensive. A daily dose can vary in price from $2.50 to $18.00 and needs to be taken over a few weeks to see results.

Light Therapy   Research suggests a link between PMS and Seasonal Affective Disorder (SAD), a type of depression that typically occurs in the fall and winter months when levels of natural light decline in countries north of the equator (Brown & Robinson, 2002; Parry et al., 1997). Exposure to full-spectrum light, including ultraviolet light, in women who are highly sensitive to light has been found to decrease the moodiness and depressive symptoms of PMS. One study found that women with severe PMS who were treated with 30 minutes of evening light therapy for two weeks during the luteal phase of their menstrual cycles experienced a significant reduction in depression and premenstrual tension (Parry et al.). It is theorized that bright light corrects disturbances in the body's internal sleep–wake cycle that are linked with PMS, or, that the light promotes the effects of the feel-good brain chemical serotonin. Light therapy may be considered a viable option for women who feel depressed all month long during the fall and winter months and experience an increased severity of premenstrual mood symptoms during these seasons. Formal light therapy should be initiated with the consultation of a psychotherapist or mental health counselor. Informally, women can brighten their world by increasing light exposure, especially to morning light. See science-based self-help books for additional recommendations (Brown & Robinson, 2002; Taylor & Colino, 2002).

CONCLUSION

Although CPPD is a term that describes the actual experiences of women and encompasses the medical diagnoses of dysmenorrhea and PMS, the definition of PMS has become a popularized entity as well as a recognized ICD classification. Biomedically, PMS has been defined as an illness experience or syndrome characterized by the repeated occurrence of behavioral, somatic, and mood symptoms severe enough to impair a woman's social and work-related functioning during the premenstrual and luteal phases of the menstrual cycle. PMDD, a severe form of PMS, is a controversial label now defined as a psychiatric diagnosis, and PMM refers to the premenstrual magnification of an underlying medical or psychiatric condition.

CPPD encompasses three diagnoses, each representing a cluster of symptoms supported by empirical research. Identifying the severity and patterns of these symptom clusters provides an evidence-based guide for sorting out whether a woman has cyclic or chronic perimenstrual pain, mild or severe perimenstrual physical or mood discomforts, premenstrual magnification, severe PMS, or a dual diagnosis. Prospective symptom self-monitoring using tracking charts or calendars combined with menstrual and health history data will provide additional diagnostic clues and is supported by good quality evidence.

According to the EBGs from ACOG and AWHONN, there is good quality evidence to recommend multimodal symptom management as a first-line treatment for cyclic perimenstrual physical and mood discomforts or for mild to moderately severe PMS, which includes the following:

- Symptom monitoring
- Dietary counseling
- Nutritional supplements
- Personal and environmental stress management
- Exercise promotion

There is also fair to good evidence to support the use of selective pharmacologic therapies, such as SSRI antidepressants, for severe PMS that does not respond to nonpharmacologic symptom management. Inconsistent evidence exists for other pharmacologic therapies such as hormonal or singular therapies. More effective than a singular therapy is a multimodal package of symptom-management strategies as outlined in the AWHONN clinical practice guidelines. They include the following:

- Exercise and dietary changes with self-monitoring
- Behavioral therapies
- Cognitive exercises
- Training in time management, role redefinition, communicating, and problem solving

A science-based self-help book for women (Taylor & Colino, 2002) complements the ACOG and AWHONN guidelines by providing step-by-step strategies for self-assessment and self-management of perimenstrual symptoms, PMS, and stress. Multimodal symptom management has been shown to be as effective as medical therapy for PMS (and without side effects). Establishing healthy dietary and exercise habits, along with personal and environmental stress management for perimenstrual symptom management may lead to lifelong improvements in health behaviors that result in chronic disease prevention or improved chronic illness symptom management.

NOTE

Beth A. Collins Sharp was an employee of the United States federal government when this work was conducted and prepared for publication. The views expressed in this chapter are those of the authors and do not necessarily reflect those of the Agency for Healthcare Research and Quality or the United States Department of Health and Human Services.

REFERENCES

American Botanical Council. (2003). *The ABC guide to herbal medicines.* Austin, TX.

American College of Obstetricians & Gynecologists. (2000). *ACOG Practice Bulletin (No. 15): Premenstrual syndrome.* Washington, DC.

American College of Obstetricians & Gynecologists. (2004). *ACOG Practice Bulletin (No. 51): Chronic pelvic pain.* Washington, DC.

American Psychiatric Association. (1987). *Diagnostic and statistical manual of mental disorders (DSM-IIIR).* Washington, DC.

American Psychiatric Association. (1994). *Diagnostic and statistical manual of mental disorders (DSM-IVR).* Washington, DC.

Angst, J., Sellaro, R., Merikangas, K., & Endicott, J. (2001). The epidemiology of perimenstrual psychological symptoms. *Acta Psychiatrica Scandinavia, 104,* 110–116.

Association of Women's Health Obstetrical & Neonatal Nursing. (2003). *Evidence-based clinical practice guideline: Nursing management for cyclic perimenstrual pain and discomfort.* Washington, DC: Author.

Backstrom, T., Sanders, G., Leask, R., Davidson, D., Warner, P., & Bancroft, J. (1983). Mood, sexuality, hormones, and the menstrual cycle: II. Hormone levels and their relationship to premenstrual syndrome. *Psychosomatic Medicine, 45,* 503–507.

Berger, D., Schaffner, W., Schrader, E., Meier, B., & Brattstrom, A. (2000). Efficacy of Vitex agnus castus L. extract Ze 440 in patients with pre-menstrual syndrome (PMS). *Archives of Gynecology & Obstetrics, 264*(3), 150–153.

Bjorn, I., Bixo, M., Nojd, K., Collberg, P., Nyberg, S., Sundstrom-Poromaa, I., et al. (2002). The impact of different doses of medroxyprogesterone acetate on mood symptoms in sequential hormonal therapy. *Gynecology and Endocrinology, 16*(1), 1–8.

Bjorn, I., Bixo, M., Nojd, K., Nyberg, S., & Backstrom, T. (2000). Negative mood changes during hormone replacement therapy: a comparison between two progestogens. *American Journal of Obstetrics and Gynecology, 183*(6), 1419–1426.

Bloch, M., Schmidt, P., Su, T., Tobin, M., & Rubinow, D. (1998). Pituitary-adrenal hormones and testosterone across the menstrual cycle in women with premenstrual syndrome and controls. *Biological Psychiatry, 43*(12), 897–903.

Bottiglieri, T. (2002). S-Adenosyl-L-methionine (SAMe): From the bench to the bedside: Molecular basis of a pleiotrophic molecule. *American Journal of Clinical Nutrition, 76*(5), 1151S–1157S.

Bressa, G. (1994). S-adenosyl-l-methionine (SAMe) as antidepressant: Meta-analysis of clinical studies. *Acta Neurol Scand Suppl., 154,* 7–14.

Brown, M. A., & Robinson, J. (2002). *When the body gets the blues.* New York: Rodale.

Brown, M., & Zimmer, P. (1986). Personal and family impact of premenstrual symptoms. *Journal of Obstetrical, Gynecological and Neonatal Nursing, 15*(1), 31–38.

Budeiri, D., Li Wan Po, A., & Dornan, J. (1996). Is evening primrose oil of value in the treatment of premenstrual syndrome? *Controlled Clinical Trials, 17*(1), 60–68.

Bulecheck, G., & McCloskey, J. (1999). *Nursing Interventions: Effective nursing treatments.* Philadelphia: Saunders.

Cahill, C. A. (1998). Differences in cortisol, a stress hormone, in women with turmoil-type premenstrual symptoms. *Nursing Research, 47,* 278–284.

Campbell, M. A., & McGrath, P. J. (1997). Use of medication by adolescents for the management of menstrual discomfort. *Archives of Pediatrics and Adolescent Medicine, 151,* 905–913.

Chapman, E., Angelica, J., Spitalny, G., & Strauss, M. (1994). Results of a study of the homeopathic treatment of PMS. *Journal of the American Institute of Homeopathy, 87,* 14–21.

Collins Sharp, B., Taylor, D., Kelly-Thomas, K., Killeen, M. B., & Dawood, M. Y. (2002). Cyclic perimenstrual pain and discomfort: The scientific basis for practice. *Journal of Obstetric, Gynecological, and Neonatal Nursing, 31,* 637–649.

Condon, M. (2004). *Women's health: Body mind and spirit.* Upper Saddle River, NJ: Prentice Hall.

Dawood, M. Y. (1990). Dysmenorrhea. *Clinical Obstetrics & Gynecology, 33*(1), 168–178.

Dawood, M. Y., McGuire, J. L., & Demers, L. M. (1985). *Premenstrual syndrome and dysmenorrhea.* Baltimore & Munich: Urban & Schwarzenberg.

Dawood & Ramos (1990). Transcutaneous electrical nerve stimulation (TENS) for the treatment of primary dysmenorrhea: A randomized, crossover comparison with placebo TENS and ibuprofen. *Obstetrics & Gynecology, 75,* 656–660.

Delle Chiaie, R., Pancheri, P., & Scapicchio, P. (2002). Efficacy and tolerability of oral and intramuscular S-adenosyl-L-methionine 1,4-butanedisulfonate (SAMe) in the treatment of major depression: Comparison with imipramine in 2 multicenter studies. *American Journal of Clinical Nutrition, 76*(5), 1172S–1176S.

Endicott, J. (2001). The epidemiology of perimenstrual psychological symptoms. *Acta Psychiatrica Scandinavica, 104,* 110–116.

Foster, S., & Tyler, V. (2000). *Tyler's honest herbal: A sensible guide to the use of herbs and related remedies.* Binghamton, NY: Haworth Press.

Freeman, E. W. (1997). Premenstrual syndrome: Current perspective on treatment and etiology. *Current Opinions in Obstetrics and Gynecology, 9,* 147–153.

Freeman, E., Kroll, R., Rapkin, A., Pearlstein, T., Brown, C., Parsey, K., et al. (2001). Evaluation of a unique oral contraceptive in the treatment of premenstrual dysphoric disorder. *Journal of Womens' Health & Gender Based Medicine, 10*(6), 561–569.

Freeman, E., Rickels, K., & Sondheimer, S. (1993). Premenstrual symptoms and dysmenorrhea in relation to emotional distress factors in adolescents. *Journal of Psychosomatic Obstetrics & Gynecology, 14,* 41–50.

Freeman, E., Rickels, K., Sondheimer, S., & Polansky, M. (1995). A double-blind trial of oral progesterone, alprazolam, and placebo in treatment of severe premenstrual syndrome. *Journal of the American Medical Association, 274*(1), 51–57.

Freeman, E., Sondheimer, S., & Rickels, K. (1988). Effects of medical history factors on symptom severity in women meeting criteria for premenstrual syndrome. *Obstetrics & Gynecology, 72,* 236–239.

Futterman, L. A., Jones, J. E., Miccio-Fonseca, L. C., & Quigley, M. E. (1992). Severity of premenstrual symptoms in relation to medical/psychiatric problems and life experiences. *Perceptual and Motor Skills, 74,* 787–799.

Gallant, S. J. (1991). The role of psychological factors in the experience of premenstrual symptoms. *Proceedings of the 9th Conference of the Society for Menstrual Cycle Research,* 139–152.

Girdler, S., Pedersen, C., & Light, K. (1995). Thyroid axis function during the menstrual cycle in women with premenstrual syndrome. *Psychoneuroendocrinology, 20*(4), 395–403.

Gise, L., Lebovits, A., Paddison, P. L., & Strain, J. J. (1990). Issues in the identification of premenstrual syndromes. *Journal of Nervous & Mental Diseases, 178*(4), 228–234.

Golding, J. M., Taylor, D. L., Menard, L., & King, M. J. (2000). Prevalence of sexual abuse history in a sample of women seeking treatment for premenstrual syndrome. *Journal of Psychosomatic Obstetrics and Gynaecology, 21*(2), 69–80.

Halbreich, U. (1997). Menstrually related disorders—towards interdisciplinary international diagnostic criteria. *Cephalalgia, 17,* 1–4.

Halbreich, U. (1999). Premenstrual syndromes: Closing the 20th century chapters. *Current Opinions in Obstetrics and Gynecology, 9,* 147–153.

Hamilton, J., Alagna, S., & Sharpe, A. (1985). Cognitive approaches to understanding and treating premenstrual depression. In H. Ofofsky (Ed.), *Premenstrual Syndrome* (pp. 69–84). Washington, DC: American Psychiatric Press.

Harlow, S. (1986). Function and dysfunction: A historical critique of the literature on menstruation and work. *Health Care for Women International, 7*(1-2), 39–50.

Harlow, S., & Park, M. (1996). A longitudinal study of risk factors for the occurrence, duration and severity of menstrual cramps in a cohort of college women. *British Journal of Obstetrics and Gynecology, 103,* 1134–1142.

Harrison, M. M. (1985). *Self-help for premenstrual syndrome* (2nd ed.). New York: Random House.

Huerta-Franco, M. R., & Malacara, J. M. (1993). Association of physical and emotional symptoms with the menstrual cycle and life-style. *Journal of Reproductive Medicine, 38,* 448–454.

Janiger, O., Riffenburgh, M., & Kersh, M. (1972). A cross-cultural study of premenstrual symptoms. *Psychosomatics, 13,* 226–235.

Jarrett, M., Heitkemper, M., & Shaver, J. (1995). Symptoms and self-care strategies in women with and without dysmenorrhea. *Health Care for Women International, 16,* 167–178.

Kendler, K., Karkowski, L., Corey, L., & Neale, M. (1998). Longitudinal population-based twin study of retrospectively reported premenstrual symptoms and lifetime major depression. *American Journal of Psychiatry, 155,* 1234–1240.

Keye, W. (1988). The clinical approach to management and treatment. In *The Premenstrual Syndrome.* Philadelphia: Saunders.

Keye, W. R., Jr. (1989). The biomedical model of premenstrual syndrome: Past, present and future. In A. Voda & R. Conover (Eds.), *Proceedings of the 8th Conference of the Society for Menstrual Cycle Research* (pp. 589–600). Salt Lake City, UT: Society for Menstrual Cycle Research.

Kinch, R., & Robinson, G. (1985). Premenstrual syndrome—current knowledge and new directions. *Canadian Journal of Psychiatry, 30*(7):467–468.

Lee, K., & Rittenhouse, C. A. (1992). Prevalence of perimenstrual symptoms in employed women. *Women & Health, 17*(3), 17–32.

Lewis, L. L., Greenblatt, E. M., Rittenhouse, C. A., Veldhuis, J. D., & Jaffe, R. B. (1995). Pulsatile release patterns of luteinizing hormone and progesterone in relation to symptom onset in women with premenstrual syndrome. *Fertility and Sterility, 64,* 288–292.

Martorano, J., Ahlgrimm, M., & Colbert, T. (1998). Differentiating between natural progesterone and synthetic progestins: Clinical implications for premenstrual syndrome and perimenopause management. *Comprehensive Therapeutics, 24*(6–7), 336–339.

Marvan, M. L., Diaz-Erosa, M., & Montesinos, A. (1998). Premenstrual symptoms in Mexican women with different educational levels. *Journal of Psychology, 132,* 517–526.

Mitchell, E. S. (1991). Identification of recurrent symptom severity patterns across multiple menstrual cycles. In *Proceedings of the 9th Conference of the Society for Menstrual Research* (pp. 73–82). Seattle, WA: Society for Menstrual Cycle Research.

Mitchell, E., Woods, N., Lentz, M., & Taylor, D. (1991). Recognizing PMS when you see it: Criteria for PMS sample selection. In D. L. Taylor & N. F. Woods (Eds.), *Menstruation, Health and Illness* (pp. 89–102). New York: Hemisphere.

Mitchell, E. S., Woods, N. F., & Lentz, M. J. (1994). Differentiation of women with three premenstrual symptom patterns. *Nursing Research, 43*(1), 25–30.

Mitchell, E. S., Woods, N. F., Lentz, M. J., Taylor, D., & Lee, K. (1992). Methodological issues in the definition of perimenstrual symptoms. In A. Dan & L. Lewis (Eds.), *Menstrual Health in Women's Lives* (pp. 7–14). Urbana: University of Illinois Press.

Moos, R. (1969). Typology of menstrual cycle symptoms. *American Journal of Obstetrics & Gynecology, 103,* 390–402.

Moynihan, R. (2004). Controversial disease dropped from Prozac product information. *British Medical Journal, 328,* 365.

O'Brien, P. M. S. (1987). Controversies in premenstrual syndrome: Etiology and treatment. In B. E. Ginsburg & B. F. Carter (Eds.), *Premenstrual syndrome: Ethical and legal implications in a biomedical perspective* (pp. 3177–3328). New York: Plenum.

Oinonen, K. A., & Mazmanian, D. (2002). To what extent do oral contraceptives influence mood and affect? *Journal of Affective Disorders, 70,* 229–240.

Parry, B. L., Udell, C., Elliott, J. A., Berga, S. L., Klauber, M. R., Mostofi, N., et al. (1997). Blunted phase-shift responses to morning bright light in premenstrual dysphoric disorder. *Journal of Biological Rhythms, 12*(5), 443–456.

Perkins, K. A., Levine, M., Marcus, M., Shiffman, S., D'Amico, D., & Miller, A. (2000). Tobacco withdrawal in women and menstrual cycle phase. *Journal of Consulting and Clinical Psychology, 68*, 176–180.

Pierce, A. (1999). *The American Pharmaceutical Association Practical Guide to Natural Medicines.* New York: William Morrow.

Praschak-Rieder, N., Willeit, M., Winkler, D., Neumeister, A., Hilger, E., Zill, P., et al. (2002). Role of family history and 5-HTTLPR polymorphism in female seasonal affective disorder patients with and without premenstrual dysphoric disorder. *European Neuropsychopharmacology, 12*(2), 129–134.

Prior, J. (2002). The ageing female reproductive axis II: Ovulatory changes with perimenopause. *Novartis Foundation Symposium, 242*, 172–192.

Prior, J., Hitchcock, C., Kingwell, E., Vigna, Y., Bishop, C., & Pride, S. (2001). Perimenopausal bone loss: More than estrogen depletion. *Journal of Bone Mineral Research, 16*(12), 2365–2366.

Reame, N., Kelch, R., Beitins, I., Yu, M., Zawacki, C., & Padmanabhan, V. (1996). Age effects of FSH and pulsatile LH secretion across the menstrual cycle of premenopausal women. *Journal of Clinical Endocrinology and Metabolism, 81*, 1512–1518.

Reame, N., Marshall, J., & Kelch, R. (1992). Pulsatile LH secretion in women with premenstrual syndrome (PMS): Evidence for normal neuroregulation of the menstrual cycle. *Psychoneuroendocrinology, 17*, 205–213.

Reid, R. L., & Yen, S. S. C. (1981). Premenstrual syndrome. *American Journal of Obstetrics & Gynecology, 139*, 85.

Ross, L. (2004). Rethinking mental health and disorder: Feminist perspectives. *Archives of Women & Mental Health, 7*(2), 151–152.

Ross, L., Sellers, E., Gilbert-Evans, S., & Romach, M. (2004). Mood changes during pregnancy and the postpartum period: Development of a biopsychosocial model. *Acta Psychiatrica Scandinavia, 109*(6), 457–466.

Ross, L., & Steiner, M. (2003). A biopsychosocial approach to premenstrual dysphoric disorder. *Psychiatric Clinics of North America, 26*, 529–546.

Rubinow, D. R., & Schmidt, P. J. (1995). The neuroendocrinology of menstrual cycle mood disorders. *Annals of the New York Academy of Sciences, 771*, 648–659.

Rubinow, D. R., Schmidt, P. J., & Roca, C. A. (1998a). Hormone measures in reproductive endocrine-related mood disorders: Diagnostic issues. *Psychopharmacology Bulletin, 34*, 289–290.

Rubinow, D. R., Schmidt, P. J., & Roca, C. A. (1998b). Estrogen-serotonin interactions: Implications for affective regulation. *Biological Psychiatry, 44*, 839–850.

Sanders, S., Graham, C., Bass, J., &, Bancroft, J. (2001). A prospective study of the effects of oral contraceptives on sexuality and well-being and their relationship to discontinuation. *Contraception, 64*(1), 51–58.

Schellenberg, R. (2001). Treatment for the premenstrual syndrome with agnus castus fruit extract: Prospective, randomised, placebo-controlled study. *British Medical Journal, 322*(7279), 134–137.

Schmidt, P., Grover, G., & Rubinow, D. (1993). Alprazolam in the treatment of premenstrual syndrome. A double-blind, placebo-controlled trial. *Archives of General Psychiatry, 50*(6), 467–473.

Schmidt, P. J., Nieman, L. K., Danaceau, M. A., Adams, L. F., & Rubinow, D. R. (1998). Differential behavioral effects of gonadal steroids in women with and in those without premenstrual syndrome. *New England Journal of Medicine, 338*, 209–216.

Shaver, J. F., & Woods, N. F. (1985). Concordance of perimenstrual symptoms across two cycles. *Research in Nursing and Health, 8*, 313–319.

Shaver, J. L., Lentz, M., Cho, S. K., Cirelli, R. A., Pollice, M., Hastie, A. T., et al. (1997). Sleep, psychological distress, and stress arousal in women with fibromyalgia. *Research in Nursing & Health, 20*, 247–257.

Smith, R. (1993). Cyclic pelvic pain and dysmenorrhea. *Obstetrics and Gynecologic Clinics of North America, 20*(4), 753–764.

Steiner, M., Korzekwa, M., Lamont, J., & Wilkins, A. (1997). Intermittent fluoxetine dosing in the treatment of women with premenstrual dysphoria. *Psychopharmacology Bulletin, 33*(4), 771–774.

Steiner, M., Romano, S., Babcock, S., Dillon, J., Shuler, C., Berger, C., et al. (2001). The efficacy of fluoxetine in improving physical symptoms associated with premenstrual dysphoric disorder. *British Journal of Obstetrics and Gynecology, 108*(5), 462–468.

Steiner, M., Steinberg, S., Stewart, D., Carter, D., Berger, C., Reid, R., et al. (1995). Fluoxetine in the treatment of premenstrual dysphoria. *New England Journal of Medicine, 332*, 1529–1534.

Stevinson, C., & Ernst, E. (2001). Complementary/alternative therapies for premenstrual syndrome: A systematic review of randomized controlled trials. *American Journal of Obstetrics & Gynecology, 185*, 227–235.

Sundell, G., Milsom, I., & Andersch, B. (1990). Factors influencing the prevalence and severity of dysmenorrhea in young women. *British Journal of Obstetrics and Gynaecology, 97*(7), 588–594.

Taylor, D. (1986). Development of perimenstrual symptom typologies. *Communicating Nursing Research, 19*, 168.

Taylor, D. (1988). *Nursing interventions for premenstrual syndrome: A longitudinal therapeutic trial.* Seattle: University of Washington.

Taylor, D. (1996a). The perimenstrual symptom management program: Elements of effective treatment. *Capsules & Comments in Perinatal/Women's Health Nursing, 2*, 140–151.

Taylor, D. (1996b). The perimenstrual symptom management program: Elements of effective treatment. *Capsules Comments Perinatal Womens Health Nursing, 2*, 140–151.

Taylor, D. (1999). Effectiveness of professional-peer group treatment: Symptom management for women with PMS. *Research in Nursing & Health, 22*(6), 496–511.

Taylor, D. (2000). More than personal change: Effective elements of symptom management. *Nurse Practitioner Forum, 11*, 79–86.

Taylor, D., & Colino, S. (2002). *Taking back the month: A personalized solution to managing PMS and enhancing your health.* New York: Perigee/Putnam-Penguin.

Taylor, D., & Woods, N. F. (Eds.). (1991). *Menstruation, health & illness.* New York: Taylor & Francis.

Taylor, D., Woods, N., Lentz, M., Mitchell, E., & Lee, K. (1991). Premenstrual negative affect: Development and testing of an explanatory model. In D. Taylor & N. Woods (Eds.), *Menstruation, health and illness.* New York: Hemisphere.

Thys-Jacobs, S. (2000). Micronutrients and the premenstrual syndrome: The case for calcium. *Journal of the American College of Nutrition, 19*, 220–227.

Ussher, J. M. (2002). Processes of appraisal and coping in the development and maintenance of premenstrual dysphoric disorder. *Journal of Community & Applied Social Psychology, 12*, 309–322.

Winter, E. J., Ashton, D. J., & Moore, D. L. (1991). Dispelling the myth: A study of PMS and relationship satisfaction. *Nurse Practitioner, 16*(5), 34, 37–38, 40, 45.

Woods, N., Dery, G., & Most, A. (1982). Stressful life events and perimenstrual symptoms. *Journal of Human Stress, 8*, 23–31.

Woods, N., Lentz, M., Mitchell, E., Heitkemper, M., & Shaver, J. (1997). PMS after 40: Persistence of a stress-related symptom pattern. *Research in Nursing & Health, 20*, 329–340.

Woods, N. F., Lentz, M., Mitchell, E. S., Heitkemper, M., Shaver, J., & Henker, R. (1998). Perceived stress, physiologic stress arousal and premenstrual symptoms: Group differences and intra-individual patterns. *Research in Nursing & Health, 21*, 511–523.

Woods, N. F., Lentz, M. J., Mitchell, E. S., Taylor, D., & Lee, K. (1992). Perimenstrual symptoms and the health-seeking process. In A. Dan & L. Lewis (Eds.), *Menstrual health in women's lives* (pp. 155–167). Urbana: University of Illinois Press.

Woods, N., Mitchell, E., & Taylor, D. (1999). From menarche to menopause: Contributions from nursing research and recommendations for practice. In I. Hinshaw, S. Feetham, & J. L. Shaver (Eds.), *Clinical Nursing Research* (Vol. 1, pp. 485–507). New York: Saunders.

Woods, N., Most, A., & Dery, G. (1982a). Estimating perimenstrual distress: A comparison of two methods. *Research in Nursing & Health, 5*, 81–91.

Woods, N., Most, A., & Dery, G. (1982b). Estimating the prevalence of perimenstrual symptoms. *American Journal of Public Health, 72*, 1257–1264.

Woods, N., Most, A., & Dery, G. (1982c). Prevalence of perimenstrual symptoms. *American Journal of Public Health, 72*, 1257–1264.

Woods, N. F., Mitchell, E. S., & Lentz, M. (1999). Premenstrual symptoms: Delineating symptom clusters. *Journal of Women's Health and Gender-Based Medicine, 8*, 1053–1062.

Woods, N. F., Mitchell, E. S., Lentz, M. J., Taylor, D., & Lee, K. (1987). Premenstrual symptoms: Another look. *Public Health Reports, Jul–Aug*(Suppl.), 106–112.

Woods, N. F., Taylor, D., Mitchell, E. S., & Lentz, M. J. (1992). Premenstrual symptoms and health-seeking behavior. *Western Journal of Nursing Research, 14*(4), 418–443.

World Health Organization. (1981). A cross-cultural study of menstruation: Implications for contraceptive development and use. *Studies in Family Planning, 12,* 3–16.

World Health Organization. (1992). *International statistical classification of diseases and related health problems* (Vol. 10). Geneva.

Wyatt, K., Dimmock, P., Jones, P., Obhrai, M., & O'Brien, S. (2001). Efficacy of progesterone and progestogens in management of premenstrual syndrome: Systematic review. *British Medical Journal, 323*(7316), 776–780.

Yakir, M., Kreitler, S., Brzezinski, A., Vithoulkas, G., Oberbaum, M., & Bentwich, Z. (2001). Effects of homeopathic treatment in women with premenstrual syndrome: A pilot study. *British Homeopathic Journal, 90,* 148–153.

Yonkers, K., & White, K. (1992). Premenstrual exacerbation of depression: One process or two? *Journal of Clinical Psychiatry, 53,* 289–292.

Chapter 20

NORMAL AND ABNORMAL UTERINE BLEEDING

MARY ANN FAUCHER
KERRI DURNELL SCHUILING

One of the goals of a feminist model of health care is to keep the woman whole with her body and to avoid medicalizing symptoms that are, in fact, representations of normal. For example, the term "dysfunctional uterine bleeding" suggests pathology and the need to fix a "problem." It is important to recognize that some of the knowledge about women's cyclicity is medicalized, socially constructed, or both. Some cases of abnormal or dysfunctional bleeding actually represent a variation of normal and signify women's bodies' physiologic passage into the next stage of development—for example, menarche or menopause. It is important to look beyond the biomedical model when providing health care. A medical model inscribes the disorder on the body, necessitating symptom interpretation from the clinician's expertise alone (Bordo, 1993).

Medical intervention, particularly surgical, should be the last resort in many cases of dysfunctional or abnormal uterine bleeding. When the uterine bleeding diagnosed as irregular or abnormal is actually a variation of normal, it may be that treatment with exercise, diet, relaxation, and stress reduction is appropriate. As more clinicians embrace the normalcy of menstrual variations, there will be less temptation to cure normal female processes (Tavris, 1992). The expert clinician is one who actively listens, values input provided by the woman, and then carefully evaluates all available information before determining if the bleeding is abnormal or a variation of normal.

A feminist approach to women's health care using a health-oriented, normalizing model allows normalcy to be validated. This paradigm enables assessment, diagnosis, and treatment that is woman-centered and that values her standpoint, background, ethnicity, and culture.

ABNORMAL AND DYSFUNCTIONAL UTERINE BLEEDING

Abnormal uterine bleeding (AUB) is one of the more common reasons women seek health care. It accounts for up to 20% of all gynecologic visits and is the indication for up to 25% of all gynecologic surgeries (Goldstein, 2003; Livingstone & Fraser, 2002; Oriel & Schrager, 1999). AUB is an all encompassing diagnosis referring to any uterine bleeding that is irregular in amount, duration, or timing. It may or may not be related to a woman's menstrual cycle. AUB can occur as a normal physiologic event such as the irregular bleeding resulting from anovulation that often accompanies menarche or is symptomatic of perimenopause, or it may signal pathologic, life-threatening conditions such as an ectopic pregnancy or endometrial cancer. Traditional terms used to describe patterns of AUB are defined in Table 20–1.

Dysfunctional uterine bleeding (DUB) is the most common type of AUB and is frequently defined as irregular uterine bleeding unrelated to organic pathology, medications, pregnancy-related disorders, systemic conditions, iatrogenic causes, or genital tract pathology (American College of Nurse Midwives [ACNM], 2002; Albers, Hull, & Wes-

TABLE 20–1   Abnormal Uterine Bleeding Terminology and Patterns

Term	Definition	Interval
Amenorrhea	Absence of menses	
Primary amenorrhea	Absence of menses by age 14 with delay in maturation of secondary sexual characteristics or absence of menses by age 16 with evidence of secondary sexual characteristics	
Secondary amenorrhea	Absence of menses for 6 months or longer in a previously menstruating woman	
Intermenstrual bleeding	Bleeding or spotting between normal menses; flow is usually light	Between normal menses
Menorrhagia	Excessive amount or prolonged duration of bleeding; in excess of 80 ml	Regular
Menometrorrhagia	Heavy, prolonged menstrual bleeding	Irregular
Metrorrhagia	Uterine bleeding that is excessive in flow or duration or both	Irregular
Oligomenorrhea	Decreased, scanty flow	>35 days
Polymenorrhea	Regular, frequent menstruation	<21–24 days

Sources: ACNM, 2002; Speroff & Fritz, 2005.

ley, 2004; Oriel & Schrager, 1999; Speroff & Fritz, 2005). AUB and DUB are sometimes used interchangeably; however, strictly speaking, they are not synonymous. Some authorities define DUB as excessively heavy uterine bleeding that is prolonged and/or frequent and is not due to pregnancy, pelvic, or systemic disease (Aeby & Frattarelli, 2003). Others suggest a diagnosis of DUB should be made only if the cycles are anovulatory (American College of Obstetricians and Gynecologists [ACOG], 2000). All definitions reach the same conclusion: DUB is a diagnosis of exclusion. It is important to emphasize that clinicians should be consistent in the definition they use in practice because the definition often guides assessment. It is equally important to define the term for the woman so she has a full understanding of the meaning of her diagnosis.

PHYSIOLOGY AND PATTERNS OF NORMAL MENSES

The physiologic basis of normal menstrual physiology and the anatomic and functional structure of the reproductive tract provide a foundation for understanding AUB (see Chapter 5). Normal menses results from a functional hypothalamic-pituitary-ovarian axis (HPOA) and a precise sequence of hormonal events that lead to ovulation. If conception does not occur and if the outflow tract is patent, menses ensues. Normal menses may vary in length, duration, and amount of flow from woman to woman and therefore normal parameters are provided as ranges (Table 20–2). It is always wise to ask women who present with a concern about abnormal bleeding "What is a normal pattern for you?" because the woman is the best authority in describing her cycles.

Menses resulting from ovulatory cycles tend to have the same interval, amount, and duration from cycle to cycle unless significant health changes occur that negatively impact the HPOA. Menses in individual women tend to have consistent patterns once ovulation is established. Women who have regular, ovulatory menstrual cycles often experience premenstrual symptoms such as bloating, fatigue, constipation, and mood changes. These symptoms (collectively called "molimina") are a result of the higher levels of progesterone. The progesterone surge in the luteal phase sustains the corpus luteum for a finite period of time and when conception does not occur, the corpus luteum atrophies with resultant withdrawal bleeding. The withdrawal of progesterone also causes the production of arachidonic acid that leads to the production of PGF2 alpha. Dysmenorrhea associated with ovulatory bleeding results from the effects of PGF2 alpha that cause vasoconstriction and contraction of smooth muscle (Mishell, 2001).

TABLE 20–2   Ranges of Normal Menstrual Cycles

PARAMETER	RANGE OF NORMAL
Cycle interval	21–34 days
Duration of flow	3–8 days
Amount of flow	30–80 ml

ETIOLOGY AND PATHOPHYSIOLOGY OF ABNORMAL AND DYSFUNCTIONAL BLEEDING

The causes of abnormal and dysfunctional bleeding can be physiologic, pathologic, or pharmacologic (Table 20–3). Disruption of endocrine function at any level of the HPOA can disrupt normal menstrual physiology and cause a disturbance of the menstrual cycle's regularity, frequency, duration, or volume. The most common cause of a bleeding pattern that is suddenly different from a woman's established menstrual pattern is a complication of pregnancy, including threatened or incomplete abortion and ectopic pregnancy (Speroff & Fritz, 2005). Therefore, clinicians treating women of childbearing age who present with AUB should always first exclude pregnancy as a cause of the bleeding.

ANOVULATORY DYSFUNCTIONAL UTERINE BLEEDING

Evidence from recent histologic and molecular studies suggests that anovulatory bleeding is a result of an increased density of abnormal vessels that have a fragile structure prone to focal rupture that is followed by the release of lysosomes (proteolytic enzymes) from surrounding epithelial and stromal cells and migratory leukocytes and macrophages (Speroff & Fritz, 2005). The lack of progesterone in the luteal phase of anovulatory cycles leads to an unstable, excessively vascular endometrium. Heavy and irregular bleeding results from an imbalance in the vasoconstricting and vasodilating properties of prostaglandins and an imbalance in platelet aggregation and inhibition (Mishell, 2001). The abnormal microvasculature is most probably the cause of the abnormal bleeding that results (Speroff & Fritz). Table 20–4 identifies physiologic and pathologic causes of anovulation.

Anovulatory bleeding, in contrast to the regular, predictable, and often painful bleeding of ovulatory cycles, often leads to abnormal cycle intervals (e.g., polymenorrhea or metrorrhagia) or abnormal amounts of bleeding (e.g., oligomenorrhea, menorrhagia, or menometrorrhagia). Anovulatory bleeding also tends to be heavy secondary to the high and sustained levels of unopposed estrogen that result in endometrial hyperplasia. Endometrial hyperplasia can also result in episodes of amenorrhea, menorrhagia, and intermenstrual bleeding. Although anovulation is the most common cause of DUB, the clinician must consider a variety of other organic (i.e., systemic, reproductive tract, or iatrogenic) causes before concluding that anovulation is the etiology involved (ACOG, 2000).

It is normal for a woman to experience irregular menstrual cycles at the beginning and end of her reproductive life cycle: menarche and perimenopause. In fact, women who are 40–59 years of age account for almost half of all DUB diagnoses (March, 1998). The HPOA is most affected by the normal life cycle transitions that occur during the first two years after menarche and three years prior to menopause (Mishell, 2001); thus irregular bleeding during this time may be a reflection of normal. The least variation in menses occurs during the childbearing years, which generally encompasses ages 20–40, although most women will experience some variation from their established normal pattern from time to time. Even though bleeding patterns may fall within the range of normal, it is

TABLE 20-3 Causes of AUB

- **Pregnancy**
  Ectopic
  Spontaneous abortion (threatened, inevitable, missed, incomplete)
- **Endocrine problems/systemic**
  Adrenal hyperplasia
  Cushings syndrome
  Diabetes
  Pituitary
  Polycystic ovarian syndrome
  Thyroid disease
- **Medications–substances–herbs**
  Amphetamines
  Anticoagulants
  Antipsychotics
  Benzodiazepines
  Corticosteroids
  Herbs (ginkgo, ginseng, soy)
  Hormone Therapy
  Isoniazide
  Selective serotonin reuptake inhibitor (SSRI) antidepressants
- **Problems with the hypothalamic-pituitary-ovarian axis**
  Systemic illness (e.g., PCOS, pituitary, thyroid)
  Premature ovarian failure
  Postmenarche
  Perimenopause
  Stress
  Eating disorders
  Severe dieting and/or weight loss
  Excessive exercise
- **Reproductive tract disease/dysfunction**
  Atrophy
  Cancer
  Endometrial hyperplasia
  Endometriosis
  Infections
  Leiomyomas (leiomyomatas, myomas, fibroids)
  Outflow tract obstruction
  Ovarian tumors
  Polyps
  Trauma
- **Systemic disease**
  Thyroid dysfunction
  Coagulation defects
  Von Willebrand's
  Leukemia
  Idiopathic thrombocytopenia

TABLE 20–4   Physiologic and Pathologic Causes of Anovulation

Causes of Anovulation

Physiologic causes
- Pregnancy
- Lactation
- Perimenarche
- Perimenopause

Pathologic causes
- Hyperandrogenic disorders/syndromes (e.g., PCOS)
- Hyperprolactinemia
- Iatrogenic
- Extreme stress (physical and psychological)

important to listen to the woman's description prior to making a diagnosis, because for her, the bleeding may be abnormal and require follow-up.

OVULATORY DYSFUNCTIONAL UTERINE BLEEDING

Ovulatory DUB occurs significantly less often than anovulatory DUB. Ovulatory DUB cycles are regular and tend to be cyclic, although the bleeding patterns are often abnormal and may include polymenorrhea, oligomenorrhea, midcycle spotting, and menorrhagia. Menorrhagia is the most frequent pattern observed with ovulatory DUB and is commonly associated with pelvic pathology such as uterine leiomyomas, adenomysosis, or endometrial polyps (Livingstone & Fraser, 2002). Menorrhagia is also frequently associated with bleeding dyscrasias, and as many as 20% of adolescents who present with menorrhagia have a bleeding disorder (Bevan et al., 2001; Claessens & Cowell, 1981).

ASSESSMENT

HISTORY

A detailed menstrual history provides the most useful information in differentiating anovulatory bleeding from other causes (Speroff & Fritz, 2005). It is critical to remember that if the woman is of reproductive age and presents with abnormal uterine bleeding, pregnancy should be ruled out prior to any other testing. Menstrual history alone often can provide enough evidence for the clinician to confidently proceed to treating the patient without incurring unnecessary laboratory evaluation or testing.

Ask the woman to describe in detail what brought her in for the visit and then obtain a detailed menstrual history. Questions should include her age at menarche and menopause (if appropriate), cycle length, duration, and estimated amount of flow. When questioning women about cycle length, duration, and flow, it is important to understand how the woman calculates each of these factors. Some women do not include the first day of spotting or may not include the days when the flow is light when determining cycle length. Teaching her the parameters of what is considered normal may also provide her with a useful guide for describing her cycles. Her observation about how the bleeding deviates from her established pattern is a valuable tool to use in the assessment.

It is particularly helpful to determine if the bleeding occurs at regular or irregular intervals. The pattern of bleeding provides clues to etiology. For example, a woman who is postmenopausal and reports that she experienced spontaneous, painless, and irregular bleeding indicates to the clinician that endometrial hyperplasia should be part of the differential diagnosis. A woman who reports she is having regular cycles that have now become heavy and are accompanied by the passage of clots, and says she has noticed a sensation of pelvic fullness, suggests to the clinician that her menorrhagia may be secondary to uterine leiomyomas (fibroids).

Studies have repeatedly demonstrated that estimation of the amount of blood loss can be highly imprecise (Chimera, Anderson, & Turnball, 1980; Halberg, Hogdahl, Nillson, & Rybo, 1966). Counting pads or tampons has not been shown to be helpful in establishing the amount of bleeding because the brands vary widely in absorption rates (Grimes, 1979; Jannsen, Scholten, & Heintz, 1995). A reliable indicator of heavy bleeding is if clots are passed and are accompanied by heavy bleeding (Mishell, 2001).

Ask her the dates of her last three menstrual periods and ask her when her last normal menses occurred. Often a calendar will assist her to answer these questions accurately. Inquire about the color and character of her flow and related signs and symptoms such as pain, odor, and postcoital spotting. Inquire whether or not hot flushes or the sensation of a racing heartbeat are present because these signs accompanied by abnormal bleeding may indicate menopause is approaching, particularly if the woman is in the perimenopausal years.

If she is currently using or has used contraception in the past, obtain information about the type, the length of use, and any side effects encountered. Contraceptive history may reveal that her abnormal bleeding is mechanically caused by an intrauterine device (IUD) or is related to the use of hormonal contraception, such as oral contraceptives or injectable depot medroxyprogesterone acetate (Depo-Provera).

The gynecologic history may reveal other episodes of abnormal bleeding. Question the woman about previous treatment for abnormal bleeding. Inquire about Papanicolaou test history, gynecologic surgeries, sexually transmitted infections, or other infections of the genital tract or organs.

A medical history or general health history, including family history, provides information that may reveal underlying medical conditions that might be the cause of the abnormal bleeding. Ask about symptoms of thyroid disorders (e.g., fatigue, hyperactivity, weight gain or loss) and hormone-secreting tumors (e.g., hair loss, changes in breast size, hirsutism). Findings in the health history may suggest the presence of a systemic disease; therefore, pay particular attention to signs and symptoms such as easy bruising, presence of petechiae, weight or appetite changes, or changes in elimination patterns. Bleeding and endocrine disorders can be inherited, so look for familial patterns. Including questions about lifestyle is important in order to ascertain the possibilities of drug use or abuse, exercise patterns, and nutrition.

PHYSICAL EXAMINATION

The physical examination provides further information about possibilities of systemic disease, particularly organic pathology. Height, weight, body mass index (BMI), vital signs, hair, and body fat distribution are important parameters to include (ACNM, 2002). Hirsutism and abdominal obesity are signs of possible androgen excess and insulin resistance, which are present in women who have polycystic ovarian syndrome (PCOS) (Reid, 2000). Tanner staging (see Chapter 2) is helpful when examining adolescents because it can validate information from the history and may help to determine ovulatory status. Observe for signs that are indicative of anemia, such as pale skin tone and delayed capillary refill. Palpating the thyroid may identify enlargement or tumors related to hypo- or hyperthyroidism. A breast examination can rule out the presence of galactorrhea, which may indicate an elevated prolactin level.

A pelvic examination is essential for a woman of any age who is (or has been) sexually active, has abdominal pain, anemia, irregular bleeding, or bleeding that is so heavy her hemodynamic stability is compromised (ACNM, 2002). However, if the patient is a young adolescent who is not sexually active and only recently began menstruating and has a normal hematocrit, a pelvic examination is most likely unnecessary. The pelvic examination should include a general assessment of the genitalia. Observe for bruising, lacerations, or evidence of infection. Clitoromegaly suggests the possibility of an endocrine disorder.

A speculum examination enables observation of the vagina and cervix for evidence of infection, trauma, or foreign objects. Cervical cultures to rule out infection and a Pap test should be obtained at this time. Clinicians who have young clients who are not sexually active but who require a pelvic examination to rule out the cause of the abnormal bleeding should use a pediatric speculum, inserting it with great care and gentleness. At times, a pelvic examination in these instances may need to be done under anesthesia in order to provide physical comfort.

A bimanual examination provides the opportunity to assess for the presence of tumors, cervical polyps, ovarian cysts, uterine tenderness or enlargement, and adnexal pain or masses. If the bimanual examination is performed on a young adolescent, the clinician should use only one digit and, again, proceed with great care and gentleness.

LABORATORY TESTING

Laboratory tests used to diagnose AUB can be invasive and expensive. Decisions regarding which tests to use should be based on the differential diagnosis and directed by the information collected during the history and physical, including the woman's age and her reproductive status (Table 20–5).

General tests to consider obtaining for all types of AUB include:

TABLE 20–5   Laboratory Testing for AUB

Test	Differential Diagnosis	Results
Urine human chorionic gonadotropin (hCG)	Pregnancy; threatened, missed, or incomplete spontaneous abortion	Positive or negative
Quantitative hCG	Ectopic or impending spontaneous abortion	Level lower than expected for gestational age and/or lack of doubling in 48 hours
CBC with platelets	Anemia, clotting abnormalities	Hemoglobin less than 10 mg/dl, platelets less than 150,000
PT, APTT, bleeding time	Von Willebrand's (VWD), leukemia, prothrombin deficiency	Bleeding time increased
Serum iron/ferritin	Iron deficiency anemia secondary to bleeding	
Follicle-stimulating hormone (FSH)	Amenorrhea due to menopause, premature ovarian failure	Levels greater than 30 mIU/ml, some texts cite 40 mIU/ml
Progesterone	Anovulatory	Levels less than 10 ng/ml
TSH	Hypothyroidism or hyperthyroidism	0.8–4 (normal values)
Pap test	Dysplasia/carcinoma	Normal epithelial cells or atypical cells suggestive of dysplasia and/or carcinoma
Prolactin	Pituitary adenoma	Levels less than 100 ng/mL usually rule out a pituitary tumor
Cultures and/or wet preps	Vaginal infection (e.g., gonorrhea, chlamydia, trichomoniasis, candidiasis)	Negative or positive

1. A pregnancy test (if the patient is of childbearing age)
   - Qualitative β-hCG
   - Serial serum quantitative β-hCG may help to diagnose specific pregnancy disorders
2. Complete blood count
   - Order only if indicated or anemia is suspected
3. Thyroid stimulating hormone (TSH)
   - Order especially if hypo- or hyperthyroidism or other thyroid abnormality is suspected
4. Pap test (unless the patient is an adolescent who is not sexually active)
5. Gonorrhea and chlamydia testing as indicated
6. Wet mount with normal saline and potassium hydroxide as indicated

TABLE 20–6   Differential Diagnosis and Laboratory Assessment of AUB

To rule out:	Labs to order:
Endocrine causes of AUB	General labs + prolactin, FSH & LH levels
Adrenal causes	
Patient is hirsute and has menorrhagia	General labs + adrenal studies, testosterone levels. Adjunct: CT scan of abdomen, cortisol levels
Hormone-producing tumor	General labs + MRI, CT scan, Cortisol levels
Structural abnormalities	General labs + ultrasound
Infection	General labs + gonorrhea and chlamydia tests + wet mount; consider need for WBC
Cervical or uterine pathology	General labs + colposcopy with biopsy, endometrial biopsy; hysteroscopy
Amenorrhea	General labs + FSH, LH, Prolactin levels, TSH, T_3, T_4
Von Willebrand's (VWD)	Ristocetin cofactor assay
Liver disease	Liver function tests
Renal disease	Renal function tests
Coagulation disorders other than VWD	PTT, PT, assessment of platelet function

Sources: American College of Nurse Midwives, 2002; Speroff & Fritz, 2005.

Additional tests should be ordered only if there are specific indications (Table 20–6). For example, if the patient says she is experiencing heavy bleeding and is passing clots greater than 1 inch in diameter and has to change her pads or tampons frequently, particularly during the night, a serum ferritin test should be considered. A recent study revealed that if the aforementioned clinical signs were accompanied by a low serum ferritin it was highly likely the woman was experiencing menorrhagia (Warner et al., 2004).

Other diagnostic tests may be required for definitive diagnosis of endometrial pathology. Transvaginal ultrasonography of the pelvis is useful for detecting polyps and submucosal leiomyomas, measuring endometrial thickness, evaluation of pregnancy complications, and ovarian masses (Albers et al., 2004; Long, 1996). If the result of transvaginal ultrasonography is abnormal, it might be prudent for the clinician to consult or refer the woman for medical management.

An endometrial biopsy is easily accomplished in the office setting and can be performed by clinicians who have had the education and training required for performing the test accurately. The sensitivity of endometrial biopsies for detecting endometrial abnormalities is quite high; yet up to 18% of local lesions, including leiomyomas and polyps, may be missed because only a small part of the endometrium is sampled at any one time (Clark et al., 2002).

Hysteroscopy is the current gold standard for evaluating the endometrium (Oriel & Schrager, 1999), although recent evidence indicates that saline-infusion sonohysterography (SIS) with endometrial biopsy offers the most complete evaluation of the endometrium with the least risk to the patient (Mihm, Quick, Brumfield, Connors, &

Finnerty, 2002; O'Connell, Fries, Zeringue, & Brehm, 1998). Both SIS and hysteroscopy are indicated when endometrial biopsy or transvaginal ultrasonography results are normal but the woman continues to be symptomatic (Bradley, 2004).

Dilatation and curettage (D & C) is used primarily for acute bleeding episodes resulting in hypovolemia and for older women if there is a high suspicion of endometrial carcinoma (March, 1998). Magnetic resonance imaging (MRI) and computerized tomography (CT) scan may be used to diagnose adnexal masses, adenomyosis, uterine leiomyomas, and pituitary adenomas (Speroff & Fritz, 2005).

None of these tests, however, are generally necessary for evaluation of an adolescent who presents with abnormal bleeding. An endometrial biopsy or hysteroscopy should, however, always be included in the assessment of abnormal bleeding in women who are perimenopausal or postmenopausal, adolescents who are obese and have had long-term (three or more years) of unexplained abnormal bleeding, or any woman whose endometrium has been exposed to unopposed estrogen.

DIFFERENTIAL DIAGNOSES OF ABNORMAL BLEEDING

The diagnosis of DUB is made after excluding all other causes of the abnormal bleeding. When all other causes of bleeding are firmly ruled out, then and only then can the diagnosis of anovulatory DUB be made.

SYSTEMIC CAUSES OF AUB

AUB can be a sign of significant systemic disease, especially if findings from the pelvic examination are normal. Systemic diseases cause AUB by impacting the HPOA or by impacting the uterine endometrium, which is the target tissue of the HPOA. Abnormal bleeding patterns with systemic etiologies typically include amenorrhea, oligomenorrhea, and menorrhagia.

The most common systemic causes of AUB are blood dyscrasias and coagulopathies such as leukemia, severe sepsis, idiopathic thrombocytopenic purpura, and hypersplenism (Brenner, 1996; Kim, 2000). Liver and renal diseases result in an inability to adequately clear estrogen, which increases biologically active, free-floating estrogen that then negatively impacts the HPOA with resultant anovulation (Kim). Von Willebrand's disease (VWD) is the most common cause of lifelong abnormal bleeding patterns in women (Kouides, 1999; Wysocki, 1999). Although the most common cause of AUB in adolescents is anovulation, the second most common cause is coagulation disorders due to VWD, platelet dysfunction, and idiopathic thrombocytopenia (Bevan et al., 2001). One of the hallmarks of VWD, a genetically inherited disease, is menorrhagia (Geil, 2003). Women presenting with a history of easy bruising, prolonged bleeding following dental work or surgery, menorrhagia, or metrorrhagia warrant further follow-up, particularly if other treatment has failed (Brenner, 1996).

Thyroid dysfunction may cause bleeding abnormalities, and therefore endocrine pathology should always be considered when evaluating a woman for AUB. Hypothyroidism can cause either amenorrhea (particularly if the hypothyroidism is chronic) or menorrhagia (if the hypothyroidism is recent) (Kim, 2000). Altered levels of TSH induce elevated levels of prolactin, which in turn inhibits ovulation. Conversely, hyperthyroidism typically causes amenorrhea (North American Menopause Society [NAMS], 2000).

Pituitary disease and some pituitary tumors may result in elevated levels of prolactin. Amenorrhea associated with elevated prolactin levels is due to prolactin inhibition of the pulsatile secretion of gonadotropin-releasing hormone (GnRH) (Speroff & Fritz, 2005). Prolactin-secreting pituitary adenomas are the most common type of pituitary tumor (Speroff & Fritz). Approximately one-third of women with elevated prolactin levels will also have galactorrhea. It is important to note that many individuals (10%) have silent pituitary masses that are not endocrinologically active and have no adverse impact on health and well-being. If there is no evidence of hormonal disturbance, no immediate action is probably necessary, although long-term surveillance is appropriate (Speroff & Fritz).

Diseases or syndromes causing insulin resistance, such as PCOS, increase circulating levels of insulin, which in turn causes an elevation in androgen production and concomitant anovulation (Seidenfeld & Rickert, 2001). The relationship between insulin and androgens is believed to be an underlying cause of PCOS (see Chapter 21 for further discussion of PCOS).

REPRODUCTIVE TRACT ETIOLOGIES

Reproductive disorders that may result in AUB include pregnancy complications such as ectopic pregnancy; threatened, missed, or incomplete abortion; subinvolution of the placental site; and trophoblastic disease (Brenner, 1996). All women of childbearing age who present with AUB should be considered pregnant until proven otherwise.

Signs of reproductive tract malignancies such as endometrial and cervical cancer include AUB, and therefore cancers of the reproductive tract should be ruled out when a woman presents with AUB. A corpus luteum is not produced when the cycle is anovulatory, and therefore the ovary fails to secrete progesterone although estrogen continues to be produced (ACOG, 2000). This results in endometrial hyperplasia and the clinical result is bleeding that is noncyclic, unpredictable, and inconsistent in volume (ACOG). All uterine bleeding that occurs in women who are postmenopausal is always considered abnormal and endometrial cancer needs to be ruled out.

Infections such as chlamydia, gonorrhea, and endometritis may cause irregular spotting due to irritation and inflammation of the tissues of the cervix or endometrium. A thorough history and physical examination (including pelvic examination) will assist in ruling out infection as a cause of the abnormal bleeding.

Leiomyomas, adenomyosis, and polyps can cause irregular or heavy abnormal uterine bleeding (see Chapter 22 for further discussion of these conditions). Leiomyomas are a frequent cause of abnormal bleeding during the reproductive years and frequently cause menorrhagia or menometrorrhagia (Mishell, 2001). Polyps are common benign growths on the cervix. They are easily visualized with a speculum and appear as smooth, deep to bright red growths that are fragile and bleed with little encouragement during examination. Women with cervical polyps may present with a concern about postcoital bleeding.

Trauma to the reproductive tract can also cause AUB. Tampons can irritate the cervix and cause spotting. Women who have been sexually assaulted may experience abnormal bleeding from lacerations and other injuries that occurred to the internal organs and genitals.

OUTFLOW TRACT CAUSES OF AUB

Normal menses depends on a normally functioning outflow tract (among other factors). Anatomic abnormalities at any level of the outflow tract can interfere with normal menstrual flow, and generally problems associated with the outflow tract result in amenorrhea. Uterine or cervical congenital and or/structural abnormalities can cause AUB. When the uterus and/or vagina have congenital structural abnormalities, it may be impossible for menses to flow properly. Rarely, segments of the Mullerian tube fail to develop, resulting in abnormalities such as imperforate hymen, lack of a vaginal orifice, lapses in the continuity of the vaginal canal, an absent uterus or cervix, an absent uterine cavity, or an absence of endometrium. Obstruction of menses may lead to painful distention due to hematometra, hematcolopos, or hemoperitoneum. Affected women are genotypically and phenotypically normal females with functioning ovaries. These abnormalities are exceedingly rare (Brunt, 1995; Engel & Rushovich, 1984). If a patient presents who is experiencing amenorrhea and whose pelvic examination and bimanual examination are normal and she has no history of infection or trauma, then an abnormality of the outflow tract is not likely.

IATROGENIC CAUSES OF AUB

Many medications predispose women to AUB, including glucocorticoids, tamoxifen, and anticoagulants (Speroff & Fritz, 2005). Ginseng, ginkgo, and soy products have been associated with alterations in estrogen levels and affecting clotting parameters (ACOG, 2001). A thorough history should reveal if a patient is on any medication that might cause AUB. It is important to clarify the regimen followed in taking the medication because sometimes taking a medication incorrectly will result in AUB. This is frequently observed in women taking oral contraceptives for the first time.

LIFESTYLE CAUSES OF AUB

Athletic women, particularly long-distance runners, gymnasts, and professional ballet dancers, are at risk for oligomenorrhea and amenorrhea as are women suffering from anorexia and other eating disorders. This type of amenorrhea occurs in a pattern referred to as hypothalamic suppression (Reid, 2000; Speroff & Fritz, 2005). Typically the amenorrhea occurs as secondary amenorrhea that follows the start of an intensive training regime, although there is documentation that when intensive training begins prior to menarche, menarche can be delayed by as much as three years and the subsequent risk of menstrual irregularity is even higher (Speroff & Fritz).

The pathophysiology of exercise-induced amenorrhea is complex and is probably due to low body fat as well as diminished secretion of GnRH. Decreased GnRH results in less luteinizing and follicle-stimulating hormone (LH and FSH) pulses, which in turn decreases the amount of estrogen produced by the ovaries. The critical weight theory hypothesizes that there is a critical weight and amount of body fat that must be maintained in order for women to experience regular menstrual cycles (Speroff & Fritz, 2005).

Illicit drugs have been shown to inhibit ovulation due to hyperprolactinemia, which results in amenorrhea. A descriptive study focusing on the endocrine profiles of women who were admitted to a substance-abuse unit found that hyperprolactinemia and macrocytosis (increased mean corpuscular volume [MCV]) was evident in up to 60% of women who were reproductive age and who abused alcohol, tranquilizers, and opiates or used illicit drugs including marijuana and cocaine (Teoh, Lex, Mendelson, Mello, & Cochin, 1992). Over 80% of the women in the study who were postmenopausal and had an alcohol dependency also had either hyperprolactinemia or increased MCV or both (Teoh et al.).

MANAGEMENT

Management goals for treating AUB are to (1) normalize the bleeding, (2) correct any anemia, (3) prevent cancer, and (4) restore quality of life. Concomitant therapy may be necessary in order to achieve these goals, particularly if the bleeding is severe and threatens hemodynamic stability. For example, a woman who presents with severe bleeding from a raw and denuded endometrium may require high-dose estrogen to stop the bleeding. The administration of estrogen to stop the acute bleeding will not address the cause of the bleeding and therefore additional treatment, such as a D & C, surgical ablation, or hysterectomy, may be required (Bayer & DeCherney, 1993; Chapple, 1999; Choung & Brenner, 1996). Additionally, if the woman is anemic from the bleeding, she will need iron therapy.

Age, desire for future fertility, and patient preference all need to be considered when determining treatment options for women with AUB. Treatment falls into two categories: treatment for acute bleeding and treatment of chronic bleeding. Women who present with excessive heavy bleeding and who have a dangerously low hematocrit require physician consultation. All episodes of acute hemorrhagic bleeding should be managed by a physician.

ACUTE LIFE-THREATENING HEMORRHAGE

Acute hemorrhage always necessitates physician referral and medical management in the hospital setting.

ACUTE NON-LIFE-THREATENING HEAVY BLEEDING

If bleeding is nonemergent, administration of high-dose estrogen usually will stop the bleeding and allow for further evaluation. Estrogen therapy stimulates rapid endometrial proliferation and resolves the bleeding from a denuded endometrium (Kim, 2000). Concomitant use of antiemetics (e.g., meclizine) is indicated when high-dose estrogen is used because of the nausea that often accompanies use of high doses of estrogen. The clinician needs to be mindful that estrogens, particularly high-dose estrogens, may precipitate thromboembolism and therefore are contraindicated in women with a history of thrombosis or family history of idiopathic venous thromboembolism. A usual dosage regimen of high-dose estrogen in these instances is 1.25 mg conjugated estrogen or 2.0 mg micronized estradiol every 4–6 hours for 24 hours. The amount of estrogen may be tapered then to once daily for 7–10 days once the bleeding is under control (Speroff & Fritz, 2005). When the bleeding stops, 2.5 mg of conjugated equine estrogens (CEE, Premarin) can be given daily followed by the addition of medroxyprogesterone acetate (MPA, Provera) 10 mg, given the last 10 days of therapy to initiate withdrawal bleeding.

A monophasic combined oral contraceptive (COC) given twice daily should also result in the reduction of bleeding within 24 hours. If the flow does not stop with 48 hours, further evaluation is indicated. The COC is typically tapered to once daily after five to seven days and continued with 21 days of active pills followed by 7 days of placebo pills or no pills. An alternative to the 21/7-day cycle pattern is an extended regime of 84 days of monophasic COCs followed by a 7-day pill-free interval (Kaunitz, Westhoff, & Leonhardt, 2002).

Three months of CEE/MPA or COC therapy should be provided, and if there is no significant improvement, then the woman should be reevaluated (Society of Obstetricians & Gynaecologists of Canada [SOGC], 2001). Women with chronic menorrhagia can be offered cyclic MPA at doses of 10 mg a day for 10–14 days. This therapy should be repeated every 30–40 days. Intramuscular injection of progesterone in oil at 100–200 mg is an alternative to cyclic MPA. Progesterone therapy is not as effective as estrogen for management of acute bleeds, but progesterone is effective for long-term management (Kim, 2000). Table 20–7 describes additional medical therapies for menorrhagia.

Nonsteroidal anti-inflammatory drugs (NSAIDs) are useful for ovulatory–idiopathic menorrhagia. The heavier the bleeding the better the effect, although the mechanism of action for NSAIDs used for menorrhagia is poorly understood. Theoretically, the NSAIDs interfere with the transformation of arachidonic acid to cyclic endoperoxidases and hence block the production of prostaglandins. This effect on the prostaglandin cascade results in a 12–50% increase in platelet aggregation (Smith, et al., 1982; Lethaby, Augood & Duckitt, 2003). Optimally, an NSAID should be initiated three days prior to the start of menses. Although only mefanamic acid has US Food and Drug Administration approval for this therapeutic indication, other NSAIDs are used in clinical practice (Table 20–8). All NSAIDs are contraindicated in women with ulcers or bronchospastic lung disease.

The levonorgestrel-releasing intrauterine system (LNG-IUS) is a particularly effective therapy for menorrhagia related to anovulation or leiomyomas (Lethaby, Cooke & Rees, 2003). Woman with myomas are candidates for the LNG-IUS if the myoma does not distort the uterine cavity and the uterus is less than 12 weeks in size. A small study demonstrated resolution of anemia in 95% of woman who used the LNG-IUS for bleeding and

TABLE 20-7   Medical Therapies for Menorrhagia

Acute bleeding	Long-term/chronic management
• Replete intravascular volume • *CEE 25 mg IV q 4–6 hrs PRN then • CEE 2.5 mg–5 mg po QID for 2–3 days then add †MPA 10 mg for 10–14 days (continue CEE) • COCs BID/TID then taper	• Cyclic MPA 10 mg/day for 10–14 days, every 30–40 days • Combined contraceptives (oral, patch, ring) • Oral micronized progesterone 300 mg for 10–14 days, every 30–40 days • Depot medroxyprogesterone acetate (Depo-Provera) 150 mg, IM, every 3 months • Levonorgestrel intrauterine system (LNG-IUS) • ‡NSAIDs

Note: High doses of estrogen may precipitate a thrombotic event and therefore are contraindicated in women with a history of thrombosis or a family history of idiopathic venous thromboembolism (Speroff & Fritz, 2005).
*CEE: conjugated equine estrogens
†MPA: medroxyprogesterone acetate
‡NSAIDs: nonsteroidal anti-inflammatory drugs

a 40% prevalence of amenorrhea after 12 months of use (Grigorieva, Chen-Mok, Tarasova, & Mikhailov, 2003). The LNG-IUS also has been compared to endometrial ablation as a therapy to resolve menorrhagia. In one study, women were referred from their primary care provider for lack of efficacy with medical therapy. One group received thermal ablation and the other group received the LNG-IUS. Both therapies were found to be equally efficacious by measurement with a pre- and postpictorial blood-loss assessment chart (Barrington, Arunkalaivannan, & Abdel-Fattah, 2003). The LNG-IUS also has been compared with hysterectomy in women with leiomyomas but not the subserosal type. At follow-up, 20% of the women with the LNG-IUS had undergone a hysterectomy, and 68% of the women were still using the LNG-IUS. Both groups reported improvement in quality of life (Hurskainen et al., 2004). Another, more recent randomized, multicenter trial in women treated with either the LNG-IUS or hysterectomy found no difference between the two groups with regard to symptom improvement. Although 42% of women in the LNG-IUS group had a hysterectomy, the LNG-IUS was found to be much less expensive (Hurskainen et al., 2004).

TABLE 20-8   NSAID Therapy for Menorrhagia

- Mefanamic acid 500 mg TID*
- Ibuprofen 600 mg TID
- Naproxen sodium 550 mg loading dose then 275 mg q 6 hours

*FDA approved

NONEMERGENT ANOVULATORY DUB

Treatment of nonemergent DUB due to anovulation can be managed by administration of COCs (March, 1998). This therapy, however, will be ineffective if the endometrium is raw and denuded. Any formulation is acceptable and therapy is one pill twice daily for 5–7 days, then one pill daily. The flow may cease within 24 hours, but the therapy is continued as prescribed. The therapy is continued for three months at which time the endometrium should be of normal height and unopposed endogenous estrogen should stimulate a withdrawal bleed of normal amount and duration. If the woman desires contraception, the COCs can be continued. If the flow does not stop, further evaluation is necessary. The combined contraceptive patch or ring may also be used. For further discussion about COCs and other types of contraception see Chapter 9.

Chronic anovulation can also be managed with cyclic progestogen therapy, given the last 10 days of the menstrual cycle (Table 20–9). In women with secondary amenorrhea due to anovulation the progestational challenge should be administered; then bleeding should commence within two to seven days after completion. Any amount of bleeding after the progestational challenge confirms adequate levels of endogenous estrogen and outflow tract patency. Generally, progestogens will not induce bleeding when the woman has hypopituitarism caused by a tumor or has profound hypothalamic suppression (Speroff & Fritz, 2005). Women who do not bleed after a progestational challenge merit further evaluation. Typically cyclic progestogen therapy is reserved for women who do not need contraception.

PROGESTIN THERAPY

Progestins can be used to treat oligomenorrhea, dysfunctional menometrorrhagia, or polymenorrhea (Table 20–9). Progestins are not as effective as estrogen in stopping acute bleeding but are effective for long-term treatment once the acute bleeding episode has been resolved. Progestins may also be the management regimen of choice if the woman has contraindications to taking estrogen. To induce normal bleeding, 5–10 mg of synthetic progestin is given for 7–12 days each month. Withdrawal bleeding should occur within 2–7 days of discontinuing the progesterone. If bleeding fails to occur or if irregular bleeding persists, diagnostic reevaluation is necessary and physician consult recommended. Do not

---

TABLE 20–9   Progestogen Therapy for Chronic Anovulation

- Medroxyprogesterone acetate (Provera) 10 mg x 10 days
- Norethindrone 5 mg BID x 10 days
- Oral micronized progesterone (Prometrium) 200 mg/day x 10 days
- Depot medroxyprogesterone acetate (Depo-Provera) 150 mg IM q 12 weeks
- Levonorgestrel-releasing IUS

use progestin therapy if the woman thinks she might be pregnant, even if her pregnancy test is negative.

SURGICAL TREATMENT

When medical therapy fails, surgical management options include endometrial ablation, uterine artery embolization, and hysterectomy. Menorrhagia and leiomyomas account for up to 75% of all hysterectomies worldwide (SGOC, 2001).

Endometrial ablation was introduced in the 1990s as an alternative to hysterectomy. Hysteroscopic resection, roller-ball, and thermal balloon are all different ablation techniques. Endometrial ablation has been best studied in women who are premenopausal and have leiomyomas less than two centimeters. Endometrial ablation compared with hysterectomy was found to have fewer complications, to cost less, and postoperative satisfaction was similar (Marjoribanks, Lethaby, & Farquhar, 2003; Pinion et al., 1994; Zupi et al., 2003). However, 30–40% of ablations require subsequent surgical intervention (i.e., re-ablation or hysterectomy) although the number of overall hysterectomies is decreased when ablation is used (Majoribanks et al.). Limitations of use include very specific candidate criteria (Table 20–10).

Some authorities do not recommend ablation in women 50 years of age or older because of the increased risk of endometrial cancer in this age group. However, this is a subject of debate and to date there is no consensus in opinion. Woman with abnormal bleeding who are considering ablation should undergo hysteroscopy before ablation to confidently rule out the presence of endometrial disease.

Because 20–50% of women have leiomyomas and many of these women are young, uterine artery embolization was introduced as a surgical intervention that provides relief but maintains the possibility of future fecundity. In one well-designed study, 200 women with a mean age of 43 years underwent uterine artery embolization. An 85–95% improvement in bleeding and a 93% improvement in overall symptoms were reported. Uterine size decreased 38% and myoma size decreased 58%. A minor complication rate of 6.3% also was reported with the occurrence of one pulmonary embolism that resolved

TABLE 20–10   Candidates and Contraindications for Endometrial Ablation

Candidates	Contraindications
• Cancer has been ruled out	• Known or suspected uterine cancer
• No previous myomectomy	• IUD
• Nondistorted uterine cavity	• Pregnancy
• Past childbearing	• Previous classical Cesarean section
• Refractory to medical therapy	• Pelvic, uterine, cervical, or vaginal infection
	• Uterus sounds to <4 cm

Sources: Adapted from Barrington et al., 2003; Pinion et al., 1994.

successfully (Spies et al., 2001). However, in 2004 ACOG released an opinion about uterine artery embolization due to concern with lack of well-designed studies, unsure efficacy and recurrence rate of myomas after the procedure, and significant risk for morbidity and mortality (ACOG, 2004). ACOG essentially recommends that all candidates for uterine artery embolization be evaluated by an obstetrician–gynecologist prior to the procedure and provide informed consent indicating an understanding about the rare but possibly deadly complications of this procedure. Clearly, more research is needed.

Hysterectomy is the only definitive treatment for women with menorrhagia. Many advantages of hysterectomy have been reported, including improved quality of life, but reports about postoperative morbidity and mortality, including post-surgical fatigue, weight change, and changes in sexual satisfaction are prevalent. Debate about post-hysterectomy sexuality is complex, due to many confounding variables, although most studies do not confirm a negative impact on sexual satisfaction (Dragisic & Milad, 2004; Maas, Weijenborg, & ter Kuile, 2003; Roussis, Waltrous, Kerr, Robertazzi, & Cabbad, 2004).

Studies have shown that women facing the decision about hysterectomy want their clinician to provide them with information that includes the physical effects of the procedure, the body parts involved, issues concerning sexuality and femininity, and the availability of support groups for dealing with some of these postoperative issues (Wade, Pletsch, Morgan, & Menting, 2000). Research demonstrates that when patients are provided with written and video information preoperatively and have an opportunity to discuss the advantages, disadvantages, and alternatives to hysterectomy, fewer women will choose hysterectomy compared with women who only receive information but do not have the opportunity to have an interview with their health care provider (Kennedy et al., 2002).

AMENORRHEA

ASSESSMENT

The management plan for woman with amenorrhea is somewhat different than for other causes of AUB; however, ruling out pregnancy is still the first step. The differential diagnosis for nonpregnant women presenting with amenorrhea is either primary amenorrhea or secondary amenorrhea, although Speroff and Fritz (2005) warn that premature categorization of amenorrhea can lead to diagnostic omissions and, frequently, unnecessary and expensive diagnostic testing.

Physiologic causes of amenorrhea include anatomic defects, ovarian failure, chronic anovulation, anterior pituitary disorders, and central nervous system disorders. Age is an important criterion in making the differential of primary versus secondary amenorrhea and is relevant in determining the types of questions to ask in the interview. Primary amenorrhea in a young woman may be indicative of HPOA or anatomical factors, such as outflow tract obstruction. If the amenorrhea is primary amenorrhea, the physical examination needs to focus on identifying the maturation of secondary sex characteristics (e.g., Tanner staging for breast development and pubic hair pattern) and establishing outflow tract patency. The clinician should ask, "Has any vaginal bleeding occurred?" Other important interview questions to consider relate to lifestyle patterns (e.g., exercise, medication, and drug use) and eating habits (e.g., investigating possible eating disorders). A family history of anatomic or genetic abnormalities should be explored.

The primary etiology of secondary amenorrhea is anovulation, but not exclusively. Premature ovarian failure, menopause, endocrine problems (e.g., PCOS, thyroid disease), anterior pituitary disorders, and central nervous system disorders all need to be considered.

Components of the interview should explore lifestyle factors that may increase the risk profile for amenorrhea due to loss of body fat and physical stress. Being in adolescence, having a family history of eating disorders, and participating in competitive athletics are risks for lifestyle stress that interrupt the function of the HPOA and lead to amenorrhea (Reid, 2000). A contraceptive history may reveal that the woman is a long-term user of hormonal contraceptives and is therefore more likely to experience amenorrhea due to endometrial atrophy (Speroff & Fritz, 2005). Changes in body weight or body distribution (e.g., large waist circumference) may suggest PCOS and chronic anovulation, whereas weight gain and temperature intolerance suggest thyroid disorders. A history of headaches and galactorrhea may be related to a prolactin-secreting tumor, or hypothyroidism. A history of hot flushes, concomitant with cessation of menses, and vaginal dryness all suggest menopause as a possible etiology for amenorrhea. The obstetric and gynecologic history might reveal a history of multiple D & Cs, significant, severe endometrial infections, or cervical treatments (e.g., cryotherapy) that indicate cervical stenosis may be the cause of the amenorrhea.

The physical examination should include an overall body assessment noting general habitus, weight, and body fat distribution and hair patterns. The thyroid should be assessed for size, presence of nodules, and tenderness. Vital signs, particularly the pulse rate and skin changes, may be helpful in diagnosing thyroid disease. Include a breast examination and note Tanner staging when doing a workup for primary amenorrhea. Assessing for the presence of galactorrhea (i.e., suggesting high prolactin levels) and performing a visual field evaluation are important to do when women present with headaches and/or galactorrhea, which are suggestive of pituitary disease.

The pelvic examination is helpful in identifying signs of estrogen depletion characterized by lack of mucus production and pale, thin, minimally rugated vaginal epithelium (Bachman, 1999). Visual inspection of the external genitalia may reveal clitoral hypertrophy and the possibility of virulization (Reid, 2000).

In young women with primary amenorrhea a sensitive and gentle approach to the pelvic examination is critical. Teaching her how to relax her vaginal muscles by first placing a well-lubricated finger into the vagina may be helpful in preparation for a gentle, nontraumatic speculum examination.

Obstruction of the vagina in the presence of a bulging, bluish colored membrane indicates imperforate hymen. An obstructed bimanual examination needs referral and fol-

TABLE 20-11   Causes of Primary and Secondary Amenorrhea

Primary Amenorrhea	Secondary Amenorrhea

• Pregnancy
• Upper genital tract causes
  o Mullerian agenesis (absence of uterus and vagina, normal secondary sex characteristics)
  o Testicular feminization (absence of uterus, blind ending vaginal pouch, normal breast development, scant pubic and maxillary hair)
• Lower genital tract causes
  o Labial agglutination
  o Imperforate hymen
  o Transverse vaginal septate
• Hypergonadotropic-hypogonadism
  o FSH > 40 mIU/L
  o Gonadal dysgenesis
  o Ovarian enzyme disorder
  o Resistant ovarian syndrome
	• Pregnancy
	• Asherman's syndrome
	• Cervical stenosis
	• Hormonal contraception
	• Hypothyroidism
	• PCOS
	• Pituitary tumor
	• Premature ovarian failure
	• Menopause
	• Hyopthalamic/CNS disorders (e.g., lifestyle stress, eating disorder, extreme athleticism)

low-up for possible presence of a vaginal septum, or a blind pouch at the end of the vagina. Both physical findings suggest the possibility of uterovaginal agenesis and should prompt a medical referral (Reid, 2000). Table 20–11 provides a list of the causes of primary and secondary amenorrhea.

MANAGEMENT

If pregnancy is excluded as the cause of the amenorrhea, a prolactin level, TSH, and a progestational challenge should be obtained. If the patient has galactorrhea, imaging of the sella turcica is also recommended (Speroff & Fritz, 2005). A progestational challenge can be accomplished by administering micronized progesterone (Prometrium) 300 mg daily or medroxyprogesterone acetate (Provera) 10 mg daily for 5 days. Withdrawal bleeding should occur within 7–10 days after the progestogen is discontinued if the level of endogenous estrogen is appropriate to produce a withdrawal bleed and the outflow tract is patent. If the patient chooses to use micronized progesterone, it is suggested she take it at bedtime because it is known to cause drowsiness in some women.

    If the response to the progestational challenge is positive (withdrawal bleeding occurs) and if the patient does not have galactorrhea and her prolactin level is normal, the possibility of a pituitary tumor is effectively ruled out (Speroff & Fritz, 2005). In this case, the diagnosis is anovulation, and the treatment is a progestogen for the first 10 days of each month or combined contraceptives. The patient should also be evaluated for PCOS. If, however, the patient does not have a positive progestational challenge, then a physician consult is warranted for further evaluation and management options.

EVIDENCE FOR PRACTICE

Level I evidence consistently demonstrates that the treatment of choice for anovulatory uterine bleeding is pharmacologic treatment with oral contraceptives. Cyclic progestogens also work well (ACOG, 2000). Recommendations that are based primarily on consensus and expert opinion (Level III) are: (1) underlying coagulopathies should be considered in all patients (particularly adolescents) with abnormal bleeding if the bleeding does not respond to treatment and is not able to explained, and (2) the efficacy of using CEE therapy in anovulatory bleeding is based on limited evidence, but it is effective in controlling the abnormal bleeding (ACOG).

SPECIAL CONSIDERATIONS

ADOLESCENTS

Nutrition has a considerable impact on the gynecologic health of adolescents. Adolescent females with eating disorders such as anorexia, bulimia nervosa, or obesity frequently have menstrual abnormalities (Seidenfeld & Rickert, 2001), and therefore history and physical assessment are important diagnostic tools. It is also important for clinicians to not assume young adolescent patients are not sexually active. It is essential to question teens about their sexual and gynecologic histories. Confidentiality is an essential part of therapeutic interactions with all teens. Most adolescents with anovulatory bleeding can be treated with medical therapy (ACOG, 2000) and nutritional counseling. Teaching patients with significant anemia about a diet rich in iron and folic acid is important, and often a short course of iron supplementation is appropriate (Aeby & Frattarelli, 2003).

PERIMENOPAUSE

The incidence of DUB increases as women approach the menopause. The onset of anovulatory cycles actually represents a continuation of declining ovarian function. Women should be educated early about health-promoting activities that offset risks associated with menopause such as osteoporosis. Women should be encouraged to exercise regularly, modify their diets to include foods rich in iron and calcium, and if they smoke they should be counseled about quitting (ACOG, 2000).

TABLE 20–12   Risk Factors for Endometrial Cancer

- Age 40 years or older
- Anovulation (PCOS)
- Family history of endometrial cancer
- New onset of heavy irregular bleeding, particularly after menopause
- Nulliparity
- Overweight
- Unopposed estrogen stimulation of endometrium
- Tamoxifen therapy

OLDER WOMEN

One of the most important goals in the assessment of DUB is to rule out endometrial cancer, particularly in older women. The risk of developing endometrial cancer increases with age. The overall incidence is 10.2 cases per 100,000 in women 19–39 years of age and increases to 36.5 cases per 100,000 in women aged 40–49 years (Albers et al., 2004). ACOG recommends endometrial evaluation in women aged 35 years and older who present with abnormal bleeding (ACOG, 2000). Estrogen stimulation resulting in endometrial hyperplasia creates a risk for the development of endometrial cancer. Symptoms of endometrial cancer include postmenopausal bleeding and, therefore, all uterine bleeding in a woman who is postmenopausal should be considered cancer until proven otherwise. Table 20–12 lists the risk factors for endometrial cancer. Chapter 23 provides further discussion about endometrial cancer.

CULTURE

Culturally, the need for regular menses seems to be an essential part of their health for many women, and therefore deviations from established regular patterns are often perceived as pathologic (Livingstone & Fraser, 2002). Previous studies have demonstrated that women will reject modes of contraception that do not produce a regular bleeding cycle (Thomas & Ellerton, 2000), although newer studies indicate women are interested in avoiding bleeding (Andrist et al., 2004). It is important for clinicians to listen to the woman who presents with a concern about abnormal bleeding and to ascertain her perception of the bleeding, to learn how her individual culture defines abnormal bleeding, and to learn what for her might be acceptable modes of management and treatment.

CONCLUSION

The clinical management of AUB is complex and requires the clinician to consider not only the physical etiology but also the individual, emotional, and economic aspects of management. Age, history, and physical examination are reliable tools that suggest etiologic factors. Always rule out pregnancy first and never assume the cause of the bleeding. Be thorough and consider cancer in the algorithm. If bleeding persists even in the face of negative or reassuring tests, re-instigate the investigation and consider consultation and referral. Order laboratory tests selectively and always involve the woman actively in the decision-making process and management plan.

REFERENCES

Aeby, T., & Frattarelli, L. (2003). Dysfunctional uterine bleeding. *eMedicine Journal, 4*(7). Retrieved November 13, 2004, from http://author.emedicine.com/ped/topic628.htm.

Albers, J., Hull, S., & Wesley, R. (2004). Abnormal uterine bleeding. *American Family Physician, 69,* 1915–1926.

American College of Nurse Midwives. (2002). Clinical Bulletin #6: Abnormal and dysfunctional uterine bleeding. *Journal of Nurse Midwifery and Women's Health, 47,* 207–213.

American College of Obstetricians and Gynecologists. (2000). Management of anovulatory bleeding. *ACOG Practice Bulletin, 14,* 1–12. Retrieved February 14, 2004, from http://www.acog.com/publications/educational_bulletins/pb014.cfm.

American College of Obstetricians and Gynecologists. (2001). Use of botanicals for management of menopausal symptoms. *ACOG Practice Bulletin, 28.* Retrieved September 15, 2004, from http://www.acog/from_home/publications/misc/pb028.htm.

American College of Obstetricians and Gynecologists. (2004). ACOG issues opinion on uterine artery embolization for treatment of fibroids. *ACOG.* Retrieved May 20, 2004, from http://www.acog.org/form_home/publications/press_release/nr01-30-04-2.cfm?printerFriend.

Andrist, L., Arias, R., Nucatola, D., Kaunitz, A., Musselman, B., Reiter, S., et al. (2004). Women's and providers' attitudes toward menstrual suppression with extended use of oral contraceptives. *Contraception, 70,* 359–363.

Bachman, G. (1999). The changing vagina: Treating atrophy and infection. *Menopause Management, 2,* 31–34.

Barrington, J., Arunkalaivannan, A., & Abdel-Fattah, M. (2003). Comparison between the levonorgestrel intrauterine system (LNG-IUS) and thermal balloon ablation in treatment of menorrhagia. *European Journal of Obstetrics & Gynecology and Reproductive Biology, 108,* 72–74.

Bayer, S., & DeCherney, A. (1993). Clinical manifestations and treatment of dysfunctional uterine bleeding. *Journal of the American Medical Association, 269,* 1823–1828.

Bevan, J., Maloney, K., Hillary, C., Gill, J., Montgomery, R., & Scott, J. (2001). Bleeding disorders: A common cause of menorrhagia in adolescents. *Journal of Pediatrics, 13,* 856–861.

Bordo, S. (1993). *Unbearable weight: Feminism, Western culture, and the body.* Berkeley: University of California Press.

Bradley, L. (2004). Assessment of abnormal uterine bleeding: 3 office-based tools. *OBG Management Online.* Retrieved August 30, 2004, from http://www.obmanagement.com/content/obg_featurexml.asp?file=2003/05/obg_0504_00.

Brenner, P. (1996). Differential diagnosis of abnormal uterine bleeding. *American Journal of Obstetrics and Gynecology, 175,* 766–769.

Brunt, M. (1995). *Endocrine disorders in women.* In P. Carr, K. Freund, & S. Somani (Eds.), *The Medical Care of Women* (pp. 168–181). Philadelphia: Saunders.

Chapple, A. (1999). Menorrhagia: Women's perception of this condition and its treatment. *Journal of Advanced Nursing, 29,* 1500–1506.

Chimera, T., Anderson, A., & Turnball, A. (1980). Relation between measured menstrual blood and patient's subjective assessment of loss during bleeding, number of sanitary towels used, uterine weight, and endometrial surface area. *British Journal of Obstetrics & Gynecology, 87,* 603–609.

Choung, C., & Brenner, P. (1996). Management of abnormal uterine bleeding. *American Journal of Obstetrics & Gynecology, 175,* 787–792.

Claessens, E., & Cowell, C. (1981). Acute adolescent menorrhagia. *American Journal of Obstetrics & Gynecology, 139,* 227–280.

Clark, T., Mann, C., Shah, N., Kahn, K., Song, F., & Gupta, J. (2002). Accuracy of outpatient endometrial biopsy in the diagnosis of endometrial cancer: A systemic quantitative review. *British Journal of Obstetrics & Gynecology, 109,* 313–321.

Dragisic, K., & Milad, M. (2004). Sexual functioning and patient expectations of sexual functioning after hysterectomy. *American Journal of Obstetrics & Gynecology, 190,* 1416–1418.

Engel, G., & Rushovich, A. (1984). True uterine diverticulum. A partial mullerian duct duplication? *Archives of Pathology and Laboratory Medicine, 180,* 734–736.

Geil, J. (2003). Von Willebrand's disease. *eMedicine Journal, 3*(5). Retrieved November 13, 2004, from http://author.emedicine.com/PED/topic2419.htm.

Goldstein, S. (2003). Diagnosing abnormal uterine bleeding. *Contemporary OB/GYN, 48*(5), 96–109.

Grigorieva, V., Chen-Mok, M., Tarasova, M., & Mikhailov, A. (2003). Use of a levonorgestrel-releasing intrauterine system to treat bleeding related to uterine leiomyomas. *Fertility and Sterility, 79,* 1194–1198.

Grimes, D. (1979). Estimating vaginal blood loss. *Journal of Reproductive Medicine, 22,* 190–192.

Halberg, L., Hogdahl, A., Nillson, L., & Rybo, G. (1966). Menstrual blood loss: A population study. *Acta Obstetrics Gynecology Scandinavia, 44,* 347–351.

Hurskainen, R., Teperi, J., Rissanen, P., Aalto, A., Grenman, S., Kivela, A., et al. (2004). Clinical outcomes and costs with the levonorgestrel-releasing intrauterine system or hysterectomy for treatment of menorrhagia: A randomized trial 5-year follow-up. *Journal of the American Medical Association, 29,* 1503–1504.

Jannsen, C., Scholten, P., & Heintz, A. (1995). A preliminary study of factors influencing perception of menstrual blood loss volume. *American Journal of Obstetrics & Gynecology, 85,* 977–982.

Kaunitz, A., Westhoff, C., & Leonhardt, K. (2002, April). Therapeutic options to reduce or halt menstruation. *Female Patient* (Suppl.), 12–16.

Kennedy, A., Sculpher, M., Coulter, A., Dwyer, N., Rees, M., Abrams, K., et al. (2002). Effects of decision aids for menorrhagia on treatment choices, health outcomes, and costs: A randomized controlled trial. *Journal of the American Medical Association, 288,* 2701–2708.

Kim, M. (2000). Dysfunctional uterine bleeding. In L. Copeland (Ed.), *Textbook of gynecology.* Philadelphia: Saunders.

Kouides, P. (1999). Von Willebrand's disease. *The Female Patient, 24,* 86–92.

Lethaby, A., Augood, C., & Duckitt, K. (2003). *Nonsteroidal anti-inflammatory drugs for heavy menstrual bleeding* (CD000400). Cochrane Database Systematic Reviews.

Lethaby, A., Cooke, I., & Rees, M. (2003). *Progesterone/progestogen releasing intrauterine systems versus either placebo or any other medication for heavy menstrual bleeding* (CD002126). Cochrane Database Systematic Reviews.

Livingstone, M., & Fraser, I. (2002). Mechanisms of abnormal uterine bleeding. *Human Reproduction Update, 8*(1), 60–67.

Long, C. (1996). Evaluation of patients with abnormal uterine bleeding. *American Journal of Obstetrics & Gynecology, 175,* 784–786.

Maas, C., Weijenborg, P., & ter Kuile, M. (2003). The effect of hysterectomy on sexual functioning. *Annual Review of Sex Research, 14,* 83–113.

March, C. (1998). Bleeding problems and treatment. *Clinical Obstetrics & Gynecology, 41,* 928–939.

Marjoribanks, J., Lethaby, A., & Farquhar, C. (2003). *Surgery versus medical therapy for heavy menstrual bleeding* (Issue 3). Oxford, UK: Update Software.

Mihm, L., Quick, V., Brumfield, J., Connors, A., & Finnerty, J. (2002). The accuracy of endometrial biopsy and saline sonohysterography in the determination of the cause of abnormal uterine bleeding. *American Journal of Obstetrics & Gynecology, 186,* 858–860.

Mishell, D. (2001). Abnormal uterine bleeding. In M. Stenchever, M. Droegemueller, A. Herbst, & D. Mishell (Eds.), *Comprehensive gynecology* (4th ed., p. 1079). St. Louis: MO: Mosby.

North American Menopause Society (2000). Clinical challenges of perimenopause: Consensus opinion of The North American Menopause Society. *Menopause: The Journal of the North America Menopause Society, 7*(1), 5–13.

O'Connell, L., Fries, M., Zeringue, E., & Brehm, W. (1998). Triage of abnormal postmenopausal bleeding: A comparison of endometrial biopsy and transvaginal sonohysterography versus fractional curettage with hysteroscopy. *American Journal of Obstetrics & Gynecology, 178,* 956–961.

Oriel, K., & Schrager, S. (1999). Abnormal uterine bleeding. *American Family Physician, 60*(5), 1371–1379.

Pinion, S., Parkin, D., Abramovich, D., Naji, A., Alexander, D., Russell, I., et al. (1994). Randomized trial of hysterectomy, endometrial laser ablation, and transcervical endometrial resection for dysfunctional uterine bleeding. *British Medical Journal, 309,* 979–983.

Reid, R. (2000). Amenorrhea. In L. Copeland (Ed.), *Textbook of gynecology.* Philadelphia: Saunders.

Roussis, N., Waltrous, L., Kerr, A., Robertazzi, R., & Cabbad, M. (2004). Sexual response in the patient after hysterectomy: Total abdominal versus supracervical versus vaginal procedure. *American Journal of Obstetrics & Gynecology, 65,* 2073–2083.

Seidenfeld, M., & Rickert, V. (2001). Impact of anorexia, bulimia and obesity on the gynecologic health of adolescents. *American Family Physician, 64,* 445–450.

Smith, S., Abel, M., Kelly, R., & Baird, D. (1982). The synthesis of prostaglandins from persistent proliferative endometrium. *Journal of Clinical Endocrinology and Metabolism, 55,* 284–289.

Society of Obstetricians & Gynaecologists of Canada [SGOC] (2001). Guidelines for the management of abnormal uterine bleeding. *SOGC Clinical Practice Guidelines, 106*(August), 1–6.

Speroff, L., & Fritz, M. (2005). *Clinical gynecologic endocrinology and infertility* (7th ed.). Philadelphia: Lippincott Williams & Wilkins.

Spies, J., Ascher, S., Roth, A., Kim, J., Levy, E., & Gomez-Jorge, J. (2001). Uterine artery embolization for leiomyomata. *Obstetrics & Gynecology, 98,* 29–34.

Tavris, C. (1992). *The mismeasure of woman.* New York: Simon & Schuster.

Teoh, S., Lex, B., Mendelson, J., Mello, N., & Cochin, J. (1992). Hyperprolactinemia and macrocytosis in women with alcohol and polysubstance abuse. *Journal of Studies on Alcohol, 53,* 176–182.

Thomas, S., & Ellerton, C. (2000). Nuisance or natural and healthy: Should monthly menstruation be optional for women? *Lancet, 355,* 922–924.

Wade, J., Pletsch, P., Morgan, S., & Menting, S. (2000). Hysterectomy: What do women need and want to know? *Journal of Obstetric, Gynecologic, and Neonatal Nursing, 29,* 33–42.

Warner, P. E., Critchley, H, Lumsden, M., Campbell-Brown, M., Douglas, A., & Murray, G. C. (2004). Menorrhagia I: Measured blood loss, clinical features, and outcome in women with heavy periods: A survey with follow-up data. *Obstetrics and Gynecology, 190*(5), 1216–1223.

Wysocki, D. (1999). Bleeding disorders in women. *The Female Patient, 24,* 15–27.

Zupi, E., Zullo, F., Marconi, D., Sbracia, M., Pellicano, P., Solima , E., et al. (2003). Hysteroscopic endometrial resection versus laparoscopic supracervical hysterectomy for menorrhagia: A prospective randomized trial. *American Journal of Obstetrics & Gynecology, 188,* 7–12.

Chapter 21

HYPERANDROGENIC DISORDERS

CHRISTINE L. ANDERSON

In the past, clinicians often regarded women with hirsutism, acne, alopecia, irregular menses, and other symptoms of hyperandrogenism as suffering from a mainly cosmetic disorder or a menstrual annoyance requiring only symptomatic treatment. The health implications of hyperandrogenism, such as hyperinsulinemia and psychological distress, were either unknown or ignored. We are now entering a new era in the understanding and management of hyperandrogenic disorders and have an opportunity to positively impact the quality and duration of life experienced by women with these conditions. It is important for clinicians to approach a patient who has symptoms of hyperandrogenism in a sympathetic and concerned manner. Hyperandrogenism is both an endocrine and a cosmetic problem. The affected woman may have concerns on many levels regarding her health, sexuality, fertility, and social acceptance. The clinician is in an excellent position to provide education about long-term risks, screen for risk factors, establish preventive treatment modalities, and make referrals as necessary. This chapter will review the symptoms, pathophysiology, diagnostic evaluation, and therapy for hyperandrogenism, along with reviewing in-depth the major cause of hyperandrogenism, polycystic ovarian syndrome, and its sequelae.

DESCRIPTION OF HYPERANDROGENIC DISORDERS

SCOPE OF THE PROBLEM

The most common cause of hyperandrogenism in reproductive-aged women is polycystic ovary syndrome (PCOS), an extremely common endocrinopathy. PCOS occurs in 5–7% of all women, and in 80–90% of women presenting with hirsutism (Goodarzi, 2001). Patients with PCOS may present with menstrual irregularity, hirsutism, acne, and infertility. Women with PCOS also have an increased risk for adverse health outcomes including, but not limited to, cardiovascular disease, endometrial carcinoma, and type 2 diabetes (Carmina & Lobo, 1999; Chang & Katz, 1999; Taylor, 1998). Women with PCOS need to have regular, comprehensive, preventive health care and education to prevent the potential long-term sequelae of the syndrome. The presence of symptoms related to PCOS is a primary focus of this chapter because PCOS is the most frequent cause of hyperandrogenism. Other causes of hyperandrogenism, such as late-onset or "nonclassical" adrenal hyperplasia or androgen-producing tumors, are rarely seen but must be included in the diagnostic evaluation of women with hyperandrogenism (Speroff & Fritz, 2005).

ETIOLOGY

Hyperandrogenism is the result of increased androgen production from the ovaries, the adrenal glands, or both. Testosterone and dehydroepiandrosterone sulfate (DHEAS) are the primary hormones responsible for symptoms of hyperandrogenism, although other androgens including dehydroepiandrosterone (DHEA), sex hormone-binding globulin (SHBG), and 5α-reductase may play a role. Although DHEAS and DHEA are produced almost exclusively by the adrenal glands, the ovaries and the adrenal glands both contribute equally to the production of androstenedione and testosterone. At midcycle the ovarian contribution increases by approximately 10–15%. Women normally produce testosterone in the range of 0.2–0.3 mg/day, 50% of which is derived from the peripheral conversion of androstenedione. The ovaries are the most common source of increased testosterone and androstenedione. Adrenal causes are rare (Speroff & Fritz, 2005). The sources of androgen production are shown in Figure 21–1.

SHBG is produced in the liver. It is suppressed by elevated production of androgens and insulin, and increased by estrogens and thyroid hormone. Therefore, more testosterone is bound making less biologically available with high levels of thyroid hormone and estrogen. It is normal for about 80% of circulating testosterone to be bound to SHBG, 19% loosely bound to albumin, and about 1% left unbound. It is mainly the unbound portion of testosterone that is responsible for androgenicity, although there is some contribution from the fraction associated with albumin. If SHBG is suppressed, or if androgen production increases, the amount of free (unbound) testosterone will increase without necessarily increasing the total testosterone level, and the woman may develop symptoms of hyperandrogenism. Thus, because of the interplay between SHBG, insulin, thyroid hormone, estrogen, and androgen production, the total testosterone concentration may remain in the normal range, with symptoms reflecting only the decreased binding capacity of the SHBG and increased percentage of unbound testosterone (Speroff & Fritz, 2005).

Although testosterone is the major circulating androgen, dihydrotestosterone (DHT) is the hormone responsible for the clinical expression of androgen stimulation in many androgen-sensitive tissues, such as the skin, the pilosebaceous unit, and the hair follicles

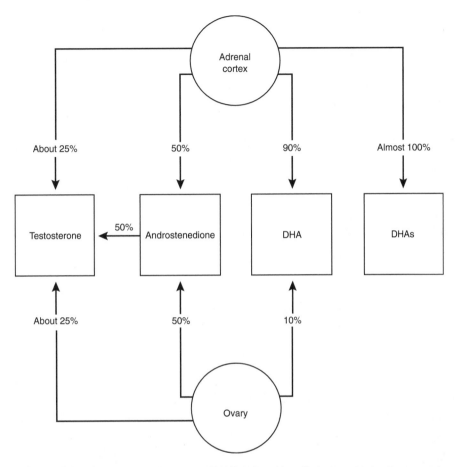

FIGURE 21–1   Sources of Androgen Production. *Note:* Dehydroepiandrosterone and dehydroepiandrosterone sulfate are abbreviated as DHA and DHAS respectively in this figure. They are abbreviated as DHEA and DHEA-S in the text of the chapter. *Source:* Reprinted with permission from Speroff, L., Glass, R.H., & Kase, N.G. (1999). *Clinical gynecologic endocrinology and infertility* (6th ed., p. 527). Baltimore: Lippincott Williams & Wilkins.

(Figure 21–2). Conversion of testosterone to DHT is accomplished by 5α-reductase, an enzyme that is present in these target tissues. There are racial and ethnic differences in the number of hair follicles present on the body and in the degree of 5α-reductase activity present in the hair follicles. The sensitivity of the hair follicle to the effect of androgens depends on the degree of 5α-reductase activity and is genetically predetermined. In women who are genetically predisposed to excessive 5α-reductase activity, normal levels of androgen can stimulate hair growth leading to idiopathic hirsutism (Speroff & Fritz, 2005).

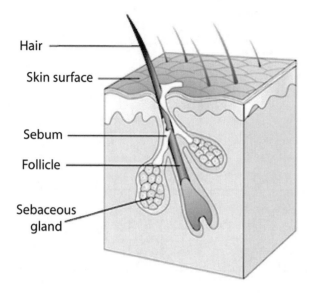

Hair

Skin surface

Sebum

Follicle

Sebaceous gland

FIGURE 21-2   Normal Pilosebaceous Unit. *Source:* Reprinted with permission from National Institute of Arthritis and Musculoskeletal and Skin Diseases. (2001). *Questions and answers about acne* (NIH Publication No. 01-4998). Bethesda, MD: Author.

As described previously, the symptoms of hirsutism, acne, alopecia, and frequently anovulation, can all be traced to an increased production in androgen levels (usually testosterone), a decreased production of SHBG, or to an increase in 5α-reductase activity in the skin and hair follicles that has caused an initial stimulus to androgen-sensitive areas and then acts to sustain continued sensitivity (Speroff & Fritz, 2005). The source of the increased androgen production is the key to determining the cause of hyperandrogenism.

BIOCHEMICAL FEATURES OF PCOS

Women with PCOS are predominantly anovulatory, and typically have a steady hormone level instead of the characteristic fluctuations of the normal menstrual cycle. The average daily production of estrogen and androgens are both increased because mean concentrations of luteinizing hormone (LH) are higher than those found in women who ovulate normally. The elevated LH levels are partly a result of an increased sensitivity of the pituitary to gonadotropin-releasing hormone (GnRH) stimulation, resulting in increased LH pulse amplitude and frequency, but mainly amplitude (Speroff & Fritz, 2005).

Follicle stimulating hormone (FSH) levels are low or at the low end of the normal range, but are not totally depressed. The FSH that is available continuously stimulates new follicular growth, but not to the point of full maturation and ovulation. Multiple follicular cysts form because full growth potential is not realized. These follicles are surrounded by hyperplastic theca cells, which are often luteinized in response to high LH levels. The accumulation of follicular tissue in varying stages of development allows for a relatively constant production of steroids in response to gonadotropin stimulation. This results in a self-sustaining condition of higher circulating levels of testosterone, androstenedione, DHEA, 17-hydroxyprogesterone (17-OHP), and estrone. A vicious cycle is created as the elevated androgens suppress SHBG synthesis, resulting in elevated estrogen levels and a two-fold increase in free testosterone. The ovaries do not secrete increased amounts of estrogen. The elevated estrogen levels are due primarily to peripheral conversion of androstenedione to estrogen, and to a reduction in SHBG. The result is the classic picture of the polycystic ovary displaying many follicles in the early stages of development with atresia and dense stromal tissue. The loss of feedback results in a hormonal steady state causing persistent anovulation with an increase in production of androgens, an increase in bioavailable estrogen, and virtually nonexistent levels of progesterone. Polycystic ovaries are thus the result of a cycle that may be initiated at any one of many entry points (Speroff & Fritz, 2005).

CLINICAL PRESENTATION

HIRSUTISM

Hirsutism is defined as excessive terminal hair growth in women, occurring in anatomic areas where the hair follicles are most androgen sensitive. Androgens cause transformation of fine, soft, unpigmented vellus hair to coarse, dark, terminal hair in androgen-dependent areas of hair growth (Goodman et al., 2001). Common sites for involvement include the face and chin, upper lip, areolae, lower abdomen, inner thighs, and perineum. The presence of significant amounts of terminal hair in these areas is considered abnormal. The degree and extent of hirsutism may be clinically evaluated by using the Ferriman–Gallwey scale (Ferriman & Gallwey, 1961) or a modified version (Figure 21–3). These scales provide a useful tool for assessment and follow-up of the response to therapy, although they are limited by subjective variability (Goodman et al.; Legro, 2003; Speroff & Fritz, 2005).

ALOPECIA

In contrast to hirsutism, prolonged exposure to circulating androgens may paradoxically cause hair loss. Elevated androgen levels are found in 15% of reproductive-aged women who have alopecia without other manifestations of hyperandrogenism (Goodman et al., 2001). Alopecia may reflect increased scalp 5α-reductase activity, so normal circulating androgen levels should not preclude treatment (Speroff & Fritz, 2005). With alopecia, the hair loss generally occurs at the frontal region, but it may affect the crown later and spread to produce a diffuse pattern of hair loss (Chang & Katz, 1999; Goodman et al.; Taylor, 1998). A careful history is necessary to rule out other factors that may be causing the alopecia, such as nutritional deficiencies, recent weight loss, anemia, thyroid dysfunction, chronic disease, or certain medications, including danazol, anabolic agents, and isotretinoin (Goodman et al.).

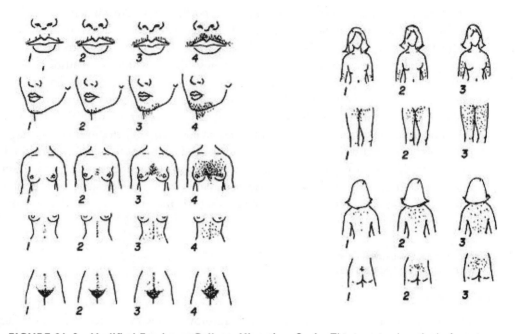

FIGURE 21-3 Modified Ferriman–Gallwey Hirsutism Scale. This is a visual method of scoring hair growth in women, modified from the original scale reported by Ferriman and Gallwey in 1961. Each of the nine areas is given a score ranging from 0 (no hair) to 4 (extensive terminal hair). The scores for each of the nine areas are totaled. Scores greater than 6–8 are generally considered to represent hirsutism. *Source:* Reprinted from *American Journal of Obstetrics and Gynecology,* Vol. 140, Hatch, Rosenfield, Kim, & Tredway, Hirsutism: Implications, etiology, and management, p. 816, 1981, with permission from Elsevier.

ACNE

Androgen stimulation of the pilosebaceous unit (PSU) can cause increased secretion of oil (seborrhea) and varying degrees of acne. Because of the genetic variability of the PSU to androgen stimulation, no correlation exists between the severity of acne and plasma levels of testosterone (Goodman et al., 2001). Acne may be caused by increased 5α-reductase activity in the PSU in up to 60% of women with acne and normal androgen levels (Speroff & Fritz, 2005). Acne is a common finding in adolescents that usually regresses by their mid-twenties. However, acne that persists beyond this time or presents in the twenties should alert the clinician to the possibility of hyperandrogenism, especially if the acne is resistant to the usual dermatologic treatment strategies and is associated with hirsutism or menstrual dysfunction (Chang & Katz, 1999; Goodman et al.; Taylor, 1998).

VIRILIZATION

Virilization is characterized by clitoral hypertrophy, severe hirsutism, deepening of the voice, increased muscle mass, breast atrophy, and male pattern baldness. It may also be associated with severe hyperinsulinemia. Virilization, particularly if it progresses rapidly and is associated with pronounced oligomenorrhea or amenorrhea, can indicate the presence of one of the less common causes of hyperandrogenism, such as adrenal or ovarian tumors, congenital adrenal hyperplasia (CAH), or hyperthecosis (Goodman et al., 2001).

MENSTRUAL IRREGULARITY AND INFERTILITY

Women with hyperandrogenism may have various degrees of ovulatory dysfunction. Menstrual irregularity is the hallmark feature of PCOS. The incidence of ovulatory dysfunction may range from sporadic episodes of oligomenorrhea to prolonged amenorrhea (Goodman et al., 2001). Bleeding is generally irregular and unpredictable with episodes occurring less than six times per year, although some patients bleed monthly. Bleeding can be heavy as a result of continuous estrogenic stimulation of the endometrium and resultant endometrial hyperplasia. Other manifestations of ovulatory dysfunction include menorrhagia, pelvic pain, and premenstrual syndrome. An awareness of the impending arrival of menses before bleeding begins is usually absent, which is a clinical indicator of anovulation. Menstrual dysfunction usually begins at the time of puberty, although some women may have relatively regular cycles with irregularity commencing with weight gain (Chang & Katz, 1999; Taylor, 1998).

Many patients with hyperandrogenism may experience infertility as a result of anovulation. Most affected women ovulate intermittently and can become pregnant, although it may take them longer to conceive. Additionally, the rate of conception after ovulation induction is lower in women with PCOS than in women with hypothalamic amenorrhea. There is also evidence that women with PCOS experience a higher incidence of spontaneous pregnancy loss. The mechanism by which this occurs is poorly understood, but is thought to be related to increased LH or plasminogen activator inhibitor type-1 (PAI-1) levels (Chang & Katz, 1999; Goodman et al., 2001; Speroff & Fritz, 2005; Taylor, 1998).

POLYCYSTIC OVARIES

Since Stein and Leventhal originally described the thickened, glistening, white, enlarged multicystic ovary in 1935, it has been clear that PCOS is associated with a classic ovarian morphology. In 2003 a consensus definition of the polycystic ovary syndrome was developed at a joint European Society of Human Reproduction and Endocrinology (ESHRE) and American Society for Reproductive Medicine (ASRM) meeting, which revised the long-standing consensus statement on PCOS sponsored by the National Institutes of Health (NIH) in 1990. At this meeting, a description of the morphology of the polycystic ovary was agreed upon. The polycystic ovary has 12 or more follicles measuring 2–9 mm in diameter, and/or increased ovarian volume of more than 10 cm^3 (Balen, Laven, Tan, & Dewailly, 2003). Only one ovary having this appearance is necessary to make the diagnosis. This definition does not apply to women who take combined oral contraceptives (COCs) because COCs modify ovarian morphology.

The previously accepted definition of the polycystic ovary as a peripheral array of eight to ten small follicles arranged in a necklace-type pattern with increased stromal echogenicity should be abandoned. Up to 23% of women with regular ovulatory cycles have polycystic-appearing ovaries on ultrasound. A woman who has polycystic ovaries without an ovulatory disorder or hyperandrogenism should not be considered to have PCOS (Balen et al., 2003; Lobo, 2003). Polycystic ovaries on ultrasound, without symptoms of PCOS, are not associated with subfecundity or subfertility (Hassan & Killick, 2003). Therefore, ultrasonography alone as a diagnostic tool for this condition is not recommended (Speroff & Fritz, 2005; Taylor, 1998).

OBESITY

Approximately half of patients with PCOS have been found to be obese. Typically the obesity occurs in the abdominal region, with an increase in waist-hip ratio (WHR), as opposed to the lower body. In some patients the onset of obesity correlates with the appearance of menstrual dysfunction. Obesity is associated with the three following alterations that interfere with normal ovulation:

1. Increased peripheral change of androgens to estrogens
2. Decreased levels of SHBG that result in increased levels of free estradiol and testosterone
3. Increased levels of insulin that stimulate ovarian stromal tissue production of androgens (Speroff & Fritz, 2005)

Obesity also increases the likelihood of metabolic complications. Patients with PCOS who are obese are more likely to develop impaired glucose tolerance, hypertension, dyslipidemias, and estrogen-dependent tumors than women with PCOS who are of normal or low weight (Goodman et al., 2001). In long-term studies, the problems of android obesity and hyperinsulinemia were observed to persist into the postmenopausal years (Speroff & Fritz).

INSULIN RESISTANCE

Perhaps the most significant advance in the study of PCOS is the finding that most, if not all, women with this condition are insulin resistant with resultant compensatory hyperinsulinemia (Dunaif, 1999). Hyperinsulinemia plays a pathogenic role in the etiology of PCOS by stimulating ovarian testosterone production, decreasing serum SHBG concentrations, and impeding ovulation. Many studies have demonstrated that women with PCOS have a form of insulin resistance that is unique and intrinsic to the disorder regardless of whether their weight is within or outside of normal ranges. Obesity further complicates the condition by increasing insulin resistance due to excess adiposity (Goodarzi & Korenman, 2003; Nestler, 1998).

Chronic hyperinsulinemia is associated with the development of type 2 diabetes because of the exhaustion of beta cells in the pancreas. It appears that hyperinsulinemia worsens spontaneously with age in adult women with PCOS, without a corresponding worsening of hyperandrogenemia (Goodarzi & Korenman, 2003). There is now clear evidence that women with PCOS have a three- to seven-fold increased risk of developing type 2 diabetes (The Rotterdam ESHRE/ASRM-Sponsored PCOS Consensus Workshop Group [The Rotterdam PCOS Consensus Group], 2004). It is estimated that 20% of women with PCOS who are obese have either impaired glucose tolerance or type 2 diabetes by the age of 40 years (Chang & Katz, 1999; Taylor, 1998). One study found that in women with PCOS who were not obese, impaired glucose tolerance and diabetes occurred in 10% and 1.5% respectively, a rate almost three times that of the normal population (Carmina & Lobo, 1999).

METABOLIC SYNDROME

As a result of the interplay between insulin resistance, hyperandrogenemia, and obesity, women with hyperandrogenism are at increased risk for cardiovascular disease and possibly cerebrovascular disease (The Rotterdam PCOS Consensus Group, 2004). Patients typically have elevated cholesterol, triglycerides, low-density lipoprotein (LDL) cholesterol, and C-peptides, and lowered high-density lipoprotein (HDL) cholesterol and apolipoprotein A-1 (Apo A-1) levels, but these findings are highly variable and depend on the degree of obesity and the woman's ethnicity. Some studies suggest that women with PCOS have a two- to seven-fold increased risk for the development of myocardial infarction (Carmina & Lobo, 1999; Chang & Katz, 1999; Nestler, 1998; Taylor, 1998). In contrast, limited epidemiologic data have not shown any increase in cardiovascular events. This may be because the women studied were under 55 years old, and the possibility that unknown factors that protect the heart in the face of other risk factors may be present in PCOS (The Rotterdam PCOS Consensus Group). Criteria for the metabolic syndrome in PCOS can be found in Table 21–1.

TABLE 21–1   Criteria for the Metabolic Syndrome in Women with PCOS

Risk Factor	Cut-off
1. Abdominal obesity (waist circumference)	> 88 cm (> 35 in)
2. Triglycerides	= 150 mg/dl
3. High-density lipoprotein cholesterol (HDL-C)	< 50 mg/dl
4. Blood pressure	= 130/ = 85 mm Hg
5. Fasting and 2 h glucose from oral glucose tolerance test (OGTT)	110–126 mg/dl and/or 2 h glucose 140–199 mg/dl
Three out of five qualify for the syndrome	

Source: The Rotterdam ESHRE/ASRM-Sponsored PCOS Consensus Workshop Group. (2004). Revised 2003 consensus on diagnostic criteria and long term health risks related to polycystic ovary syndrome (PCOS). *Human Reproduction, 19*(1), 41–47. ©European Society of Human Reproduction and Embryology. Reproduced by permission of Oxford University Press/Human Reproduction.

PSYCHOLOGICAL IMPACT

The expression of hyperandrogenism (hirsutism, alopecia, and acne), the annoyance and unpredictability of irregular menstrual bleeding, and the pain of infertility can have significant negative impacts on psychological health and well-being. There is evidence that women with hyperandrogenism have an increased rate of reactive depression and minor psychological abnormalities, possibly because of an increased catecholamine release secondary to provoked stress (Carmina & Lobo, 1999). Additionally, the frequent occurrence of obesity with hyperandrogenism can have a further negative effect on self-esteem and self-image. Fear of social rejection as a result of appearance may cause some women to become reclusive and may slow their development of social skills and confidence (Goodman et al., 2001). A study done in Germany by Elsenbruch et al. (2003) found that women with PCOS reported negative emotions of frustration, anxiety, and, to a lesser extent, sadness with PCOS as a result of the accompanying clinical symptoms and long-term complications associated with the condition. Women with PCOS also found themselves significantly less sexually attractive as a result of disease-related changes in appearance, particularly hirsutism, acne, and obesity. They were significantly less satisfied with their sex lives and felt that their partners were also less satisfied. It is thought that because PCOS often manifests at a time when finding a partner, sexual activity, and marriage are important, the cosmetic and psychosexual implications can cause profound emotional distress in affected women. Thus, quality of life for these women may be seriously compromised.

Eating disorders are more prevalent among women with PCOS. One study of women with PCOS found that one-third of patients had abnormal bulimia investigation scores. Also, subclinical eating disorders such as binge eating and fasting were more common in these women (McCluskey, Evan, Lacey, Pearce, & Jacobs, 1991). The cause of this association is unknown, but is thought to be related either to an association between insulin and leptin levels, or to the maintenance of blood glucose at lower than normal levels that can stimulate a constant drive to eat (Balen, 1999; Cortet-Rudelli & Dewailly, 1998; Holte, 1998).

CANCER RISKS

Women with PCOS are at a three-fold increased risk of endometrial cancer because of chronic, unopposed estrogen stimulation of the endometrium. Women who are obese are thought to have the greatest risk of endometrial cancer because of the peripheral conversion of androgens to estrogen in adipose tissue (The Rotterdam PCOS Consensus Group, 2004). Ovarian cancer is also increased two- to three-fold in women with PCOS. The risk of ovarian cancer is greater in those who are not obese and in those who have never used COCs (Carmina & Lobo, 1999). It is unclear if women with PCOS have an increased risk of breast cancer, partially because of confounding factors such as obesity and nulliparity. A few studies have found that chronic anovulation during the reproductive years is linked with a three- to four-fold increased risk of breast cancer appearing during the postmenopausal years, but these studies were limited by small numbers (De Leo, la Marca, & Petraglia, 2003; Marantides, 1997). The Nurses' Health Study found that women with the most irregular menstrual cycles (presumably anovulatory) actually had a reduced risk of breast cancer (Speroff & Fritz, 2005).

ASSESSMENT

Women with hyperandrogenism are prone to develop a range of clinical problems. Therefore, appropriate diagnosis, therapeutic management, and follow-up are essential for all women with hyperandrogenism (Speroff & Fritz, 2005). A thorough history and physical examination will give clues to the etiology of hyperandrogenism.

HISTORY

The history should include details about the patient's age at thelarche, adrenarche, and menarche, and the menstrual pattern since menarche. A reproductive history, including time to conceive and history of miscarriages, should be taken. The patient should be questioned about the age of onset and progression of obesity, hirsutism, seborrhea, acne, and alopecia, along with the success or failure of any treatments for these conditions. A complete medication history is important to seek a pharmacologic cause of the symptoms. Medications that have been associated with hyperandrogenism include testosterone, anabolic steroids, danazol, certain progestins, minoxidil, valproate, phenobarbital, phenytoin, phenothiazines, diazoxide, and metyrapone. A family history should be taken to determine the presence of hirsutism, acne, infertility, diabetes mellitus, cardiovascular disease, dyslipidemia, premature balding (before the age of 35 years) in male relatives, or obesity in family members (Goodarzi, 2001; Goodman et al., 2001).

Especially important in the history is the rapid development of symptoms of hirsutism after the age of 25 years and any rapid progression to virilization over the course of several months. Ask the patient if she has experienced increased libido, increased muscle bulk, voice deepening, breast atrophy, or clitoromegaly. Although rare, this should raise the suspicion of an androgen-producing tumor (Goodarzi, 2001; Speroff & Fritz, 2005).

PHYSICAL EXAMINATION

The physical examination should be geared toward establishing the degree of severity of hyperandrogenism and its related symptoms. In addition to assessing height and weight, waist circumference and the body mass index (BMI—see Chapter 6) are important in assessing the degree of obesity in women with hyperandrogenism. Abnormalities may indicate an increased risk for morbidity and mortality related to the metabolic syndrome.

A thorough skin examination should be completed, with particular attention given to the presence of hirsutism, acne, and alopecia. The degree of hirsutism may be evaluated using a grading tool such as the modified Ferriman–Gallwey scale (Figure 21-3). Racial, familial, genetic, and hormonal influences that affect body hair distribution and amount should be considered. Northern Europeans, natives of North and South America, and African-Americans generally have less hair than those of Mediterranean descent. East Asians tend to have less hair than Euro-Americans, with no difference in testosterone levels (Goodman et al., 2001). In addition, look for signs of Cushing's syndrome, such as violaceous striae, telangiectasias, thinned skin, and ecchymoses. Acanthosis nigricans and skin tags may be present with hyperandrogenism, usually in the neck area, and may be associated with states of severe insulin resistance. A thyroid examination and breast examination should be completed to evaluate for thyroid conditions or evidence of galactorrhea (Goodarzi, 2001; Goodman et al.).

A complete pelvic examination should include evaluation of the clitoris for hypertrophy and the cervix for degree of dilatation of the os and the presence and type of cervical mucus. A bimanual examination should be completed to determine the size of the uterus and adnexae, and the presence of masses. In a woman who is obese, bimanual examination may be limited and a pelvic ultrasound is imperative to identify pathologic changes in the pelvic organs (Goodman et al., 2001).

DIAGNOSTIC TESTING

Laboratory Studies Laboratory tests for patients with evidence of hyperandrogenism should be selected based on the individual patient's history and physical examination. Although there is some disagreement in the literature regarding which tests are essential and which are superfluous, a general recommendation for laboratory studies to be completed during the initial assessment of hyperandrogenism is as follows:

1. Measure total and free testosterone. Total testosterone is often normal in patients with PCOS, thus a screen for total and free testosterone is more sensitive at detecting the presence of SHBG deficiency (Goodarzi, 2001). Caution should be exercised, however, to select a laboratory known to be proficient in androgen determinations. There is much variability among different laboratories' normal ranges for testosterone, and studies have shown that the same testosterone value may be designated as normal to abnormally high when measured by different laboratories and compared with the supplied reference ranges (Azziz, 2003a; Lobo, 2003). Extremely elevated testosterone levels (above 200 ng/dL) may, but do not necessarily, indicate an androgen-secreting tumor. Recent data suggest the best predictor for these neoplasms is the history and physical examination (Goodarzi; Goodman et al., 2001; Speroff & Fritz, 2005; The Rotterdam PCOS Consensus Group, 2004).
2. Measure DHEA-S to assess adrenal gland function (Goodman et al.; Goodarzi). A DHEA-S level of 700 µg/dL has been established as a marker for abnormal adrenal

function. However, this level is encountered so rarely that Speroff and Fritz no longer recommend a screening DHEA-S level. Instead, they recommend doing an imaging assessment of the adrenal glands whenever a markedly elevated testosterone level is encountered, as this will be more cost-effective than measuring DHEA-S in all women with hirsutism.

3. Measurement of plasma 17-OHP level to rule out nonclassical congenital adrenal hyperplasia (NCAH). This syndrome is a result of a mild deficiency in 21-hydroxylase. It affects about 1–5% of patients with hirsutism and is clinically indistinguishable from PCOS. 17-OHP should be measured in the morning and during the follicular phase if this can be determined from the menstrual cycle pattern. Levels less than 200 ng/dL rule out NCAH. Levels above 200 ng/dL require referral to an endocrinologist for adrenocorticotropic hormone (ACTH) stimulation testing. Levels above 800 ng/dL are usually diagnostic of NCAH (Goodarzi; Goodman et al.; Speroff & Fritz).

4. All women who have hyperandrogenism with ovulatory dysfunction should have an evaluation of FSH, LH, prolactin, thyroid stimulating hormone (TSH), glucose, and lipid levels to screen for abnormalities. Women who have hirsutism with regular menstrual cycles should be evaluated for ovulatory dysfunction by charting basal body temperature (see Chapter 16), and obtaining a serum progesterone in the luteal phase (days 20–24) of the menstrual cycle. If a luteal phase progesterone level is less than 3–5 ng/mL, or obvious menstrual irregularities are noted on the basal body temperature chart, PCOS or hyperandrogenism (HA) insulin resistance (IR) acanthosis nigricans (AN) or HAIR-AN syndrome should be considered (Azziz, 2003b).

5. A 2-hour glucose tolerance test should be ordered for all women with a BMI greater than 27, for all women who are anovulatory, and for those with risk factors for diabetes such as family history (Legro, Castracane, & Kauffman; Speroff & Fritz; The Rotterdam PCOS Consensus Group). Opinions differ on the need to screen for insulin resistance because there is no currently validated clinical test for detecting insulin resistance. Although a test of insulin resistance is not considered necessary to make the diagnosis of PCOS, a screen for insulin resistance in women suspected to have HAIR-AN syndrome or with risk factors for diabetes should be considered (The Rotterdam PCOS Consensus Group). A fasting insulin level above 80 µU/mL with normal fasting glucose is suggestive of HAIR-AN syndrome and requires referral to an endocrinologist (Goodarzi). Speroff and Fritz also recommend screening all anovulatory women who have symptoms of hyperandrogenism for insulin resistance during the 2-hour glucose tolerance test by measuring the 2-hour insulin response after a 75 gram glucose load. Insulin resistance is very likely at levels of 100–150 µU/mL, is present at levels of 151–300 µU/mL, and is severe at levels greater than 300 µU /mL.

Based on the results of the initial testing, history, and physical examination, further testing may be indicated. If Cushing's syndrome is suspected, perform a 24-hour urinary free cortisol determination, or a 1 mg overnight dexamethasone suppression test. To perform the overnight dexamethasone suppression test, 1 mg of dexamethasone is given orally at 11 PM, and a plasma cortisol is drawn at 8 AM the next morning. A level below 5 µg/dL rules out Cushing's syndrome. If the level of urinary free cortisol is elevated above 90 µg/day, or if the serum cortisol level is not suppressed below 5 µg/dL, referral to an endocrinologist for further testing is advised (Goodarzi; Speroff & Fritz).

Imaging Studies and Endometrial Biopsy Pelvic ultrasonography may help to identify endometrial hyperplasia in women who are oligomenorrheic or amenorrheic. An endometrial biopsy is recommended for any patient who has long-standing anovulation because of the risk for endometrial carcinoma. The decision to perform an endometrial biopsy should not be based on a woman's age because endometrial cancer can be encountered in young women who are anovulatory. It is the duration of exposure to unopposed estrogen that is critical rather than the patient's age (Ehrmann & Rychlik, 2003; Speroff & Fritz, 2005).

If a virilizing tumor is suspected but an adnexal mass is not palpable, imaging of the ovaries and adrenal glands is indicated. Computed tomography (CT) scanning is more sensitive for adrenal imaging than magnetic resonance imaging (MRI) or ultrasonography, and transvaginal ultrasound is the method of choice for ovarian imaging (Speroff & Fritz, 2005). Goodarzi (2001) suggests considering selective venous catheterization of the ovarian and adrenal veins if the clinical picture suggests a virilizing tumor and ovarian and adrenal imaging is negative.

MAKING THE DIAGNOSIS OF PCOS

If history, physical examination, and laboratory testing rule out all other possible causes of hyperandrogenism, the most likely diagnosis is PCOS. According to The Rotterdam PCOS Consensus Group (2004), the exclusion of other etiologies and two out of three of the following criteria must be present to make the diagnosis of PCOS:

1. Oligo- or anovulation
2. Clinical and/or biochemical signs of hyperandrogenism
3. Polycystic ovaries

Finally, it is important to remember that PCOS is a syndrome, and no single diagnostic criterion is sufficient for clinical diagnosis. Women with regular menstrual cycles, polycystic ovaries, and hyperandrogenism may have PCOS. Women may also have ovulatory dysfunction and polycystic ovaries, but no symptoms of hyperandrogenism.

DIFFERENTIAL DIAGNOSES

The differential diagnoses for hyperandrogenism include PCOS, CAH, HAIR-AN syndrome, virilizing ovarian or adrenal tumors, idiopathic hirsutism, Cushing's syndrome, thyroid disorders, androgenic medications, pregnancy, and hyperprolactinemia. The most likely of these is PCOS. Key points for each differential diagnosis can be found in Table 21–2.

MANAGEMENT

The initial goals of treatment are to lower the androgen levels and ameliorate long-term sequelae of hyperandrogenism. Androgen levels are usually decreased during the first two to three months of therapy. Once these goals have been achieved, further therapy should be directed to returning the function of any organs initially affected by the hyperandrogenism. Management of nontumor-related hyperandrogenism requires long-term therapy and monitoring of symptoms, and should be carried out in collaboration with an endocrinologist (Goodman et al., 2001). The secondary goals of treatment are to improve or relieve any cosmetic manifestations of hyperandrogenism the patient finds distressing, and to help alleviate the psychological stress associated with these symptoms.

NONPHARMACOLOGIC

Weight Loss   Weight loss should be the first line of treatment for women with hyperandrogenism who are obese, whether or not they have PCOS. Weight loss, even in relatively small amounts, decreases androgen levels, increases SHBG, and may reduce the risk of the metabolic syndrome (The Rotterdam PCOS Consensus Group, 2004). Additional benefits include reduction of circulating levels of insulin, resumption of ovulation, and improved pregnancy rates. Hirsutism may also improve in some women simply by losing weight (Ehrmann, 1999; Holte, 1998; Moghetti & Castello, 1998; Pasquali & Filicori, 1998; Toscano, 1998; Utiger, 1996; van Montfrans, van Hooff, Hompes, & Lambalk, 1998).

A weight loss of 5–10% of total body weight can have a beneficial impact on insulin resistance and cardiovascular hemodynamic function, with a reduction of PAI-1 levels. A body mass index (BMI) of less than 27 is a goal for weight loss that correlates with a reduction in insulin resistance and a decrease in free testosterone levels. In women without hyperandrogenism, insulin resistance is rarely detected below a BMI of 27. However, women with PCOS can still manifest some degree of insulin resistance despite weight loss, as women with PCOS who are both obese and of normal weight have been found to be insulin resistant (Speroff & Fritz, 2005). In addition, weight loss in women with PCOS may be very difficult to accomplish because of this insulin resistance and the impaired lipolysis that accompanies it (Carmina & Lobo, 1999).

There are currently no specific strategies for weight loss in women with PCOS (Ehrmann, 1998). A consultation with a dietician versed in type 2 diabetes and refractory obesity may be beneficial along with a structured diet and exercise program with appropriate dietary modifications for women with hyperlipidemia (Kidson, 1998). These diet modifications may consist of a modest calorie reduction of 500 kcal/day, a fat intake that is less than 35% of total calories, and an increase in fiber intake to 30g/day (Cortet-

TABLE 21–2   Differential Diagnoses for Hyperandrogenism

PCOS	• Most common cause of hyperandrogenism, accounts for 75–90% of cases • Clinical and/or biochemical evidence of hyperandrogenism • Oligo- and/or anovulation • Polycystic ovaries • Exclusion of other etiologies
CAH—late onset/nonclassic	• Occurs in 1–5% of women with hirsutism • Clinically indistinguishable from PCOS • Elevated 17-OHP above 200 ng/dL
HAIR-AN syndrome	• Occurs in 3% of cases • Severe hyperandrogenism, possible virilization • Acanthosis nigricans • Severe hyperinsulinemia/insulin resistance
Virilizing tumors (ovarian or adrenal)	• Very rare (occurring in 1/300 to 1/1000 patients with hirsutism) • Acute rapid course of virilizing symptoms • Testosterone usually elevated above 200 ng/dL in premenopausal women, or 100 ng/dL in postmenopausal women • Palpable adnexal mass, or mass on imaging of ovaries and/or adrenal glands
Idiopathic hirsutism	• Occurs in 5–15% of cases • Biochemical hyperandrogenism is not present • Normal ovulation by basal body temperature charting or luteal phase progesterone measurements
Cushing's syndrome	• Frequent referral diagnosis, one of the least common final diagnoses • Evidence of striae over abdomen, central weight distribution, muscle weakness, altered mood, easy bruisability • Elevated 24-hour urinary cortisol or failure of cortisol suppression after overnight dexamethasone suppression test
Thyroid disorders	• Palpable thyroid enlargement or mass • Elevated TSH • Suspect with presence of alopecia
Androgenic medication use	• May be systemic or topical • Hirsutism
Pregnancy	• Virilization occurs during pregnancy • Possible luteoma or theca-lutein cyst
Hyperprolactinemia	• Galactorrhea • Elevated PRL

Sources: Goodarzi & Korenman, 2003; Goodman et al., 2001; The Rotterdam ESHRE/ASRM-Sponsored PCOS Consensus Workshop Group, 2004; Speroff & Fritz, 2005.

Rudelli & Dewailly, 1998). Before beginning dietary treatment, women who have PCOS and are obese should be screened for abnormal eating behaviors because of their higher prevalence of eating disorders (McCluskey et al., 1991). No direct reference to low carbohydrate diets as a strategy for weight loss was found in medical or nursing literature at the time this chapter was written. However, low carbohydrate diets have been cited extensively as effective in the treatment of hyperinsulinism in lay literature, and are recommended in nearly every Internet site dedicated to PCOS. Research on the efficacy of this diet in the treatment of PCOS is necessary before it can be officially recommended; until that time it is the responsibility of each clinician to become familiar with the pros and cons of the low carbohydrate diet, as it is certain to be a frequently encountered question posed by patients.

Mechanical Hair Removal   Contrary to popular belief, mechanically removing hair by shaving, plucking, waxing, or depilatories does not stimulate further hair growth. These methods may be used in conjunction with pharmacologic therapy to remove hair as needed. Electrolysis and laser therapy require several sessions of treatment, but eventually provide permanent results (Goodarzi, 2001).

PHARMACOLOGIC

Insulin Sensitizing Agents   As stated previously, weight reduction is an initial treatment for women with PCOS who are obese. Because of the difficulty in accomplishing this, the use of insulin sensitizing agents may offer great benefit in breaking the pathogenetic link between hyperinsulinemia and the hormonal and metabolic alterations in patients with PCOS. Even without inducing weight loss, long-term therapy with these agents may significantly reduce the risk of diabetes and cardiovascular disease associated with hyperinsulinemia, and should be considered an important component of the health care of women with PCOS (De Leo et al., 2003; Kidson, 1998; Pasquali, Pelusi, Genghini, Cacciari, & Gambineri, 2003; Speroff & Fritz, 2005; Toscano, 1998). Insulin sensitizing agents include metformin, D-chiro-inositol, and the thiazolidinediones.

Metformin is an oral antihyperglycemic agent whose primary mechanism of action is to reduce hepatic glucose output, with a modest improvement in glucose disposal. It has been shown to increase ovulatory frequency, reduce plasma insulin levels, increase SHBG, and improve androgen profiles in women with PCOS regardless of their weight, including those without evidence of insulin resistance (Dunaif, 2003; Goodarzi & Korenman, 2003; Perloe, 2003). Metformin may help to facilitate weight loss in some women (Pasquali et al., 2003). The usual dose is 500 mg tid, or 850 mg bid. It is contraindicated in cases of impaired renal function, congestive heart failure, hepatic dysfunction, sensitivity to metformin, or any state of metabolic acidosis. The most serious side effect of metformin is the development of lactic acidosis. Vitamin B_{12} deficiency may develop with long-term use (Azziz, 2003c). Minor side effects that are common when beginning treatment include nausea, abdominal discomfort, diarrhea, and anorexia. The starting dose may be titrated on a weekly basis to reduce the frequency of unpleasant side effects and increase tolerance (Goodman et al., 2001; Lord, Flight & Norman, 2003; Wei & Pritts, 2003).

Metformin has also been used as an adjuvant to clomiphene citrate for ovulation induction in the treatment of infertility associated with PCOS. When added to clomiphene citrate in women who were previously resistant to clomiphene, metformin increases the rate of spontaneous ovulation and may improve the pregnancy rate (Costello & Eden, 2003; Ehrmann & Rychlik, 2003; Goodarzi & Korenman, 2003; Homburg, 2003; Lord et al., 2003). There is also evidence that metformin may reduce the high rate of first trimester spontaneous abortion by reducing levels of PAI-1. Although clinical use of metformin in pregnancy is limited, early studies indicate that in addition to reducing the incidence of first trimester spontaneous abortion, continuing metformin into later pregnancy may reduce the risk of gestational diabetes. There has been no evidence to date of teratogenicity (Goodarzi & Korenman; McCarthy, Walker, McLachlan, Boyle, & Permezel, 2004; Pasquali et al., 2003).

D-chiro-inositol is currently under investigation as an insulin-sensitizing agent that mediates insulin action through mechanisms involving rate-limiting enzymes of nonoxidative and oxidative glucose disposal. A deficiency in this substance in the body may contribute to the development of insulin resistance. A recent study demonstrated that this drug could reduce insulin, increase SHBG, reduce free testosterone levels, and restore spontaneous ovulation (Pasquali et al., 2003).

The thiazolidinediones increase insulin sensitivity by improving the action of insulin in the liver, skeletal muscles, and adipose tissue directly, with a major impact on the glucose disposal rate, and a modest impact on hepatic glucose output (Ehrmann, 1999; Wei & Pritts, 2003). Most studies on this class of drugs used troglitazone at 400 mg once daily and showed reductions in insulin, androgens, and LH, with improvements in insulin sensitivity and PAI-1 levels. The studies did not assess ovulation, but some women resumed menses spontaneously without a decrease in BMI (Dunaif, Scott, Finegood, Quintana, & Whitcomb, 1996; Ehrmann, 1998; Ehrmann et al., 1997). Troglitazone was withdrawn from the market because it can cause significant hepatocellular toxicity. Two related drugs, rosiglitazone and pioglitazone have not been associated with hepatocellular toxicity and may be of some benefit. However, because this class of drugs tends to cause weight gain and fluid retention, metformin remains the insulin sensitizer drug of choice at this time (Goodarzi & Korenman, 2003).

Progestins Administration of medroxyprogesterone acetate at regular intervals causes withdrawal bleeding and prevents endometrial hyperplasia and carcinoma (Speroff & Fritz, 2005; Taylor, 1998; van Montfrans et al., 1998). A dose of 5–10 mg daily for the first 14 days of each month interrupts the hormonal steady state on the endometrium and the breast. Duration of therapy for 14 days has been demonstrated in clinical trials to be essential to protect the endometrium from cancer in postmenopausal women on estrogen therapy. According to Speroff and Fritz, "until specific clinical data are available, it seems logical that young, anovulatory women also require at least 14 days of progestational exposure every month" (p. 486). Progestational therapy alone is appropriate for women who do not wish to become pregnant, do not have hirsutism, and do not require reliable contraception. If these three criteria do not apply, continuous hormonal suppression with COCs, or the transdermal or transvaginal methods may be a more desirable alternative (Ehrmann & Rychlik, 2003; Speroff & Fritz).

Combined Oral Contraceptives   Combined oral contraceptives (COCs) have traditionally been recommended as first-line pharmacologic treatment for hyperandrogenism (Ehrmann & Rychlick, 2003; Goodarzi, 2001; Taylor, 1998; Wei & Pritts, 2003). COCs provide cosmetic relief of acne and hirsutism by inhibiting LH secretion and subsequently LH-dependent ovarian androgen production. They raise the concentration of SHBG, which binds free testosterone. COCs also decrease DHEA-S levels, possibly by reducing adrenocorticotrophic (ACTH) levels (Ehrmann & Rychlick). COCs provide protection against endometrial carcinoma by interrupting the steady state of estrogen stimulation on the uterus and by inducing a monthly withdrawal bleed. The increased risk of cardiovascular disease, which is related both to direct atherogenic action of increased PAI-1 and to the adverse lipid profiles induced by high androgen levels, is of additional concern in women with PCOS. COCs that have a positive effect on lipid profiles can help reduce the long-term risk of cardiovascular disease by improving adverse lipid profiles (Speroff & Fritz, 2005; Taylor).

A COC with a low dose of estrogen (less than 50 μg) and a nonandrogenic progestin component is recommended. Formulations containing levonorgestrel and norgestrel should be avoided because these progestins have higher androgenic activities. Triphasic COC formulations are also discouraged because the early dose of estrogen is often too low to inhibit dominant follicle selection, and they have the potential to increase rather than reduce the number of ovarian cysts (Kidson, 1998). Generally, COCs containing the newer third-generation progestins desogestrel and norgestimate are recommended. These progestins are minimally androgenic, may have less adverse effects on the serum lipid profiles, and may be more effective for the treatment of hirsutism (Dickey, 2002; Ehrmann & Rychlik, 2003; Goodman et al., 2001; Speroff & Fritz, 2005; Taylor, 1998). The progestin drospirenone may also be beneficial in the treatment of hyperandrogenism. Drospirenone is an analogue of spironolactone. The maximal effect of COCs on acne is usually observed within two months. In contrast, maximal effect on hair growth may take as long as 9–12 months because of the length of the hair growth cycle (Ehrmann & Rychlik).

In the past there was concern that higher-dose COCs (greater than 35 μg estrogen) increased insulin resistance and that these COCs should be avoided in women who are anovulatory and overweight. It is now thought that the newer low-dose COCs (35 μg or less estrogen) have little effect on carbohydrate metabolism. The majority of women with hyperandrogenism and hyperinsulinemia can be expected to respond favorably to low-dose COCs (Speroff & Fritz, 2005). Most long-term studies have failed to detect any increase in the incidence of diabetes or impaired glucose tolerance in past users of COCs (Pasquali et al., 1999; Speroff & Fritz; Wei & Pritts, 2003). Combination therapy with COCs and metformin may help reduce any increased risk (Speroff & Fritz; Wei & Pritts).

Antiandrogens Antiandrogens are effective in the treatment of hirsutism. They should always be used in combination with contraception in a woman who is sexually active because of their potential for teratogenic effects on the fetus. COCs are generally used as a first-line treatment for hirsutism, but for women with moderate to severe hirsutism refractory to COC use, the addition of an antiandrogen medication may be more effective than either agent alone. Medications for hirsutism should be tried for at least six to eight months because of the long hair growth cycle (Goodarzi, 2001). The antiandrogens include spironolactone, flutamide, finasteride, and cyproterone acetate.

Spironolactone is the only antiandrogen that is Food and Drug Administration (FDA)-approved for the treatment of hirsutism. It is also effective in the treatment of androgenic alopecia. It works by inhibiting testosterone from binding to its receptors, therefore inhibiting its action. The usual dose is 50–100 mg twice daily, but the effects are dose dependent and larger doses are sometimes required. Effectiveness ranges from 60–70%. Side effects may include lightheadedness, fatigue, mood swings, reduced libido, headaches, mastalgia, and a risk of hyperkalemia. It may cause polymenorrhea when used as monotherapy. Combination therapy with COCs reduces this side effect, and improves clinical response (Goodman et al., 2001; Speroff & Fritz, 2005).

Flutamide is another antiandrogen that has shown some benefit in treating hirsutism and hyperandrogenic alopecia (Carmina & Lobo, 2003). However, flutamide is not FDA approved for use in hirsutism, and is not recommended because of hepatotoxicity at necessary doses (usually 250 mg daily) (Speroff & Fritz, 2005). Flutamide should only be used in the most severe cases that are resistant to other forms of treatment (Goodman et al., 2001).

Finasteride inhibits 5α-reductase activity, which blocks the conversion of testosterone to dihydrotestosterone (DHT) in the skin. A dose of 5–7.5 mg per day is effective in decreasing hirsutism without adverse effects. In studies comparing finasteride to spironolactone, it proved slightly less or equally efficacious than spironolactone in doses of 100 mg daily. The major benefit of finasteride is its lack of side effects. Women who are treated with finasteride should be aware that this medication can adversely affect the development of the genital tract in male fetuses, and must be counseled to use an effective contraceptive method (Goodman et al., 2001; Speroff & Fritz, 2005).

Cyproterone acetate is approximately 70% effective in the treatment of hirsutism, but is not available in the United States. Side effects of cyproterone acetate include irregular uterine bleeding, nausea, headaches, fatigue, weight gain, edema, mastalgia, and decreased libido (Ehrmann & Rychlik, 2003; Goodman et al., 2001; Speroff & Fritz, 2005; Taylor, 1998).

GnRH analogs Gonadotropin-releasing hormone (GnRH) analogs, such as leuprolide, have been used in the treatment of hirsutism and infertility. GnRH analogs work by inhibiting gonadotropin secretion and subsequent ovarian hormone secretion, which results not only in a slowing of hair growth, but also in estrogen deficiency. Administration with COCs eliminates this side effect. GnRH treatment may be considered for women whose hirsutism has not responded adequately to COC and antiandrogen treatment; however these drugs are much more expensive than antiandrogens and may not be more effective (Taylor, 1998). In addition, GnRH analogs have shown no benefit in reducing hyperinsulinemia (Goodman et al., 2001).

Glucocorticoids   Glucocorticoids (prednisone, dexamethasone) have the ability to suppress adrenal androgen production and are indicated in patients with NCAH to suppress ACTH and thus adrenal output. Dexamethasone is usually given in doses of 0.25–0.5 mg orally before bedtime. Prednisone may be administered in doses of 5–7.5 mg orally before bedtime. These medications are initially given for two to three months. If the androgen levels are normalized, the dose is lowered to 0.25 mg of dexamethasone or 5 mg of prednisone for an additional two to three months. At that time the dose may be halved or discontinued. Periodic monitoring for recurrence of hyperandrogenemia is indicated every three to four months for one year. In most cases, DHEA-S levels remain suppressed indefinitely, although elevated testosterone levels may recur (Goodman et al., 2001; Speroff & Fritz, 2005). Glucocorticoids may also be useful in the treatment of PCOS with an adrenal component (Thatcher, 1999); however, this therapy is usually not recommended because of the effectiveness of antiandrogen medications and the frequency of Cushingoid side effects (Taylor, 1998; Thatcher).

Topical Preparations   Eflornithine HCl 13.9% (Vaniqa) is a topical cream approved for the treatment of facial hirsutism. It has been shown to slow facial hair growth in 20–40% of women. It is applied to affected areas twice daily. Improvement may be noted in four to eight weeks. Its primary mechanism of action is inhibition of the enzyme ornithine decarboxylase in human skin, which inhibits cell growth, polyamine synthesis, and ultimately the rate of hair growth. It is not a depilatory, and hair growth returns after discontinuation of the cream. Its main side effect is skin irritation (Ehrmann & Rychlik, 2003; Goodarzi, 2001; Wei & Pritts, 2003).

Additional Medications   Bromocriptine, a dopamine receptor agonist, is indicated for women with hyperprolactinemia. Divided doses of 5–7.5 mg are taken daily with meals. Bromocriptine helps to improve menstrual cyclicity and hirsutism in women with PCOS and hyperprolactinemia. No data indicate that bromocriptine is indicated in the treatment of hyperandrogenism without evidence of hyperprolactinemia. Treatment should be initiated gradually to minimize initial side effects, such as lightheadedness, hypotension, and nausea (Goodman et al., 2001).

Ketoconazole is an antifungal agent that has shown some effectiveness in treating the symptoms of androgen excess at doses of 200–400 mg daily. The potential for significant hepatotoxicity limits the use of this drug (Goodarzi, 2001; Goodman et al., 2001).

ALTERNATIVE AND COMPLEMENTARY

The literature is scarce on alternative and complementary therapies for hyperandrogenic disorders. As of this writing, one nonrandomized study of a Japanese herb called shakayaku-kanzo-to was able to be located. The herb was given to 34 Japanese women with PCOS and resulted in a significant decrease in total and free testosterone. The effects of this herb on hirsutism were not described (Takahashi & Kitao, 1994).

FOLLOW-UP

PCOS is a common endocrinopathy that is increasingly recognized as having negative long-term sequelae. With awareness of these potential sequelae on the part of the clinician, the majority of women with PCOS may be managed in the primary care setting. Patient education and comprehensive woman-centered care are crucial to the successful management of PCOS. For patients with chronic hyperandrogenic conditions, long-term follow up is appropriate. The patient should be seen every three to six months to monitor response to treatment and side effects of medications. Screening for evidence of development of metabolic consequences must be undertaken at regular intervals. Diabetes mellitus, hypertension, dyslipidemia, or atherosclerosis should be promptly treated upon diagnosis. See Table 21–1 for criteria for the metabolic syndrome in PCOS. Kidson (1998) recommends an oral glucose tolerance test with measurement of serum insulin at diagnosis and at 5-year intervals thereafter. He also recommends that fasting lipids be measured at diagnosis and at 2- to 3-year intervals, with the exception of a woman aged less than 20 years who is not overweight and does not have a family history of diabetes mellitus, gestational diabetes, or large birth weight.

Both Kidson (1998) and Speroff and Fritz (2005) recommend glucose tolerance tests and insulin evaluation of family members of already diagnosed patients because of the probable inherited susceptibility of anovulation and insulin resistance. Genetic counseling for patients with PCOS and their family members should be considered because of growing evidence that PCOS is genetically inherited in an autosomal dominant pattern. Speroff and Fritz assert that 50% of sisters and daughters of women with PCOS have a chance of having the condition, but the actual expression may be closer to 20–40% as a result of modification by both genetic and environmental factors. In the future, further definition of the genetics of PCOS may permit family screening with advice on prevention (Balen, 1999).

WHEN TO REFER

Life-Threatening Conditions   Acute treatment is not indicated for hyperandrogenism, unless the diagnosis is a life-threatening disorder, such as a metastatic ovarian or adrenal tumor. Referral for immediate surgical excision is then indicated.

Rare Endocrinopathies   In the event diagnostic testing reveals NCAH, HAIR-AN syndrome, Cushing's syndrome, hyperprolactinemia, acromegaly, or virilizing tumors, the patient should be referred to an endocrinologist. An endocrinology consultation should be considered for patients who are refractory to treatment with COCs, insulin sensitizers, and spironolactone, either alone, or in combination therapy (Goodarzi, 2001).

Treatment of Infertility   Women with PCOS can be advised that ovulation can be induced by the administration of clomiphene citrate about 80% of the time; however, only about 50% of patients actually conceive using clomiphene. The addition of metformin or GnRH agonists increases the effectiveness of clomiphene and may increase the rate of conception (Homburg, 2003; Kidson, 1998). These medications can cause ovarian hyperstimulation in patients with PCOS, therefore these women may be good candidates for in vitro fertilization which allows for control of multiple gestations. As a rule, the treatment of infertility in women with PCOS is complex and best carried out by specialists (Taylor, 1998).

EMERGING EVIDENCE FOR THE PRACTICE

Research in all areas of PCOS is ongoing. It is the hope of researchers that a more complete understanding of the genetic inheritance of PCOS will lead to strategies to prevent the development of this disorder. Much remains to be done before the causes of PCOS are identified and eliminated. Additionally, more research is needed to assess the level of risk associated with PCOS, to identify those who are at risk, to longitudinally follow women with PCOS into their sixties and beyond, and to determine the appropriate place, timing, and efficacy of interventional measures (The Rotterdam PCOS Consensus Group, 2004).

SPECIAL CONSIDERATIONS

ADOLESCENTS

Unfortunately, the symptoms of hyperandrogenism are not usually brought to the attention of health care providers until the patient is in her late teens, early twenties, or even older. However, the most common causes of hyperandrogenism begin in early adolescence. Premature adrenarche may be a consequence of hyperinsulinemia. These teenagers go on to develop polycystic ovaries, hyperandrogenism, and/or irregular menses for which they often are treated symptomatically without undergoing a thorough assessment of the causes of symptoms. Every attempt should be made to diagnose and treat hyperandrogenic conditions as early as possible because early treatment may help ameliorate symptoms and prevent the development of adverse sequelae and psychological dysfunction (Goodman et al., 2001; Speroff & Fritz, 2005). A few recent studies have suggested that early intervention in adolescent women with PCOS using combination flutamide–metformin therapy (flutamide 62.5–250 mg/d and metformin 1275 mg/d), with or without a third-generation COC, reversed the endocrine–metabolic abnormalities, increased lean body mass, and reduced total fat mass. The same benefits were demonstrated in adult women, but adolescents showed a better response overall. In addition, abdominal fat was reduced in adolescents but not in adult women. These results suggest that early intervention may correct the adiposity of women with PCOS, and this combination therapy has promise as a treatment of choice with potential benefits for long-term prevention of cardiovascular disease (Ibanez & de Zegher, 2003). It is the responsibility of those who care for adolescents to identify patients with hyperandrogenism and diagnose and treat their symptoms appropriately (Goodman et al.).

PREGNANT WOMEN

Virilization presenting in pregnancy should raise the suspicion of a luteoma, which is an exaggerated reaction of the ovarian stroma to normal levels of chorionic gonadotropin and not a true tumor. The solid luteoma is associated with a normal pregnancy and is usually unilateral. Maternal virilization occurs in 35% of pregnancies affected by a luteoma. If the mother is virilized as a result of the luteoma, there is an 80% chance that her female fetus will show some signs of masculinization. The luteoma does not cause other maternal effects and regresses postpartum. Subsequent pregnancies are usually normal, but virilization may be recurrent (Speroff & Fritz, 2005). In contrast, a theca-lutein cyst or hyperreactio luteinalis is usually bilateral and is seen with trophoblastic disease or with the high human chorionic gonadotropin (hCG) levels of a multiple gestation. Maternal virilization will occur in 30% of pregnancies affected with a theca lutein cyst, but no risk of fetal masculinization is noted (Speroff & Fritz).

Androgen-secreting tumors are very rarely encountered in pregnancy because ovulation is usually suppressed by high levels of androgens. If a woman is experiencing virilization during pregnancy, a pelvic ultrasound is very helpful in making the diagnosis. If a solid unilateral ovarian lesion is present, malignancy is likely (Speroff & Fritz, 2005).

Women being treated for hyperandrogenism who become pregnant should be aware of the benefits and risks of any medications they are taking. Although metformin is not universally accepted as a safe medication during pregnancy, the benefits may outweigh the risks for some women. Some medications, such as finasteride, flutamide, and spironolactone are contraindicated in pregnancy and should be discontinued immediately (Speroff & Fritz, 2005).

TALKING WITH THE PATIENT

Clinicians should provide informed consent to all women presenting for evaluation or treatment of hyperandrogenic disorders. The information required includes the risks and benefits of the proposed treatment, the alternative treatments available, their advantages and disadvantages, and the consequences of not receiving treatment at all. Clinicians should be careful to mention any important side effects of treatment or medication of which the patient should be aware. Document in the patient's chart that the risks and benefits of treatment have been explained. Consider giving the patient printed information about the condition or medication to supplement the amount of information that can be verbally communicated in the time constraints of typical clinical practice (Starr, 2004).

REFERENCES

Azziz, R. (2003a). Androgen excess is the key element in polycystic ovary syndrome. *Fertility and Sterility, 80*(2), 252–251.

Azziz, R. (2003b). The evaluation and management of hirsutism. *Obstetrics & Gynecology, 101*(5, Pt. 1), 995–1007.

Azziz, R. (2003c). We should avoid the indiscriminate use of insulin sensitizers in women with polycystic ovary syndrome. *Fertility and Sterility, 80*(2), 264–265.

Balen, A. (1999). Pathogenesis of polycystic ovary syndrome: The enigma unravels? *The Lancet, 354,* 966–67.

Balen, A. H., Laven, J. S., Tan, S., & Dewailly, D. (2003). Ultrasound assessment of the polycystic ovary: International consensus definitions. *Human Reproduction Update, 9*(6), 505–514.

Carmina, E., & Lobo, R. A. (1999). Polycystic ovary syndrome (PCOS): Arguably the most common endocrinopathy is associated with significant morbidity in women. *Journal of Clinical Endocrinology & Metabolism, 84*(6), 1897–1899.

Carmina, E., & Lobo, R. A. (2003). Treatment of hyperandrogenic alopecia in women. *Fertility and Sterility, 79*(1), 91–95.

Chang, R. J., & Katz, S. E. (1999). Diagnosis of polycystic ovary syndrome. *Endocrinology and Metabolism Clinics of North America, 28*(2), 397–408.

Cortet-Rudelli, C., & Dewailly, D. (1998). How actual is the dietary treatment in overweighting patients with polycystic ovary syndrome? *Journal of Endocrinological Investigation, 21,* 636–640.

Costello, M. F., & Eden, J. A. (2003). A systematic review of the reproductive system effects of metformin in patients with polycystic ovary syndrome. *Fertility and Sterility, 79*(1), 1–13.

De Leo, V., la Marca, A., & Petraglia, F. (2003). Insulin-lowering agents in the management of polycystic ovary syndrome. *Endocrine Reviews, 24*(5), 633–667.

Dickey, R. P. (2002). *Managing contraceptive pill patients* (11th ed.). New Orleans, LA: EMIS.

Dunaif, A., Scott, D., Finegood, D., Quintana, B., & Whitcomb, R. (1996). The insulin-sensitizing agent troglitazone improves metabolic and reproductive abnormalities in the polycystic ovary syndrome. *Journal of Clinical Endocrinology and Metabolism, 81*(9), 3299–3306.

Dunaif, A. (1999). Insulin action in the polycystic ovary syndrome. *Endocrinology and Metabolism Clinics of North America, 28*(2), 341–358.

Dunaif, A. (2003), Hyperandrogenemia is necessary but not sufficient for polycystic ovary syndrome. *Fertility and Sterility, 80*(2), 262–263.

Ehrmann, D. A. (1998). Attenuation of hyperinsulinemia in polycystic ovary syndrome: What are the options? *Journal of Endocrinological Investigation, 21,* 632–635.

Ehrmann, D. A. (1999). Insulin-lowering therapeutic modalities for polycystic ovary syndrome. *Endocrinology and Metabolism Clinics of North America, 28*(2), 423–438.

Ehrmann, D. A., & Rychlik, D. (2003). Pharmacologic treatment of polycystic ovary syndrome. *Seminars in Reproductive Medicine, 21*(3), 277–283.

Ehrmann, D. A., Schneider, D. J., Sobel, B. E., Cavaghan, M. K., Imperial, J., Rosenfield, R. L., et al. (1997). Troglitazone improves defects in insulin action, insulin secretion, ovarian steroidogenesis, and fibrinolysis in women with polycystic ovary syndrome. *Journal of Clinical Endocrinology and Metabolism, 82*(7), 2108–2116.

Elsenbruch, S., Hahn, S., Kowalski, D., Offner, A. H., Schedlowski, M., Mann, K., et al. (2003). Quality of life, psychosocial well-being, and sexual satisfaction in women with polycystic ovary syndrome. *Journal of Clinical Endocrinology and Metabolism, 88*(12), 5801–5807.

Ferriman, D., & Gallwey, J. D. (1961). Clinical assessment of body hair growth in women. *Journal of Clinical Endocrinology and Metabolism, 21,* 1440–1447.

Goodarzi, M. O. (2001). Hirsutism. *Best Practice of Medicine.* Retrieved September 25, 2004, from http://merck.micromedex.com/index.asp?page=b pm_brief&article_id=BPM01EN01&hilight=pol ycysticlovarian

Goodarzi, M. O., & Korenman, S. G. (2003). The importance of insulin resistance in polycystic ovary syndrome. *Fertility and Sterility, 80*(2), 255–258.

Goodman, N. F., Bledsoe, M. B., Futterweit, W., Goldzieher, J. W., Petak, S. M., Smith, K. D., et al. (2001). American Association of Clinical Endocrinologists medical guidelines for clinical practice for the diagnosis and treatment of hyperandrogenic disorders. *Endocrine Practice, 7*(2), 120–134.

Hassan, A. M., & Killick, S. R. (2003). Ultrasound diagnosis of polycystic ovaries in women who have no symptoms of polycystic ovary syndrome is not associated with subfecundity or subfertility. *Fertility and Sterility, 80*(4), 966–975.

Holte, J. (1998). Polycystic ovary syndrome and insulin resistance: Thrifty genes struggling with over-feeding and sedentary life style? *Journal of Endocrinological Investigation, 21,* 589–601.

Homburg, R. (2003). The management of infertility associated with polycystic ovary syndrome. *Reproductive Biology and Endocrinology, 1*(1), 109. Retrieved September 12, 2004, from http://www.rbej.com/content/1/1/109.

Ibanez, L., & de Zegher, F. (2003). Flutamide-metformin therapy to reduce fat mass in hyperinsulinemic ovarian hyperandrogenism: Effects in adolescents and in women on third-generation oral contraception. *Journal of Clinical Endocrinology and Metabolism, 88*(10), 4720–4724.

Kidson, W. (1998). Polycystic ovary syndrome: A new direction in treatment [Electronic version]. *The Medical Journal of Australia, 169,* 537–540.

Legro, R. S. (2003). Diagnostic criteria in polycystic ovary syndrome. *Seminars in Reproductive Medicine, 21*(3), 267–275.

Legro, R. S., Castracane, V. D., & Kauffman, R. P. (2004). Detecting insulin resistance in polycystic ovary syndrome: Purposes and pitfalls. *Obstetrical and Gynecological Survey, 59*(2), 141–154.

Lobo, R. A. (2003). What are the key features of importance in polycystic ovary syndrome? *Fertility and Sterility, 80*(2), 259–261.

Lord, J. M., Flight, I. H., & Norman, R. J. (2003). Metformin in polycystic ovary syndrome: Systematic review and meta-analysis. *British Medical Journal, 327*(7421), 951–953.

Marantides, D. (1997). Management of polycystic ovary syndrome. *The Nurse Practitioner, 22*(12), 34–41.

McCarthy, E. A, Walker, S. P., McLachlan, K., Boyle, J., & Permezel, M. (2004). Metformin in obstetric and gynecologic practice: A review. *Obstetrical and Gynecological Survey, 59*(2), 118–127.

McCluskey, S., Evan, C., Lacey, J. H., Pearce, J. M., & Jacobs, H. (1991). Polycystic ovary syndrome and bulimia. *Fertility and Sterility, 55*(2), 287–291.

Moghetti, P., & Castello, R. (1998). New routes in the polycystic ovary syndrome labyrinth: A way out? *Journal of Endocrinological Investigation, 21,* 648–655.

Nestler, J. E. (1998). Polycystic ovary syndrome: A disorder for the generalist. *Fertility and Sterility, 70*(5), 811–12.

Pasquali, R., & Filicori, M. (1998). Insulin sensitizing agents and polycystic ovary syndrome. *European Journal of Endocrinology, 138,* 253–254.

Pasquali, R., Gambineri, A., Anconetani, B., Vicennati, V., Colitta, D., Caramelli, E., et al. (1999). The natural history of the metabolic syndrome in young women with the polycystic ovary syndrome and the effect of long term oestrogen-progestagen treatment. *Clinical Endocrinology, 50,* 517–527.

Pasquali, R., Pelusi, C., Genghini, S., Cacciari, M., & Gambineri, A. (2003). Obesity and reproductive disorders in women. *Human Reproduction Update, 9*(4), 359–372.

Perloe, M. (2003). Polycystic ovary syndrome: Treatment with insulin lowering medications. *Georgia Reproductive Specialists.* Retrieved September 25, 2004, from http://www.ivf.com/pcostreat.html.

The Rotterdam ESHRE/ASRM-Sponsored PCOS Consensus Workshop Group. (2004). Revised 2003 consensus on diagnostic criteria and long term health risks related to polycystic ovary syndrome (PCOS). *Human Reproduction, 19*(1), 41–47.

Speroff, L., & Fritz, M. (2005). *Clinical gynecologic endocrinology and infertility* (7th ed.). Baltimore: Lippincott Williams & Wilkins.

Starr, D. S. (2004, April). The duties of informed consent. *The Clinical Advisor,* 83.

Takahashi, K., & Kitao, M. (1994). Effect of TJ-68 (shakayaku-kanzo-to) on polycystic ovarian disease. *International Journal of Fertility and Menopausal Studies, 39*(2), 69–76.

Taylor, A. E. (1998). Polycystic ovary syndrome. *Endocrinology and Metabolism Clinics of North America, 27*(4), 877–902.

Thatcher, S. S. (1999). *What is polycystic ovarian syndrome (PCOS)?* Retrieved September 12, 2004, from http://

www.obgyn.net/displayarticle.asp?page=/pcos/articles/whatispcos.

Toscano, V. (1998). Polycystic ovary syndrome: What is it? Pathogenetic enigma and therapeutic dilemma. *Journal of Endocrinological Investigation, 21*, 546–550.

Utiger, R. D. (1996). Insulin and the polycystic ovary syndrome. *The New England Journal of Medicine, 335*(9), 657–8.

van Montfrans, J. M., van Hooff, M. H. A., Hompes, P. G. A., & Lambalk, C. B. (1998). Treatment of hyperinsulinemia in polycystic ovary syndrome? *Human Reproduction, 13*(1), 5–8.

Wei, A. Y., & Pritts, E. A. (2003). Therapy for polycystic ovarian syndrome. *Current Opinion in Pharmacology, 3*, 678–682.

Chapter 22

BENIGN GYNECOLOGIC CONDITIONS

CAROL A. VERGA

This chapter addresses a variety of conditions commonly encountered in gynecologic care including vulvar dermatoses, nabothian cysts, cervical polyps, uterine fibroids, adenomyosis, endometriosis, and ovarian cysts. These conditions, although usually not malignant (with exceptions as noted), are still significant to the woman experiencing them. Some of these conditions are associated with physical symptoms that can be severe, and all of them have the potential to cause women distress and anxiety. Therefore, emotional support is an essential component of care. Many of the conditions in this chapter are chronic and require ongoing, long-term care. Thorough patient education about the clinical course and treatment options is imperative, and the provider should act in partnership with the woman to develop management plans that meet her individual needs.

VULVAR DERMATOSES

The vulva is composed of skin and mucous membrane (see Chapter 5). Most dermatoses that affect either the skin or mucous membranes can appear on the vulva. This section presents the general assessment of vulvar dermatoses and the specific assessment and management of some of the more common benign vulvar dermatoses: primary irritant and allergic dermatitis, lichen sclerosus, lichen planus, squamous cell hyperplasia, and psoriasis. Vulvar cancer is addressed in Chapter 23. A list of vulvar dermatology resources is provided at the end of the chapter for the many conditions that are beyond the scope of this text. Many of these resources contain color photographs, and reviewing these can improve a provider's ability to recognize the many lesions that can occur on the vulva.

Vulvar dermatoses cause physical symptoms and can have significant psychological consequences. A woman may have suffered for years with her condition and may present for care feeling frustrated and hopeless. It is important for a clinician to convey realistic expectations for treatment and to explain to the woman that more than one therapy may be needed to effect resolution, or at least relief. At the same time, the clinician can express a commitment to helping the woman obtain relief of her symptoms. Women may have cosmetic concerns related to the physical changes caused by their dermatosis. These concerns, particularly in conjunction with physical symptoms, can interfere with sexual functioning and cause distress for the woman and her partner. Asking the woman about the psychological impact of her condition and providing emotional support are crucial components of care. In addition, women with chronic dermatoses may benefit from support groups, either locally or online.

ASSESSMENT OF VULVAR DERMATOSES

Many of the benign diseases of the vulva share similar appearances, symptoms, and even therapies. Having the precise diagnosis is essential for accurate client education, monitoring of therapy, and prevention of complications. In addition, malignancy must be ruled out. A systematic approach to assessment is essential for accurate diagnosis.

History   The clinician needs to identify when the woman first became aware of the lesion. Ask about associated symptoms including pruritis, pain, burning, bleeding, and vaginal discharge, and if there are aggravating or alleviating factors. Identify treatments that have already been tried and whether they were successful or not. Ask if the woman has any history of dermatologic disease as well as any skin changes elsewhere on her body. Obtain a sexual history with specific attention to dyspareunia, changes in sexual activity related to the condition, and whether or not her partner has symptoms. Note family history of dermatologic disease or malignancy. Complete gynecologic and general health histories should also be obtained.

Physical Examination   Carefully examine the external genitalia using a good light source. Speculum examination should be performed because some vulvar conditions have vaginal manifestations. General inspection of the skin can be useful for detecting systemic dermatologic conditions. Additional examination should be directed by the history and genital findings.

Diagnostic Testing   Microscopic evaluation of vaginal discharge should be performed to rule out vaginitis. The definitive diagnostic technique for vulvar dermatoses is biopsy, which is relatively simple to perform (Box 22–1). Biopsy should be performed liberally when vulvar lesions are present to avoid delayed diagnosis of malignancy (Foster, 2002). Colposcopy may be warranted to more closely examine the vulva and to direct biopsy. Additional evaluations, such as testing for sexually transmitted infections, may be appropriate depending on the history and physical examination findings (see Chapter 18).

DIFFERENTIAL DIAGNOSIS

The differential diagnoses for vulvar lesions are identified in Box 22–2.

BOX 22-1   TECHNIQUE FOR VULVAR BIOPSY

Begin by identifying the best location for the biopsy. This may be the entire lesion or a portion, depending on the size. Do not be reluctant to take more than one biopsy if needed to sample all the variations of the presenting lesion(s). Consider desensitizing the area by applying ice or a topical anesthetic before injecting the local anesthetic. Seldom is any medication stronger than 1% lidocaine with epinephrine needed, though 0.5% bupivacaine lasts longer after the procedure. Use the smallest dose needed for anesthesia to prevent skin distention and more discomfort. The usual needle size is 27 or 30 gauge, the length should fit the area to be anesthetized, and medication is injected with the bevel up. Only a small amount of medication is usually needed, but the size of the biopsy must be considered in determining how much to use.

Punch biopsy can be done with either a disposable or reusable unit; if the latter is used, be certain it has been sterilized and is still sharp. A sharp instrument assures the least pain, the least bleeding, and the most reliable specimen. Most of the vulva is soft tissue; therefore, be sure to provide support for the tissue as the sharp edge is gently twisted and pushed into the area being biopsied. Other tissue sampling devices include biopsy forceps used for colposcopy. Explain to the woman that the major portion of larger instruments is the handle, as their size can be intimidating.

Specimens of 3 mm or under often do not require suturing for closure. Drysol (20% aluminum chloride) or silver nitrate may be used to stop bleeding. The biopsy will heal readily and care after biopsy is simply good personal hygiene; most biopsies do not require topical or oral antibiotic therapy. When sutures are needed, small dissolvable suture material (e.g., 4–0 or 5–0 chromic) is used and usually only one or two sutures are required. If the woman has a known sensitivity to chromic, or if the sutures will need to be in for more than five to seven days because of the site of biopsy, use inert suture material (e.g., Monopril, Dermalon, etc.). Sutures should be removed in 5 to 14 days depending on their site.

PRIMARY IRRITANT AND ALLERGIC DERMATITIS

Primary irritant and allergic dermatitis are often referred to collectively as contact dermatitis, but there are distinctions between these two forms of dermatitis. The etiology is nonimmunologic in primary irritant dermatitis and immunologic in allergic dermatitis. Typically symptoms of primary irritant dermatitis appear quickly following exposure to the irritant, while allergic dermatitis can take 36–48 hours to manifest after allergen exposure. Primary irritant dermatitis also resolves more quickly than allergic dermatitis (Stenchever, Droegmueller, Herbst, & Mishell, 2001). A detailed history to identify the irritant or allergen is necessary.

Primary Irritant Dermatitis   Exposure of the vulva to an irritant can result in burning, pruritis, and pain. Potential irritants include perfumed soaps, feminine hygiene sprays and

BOX 22-2   DIFFERENTIAL DIAGNOSES FOR VULVAR LESIONS

Acanthosis nigricans
Acrochordon (skin tags)
Allergic dermatitis
Aphthosis
Atrophic vaginitis
Basal cell carcinoma
Behçet's
Bullous pemphigoid
Candidiasis
Chancroid
Cicatricial pemphigoid
Condyloma acuminata (genital warts)
Crohn's disease
Desquamative inflammatory vaginitis
Eczema
Epidermal cysts
Erythema multiforme
Folliculitis
Granuloma inguinale
Hemangiomas
Herpes simplex virus
Herpes zoster
Hidradenitis suppurativa
Impetigo
Intertrigo
Lentigo

Lichen planus
Lichen sclerosus
Lichen simplex chronicus
Lupus
Lymphogranuloma venereum
Melanoma
Molloscum contagiosum
Nevi (moles)
Pityriasis versicolor
Paget's disease
Pemphigus vulgaris
Primary irritant dermatitis
Psoriasis
Pyoderma gangrenosum
Scabies
Seborrheic dermatitis
Squamous cell carcinoma
Squamous cell hyperplasia
Steroid-rebound dermatitis
Stevens-Johnson syndrome
Syphilis
Vitiligo
Vulvar intraepithelial neoplasia (VIN)
Vulvar vestibulitis
Vulvodynia

deodorants, bath bubbles and oils, colored or scented toilet paper, laundry detergents, sanitary napkins, tampons, spermicides, riding a bicycle or horse, tight clothing including thong underwear, and trapped moisture as a result of wearing synthetic fabrics. A detailed history of contact with potential irritants is crucial. Physical examination will typically reveal erythema of the involved skin, and there may be excoriation, ulceration, and edema (Larrabee & Kylander, 2001; Star, 1995).

Allergic Dermatitis   Known allergens that can cause vulvar dermatitis include pollen, foods, topical and oral medications, latex, poison ivy and poison oak, and semen. Allergic dermatitis may also occur with generalized allergy symptoms in women who have a hereditary tendency to allergic reactions (atopic individual). Physical examination find-

TABLE 22–1 Topical Corticosteroid Ointments Used for Vulvar Dermatoses

Potency	Medication	Strength
Low	Alclometasone diproprionate (Aclovate)	0.05%
	Desonide (Desowen)	0.05%
	Hydrocortisone (Hytone)	2.5%
Medium	Fluticasone proprianate (Cutivate)	0.005%
	Triamcinolone (Aristocort, Kenalog)	0.025%, 0.1%
	Mometasone furoate (Elocon)	0.1%
High/Potent	Betamethasone dipropionate (Diprosone, Maxivate)	0.05%,
	Desoximetasone (Topicort)	0.05%, 0.25%
	Fluocinonide (Lidex)	0.05%
	Halcinonide (Halog)	0.1%
Very high/Super potent*	Betamethasone dipropionate (Diprolene)	0.05%
	Clobetasol (Temovate)	0.05%
	Diflorasone diacetate (Psorcon)	0.05%
	Halobetasol propionate (Ultravate)	0.05%

*Avoid the use of occlusive dressings with this potency.

ings may be similar to those of primary irritant dermatitis, but may also include dryness, scaling, and excoriations (Larrabee & Kylander, 2001; Stenchever et al., 2001).

Management Identification of the irritant or allergen and avoidance of further contact is essential to treatment. Topical corticosteroids are the mainstay of pharmacologic therapy and are typically used for 4–10 days after the dermatitis resolves (Table 22–1). Cool sitz baths and wet dressings with Burow's solution (Domeboro) can be used to reduce discomfort. If symptoms are severe, systemic corticosteroids and/or oral antihistamines may be warranted (Larrabee & Kylander, 2001; Star, 1995).

LICHEN SCLEROSUS

Lichen sclerosus (LS) is a benign, chronic, progressive disease of the skin characterized by inflammation, epithelial thinning, and distinctive dermal changes. It can occur on the trunk, neck, forearms, axillae, and under the breasts, as well as on the vulva. LS is most common in postmenopausal women, but it can occur as early as childhood. The exact etiology of LS is unknown, but there is a familial association (Black, McKay, & Braude, 1995). There is an increased risk of vulvar cancer for women with LS (see Chapter 23).

Clinical Presentation   Vulvar pruritis is the most common presenting symptom of LS. The pruritis may be so intense as to interrupt sleep. Anorectal symptoms, including pruritis ani, painful defecation, anal fissures, and rectal bleeding, may also occur. For some women a dull, nonspecific vulvar discomfort is a prodrome to LS. Dyspareunia is a later symptom occurring from small lacerations or introital stenosis. Phimosis of the labia minora over the clitoris may lead to diminished sexual sensation. Dysuria may occur if there is fusion of the minora over the urethra. Some women may be asymptomatic leading to a delay of diagnosis of LS until routine examination.

Physical Examination Findings   Lichen sclerosus involves both the skin and mucosal surfaces of the vulva and perianal area. Initially lesions are macular becoming macular–papular with a flat surface. Most often they eventually coalesce into plaques. A classic figure-eight formation surrounds the vulva and perianal area. Over time the skin thins, and takes on a wrinkled, "cigarette paper" appearance. Normal architecture of both the dermis and mucosa are lost. Eventually the labia minora atrophy and are assumed into the labia majora completely or partially by a process called agglutination. There may be phimosis over the clitoris and possibly the urethra. Introital stenosis is common in advanced disease but, unlike the complete stenosis of the vagina itself seen in lichen planus, LS causes no reduction in the vaginal caliber (diameter).

Management   The goals of LS treatment are relief of symptoms and discomfort, prevention of further architectural distortion, and theoretical reduction in the incidence of malignancy (Funaro, 2004). Prior to initiating therapy for LS, any concomitant vaginitis (particularly vulvovaginal candidiasis) should be treated. Medium potency corticosteroids used in a tapering protocol will usually control mild or early LS. High- or very high-potency steroids are needed for control and hopefully some reversal of advanced disease (Zellis & Pincus, 1996). Further information about corticosteroid therapy can be found in Table 22–1 and Box 22–3. Intralesion injection of 5–20 mg of triamcinolone hexacetonide directly into thickened lesions can be used when LS is not responding to topical corticosteroids (Mazdisnian, Degregorio, Mazdisnian, & Palmieri, 1999).

The most recent innovation in the treatment of LS is the use of tacrolimus topical ointment, 0.03% or 0.1% twice daily about 12 hours apart, which may be decreased to once daily when symptoms improve (Assman, Becker-Wegerich, Grewe, Megahed, & Ruzicka, 2003; Kunstfeld, Kirnbauer, Stingl, & Karlhofer, 2003). Persistent vulvar burning despite appropriate therapy may indicate that vulvodynia is present (see Chapter 14). Surgery is used only as treatment for release of phimosis, introital stenosis, or for the excision of malignancy. These procedures should not be performed until the disease is stable and all evidence of inflammation is well-controlled by the use of steroids. All women being treated for LS should be examined at least yearly to be sure their symptoms are not returning, to evaluate the effect of any ongoing steroid use, and to monitor for the appearance of vulvar dysplasia.

BOX 22-3   GUIDELINES FOR TOPICAL CORTICOSTEROID THERAPY

- Rule out or treat vulvovaginal infections, especially candidiasis, prior to initiating corticosteroid therapy, as steroids can worsen candidal infection.
- Corticosteroid use during pregnancy should be avoided or limited.
- Ointments should be used as creams contain alcohol, which is irritating to mucosal tissue.
- A taper protocol should be titrated to the amount of disease present and to the extent of symptoms at the onset of therapy.
- A sample tapering protocol is twice daily application of medication for two to four weeks, then use of medication once daily for 4–12 weeks, followed by use every other day for one or more months.
- The woman should be reevaluated 8–12 weeks after beginning therapy to assess her response to the medication and to determine if vulvar atrophy is developing.
- Once the desired response is achieved, the woman should be switched to a lower potency corticosteroid for maintenance, if possible. Some women will require high- or very high-potency steroids for maintenance.
- Maintenance dosing is usually one to three times weekly.
- It is important to limit the quantity of medication prescribed and to have follow-up visits prior to providing refills.
- Ongoing assessment for vulvar atrophy should occur at least annually.
- Referral should be considered when symptoms are severe or unresponsive to therapy, or if management involves medications with which the clinician is unfamiliar.

LICHEN PLANUS

Lichen planus (LP) is an inflammatory condition of the skin, nails, and mucous membranes. Lesions may be isolated to the vulva or occur with other skin manifestations of LP. Onset is usually between 30 and 60 years of age (Ball & Wojnarowska, 1998).

Clinical Presentation   An irritating vaginal discharge is often the presenting symptom of LP. Other symptoms are vulvar pruritis (which may be intense), vulvar pain and burning, vaginal soreness or discharge, dyspareunia, and postcoital bleeding (Lewis, 1998). The onset may be abrupt or gradual, and symptoms may be intermittent for years.

Physical Examination Findings   There are three major classifications for vulvar LP: papulosquamous, erosive, and hypertrophic. Papulosquamous LP presents as small, intensely pruritic papules with a violaceous hue that arise on keratinized and perianal skin. There may be milky striae on the inner aspects of the labia (Ridley, 1999). Hyperpigmentation often follows resolution of the papulosquamous lesions (Ball & Wojnarowska, 1998). Erosive LP is associated with brightly erythematous vulvar mucosa erosions with white striae or borders (Wickham's striae). The lesions of erosive LP are usually glassy or shiny in appearance. They can occur on the labia minora and vestibule as isolated lesions on otherwise normal-appearing tissue, or they can cause marked architectural distortion including loss of the labia minora. Small isolated lesions on the labia majora are uncommon (Lewis, 1998). Hypertrophic LP exhibits hyperkeratotic, rough lesions of the perineum and the perianal area, and is the rarest form of LP (Lewis).

Up to 70% of women with LP will have vaginal involvement. This contrasts with LS, in which vaginal involvement is unusual (Ridley, 1990). The vaginal epithelium of women with LP bleeds easily with vaginal penetration by a speculum or with attempts at coitus. The tissue appears denuded, and a seropurulent exudate, pseudomembrane or serosanguinous vaginal discharge may occur (Mann & Kaufman, 1991; Lewis, 1998). In severe cases, adhesions may develop leading to stenosis or even obliteration of the vagina (Pelisse, 1996). Anal involvement may also occur. Vulvo-vaginal-gingival syndrome is a variant of erosive LP that involves all three areas, not always concurrently. This form of LP is the most resistant to therapy and requires referral to a physician (Eisen, 1994; Pelisse, 1989).

Management   Medium potency topical steroids with occlusion are very effective. Oral antihistamines, such as hydroxyzine, may be needed if intractable pruritis is causing severe insomnia. Other therapies that can be used are intralesional injection of methylprednisolone, vaginal hydrocortisone suppositories, and prednisolone suppositories. These medications can all cause mucosal thinning and vaginal atrophy and therefore should only be prescribed by providers experienced in their use. Cyclosporine can be used in very resistant cases but is best left to the specialist.

Therapy with progressively sized vaginal dilators may be needed if there is vaginal stenosis or closure. The dilator is coated with a steroid ointment and retained in the vagina overnight by use of snug-fitting underwear. Begin with the smallest dilator that the woman can tolerate comfortably and gradually increase the size. The largest dilator may need to be used weekly for maintenance of vaginal patency (Stewart, 2004). If vaginal adhesions are severe, surgical excision may be needed before the steroid-coated dilators can be used.

SQUAMOUS CELL HYPERPLASIA

Squamous cell hyperplasia (SCH), formerly called hyperplastic dystrophy or leukoplakia, is a description of a morphologic alteration of vulvar skin rather than a distinct entity, and is most common prior to menopause (Sideri, 2004; Star, 1995). SCH usually begins with a benign disorder that causes pruritis. As scratching and itching persist, eventually keratosis and hyperproliferation of the cells (lichenification) occur and hyperplasia becomes apparent. As the tissue continues to thicken and blood flow is further compromised, itching becomes almost intractable and the scratch–itch cycle progresses more rapidly. The thickening tissue becomes white as the vascular layer is covered by additional hyperplastic tissue. SCH has been associated with invasive cancer, but this risk appears minimal unless intraepithelial neoplasia is also present (Sideri).

Clinical Presentation   Many women present with a history of what they think are chronic yeast infections and describe recurrent pruritis that is relieved by topical therapies. However, the pruritis returns within days to weeks after treatment. This cycle may have been present for years. The pruritis of SCH can be distinguished from candidiasis during the history by report of the location. Pruritis with SCH is typically localized, while pruritis with candidiasis is usually generalized. In addition, the pruritis of candidiasis is usually relieved by scratching, but with SCH the scratching must often be hard enough to create a sensation of pain to allow the itching to diminish briefly.

Physical Examination Findings   Early in the disease process there is localized edema with erythema and mild exaggeration of the skin architecture. Fissures and excoriation may also be present. As the disease progresses, the hyperplastic changes are visible and, if present, the whiteness of the tissue is evident. SCH can develop within an LS lesion if untreated pruritis has led to intensive scratching. Because these two dermatoses can occur simultaneously, colposcopic examination is recommended for women with excoriations that do not heal with topical therapy, white on white areas of disease, and for those with areas of both thinning and thickening on visual examination. Concomitant LS and SCH are associated with a higher risk for invasive vulvar cancer (Sideri, 2004).

Management   Medium- to very high-potency corticosteroid ointments can be used for initial treatment of SCH depending on the severity of the condition (Table 22–1 and Box 22–3). These medications can both relieve the pruritis and reverse the skin changes of SCH (Bergman, Karram, & Bhatia, 1988). SCH, either alone or in conjunction with LS, responds less quickly and completely to corticosteroid therapy than does LS by itself (Clark, Etherington, & Luesley, 1999).

PSORIASIS

Psoriasis is a chronic, immune-mediated, genetic disease that manifests in the skin and joints. Peak incidence is in adolescence through one's twenties, but it can develop at any age. The most common form of psoriasis is characterized by papules or plaques that are covered with silvery–white scales, and are most frequently found on the knees, elbows, and scalp. Vulvar psoriasis can occur as an isolated manifestation of the disease or can coexist with psoriasis at other sites on the body. The major clinical variation noted in the vulvar form of psoriasis is that erythema is more common and scaling is finer with thick plaque seldom seen. Topical corticosteroids are the mainstay of therapy for psoriasis (Table 22–1 and Box 22–3). Referral is indicated if vulvar psoriasis is unresponsive to corticosteroids.

NABOTHIAN CYSTS

Nabothian cysts of the cervix are a common finding. The exact incidence of nabothian cysts is unknown because they are rarely symptomatic. Nabothian cysts occur as a result of metaplasia. The cervical canal glandular or columnar mucosa is always in the process of transformation to the pink, smooth, squamous cells that compose the ectocervix at the active transformation zone of the cervix. As the squamous tissue evolves toward the canal, occasionally the glandular cells remain active and continue to secrete mucus while becoming trapped under the more dense squamous tissue. The secretions usually stop over time, but if they do not, mucus collects, creating the smooth, often shiny bulge on the cyst (Goldstein, 2004). Usually the mucus is clear, but it can be cloudy and give a more opaque appearance to the cyst. Blood vessels parallel to the surface can frequently be seen in the overlying tissue. These vessels are long, usually curve over the surface of the cyst, and do not bleed on contact. Nabothian cysts are usually an incidental finding on visual examination of the cervix, but occasionally a woman presents having felt one of the larger cysts during self-examination.

ASSESSMENT

Diagnosis of a nabothian cyst is made by physical examination. No laboratory testing is needed unless the cyst seems atypical. If the blood vessels seem short, comma-like, or corkscrew shaped, and bleed on contact, colposcopy should be performed because these findings may represent malignant or premalignant cervical changes.

DIFFERENTIAL DIAGNOSIS

An atypical-appearing nabothian cyst can represent cervical neoplasia, as noted previously. A mucin-producing carcinoma of the cervix can appear somewhat similar to a nabothian cyst, but would have visible abnormal blood vessels and bleeding on contact. This type of cancer is extremely rare. Magnetic resonance imaging (MRI) is used to differentiate carcinoma from the common nabothian cyst (Li et al., 1999).

MANAGEMENT

A nabothian cyst will frequently resolve on its own with further evolution of the transformation zone and therefore no treatment is required. The evolution of the transformation zone may take up to 12 weeks. Nabothian cysts may rupture or extrude their contents during labor or with deep penetration at intercourse. The cyst is rarely so large that obtaining a thorough Pap test is difficult. If the cyst is so large that it precludes access to the cervix, the clinician may puncture the cyst with a 21 gauge needle and extrude the mucinous material with pressure from a cotton-tipped swab. The cyst may resolve or recur. Cryotherapy has also been used to treat nabothian cysts but is rarely necessary (Kourounis et al., 1999). Referral is indicated if the clinician is unsure of the benign nature of the observed cyst, or if the cyst seems atypical or bleeds on contact.

CERVICAL POLYPS

Cervical polyps occur in 2–5% of women, and approximately 1.7% of these polyps have cancerous changes (Omrani, Schnatz, Qi, Greene, & Curry, 2004). The etiology of cervical polyps is unknown, but hormones and inflammation of the cervical canal seem to play a role in their development (Goldstein, 2004). Mucosal polyps are a result of benign hyperplasia of glandular tissue arising from the mucosa itself. Mucosal polyps may arise anywhere on the body that has glandular mucosa, including the cervix. They often form on a pedicle or stalk. Cervical polyps can become malignant when infected by human papillomavirus and may become dysplastic with infection of either high- or low-risk virus. Cervical polyps are often asymptomatic and thus incidentally diagnosed during a speculum examination done for another purpose. If symptoms occur, they are most likely to be postcoital or intermenstrual spotting or bleeding.

ASSESSMENT

On speculum examination, cervical polyps appear moist, red, and glandular. They range in size from barely visible to greater than 5 centimeters, and arise from a stalk in the cervical canal. Note the size of the polyp, location on the cervix, color, friability, and if the base arises from within the cervical canal. A Pap test is performed to rule out dysplasia or malignancy. Any polyp with an atypical appearance should be biopsied. Atypical findings would include necrosis, contact bleeding, or change in color. These findings could indicate dysplasia or malignancy. Histologic testing is the final confirmation of the benign or malignant nature of a cervical polyp.

DIFFERENTIAL DIAGNOSIS

Endometrial polyps appear very similar to those of cervical origin. If the base is not clearly seen or is too broad to allow visualization, biopsy should not be performed. As many as 8% of polyps that appear cervical may in fact be endometrial, and this could lead to significant bleeding if biopsy were performed in the office setting (Spiewankiewicz, Stelmachow, Sawicki, Cendrowski, & Kuzlik, 2003). Ultrasound to rule out endometrial origin should be performed if the base of the polyp cannot be clearly identified.

MANAGEMENT

Historically, all cervical polyps were removed whether they were symptomatic or not. Fewer clinicians are now removing benign, asymptomatic polyps because of the cost and potential discomfort to the patient for a harmless finding. When a polyp is not removed, the woman should be advised to report irregular bleeding or bleeding after intercourse.

Polyps that are bothersome or atypical should be removed. The technique for removal is to first clearly visualize the base of the stalk, then to cross clamp the stalk with a curved instrument, such as a Kelly clamp or uterine sponge forcep. Moderately firm clamping pressure for one to three minutes should assure hemostasis but not tear the polyp. Using the same clamp, twist the polyp in the canal with gentle traction until the stalk is separated. The specimen is placed in a formalin laboratory jar and sent for histology. Bleeding from the base of the lesion can be treated using a silver nitrate stick, or it can be covered with Monsel's paste if there is too much bleeding for silver nitrate alone. Atypical or broad-based polyps may need to be removed by operative hysteroscopy, which facilitates assessment and treatment of any concurrent intrauterine pathology (Spiewankiewicz et al., 2003).

SPECIAL CONSIDERATIONS

Pregnant Women   Pregnant women have increased blood flow to the cervix that can cause significant bleeding with polyp biopsy or removal. Biopsy or removal of a cervical polyp should only be performed during pregnancy for indications that are too urgent to be postponed until after the woman gives birth, and referral for biopsies in pregnancy should be considered.

UTERINE FIBROIDS

Uterine fibroids, also known as myomas or leiomyomatas, are benign growths that arise from the smooth muscle of the uterus. Fibroids are classified by the uterine layer most involved in their location (see Chapter 5 for uterine anatomy) and can be located on the external surface of the uterus (subserosal), completely within the myometrium (intramural or myometrial), or can have contact with the endometrial layer (submucosal). Fibroids may be pedunculated off the serosal surface and sometimes prolapse into the cervical canal. They range in size from microscopic to large tumors weighing several pounds. Multiple fibroids are common, but they also occur singularly.

INCIDENCE

The exact incidence of fibroids is unknown because they are often asymptomatic. They may be clinically apparent in 25–50% of women and have been found in as many as 77% of surgical specimens (Buttram & Reiter, 1981; Cramer & Patel, 1990). The incidence of fibroids increases with age, and they are two to three times more prevalent in black women (Marshall et al., 1997).

ETIOLOGY AND PATHOPHYSIOLOGY

Uterine fibroids develop when a normal myocyte becomes abnormal and grows into a tumor. This growth occurs by clonal expansion from a single abnormal cell (Mashall et al., 1994). Growth factor abnormalities, injury, and genetic origins are some of the proposed causes of the conversion of the myocyte from normal to abnormal (Stewart & Nowak, 1998). Less than 1% of women with fibroids have malignant leiomyosarcoma (Parker, Fu, & Berek, 1994).

PRESENTATION

The majority of fibroids do not cause symptoms, and thus fibroids are commonly identified as an incidental finding on examination, ultrasound, or surgery. Increased uterine bleeding at menses is the most frequent symptom of fibroids. Menses are typically heavier and longer, and intermenstrual or postcoital bleeding may also occur. The second and third most common symptoms are pelvic pressure or pain and reproductive difficulties, including infertility and pregnancy complications (Stewart, 2001). Pain related to a uterine fibroid may be chronic and mild in nature or severe and acute as occurs in the event of torsion or necrosis. Other possible symptoms are increased abdominal girth, urinary symptoms, and rectal pain or pressure. Peritoneal signs will be present if there is bleeding into the abdominal cavity, necrosis, or infection.

ASSESSMENT

History   Anytime a woman presents with abnormal uterine bleeding, pelvic pain or pressure, or other symptoms that may be related to uterine fibroids, a detailed menstrual history should be obtained. If alterations in the menstrual pattern have occurred, identify when these began and what the specific changes have been. If there is intermenstrual bleeding, ask the woman if it is related to intercourse. If she is experiencing pain or pressure, ask about the onset, location, frequency, quality, intensity, and aggravating and alleviating factors. Obtain a detailed obstetric history with particular attention to complications of pregnancy and infertility. Ask if any female relatives have had fibroids, as there is a familial predisposition. Complete general health and gynecologic histories should also be obtained.

Physical Examination   Abdominal and pelvic examinations should be performed. The uterus may be palpable abdominally if the fibroid is very large. Guarding or rebound tenderness can indicate irritation of the peritoneum. Whether or not fibroids are palpable depends on their location and size. The bimanual examination can be normal even though fibroids are present. Palpable subserosal fibroids most often feel like smooth cobbles on the uterine serosal surface. Pedunculated subserosal fibroids may be palpated as a firm mass in the adnexae, posterior or anterior to the uterus, or in the uterine ligaments. Intramural and submucosal fibroids may not be palpable but can be noted as generalized enlargement or asymmetry of the uterus on bimanual examination. Fibroids are typically nontender.

Diagnostic Testing   Definitive diagnosis of fibroids is usually made by ultrasound. There are no specific laboratory tests for uterine fibroids. If a woman is experiencing frequent and heavy bleeding, a hematocrit or hemoglobin should be obtained in order to evaluate the extent of blood loss. A complete blood count is warranted if infection is suspected. A C-reactive protein or erythrocyte sedimentation rate may be useful to determine the presence of inflammation.

DIFFERENTIAL DIAGNOSIS

There are numerous causes of abnormal uterine bleeding, and the most important to rule out is endometrial cancer (see Chapters 20 and 23). Symptoms of endometriosis and adenomyosis can be similar to those caused by uterine fibroids. Pelvic pressure symptoms can be caused by constipation, irritable bowel syndrome and other gastrointestinal disorders, urinary tract disorders, ovarian masses and other neoplasia of the abdomen or pelvis, and ascites.

MANAGEMENT

Asymptomatic uterine fibroids can be managed expectantly, particularly in women who do not plan future childbearing. Treatment options include medical therapy, surgery, and uterine artery embolization. The timing and type of treatment depends on the number, size, and location of fibroids; type and severity of symptoms; the woman's age or proximity to menopause; and her future childbearing plans (American College of Obstetricians and Gynecologists [ACOG], 2000). Treatment today is aimed more at sparing the uterus than therapy was in the past.

Medical Therapy Gonadotropin-releasing hormone (GnRH) agonists are used to reduce the size of the uterine fibroid prior to surgery or attempts at pregnancy (Table 22–2). GnRH treatment not only reduces fibroid volume, but also increases the woman's blood

TABLE 22–2 Gonadatropin-Releasing Hormone Agonists

Product Name	Approved Indications	Route of Administration	Dosage
Leuprolide (Lupron)	Endometriosis and uterine fibroids	Intramuscular injection	3.75 mg monthly or 11.25 mg every three months
Nafarelin (Synarel)	Endometriosis	Nasal spray, 200 mcg per spray	400–800 mcg per day 400 mcg: one spray in one nostril in the morning and one spray in the other nostril in the evening, 800 mcg: one spray in each nostril twice a day
Goserelin (Zoladex)	Endometriosis	Subcutaneous injection in the upper abdomen	3.6 mg monthly

Note: These medications are contraindicated in pregnancy and must be used in conjunction with contraception. See prescribing reference for full information on doses, side effects, contraindications, and cautions.

volume, thus lowering the risk of surgery by reducing fibroid size and decreasing surgical blood loss (Lethaby, Vollenhoven, & Sowter, 2002). Reduction of fibroid size by 35–60% occurs within three months of initiating therapy (Carr et al., 1993). Vasomotor symptoms and decrease in bone density are the major concerns with the use of GnRH agonists. These side effects can be ameliorated by "add-back therapy" or giving estrogen and/or progestin in addition to the GnRH agonist. The disadvantage of GnRH agonists is that the effects are usually reversed within months of discontinuation, thus surgery or pregnancy attempts must ensue shortly after therapy to maximize the benefits.

The levonorgestrel intrauterine system (LNG-IUS, Mirena) is a newer treatment option for women whose fibroids are relatively small and do not distort the uterine cavity significantly (Grigorieva, Chen-Mok, Tarasova, & Mikhailov, 2003). The uterus should be less than 12-week gestational size or sound to less than 12 centimeters to use this treatment for uterine fibroids. Menorrhagia is greatly reduced, although it is uncertain if the LNG-IUS has its effect only on the endometrium or if there is also some effect on fibroid growth (Grigorieva et al.). Further information about the LNG-IUS can be found in Chapter 9. Other medical therapies used in the management of fibroids include progestins, combined oral contraceptives (COCs), and nonsteroidal anti-inflammatory drugs (NSAIDs). These appear to provide symptom relief rather than actually altering the fibroids.

Surgery   Surgical options for the treatment of fibroids include myomectomy and hysterectomy. Myomectomy is usually performed laparoscopically or abdominally, can be used for removal of one or multiple fibroids, and may involve partial or full thickness of the myometrium. Hysteroscopic myomectomy, which approaches the fibroid through the cervix, is also possible and results in high postoperative fertility rates because full-thickness myometrial incision is not required (Ubaldi et al., 1995). Myomectomy will not prevent growth of new lesions, and 11–26% of women will require a second procedure within 5 years of the initial surgery (Fedele et al., 1995; Malone, 1969). Treatment with GnRH agonists before surgery often leads to successful preservation of uterine function for pregnancy, but cesarean section is indicated after myomectomy because of the risk of uterine rupture. Myomectomy can also be performed in conjunction with a cesarean section though this is controversial because of the potential for excessive blood loss. Hysterectomy is the definitive therapy for symptomatic fibroids, which remain the most frequent indication for hysterectomy. Laparoscopically assisted vaginal hysterectomy, which reduces postoperative recovery time, is possible for many women with fibroids. Hysterectomy is the final resort when other therapies have failed.

Uterine Artery Embolization   Uterine artery embolization (UAE) is performed by an interventional radiologist and involves injecting polyvinyl alcohol particles into the uterine arteries. The therapy is based on the belief that control of arterial blood flow to the fibroid will control symptoms (Spies et al., 2001). In short-term follow-up studies of women who had UAE, 83–84% experienced reduced menorrhagia and 77–79% reported less dysmenorrhea. Pelvic pressure and urinary symptoms were also reduced (Pron et al., 2003; Walker & Pelage, 2002). UAE is used for women who have completed their childbearing as there is potential for loss of fertility and there are only limited data about pregnancy outcomes after this procedure.

When to Refer Acute torsion of a uterine fibroid is a surgical emergency requiring immediate referral. Most uterine fibroids present as a chronic condition, but acute hemorrhage can occur and is usually unresponsive to medical therapy. Collaborative management is often warranted in determining a plan for medical therapy, and referral is indicated when surgical options are being considered.

EMERGING EVIDENCE THAT MAY CHANGE MANAGEMENT

Mifepristone (formerly known as RU-486) has effectiveness comparable to GnRH agonists, but the dosages used (5–50 mgs) are not available in the United States at this time (Murphy, Morales, Kettel, & Yen, 1995; Eisinger, Meldrum, Fiscella, le Roux, & Guzick, 2003). Raloxifene decreased fibroid size in one trial of postmenopausal women but was not successful in a separate study of premenopausal women (Palomba, Sammartino, et al., 2001; Palomba et al., 2002). Medical therapy with aromatase inhibitors and MRI-guided thermoablation are also being investigated (Karaer, Oruc, & Koyuncu, 2004; Visvanathan, Connell, Hall-Craggs, Cutner, & Bown, 2002).

SPECIAL CONSIDERATIONS

Pregnant Women According to ultrasound measurements most fibroids are stable or reduced in size during pregnancy, but some may show growth (Strobelt et al., 1994; Rosati, Exacoustos, & Mancuso, 1992). Larger fibroids can make assessment of fetal size difficult. Potential complications of fibroids during pregnancy include failed implantation, spontaneous abortion, preterm labor, fetal growth restriction, placental abruption, malpresentation, arrested labor or descent as a result of obstruction of the lower uterine segment or cervix, and retained placenta (Coronado, Marshall, & Schwartz; 2000; Exacoustos & Rosati, 1993; Rice, Kay, & Mahony, 1989). Rapid fibroid growth during pregnancy can lead to infarction with bleeding into the fibroid itself rather than vaginally (red infarction or red fibroids), necrosis, and hemorrhage. In the postpartum period, rapid estrogen loss and vasculature reduction can lead to fibroid degeneration with attendant bleeding and pain.

Older Women The spontaneous decrease in hormones at menopause often leads to a reduction in uterine fibroid size. Exogenous hormone therapy (HT, see Chapter 11) after menopause can cause stimulation of uterine fibroids leading to abnormal growth, and fibroid location seems to play a role in whether or not HT will lead to abnormal bleeding (Akkad, Habiba, Ismail, Abrams, & al-Azzawi, 1995). Transdermal estrogen was associated with postmenopausal fibroid growth in one study but not in another; therefore, it is unclear whether oral or transdermal estrogen is preferable (Polatti, Viazzo, Colleoni, &

Nappi, 2000; Palomba, Sena, et al., 2001). Leiomyosarcoma should be considered in postmenopausal women who present with an enlargening pelvic mass accompanied by vaginal bleeding (Leibsohn, d'Ablaing, Mishell, & Schlaerth, 1990).

Influences of Culture   Abnormal bleeding can cause significant sexual difficulties for women from cultures in which sex during bleeding is taboo. The lack of proven alternative therapies for treatment of uterine fibroids and the potential need for surgery may cause cultural difficulty for those who prefer to avoid allopathic medicine. The effects of surgeries that cause loss of reproductive capability in women from cultures where fertility is equated with value should be considered, and medical therapies may be more appropriate. Aspects of these cultural influences also apply to the conditions discussed in the remainder of this chapter: adenomyosis, endometriosis, and ovarian cysts.

ADENOMYOSIS

Adenomyosis is the presence of endometrial tissue in the myometrium. Adenomyosis can be divided into two types of lesions: diffuse and nodular. The diffuse lesions, sometimes referred to as endometriosis interna, involve both anterior and posterior myometrium and are not encapsulated. The nodular or local and discrete adenomyosis lesions within the myometrium are called adenomyomas (Johnson, 2003).

INCIDENCE

The estimated incidence of adenomyosis varies because the final diagnosis can only be made from microscopic examination of the uterine musculature. It is estimated that 20% of women who are 40 to 50 years of age have adenomyosis, although one study of operative specimens revealed a 60% occurrence (McElin & Bird, 1974). Adenomyosis is thought to be underdiagnosed as a result of being mistaken for small uterine fibroids on ultrasound (Johnson, 2003). Adenomyosis occurs more often in women who have had children than in those who have not, but a greater number of pregnancies does not increase the incidence of adenomyosis (McElin & Bird; Molitor, 1971).

ETIOLOGY AND PATHOPHYSIOLOGY

The exact etiology of adenomyosis is unknown. The prevailing theory is that the endometrial glandular and basalis layers invaginate the myometrium. The mechanism that causes the endometrium to grow into the myometrium has not been determined (Ferenczy, 1998).

CLINICAL PRESENTATION

The most common symptoms of adenomyosis are pelvic pain and menorrhagia. Pain with intercourse during deep penetration is common, and women will often report an increase in clotting with menses. As with uterine fibroids, the majority of women who have adenomyosis are asymptomatic or experience only mild changes that are usually attributed to aging or perimenopause. Therefore, to make a timely diagnosis and institute management, it is important to maintain a high index of suspicion for adenomyosis.

ASSESSMENT

History   Obtain a detailed menstrual history and information about pain, including onset, location, frequency, quality, intensity, and aggravating and alleviating factors. If alterations in the menstrual pattern have occurred, identify when these began and what the specific changes have been. Ask if there is dyspareunia and if so, note the onset and location (e.g., at the introitus, deep in the pelvis). Inquire about previous evaluation or treatment for the symptoms she is experiencing. Complete general health and gynecologic histories should also be obtained.

Physical Examination   Inspect and palpate the abdomen, then perform a complete pelvic examination. Bimanual examination with adenomyosis typically reveals a diffusely larger-than-average uterus that is somewhat boggy and tender to palpation. If the adenomyosis is of the nodular type, the uterus may be asymmetrical. Unlike fibroids, distinct, firm, raised lesions are not palpable.

Diagnostic Testing   Laboratory testing cannot be used to diagnose adenomyosis, but measurement of hemoglobin or hematocrit should be performed to assess the severity of any irregular bleeding. Assessment for adenomyosis is generally performed as part of ruling out the differential diagnoses, and additional testing may be warranted if another condition is suspected and has not been excluded. In particular, endometrial biopsy should be strongly considered in the evaluation of women 35 years and older who present with menorrhagia.

Ultrasound is the most commonly used diagnostic tool, but it has limitations. Diffuse adenomyosis lesions often appear only as an enlarged uterus, and the nodular form of adenomyosis can be difficult to differentiate from small uterine fibroids (Atri, Reinhold, Mehio, Chapman, & Bret, 2000). Color Doppler ultrasound can be helpful for making this distinction. MRI gives a more definitive picture of adenomyosis and is useful in distinguishing it from fibroids and malignancy, but cost limits its use (Byun et al., 1999; Reinhold et al., 1999).

DIFFERENTIAL DIAGNOSIS

Uterine fibroids, endometrial hyperplasia and malignancy (see Chapter 23), abnormal uterine bleeding (see Chapter 20), and other causes of chronic pelvic pain (see Chapter 25) should be considered in the differential diagnosis. It is important to differentiate adenomyosis from uterine fibroids because the treatments for fibroids can make the symptoms of adenomyosis worse, or at least delay proper management. The presence of pain on examination helps distinguish fibroids and adenomyosis. Fibroids are generally only painful at times of rapid growth or if degenerating, while tenderness to uterine palpation is usually present with adenomyosis.

MANAGEMENT

Medical   Analgesics and contraceptives may be useful in the early management of adenomyosis when changes are still mild and for women who are not ready for definitive surgery. NSAIDs or narcotics may be used for dysmenorrhea, though they do not control the pain of adenomyosis as well as they do other causes of menstrual pain. Combined oral contraceptives can temporarily control the heavy menses of adenomyosis, but they will become ineffective as the lesions multiply or become larger. There is very limited evidence of successful treatment of adenomyosis with the LNG-IUS (Fedele, Bianchi, Raffaelli, Portuese, & Dorta, 1997; Fong & Singh, 1999). The depot medroxyprogesterone acetate (Depo-Provera) injection should be avoided because it can make menorrhagia worse.

Surgical   Hysterectomy is the definitive treatment for adenomyosis. Removal of the ovaries is not essential for control of adenomyosis (as it is with endometriosis), because the lesions do not respond to hormonal fluctuations. Endometrial ablation or resection is only likely to be effective if adenomyosis is superficial (McCausland & McCausland, 1998; Wood, 1998).

ENDOMETRIOSIS

Endometriosis is the presence of endometrial glands and stroma outside of the uterus. The most common sites for endometrial implants are, in decreasing order of frequency, the ovaries, anterior and posterior cul-de-sac, posterior broad ligaments, uterosacral ligaments, fallopian tubes, sigmoid colon, appendix, and round ligaments (Jenkins, Olive, & Haney, 1986). Endometrial implants have also been found in the vagina, vulva, cervix, perineum, inguinal canal, urinary system, gastrointestinal tract locations other than those noted previously, pulmonary structures, extremities, skin, and central nervous system (Honoré, 1999). The appearance and size of implants is widely variable. Endometriomas are cystlike structures that contain endometrial tissue and are often found on the ovaries (see section on ovarian cysts for further information).

INCIDENCE

The true incidence of endometriosis is unknown. Prevalence estimates for endometriosis are 5–20% in women with pelvic pain, 20–40% in women with infertility, and 3–10% in the general population of reproductive-aged women (Speroff & Fritz, 2005). Among adolescents who undergo laparoscopy for pelvic pain unrelieved by medical therapy, 50–70% will have endometriosis (Laufer, Sanfilippo, & Rose, 2003). The condition is six to seven times more prevalent among women who have a first-degree relative with endometriosis as compared to the general population (Simpson, Elias, Malinak, & Buttram, 1980; Speroff & Fritz). Early menarche, short menstrual cycles, and menses longer than seven days have also been associated with increased risk of endometriosis. Endometriosis is rare in premenarcheal girls and postmenopausal women.

ETIOLOGY AND PATHOPHYSIOLOGY

There are several theories for the pathogenesis of endometriosis, and no single theory explains all cases of the condition. The retrograde menstruation theory proposes that reverse flow of menses out of the fallopian tubes allows endometrial cells to enter the pelvis and implant on the pelvic organs or peritoneal surface. The coelomic metaplasia theory proposes that endometriosis develops from spontaneous metaplasia of cells derived from the coelomic epithelium. The induction theory, which is related to the coelomic metaplasia theory, proposes that endogenous biochemical or immunologic factors stimulate cells to differentiate into endometrial tissue. The theory that endometrial cells can be directly implanted during surgery or episiotomy repair best explains finding endometriosis in surgical scars and the perineum. Endometriosis outside the pelvis is explained by the theory that cells are carried to distant sites in the lymphatic system or blood vessels. The most widely accepted theory for the origin of endometriosis is retrograde menstruation, which occurs in 76–90% of women. However, other factors must be involved in the development of endometriosis because the actual prevalence of endometriosis is much lower. Potential contributing factors include immunologic and hormonal abnormalities, heredity, and environmental toxins (Seli, Berkkanoglu, & Arici, 2003; Speroff & Fritz, 2005). Recent research indicates that endometriosis is associated with an increased risk of ovarian cancer, which is thought to be a result of exposure to unopposed estrogen (Brinton et al., 2004; Modugno et al., 2004).

CLINICAL PRESENTATION

Endometriosis is often asymptomatic, but it can be a severe and debilitating condition. The most common symptoms of endometriosis are pelvic pain, dysmenorrhea, dyspareunia, abnormal menstrual bleeding, and infertility. Unfortunately these same symptoms occur with many other conditions, which can lead to a delay in the diagnosis of endometriosis (Husby, Haugen, & Moen, 2003). Other symptoms include pressure and pain in the rectum (especially with sitting), nausea and sometimes vomiting with menses, and diarrhea at the time of menses. Pain can radiate to the legs and lower back, and can be so intense that syncope occurs. The extent of disease and severity of pain do not necessarily correlate (Gruppo Italiano per lo Studio dell'Endometriosi, 2001; Porpora et al., 1999; Vercellini et al., 1996). Women with mild disease can have significant pain, and women with advanced disease can have minimal or no pain. However, there does appear to be a correlation between the severity of disease and the incidence of decreased fertility (Speroff & Fritz, 2005).

ASSESSMENT

History   Obtain a detailed history about any pelvic pain that includes the onset, location, frequency, quality, intensity, and aggravating and alleviating factors. If dyspareunia is present, identify the location. Ask about menstrual cycle patterns, symptoms with menses (e.g., dysmenorrhea, nausea and vomiting, and diarrhea), and infertility. Note specifically if there have been any time periods when the woman was having intercourse without using contraception and didn't become pregnant to assess for undiagnosed infertility. Document any family history of endometriosis. Complete general health and gynecologic histories should also be obtained.

Physical Examination   Abdominal and pelvic examinations should be performed with particular attention to the bimanual examination. Findings on physical examination may be limited, if present at all. The most common finding is pain during palpation of the posterior fornix. Tenderness or induration of the uterosacral ligaments, palpation of nodules in the cul-de-sac or on the rectovaginal septum, tenderness with uterine motion, and a tender enlarged adnexal mass may also be present. If the disease is extensive, the uterus may be fixed, and is most often in a retroflexed position.

Diagnostic Testing   There are no specific laboratory tests for endometriosis. Ultrasound can identify endometriomas but will not demonstrate adhesive changes. MRI can also identify endometriomas and may detect some endometrial implants, but it is not sufficiently sensitive for diagnosis. Hysterosalpingography may demonstrate tubal obstruction secondary to adhesive disease.

Laparoscopy with biopsy is the gold standard for the diagnosis of endometriosis. Laparoscopic findings can be used to stage the disease according to the classification system developed by the American Society for Reproductive Medicine (ASRM, 1997). Disease stages I to IV are based on the site(s) and severity of endometrial implants and adhesions (ASRM). This classification system can be helpful for reporting operative findings and interpreting study results, but it does not correlate well with a woman's symptoms or prognosis for fertility (ACOG, 1999; Guzick et al., 1997).

DIFFERENTIAL DIAGNOSIS

Differential diagnoses include other gynecologic and nongynecologic causes of chronic pelvic pain (see Chapter 25). The woman may also be experiencing menstrual pelvic pain and discomfort (see Chapter 19), infertility caused by another etiology (see Chapter 16), or abnormal uterine bleeding related to other causes (see Chapter 20).

MANAGEMENT

Treatment options for endometriosis include expectant management, medical therapy, and surgery. The woman's disease stage, level of pain, and desire for pregnancy should be considered in developing the management plan (ACOG, 1999). Additional considerations used in the management of endometriosis-associated infertility are discussed later in the Special Considerations section.

Medical Therapy Options for medical therapy of endometriosis include progestins, combined oral contraceptives, GnRH agonists, and danazol. The rationale for their use is to eliminate or reduce menses and thus the potential for retrograde menstruation. There is no evidence that any of these medications improve fertility, and they are all equally effective for pain relief (ACOG, 1999; Practice Committee of the ASRM, 2004; Speroff & Fritz, 2005). Recurrence of symptoms may occur after discontinuation of medical therapy. Medical therapy may be used as the primary treatment, or it may be used after surgery to prevent recurrence of endometriosis.

Medroxyprogesterone acetate is the progestin most widely used for the treatment of endometriosis, and it can be taken orally (20–100 mg daily) or given via intramuscular injection (150 mg every three months). Side effects of progestins include irregular menstrual bleeding, breast tenderness, fluid retention, and depression or mood instability. Combined oral contraceptives are also used for treatment, and continuous dosing of active pills may be more effective in the control of pain than cyclic dosing (Vercellini, Frontino, De Giorgi, Pietropaolo, et al., 2003). Combined oral contraceptives can substantially decrease the risk of ovarian cancer in women with endometriosis (Modugno et al., 2004).

GnRH agonists (Table 22–2) and danazol can decrease the size of endometriomas in addition to relieving pain, but do not eliminate them. Reduction in size prior to surgery can be helpful (Rana, Thomas, Rotman, & Dmowski, 1996). Both GnRH agonists and danazol have significant side effects. GnRH agonists can cause vasomotor symptoms and bone loss. "Add-back" therapy is given to attenuate these effects. Estrogen-only add-back therapy is not recommended for women with endometriosis, as it may increase their pain (Hurst, Gardner, Tucker, Awoniyi, & Schlaff, 2000). Either progestin or a combination of estrogen and progestin can be used (Makarainen, Ronnberg, & Kauppila, 1996; Moghissi, Schlaff, Olive, Skinner, & Yin, 1998; Surrey & Hornstein, 2002). Other medications that can be used in add-back therapy to prevent bone loss include parathyroid hormone, calcitonin, and biphosphonates, as well as adequate doses of calcium carbonate or citrate with vitamin D (Finkelstein et al., 1998; Roux et al., 1995; Surrey, Voigt , Fournet, & Judd, 1995). Discontinuation of GnRH therapy is usually followed by active attempts at pregnancy or with suppression of menses by continuous use of combined oral contraceptives. Otherwise, menses usually returns within 60 to 90 days after discontinuation of therapy. Danazol is given orally at 600–800 mg per day (Speroff & Fritz, 2005). Danazol has both hypoestrogenic and androgenic side effects, including weight gain, muscle cramps, decreased breast size, acne, hirsutism, oily skin, hot flashes, mood changes, and depression.

Surgery Surgery for endometriosis is indicated for severe or debilitating symptoms, symptoms that have not been controlled by medical therapy, anatomic distortion, urinary or bowel obstruction, and otherwise advanced disease. Surgery may also be indicated during infertility treatment (Practice Committee of the ASRM, 2004). Surgery can be conservative or definitive. The goal of conservative surgery, which is usually done laparoscopically, is to treat the endometriosis while preserving the uterus and as much ovarian tissue as possible. Ablation, laser vaporization, or fulgarization of implants and adhesions are all performed. Up to 90% of women experience pain relief with conservative surgery, but the risk of recurrence of implants or adhesions is as high as 40% at five years (Wheeler & Malinak, 1983). The definitive surgery for endometriosis is a hysterectomy, with or without salpingo-oopherectomy. Hysterectomy is indicated when significant disease is present and future fertility is not desired, when incapacitating symptoms persist despite medical therapy or conservative surgery, and if coexisting pelvic pathology requires hysterectomy. Conservation of the ovaries is attempted, especially in younger women who are remote from menopause, but is not possible if disease is extensive as the implants will cyclically respond as before the uterine surgery.

EMERGING EVIDENCE THAT MAY CHANGE MANAGEMENT

Three small trials have examined LNG-IUS use after conservative surgery. Participants in the first study had reduced blood loss and dysmenorrhea (Vercellini et al., 1999). The second study found that women with rectovaginal endometriosis had reduced pain with a small but significant decrease in lesion volume (Fedele, Bianchi, Zanconato, Portuese, & Raffaelli, 2001). The third study demonstrated lower recurrence of moderate or severe dysmenorrhea at one year after surgery when the LNG-IUS was placed after surgery, as compared with expectant management (Vercellini, Frontino, De Giorgi, Aimi, et al., 2003). A fourth study used the LNG-IUS as primary therapy for mild to moderate endometriosis, and participants had reduced pain as well as improvement of disease stage on follow-up laparoscopic examination (Lockhat, Emembolu, & Konje, 2004). Aromatase inhibitors are another potential therapy for endometriosis (Bulun, Zeitoun, Takayama, & Sasano, 2000).

SPECIAL CONSIDERATIONS

Adolescents   Combined oral contraceptives and NSAIDs are the main treatments for adolescents (Laufer et al., 2003). Some families object to adolescent use of contraception. They may fear that sexual activity will be encouraged or that their daughter's ability to have children will be harmed; however, lack of treatment can pose a more severe risk to future fertility. It is important to include the family (with the patient's permission) when planning management, and to find balance in explaining the necessity of long-term treatment without promoting unnecessary fear. Diagrams to demonstrate anatomy and physiology and handouts that can be reviewed at home may be particularly helpful when caring for adolescents. Regardless of age, patients who do not respond to medical therapy should be referred for diagnostic laparoscopy (Laufer et al.).

Infertility   Despite the clear association between endometriosis and infertility, the mechanisms of this relationship are unclear. In addition, there is not universal agreement on the indications for surgical evaluation and therapy during infertility treatment. Age, duration of infertility, family history, pelvic pain, and stage of endometriosis should be taken into account when determining the management plan. For Stages I and II endometriosis, treatment may include ovulation induction with intrauterine insemination or in vitro fertilization (see Chapter 16) prior to or after laparoscopy. Expectant management after laparoscopy is also an option for women under 35 years of age. Conservative surgical treatment is indicated for women with Stages III and IV endometriosis. In vitro fertilization may be necessary if pregnancy does not occur after surgery (Practice Committee of the ASRM, 2004).

OVARIAN CYSTS

Ovarian cystic structures can arise from all of the differentiated tissues of the ovary. Benign cysts are classified as functional or organic, depending on their etiology. This section focuses on ovarian cysts that are most likely benign, and ovarian malignancies are discussed further in Chapter 23. Ovarian cysts can cause women to have significant anxiety that may remain unspoken. When accurate, reassuring a woman of the nonmalignant nature of her condition or the unlikely loss of her fertility can be supportive.

INCIDENCE

The actual incidence of ovarian cysts is difficult to estimate because many are asymptomatic and never diagnosed. Pathology reports of ovarian cysts requiring surgery demonstrate that 25% are functional and 75% are organic, with approximately 1–4% of supposedly benign cysts found to be malignant at the time of surgery (Demont, Fourquet, Rogers, & Lansac, 2001).

ETIOLOGY AND PATHOPHYSIOLOGY

Functional ovarian cysts, also called simple cysts because of their appearance on ultrasound, are classified by whether they occur in the follicular or luteal phase of the menstrual cycle. Follicular phase cysts are more common and are usually asymptomatic and undiagnosed unless they spontaneously rupture or cause pain with ovulation (mittelschmerz). If ovulation does not occur, the follicular cyst may continue to grow with the risk of torsion or rupture increasing with size of the cyst. With consistent anovulation, the ovary takes on a polycystic appearance on ultrasound (see Chapter 21). A luteal ovarian cyst or corpus luteum is normally formed with each menstrual cycle after ovulation occurs. The corpus luteum is a transient, functional gland producing progesterone to maintain the lining of the uterus in the event of pregnancy. If pregnancy does not occur, the cyst should undergo luteolysis and regress with the onset of menses (Davis & Rueda, 2002).

Organic cysts may be referred to as complex cysts because of their appearance on ultrasound. Mucinous or serous cysts arise from mucinous or secretory ovarian glandular cells and can become very large, though they usually grow slowly. These borderline tumors or tumors of low malignancy potential generally have a good prognosis, but approximately 10–20% of them can behave like a carcinoma and have an unfavorable prognosis (Trimble & Trimble, 2001; Dietel & Hauptmann, 2000). Teratomas, also known as "dermoid cysts", and endometriomas may be cystic or have a cystic component but are most often solid tumors. Teratomas arise from the ovarian germ cell, grow rapidly, and can become very large. Endometriomas are caused by endometriosis. Teratomas and endometriomas are very rarely malignant (Templeman et al., 2000; Prefumo, Todeschini, Fulcheri, & Venturini, 2002).

CLINICAL PRESENTATION

The presentation of ovarian cysts varies greatly because there are diverse etiologies with different clinical courses, and cysts can range in size from a few cm to several pounds. All ovarian cysts can be asymptomatic, though this is more likely with cysts that are functional and/or small in size. Functional cysts may cause pain but are often an incidental finding on examination or ultrasound. Organic cysts may present as a unilateral or bilateral pelvic mass or with abdominal pain or pressure. Pain may be intermittent or persistent and have a gradual or abrupt onset. Usually pain with abrupt onset represents bleeding or spilling of cystic fluid into the abdomen with resultant peritoneal irritation. Pain can also occur with ovarian torsion. When cysts become large, abdominal girth can increase from the tumor or ascites and may be mistaken for pregnancy. Urinary frequency without dysuria can occur if a large cyst presses on the bladder.

ASSESSMENT

History   Obtain a detailed history of any symptoms the woman is experiencing, including onset, location, frequency, quality, intensity, and aggravating and alleviating factors. Note the last menstrual period and whether or not the menstrual cycles are regular. The menstrual history can help differentiate follicular and luteal cysts and identify irregular menstrual patterns that may result from functional cysts. Complete general health and gynecologic histories should also be obtained.

Physical Examination   Vital signs and weight should be obtained. Infection and thus fever are unlikely with ovarian cysts, but heart rate and blood pressure changes may occur with significant pain. A disproportionate change in abdominal girth without a concomitant weight gain may indicate large tumor growth. The abdomen should be inspected, auscultated, and palpated. Large masses may cause visible changes in the abdomen or may be palpable abdominally. Guarding or rebound tenderness can indicate irritation of the peritoneum. A complete pelvic examination should be performed. Assess the location, size, shape, texture, mobility, and tenderness of any palpable mass.

Diagnostic Testing Pregnancy testing should be performed in all women of reproductive age to rule out ectopic pregnancy. Gonorrhea and chlamydia testing are warranted if a tubo-ovarian abscess is suspected. Additional laboratory testing can be deferred until after ultrasound if a functional cyst is the most likely diagnosis based on menstrual timing, age, and examination. Other tests to consider include complete blood count, C-reactive protein, and erythrocyte sedimentation rate. Tumor markers, such as the CA125, alpha fetoprotein (AFP), and human chorionic gonadotropin (hCG), should also be measured if there is a strong suspicion of a malignant mass (Ind & Shepherd, 2003). Many of these tests are expensive and should be avoided unless findings are highly suspicious for malignancy.

An ultrasound should be performed. Functional or simple cysts are readily identified by ultrasound. Their appearance may be complex if there is spontaneous bleeding into the cyst. Organic cysts can include cystic areas, papillary projections, nodules, and solid areas. The accurate diagnosis of complex cysts is enhanced by color flow Doppler ultrasound (Jermy, Luise, & Bourne, 2001). MRI is useful in determining if a solid tumor is at high risk for malignancy.

DIFFERENTIAL DIAGNOSIS

Ectopic pregnancy, tubo-ovarian abscess, and ovarian cancer are the most likely other causes of an ovarian mass. Polycystic ovarian syndrome should be considered if multiple follicular cysts are present on ultrasound (see Chapter 21). There are numerous other gynecologic and nongynecologic causes of acute and chronic pelvic pain. If the pain is acute, pelvic inflammatory disease and appendicitis particularly warrant consideration. Differential diagnoses for chronic pelvic pain can be found in Chapter 25.

MANAGEMENT

Functional Cysts Functional ovarian cysts will spontaneously resolve in approximately 65% of cases without any therapy (Christensen, Boldsen, & Westergaard, 2002). Simple cysts require no therapy unless they are greater than 8 centimeters, rupture, or lead to ovarian torsion, in which case surgical intervention is required. Minor pain at ovulation or from a persistent cyst less than 5 cm can be treated with oral pain medication until the cyst spontaneously resolves. Repeat ultrasound after one to three menstrual cycles can be performed but is not mandatory unless symptoms persist. Cysts between 5 and 8 cm should be followed for further growth, and the woman should be cautioned to call for any significant increase in pain that might represent rupture or torsion. A CA125 should be performed while following these larger masses. Repeated episodes of functional cysts can be reduced by using contraceptives to suppress ovulation. Contraceptives do not promote resolution of simple or complex cysts that are already formed.

Complex Cysts Complex ovarian cysts will usually require careful ultrasound and MRI to determine if the complexity is merely blood in a simple cyst, or if this a serous cyst or solid tumor with cystic components. Small cysts with some complexity on ultrasound, which may represent bleeding into the cyst, can be followed with repeat ultrasound in four to six weeks if the CA125 is negative. Indications for removal of a complex cyst are size greater than 8 cm regardless of the results of tumor markers, or elevated CA125 regardless of size. All solid tumors must be removed regardless of the CA125. A complex cyst of any size with an elevated CA125 and all solid tumors are presumed malignant until proven otherwise. The CA125 is helpful in determining the type of surgical incision that will be performed. Generally a complex or solid cyst with a negative CA125 can be approached with laparoscopy, but a laparotomy is necessary if the CA125 is elevated.

SPECIAL CONSIDERATIONS

Adolescents   Functional cysts, both follicular and luteal, are common in adolescents. Their immature pituitary-hypothalamic-ovarian axis allows more anovulatory cycles leading to more persistent simple cysts. Early evidence of polycystic ovarian syndrome may also manifest in this age group (see Chapter 21). Teratomas are occasionally found in adolescents and are usually surgically removed with an effort to save as much functional ovarian tissue as possible.

Pregnant Women   More ovarian cysts are being diagnosed during early pregnancy with the current trend of increasing use of first trimester ultrasound. Corpus luteum cysts will generally resolve by the end of the first trimester. Rupture of a corpus luteum cyst in the first trimester with subsequent surgery and loss of the cyst's functional capacity to produce progesterone leads to a high rate of early pregnancy loss. The use of exogenous progesterone has helped to reduce the rate of loss (Sergent, Verspyck, & Marpeau, 2003). Organic cysts are most commonly seen after 16 weeks gestation. These are usually teratomas and are removed during pregnancy only if they are larger than 6 cm because of the risk for torsion, intracystic bleeding or rupture which could lead to pregnancy loss. Incidence of teratomas requiring surgery during pregnancy is 0.5–2 per 1000 pregnancies (Sergent et al.). The beginning of the second trimester is considered the ideal time for removal of ovarian cysts as earlier removal is associated with a higher rate of pregnancy loss.

Older Women   Cysts that occur in postmenopausal women are regarded seriously because of the increased incidence of ovarian cancer in this population and the less likely occurrence of benign functional cysts. Studies have shown that unilocular cysts under 5 cm and with a negative CA125 can be followed with serial ultrasound. If the cyst increases in size or if the CA125 is elevated, the cyst should be removed (Hartge et al., 2000).

REFERENCES

Akkad, A. A., Habiba, M. A., Ismail, N., Abrams, K., & al-Azzawi, F. (1995). Abnormal uterine bleeding on hormone replacement: The importance of intrauterine structural abnormalities. *Obstetrics and Gynecology, 86*(3), 330–334.

American College of Obstetricians and Gynecologists. (1999). *Medical management of endometriosis* (Practice Bulletin 11). Washington, DC: Author.

American College of Obstetricians and Gynecologists. (2000). *Surgical alternatives to hysterectomy in the management of leiomyomas* (Practice Bulletin 16). Washington, DC: Author.

American Society for Reproductive Medicine. (1997). Revised American Society for Reproductive Medicine classification of endometriosis: 1996. *Fertility and Sterility, 67*(5), 817–821.

Assmann, T., Becker-Wegerich, P., Grewe, M., Megahed, M., & Ruzicka, T. (2003). Tacrolimus ointment for the treatment of vulvar lichen sclerosus. *Journal of the American Academy of Dermatology, 48*(6), 935–937.

Atri, M., Reinhold, C., Mehio, A. R., Chapman, W. B., & Bret, P. M. (2000). Adenomyosis: US features with histologic correlation in an in-vitro study. *Radiology, 215*(3), 783–790.

Ball, S. B., & Wojnarowska, F. (1998). Vulvar dermatoses: Lichen sclerosus, lichen planus, and vulval dermatitis/lichen simplex chronicus. *Seminars in Cutaneous Medicine and Surgery, 17*(3), 182–188.

Bergman, A., Karram, M., & Bhatia, N. N. (1988). Local steroid application for hyperplastic dystrophy of the vulva. Clinical and pathologic evaluation. *Journal of Reproductive Medicine, 33*(6), 542–544.

Black, M. M., McKay, M., & Braude, P. (1995). *Color atlas and text of obstetric and gynecologic dermatology.* London: Mosby-Wolfe.

Brinton, L. A., Lamb, E. J., Moghissi, K. S., Scoccia, B., Althuis, M. D., Mabie, J. E., et al. (2004). Ovarian cancer risk associated with varying causes of infertility. *Fertility and Sterility, 82*(2), 405–414.

Bulun, S. E., Zeitoun, K. M., Takayama, K., & Sasano, H. (2000). Molecular basis for treating endometriosis with aromatase inhibitors. *Human Reproduction Update, 6*(5), 413–418.

Buttram, V. C., Jr., & Reiter, R. C. (1981). Uterine leiomyomata: Etiology, symptomatology, and management. *Fertility and Sterility, 36*(4), 433–445.

Byun, J. Y., Kim, S. E., Choi, B. G., Ko, G. Y., Jung, S. E., & Choi, K. H. (1999). Diffuse and focal adenomyosis: MR imaging findings [Special Issue]. *Radiographics, 19*, S161–S170.

Carr, B. R., Marshburn, P. B., Weatherall, P. T., Bradshaw, K. D., Breslau, N. A., Byrd, W., et al. (1993). An evaluation of the effect of gonadotropin-releasing hormone analogs and medroxyprogesterone acetate on uterine leiomyomata volume by magnetic resonance imaging: A prospective, randomized, double blind, placebo-controlled, crossover trial. *Journal of Clinical Endocrinology and Metabolism, 76*(5), 1217–1223.

Christensen, J. T., Boldsen, J. L., & Westergaard, J. G. (2002). Functional ovarian cysts in premenopausal and gynecologically healthy women. *Contraception, 66*(3), 153–157.

Clark, T. J., Etherington, I. J., & Luesley, D. M. (1999). Response of vulvar lichen sclerosus and squamous cell hyperplasia to graduated topical steroids. *Journal of Reproductive Medicine, 44*(11), 958–962.

Coronado, G. D., Marshall, L. M., & Schwartz, S. M. (2000). Complications in pregnancy, labor, and delivery with uterine leiomyomas: A population-based study. *Obstetrics and Gynecology, 95*(5), 764–769.

Cramer, S. F., & Patel, A. (1990). The frequency of uterine leiomyomas. *American Journal of Clinical Pathology, 94*(4), 435–438.

Davis, J. S., & Rueda, B. R. (2002). The corpus luteum: An ovarian structure with maternal instincts and suicidal tendencies. *Frontiers in Bioscience, 7*, d1949–d1978.

Demont, F., Fourquet, F., Rogers, M., & Lansac, J. (2001). Epidemiology of apparently benign ovarian cysts. *Journal de Gynecologie, Obstetrique et Biologie de la Reproduction, 30*(Suppl. 1), S8–S11.

Dietel, M., & Hauptmann, S. (2000). Serous tumors of low malignant potential of the ovary. 1. Diagnostic pathology. *Virchows Archiv, 436*(5), 403–412.

Eisen, D. (1994). The vulvovaginal-gingival syndrome of lichen planus. The clinical characteristics of 22 patients. *Archives of Dermatology, 130*(11), 1379–1382.

Eisinger, S. H., Meldrum, S., Fiscella, K., le Roux, H. D., & Guzick, D. S. (2003). Low-dose mifepristone for uterine leiomyomata. *Obstetrics and Gynecology, 101*(2), 243–250.

Exacoustos, C., & Rosati, P. (1993). Ultrasound diagnosis of uterine myomas and complications in pregnancy. *Obstetrics and Gynecology, 82*(1), 97–101.

Fedele, L., Bianchi, S., Raffaelli, R., Portuese, A., & Dorta, M. (1997). Treatment of adenomyosis-associated menorrhagia with a levonorgestrel-releasing intrauterine device. *Fertility and Sterility, 68*, 426–429.

Fedele, L., Bianchi, S., Zanconato, G., Portuese, A., & Raffaelli, R. (2001). Use of a levonorgestrel-releasing intrauterine device in the treatment of rectovaginal endometriosis. *Fertility and Sterility, 75*(3), 485–488.

Fedele, L., Parazzini, F., Luchini, L., Mezzopane, R., Tozzi, L., & Villa, L. (1995). Recurrence of fibroids after myomectomy: A transvaginal ultrasonographic study. *Human Reproduction, 10*(7), 1795–1796.

Ferenczy, A. (1998). Pathophysiology of adenomyosis. *Human Reproduction Update, 4*(4), 312–322.

Finkelstein, J. S., Klibanski, A., Arnold, A. L., Toth, T. L., Hornstein, M. D., & Neer, R. M. (1998). Prevention of estrogen deficiency-related bone loss with human parathyroid hormone-(1-34): A randomized controlled trial. *Journal of the American Medical Association, 280*(12), 1067–1073.

Fong, Y. F., & Singh, K. (1999). Medical treatment of a grossly enlarged adenomyotic uterus with the levonorgestrel-releasing intrauterine system. *Contraception, 60*(3), 173–175.

Foster, D. C. (2002). Vulvar disease. *Obstetrics and Gynecology, 100*(1), 145–163.

Funaro, D. (2004). Lichen sclerosus: A review and practical approach. *Dermatologic Therapy, 17*(1), 28–37.

Goldstein, D. P. (2004). Congenital cervical anomalies and benign cervical lesions. In B. D. Rose (Ed.), *UpToDate*. Wellesley, MA: UpToDate.

Grigorieva, V., Chen-Mok, M., Tarasova, M., & Mikhailov, A. (2003). Use of a levonorgestrel-releasing intrauterine system to treat bleeding related to uterine leiomyomas. *Fertility and Sterility, 79*(5), 1194–1198.

Gruppo Italiano per lo Studio dell'Endometriosi. (2001). Relationship between stage, site and morphological characteristics of pelvic endometriosis and pain. *Human Reproduction, 16*(12), 2668–2671.

Guzick, D. S., Silliman, N. P., Adamson, G. D., Buttram, V. C., Jr., Canis, M., Malinak, L. R., et al. (1997). Prediction of pregnancy in infertile women based on the American Society for Reproductive Medicine's revised classification of endometriosis. *Fertility and Sterility, 67*(5), 822–829.

Hartge, P., Hayes, R., Reding, D., Sherman, M. E., Prorok, P., Schiffman, M., et al. (2000). Complex ovarian cysts in postmenopausal women are not associated with ovarian cancer risk factors: Preliminary data from the prostate, lung, colon, and ovarian cancer screening trial. *American Journal of Obstetrics and Gynecology, 183*(5), 1232–1237.

Honoré, G. M. (1999). Extrapelvic endometriosis. *Clinical Obstetrics and Gynecology, 42*(3), 699–711.

Hurst, B. S., Gardner, S. C., Tucker, K. E., Awoniyi, C. A., & Schlaff, W. D. (2000). Delayed oral estradiol combined with leuprolide increases endometriosis-related pain. *Journal of the Society of Laparoendoscopic Surgeons, 4*(2), 97–101.

Husby, G. K., Haugen, R. S., & Moen, M. H. (2003). Diagnostic delay in women with pain and endometriosis. *Acta Obstetricia et Gynecologica Scandinavica, 82*(7), 649–653.

Ind, T., & Shepherd, J. (2003). Pelvic tumours in adolescence. *Best Practice and Research: Clinical Obstetrics and Gynaecology, 17*(1), 149–168.

Jenkins, S., Olive, D. L., & Haney, A. F. (1986). Endometriosis: Pathogenetic implications of the anatomic distribution. *Obstetrics and Gynecology, 67*(3), 335–338.

Jermy, K., Luise, C., & Bourne, T. (2001). The characterization of common ovarian cysts in premenopausal women. *Ultrasound in Obstetrics and Gynecology, 17*(2), 140–144.

Johnson, K. (2003). Differentiating adenomyosis and fibroids. *Medscape Ob/Gyn & Women's Health, 8*(2). Retrieved August 18, 2004, from http://www.medscape.com/viewarticle/459772.

Karaer, O., Oruc, S., & Koyuncu, F. M. (2004). Aromatase inhibitors: Possible future applications. *Acta Obstetricia et Gynecologica Scandinavica, 83*(8), 699–706.

Kourounis, G., Iatrakis, G., Diakakis, I., Sakellaropoulos, G., Ladopoulos, I., & Prapa, Z. (1999). Treatment results of liquid nitrogen cryotherapy on selected pathologic changes of the uterine cervix. *Clinical and Experimental Obstetrics & Gynecology, 26*(2), 115.

Kunstfeld, R., Kirnbauer, R., Stingl, G., & Karlhofer, F. M. (2003). Successful treatment of vulvar lichen sclerosus with topical tacrolimus. *Archives of Dermatology, 139*(7), 850–852.

Larrabee, R., & Kylander, D. J. (2001). Benign vulvar disorders. Identifying features, practical management of nonneoplastic conditions and tumors. *Postgraduate Medicine, 109*(5), 151–154, 157–159, 163–154.

Laufer, M. R., Sanfilippo, J., & Rose, G. (2003). Adolescent endometriosis: Diagnosis and treatment approaches. *Journal of Pediatric and Adolescent Gynecology, 16*(Suppl. 3), S3–S11.

Leibsohn, S., d'Ablaing, G., Mishell, D. R., Jr., & Schlaerth, J. B. (1990). Leiomyosarcoma in a series of hysterectomies performed for presumed uterine leiomyomas. *American Journal of Obstetrics and Gynecology, 162*(4), 968–974.

Lethaby, A., Vollenhoven, B., & Sowter, M. (2002). Efficacy of pre-operative gonadotrophin hormone releasing analogues for women with uterine fibroids undergoing hysterectomy or myomectomy: A systematic review. *British Journal of Obstetrics and Gynecology, 109*(10), 1097–1108.

Lewis, F. M. (1998). Vulval lichen planus. *British Journal of Dermatology, 138*(4), 569–575.

Li, H., Sugimura, K., Okizuka, H., Yoshida, M., Maruyama, R., Takahashi, K., et al. (1999). Markedly high signal intensity lesions in the uterine cervix on T2-weighted imaging: Differentiation between mucin-producing carcinomas and nabothian cysts. *Radiation Medicine, 17*(2), 137–143.

Lockhat, F. B., Emembolu, J. O., & Konje, J. C. (2004). The evaluation of the effectiveness of an intrauterine-administered progestogen (levonorgestrel) in the symptomatic treatment of endometriosis and in the staging of the disease. *Human Reproduction, 19*(1), 179–184.

Makarainen, L., Ronnberg, L., & Kauppila, A. (1996). Medroxyprogesterone acetate supplementation diminishes the hypoestrogenic side effects of gonadotropin-releasing hormone agonist without changing its efficacy in endometriosis. *Fertility and Sterility, 65*(1), 29–34.

Malone, L. J. (1969). Myomectomy: Recurrence after removal of solitary and multiple myomas. *Obstetrics and Gynecology, 34*(2), 200–203.

Mann, M. S., & Kaufman, R. H. (1991). Erosive lichen planus of the vulva. *Clinical Obstetrics and Gynecology, 34*(3), 605–613.

Marshall, L. M., Spiegelman, D., Barbieri, R. L., Goldman, M. B., Manson, J. E., Colditz, G. A., et al. (1997). Variation in the incidence of uterine leiomyoma among premenopausal women by age and race. *Obstetrics and Gynecology, 90*(6), 967–973.

Mashall, R. D., Fejzo, M. L., Friedman, A. J., Mitchner, N., Nowak, R. A., Rein, M. S., et al. (1994). Analysis of androgen receptor DNA reveals the independent clonal origins of uterine leiomyomata and the secondary nature of cytogenetic aberrations in the development of leiomyomata. *Genes, Chromosomes, and Cancer, 11*(1), 1–6.

Mazdisnian, F., Degregorio, F., Mazdisnian, F., & Palmieri, A. (1999). Intralesional injection of triamcinolone in the treatment of lichen sclerosus. *Journal of Reproductive Medicine, 44*(4), 332–334.

McCausland, V., & McCausland, A. (1998). The response of adenomyosis to endometrial ablation/resection. *Human Reproduction Update, 4*(4), 350–359.

McElin, T. W., & Bird, C. C. (1974). Adenomyosis of the uterus. *Obstetrics and Gynecology Annual, 3*(0), 425–441.

Modugno, F., Ness, R. B., Allen, G. O., Schildkraut, J. M., Davis, F. G., & Goodman, M. T. (2004). Oral contraceptive use, reproductive history, and risk of epithelial ovarian cancer in women with and without endometriosis. *American Journal of Obstetrics and Gynecology, 191*(3), 733–740.

Moghissi, K. S., Schlaff, W. D., Olive, D. L., Skinner, M. A., & Yin, H. (1998). Goserelin acetate (Zoladex) with or without hormone replacement therapy for the treatment of endometriosis. *Fertility and Sterility, 69*(6), 1056–1062.

Molitor, J. J. (1971). Adenomyosis: A clinical and pathological appraisal. *American Journal of Obstetrics and Gynecology, 110*(2), 275–284.

Murphy, A. A., Morales, A. J., Kettel, L. M., & Yen, S. S. (1995). Regression of uterine leiomyomata to the antiprogesterone RU486: Dose-response effect. *Fertility and Sterility, 64*(1), 187–190.

Omrani, A., Schnatz, P. F., Qi, J., Greene, J. F., & Curry, S. L. (2004). Lung cancer metastatic to a cervical polyp. *Gynecologic Oncology, 92*(1), 22–24.

Palomba, S., Orio, F., Jr., Morelli, M., Russo, T., Pellicano, M., Zupi, E., et al. (2002). Raloxifene administration in premenopausal women with uterine leiomyomas: A pilot study. *Journal of Clinical Endocrinology and Metabolism, 87*(8), 3603–3608.

Palomba, S., Sammartino, A., Di Carlo, C., Affinito, P., Zullo, F., & Nappi, C. (2001). Effects of raloxifene treatment on uterine leiomyomas in postmenopausal women. *Fertility and Sterility, 76*(1), 38–43.

Palomba, S., Sena, T., Noia, R., Di Carlo, C., Zullo, F., & Mastrantonio, P. (2001). Transdermal hormone replacement therapy in postmenopausal women with uterine leiomyomas. *Obstetrics and Gynecology, 98*(6), 1053–1058.

Parker, W. H., Fu, Y. S., & Berek, J. S. (1994). Uterine sarcoma in patients operated on for presumed leiomyoma and rapidly growing leiomyoma. *Obstetrics and Gynecology, 83*(3), 414–418.

Pelisse, M. (1989). The vulvo-vaginal-gingival syndrome. A new form of erosive lichen planus. *International Journal of Dermatology, 28*(6), 381–384.

Pelisse, M. (1996). Erosive vulvar lichen planus and desquamative vaginitis. *Seminars in Dermatology, 15*(1), 47–50.

Polatti, F., Viazzo, F., Colleoni, R., & Nappi, R. E. (2000). Uterine myoma in postmenopause: A comparison between two therapeutic schedules of HRT. *Maturitas, 37*(1), 27–32.

Porpora, M. G., Koninckx, P. R., Piazze, J., Natili, M., Colagrande, S., & Cosmi, E. V. (1999). Correlation between endometriosis and pelvic pain. *Journal of the American Association of Gynecologic Laparoscopists, 6*(4), 429–434.

Practice Committee of the American Society for Reproductive Medicine. (2004). Endometriosis and infertility. *Fertility and Sterility, 82*(Suppl. 1), S40–S45.

Prefumo, F., Todeschini, F., Fulcheri, E., & Venturini, P. L. (2002). Epithelial abnormalities in cystic ovarian endometriosis. *Gynecologic Oncology, 84*(2), 280–284.

Pron, G., Bennett, J., Common, A., Wall, J., Asch, M., & Sniderman, K. (2003). The Ontario Uterine Fibroid Embolization Trial. Part 2. Uterine fibroid reduction and symptom relief after uterine artery embolization for fibroids. *Fertility and Sterility, 79*(1), 120–127.

Rana, N., Thomas, S., Rotman, C., & Dmowski, W. P. (1996). Decrease in the size of ovarian endometriomas during ovarian suppression in stage IV endometriosis. Role of preoperative medical treatment. *Journal of Reproductive Medicine, 41*(6), 384–392.

Reinhold, C., Tafazoli, F., Mehio, A., Wang, L., Atri, M., Siegelman, E. S., et al. (1999). Uterine adenomyosis: Endovaginal US and MR imaging features with histopathologic correlation [Special issue]. *Radiographics, 19*, S147–S160.

Rice, J. P., Kay, H. H., & Mahony, B. S. (1989). The clinical significance of uterine leiomyomas in pregnancy. *American Journal of Obstetrics and Gynecology, 160*(5, Pt. 1), 1212–1216.

Ridley, C. M. (1990). Chronic erosive vulval disease. *Clinical and Experimental Dermatology, 15*(4), 245–252.

Ridley, C. M., (1999). Non-infective cutaneous conditions of the vulva. In C. M. Ridley & S. M. Neill (Eds.), *The vulva.* Oxford, UK: Blackwell Science.

Rosati, P., Exacoustos, C., & Mancuso, S. (1992). Longitudinal evaluation of uterine myoma growth during pregnancy. A sonographic study. *Journal of Ultrasound in Medicine, 11*(10), 511–515.

Roux, C., Pelissier, C., Listrat, V., Kolta, S., Simonetta, C., Guignard, M., et al. (1995). Bone loss during gonadotropin releasing hormone agonist treatment and use of nasal calcitonin. *Osteoporosis International, 5*(3), 185–190.

Seli, E., Berkkanoglu, M., & Arici, A. (2003). Pathogenesis of endometriosis. *Obstetrics and Gynecology Clinics of North America, 30*(1), 41–61.

Sergent, F., Verspyck, E., & Marpeau, L. (2003). Management of an ovarian cyst during pregnancy. *Presse Medicale, 32*(22), 1039–1045.

Sideri, M. (2004). *Squamous hyperplasia.* Retrieved November 5, 2004, from http://asccp.org/edu/practice/vulva/squamous.shtml.

Simpson, J. L., Elias, S., Malinak, L. R., & Buttram, V. C., Jr. (1980). Heritable aspects of endometriosis. I. Genetic studies. *American Journal of Obstetrics and Gynecology, 137*(3), 327–331.

Speroff, L., & Fritz, M. (2005). *Clinical gynecologic endocrinology and infertility* (7th ed.). Baltimore: Lippincott Williams & Wilkins.

Spies, J. B., Ascher, S. A., Roth, A. R., Kim, J., Levy, E. B., & Gomez-Jorge, J. (2001). Uterine artery embolization for leiomyomata. *Obstetrics and Gynecology, 98*(1), 29–34.

Spiewankiewicz, B., Stelmachow, J., Sawicki, W., Cendrowski, K., & Kuzlik, R. (2003). Hysteroscopy in cases of cervical polyps. *European Journal of Gynaecological Oncology, 24*(1), 67–69.

Star, W. L. (1995). Vulvar disease. In W. L. Star, L. L. Lommel, & M. T. Shannon (Eds.), *Women's primary health care: Protocols for practice* (pp. 12-218–12-262). Washington, DC: American Nurses Association.

Stenchever, M.A., Droegmueller, W., Herbst, A. L., & Mishell, D. R. (2001). *Comprehensive gynecology* (4th ed.). St. Louis, MO: Mosby.

Stewart, E. A. (2001). Uterine fibroids. *Lancet, 357*(9252), 293–298.

Stewart, E. A., & Nowak, R. A. (1998). New concepts in the treatment of uterine leiomyomas. *Obstetrics and Gynecology, 92*(4, Pt. 1), 624–627.

Stewart, E. A. (2004). Vulval lichen planus. In B. D. Rose (Ed.), *UpToDate*. Wellesley, MA: UpToDate.

Strobelt, N., Ghidini, A., Cavallone, M., Pensabene, I., Ceruti, P., & Vergani, P. (1994). Natural history of uterine leiomyomas in pregnancy. *Journal of Ultrasound in Medicine, 13*(5), 399–401.

Surrey, E. S., & Hornstein, M. D. (2002). Prolonged GnRH agonist and add-back therapy for symptomatic endometriosis: Long-term follow-up. *Obstetrics and Gynecology, 99*(5, Pt. 1), 709–719.

Surrey, E. S., Voigt, B., Fournet, N., & Judd, H. L. (1995). Prolonged gonadotropin-releasing hormone agonist treatment of symptomatic endometriosis: The role of cyclic sodium etidronate and low-dose norethindrone "add-back" therapy. *Fertility and Sterility, 63*(4), 747–755.

Templeman, C. L., Fallat, M. E., Lam, A. M., Perlman, S. E., Hertweck, S. P., & O'Connor, D. M. (2000). Managing mature cystic teratomas of the ovary. *Obstetrical and Gynecological Survey, 55*(12), 738–745.

Trimble, E. L., & Trimble, C. L. (2001). Ovarian tumors of low malignant potential. *Current Treatment Options Oncology, 2*(2), 103–108.

Ubaldi, F., Tournaye, H., Camus, M., Van der Pas, H., Gepts, E., & Devroey, P. (1995). Fertility after hysteroscopic myomectomy. *Human Reproduction Update, 1*(1), 81–90.

Vercellini, P., Aimi, G., Panazza, S., De Giorgi, O., Pesole, A., & Crosignani, P. G. (1999). A levonorgestrel-releasing intrauterine system for the treatment of dysmenorrhea associated with endo-metriosis: A pilot study. *Fertility and Sterility, 72*(3), 505–508.

Vercellini, P., Frontino, G., De Giorgi, O., Aimi, G., Zaina, B., & Crosignani, P. G. (2003). Comparison of a levonorgestrel-releasing intrauterine device versus expectant management after conservative surgery for symptomatic endometriosis: A pilot study. *Fertility and Sterility, 80*(2), 305–309.

Vercellini, P., Frontino, G., De Giorgi, O., Pietropaolo, G., Pasin, R., & Crosignani, P. G. (2003). Continuous use of an oral contraceptive for endometriosis-associated recurrent dysmenorrhea that does not respond to a cyclic pill regimen. *Fertility and Sterility, 80*(3), 560–563.

Vercellini, P., Trespidi, L., De Giorgi, O., Cortesi, I., Parazzini, F., & Crosignani, P. G. (1996). Endometriosis and pelvic pain: Relation to disease stage and localization. *Fertility and Sterility, 65*(2), 299–304.

Visvanathan, D., Connell, R., Hall-Craggs, M. A., Cutner, A. S., & Bown, S. G. (2002). Interstitial laser photocoagulation for uterine myomas. *American Journal of Obstetrics and Gynecology, 187*(2), 382–384.

Walker, W. J., & Pelage, J. P. (2002). Uterine artery embolisation for symptomatic fibroids: Clinical results in 400 women with imaging follow up. *British Journal of Obstetrics and Gynecology, 109*(11), 1262–1272.

Wheeler, J. M., & Malinak, L. R. (1983). Recurrent endometriosis: Incidence, management, and prognosis. *American Journal of Obstetrics and Gynecology, 146*(3), 247–253.

Wood, C. (1998). Surgical and medical treatment of adenomyosis. *Human Reproduction Update, 4*(4), 323–336.

Zellis, S., & Pincus, S. H. (1996). Treatment of vulvar dermatoses. *Seminars in Dermatology, 15*(1), 71–76.

VULVAR DERMATOLOGY RESOURCES

American Society for Colposcopy and Cervical Pathology. (2004). *The vulva*. Retrieved November 5, 2004, from http://asccp.org/edu/practice/vulva.shtml.

Black, M. M., McKay, M., Braude, P. R., Vaughan-Jones, S., & Margesson, L. J. (2001). *Obstetric and gynecologic dermatology* (2nd ed.). London: Mosby.

Epstein, E. (2002). *Common skin disorders* (5th ed.). Philadelphia: W. B. Saunders.

Habif, T. P., Campbell, J. L., Quitadamo, M. J., & Zug, K. A. (2001). *Skin disease: Diagnosis and treatment*. St. Louis, MO: Mosby.

Haefner, H. K., & Kaufman, R. H. (1998). *A classical approach to vulvar disease* [CD]. Washington,

DC: American College of Obstetricians and Gynecologists.

International Society for the Study of Vulvovaginal Disease. (n.d.). Retrieved November 5, 2004, from http://www.issvd.org.

Kaufman, R. H., Faro, S., & Brown, D. (2004). *Benign diseases of the vulva and vagina* (5th ed.). St. Louis, MO: Mosby.

Lawrence, C. M., & Cox, N. H. (2002). *Physical signs in dermatology* (2nd ed.). London: Mosby.

Leibowitch, M., Staughton, R., Neill, S., Barton, S., & Marwood, R. (1997). *An atlas of vulval disease: A combined dermatological, gynaecological, and venereological approach* (2nd ed.). London: Martin Dunitz.

National Lichen Sclerosus Support Group. (2004). Retrieved November 5, 2004, from http://www.lichensclerosus.org.

The National Psoriasis Foundation. (2004). Retrieved November 5, 2004, from http://www.psoriasis.org.

Reeves, J. R. T., & Maibach, H. (1991). *Clinical dermatology illustrated: A regional approach* (2nd ed.). Philadelphia: F. A. Davis.

Ridley, C. M., & Neill, S. M. (Eds.). (1999). *The vulva.* Oxford UK: Blackwell Science.

Ridley, C. M., Robinson, A. J., & Oriel, J. D. (2000). *Vulval disease: A practical guide to diagnosis and management.* London: Arnold.

Stewart, E. G. (2002). *The V book: A doctor's guide to complete vulvovaginal health.* New York: Bantam Books.

Wolverton, S. W. (Ed.). (2001). *Comprehensive dermatologic drug therapy.* Philadelphia: W. B. Saunders.

Chapter 23

GYNECOLOGIC CANCERS

MARY WALLACE
ANNA SANFORD

Gynecologic cancers are serious, life-threatening diseases. Many symptoms of these diseases are vague and subtle, making early diagnosis, treatment, and successful recovery difficult. A humanistic approach that integrates medical and sociopsychological perspectives and that is patient centered serves to equalize the power imbalance between a woman and her provider. Clinicians using this approach actively listen to their patients and assess them in the context of their lived experiences, ethnicity, culture, and socioeconomic class. These clinicians are less likely to miss hearing a woman as she describes vague symptoms that may be warnings of underlying disease, and instead encourage her to provide more information that may be helpful in making an accurate diagnosis. Clinicians using a humanistic approach are cautious, thoughtful, and think critically, using the most recent evidence in assessing and formulating treatment for the disease. They arm their patients with information that is critical to informed consent and decision making. Sensitive clinicians that use good listening skills are the ones who have helped decrease the number of cancer deaths in women who were misdiagnosed when their voices were ignored.

The focus of this chapter is gynecologic cancers. Gynecologic cancers account for about 77,500 new cases of cancer each year. All gynecologic cancers are curable if diagnosed in the early stages (American Cancer Society [ACS], 2004a). Preventative health then is the primary goal of clinicians who provide health care for women. Genetic, behavioral, and environmental factors influence the risk of developing a gynecologic malignancy.

VULVAR CANCERS

SCOPE OF THE PROBLEM

Vulvar cancer accounts for about 4% of all reproductive organ cancers in women (ACS, 2004a). If detected, vulvar cancer is usually curable (ACS). The overall 5-year survival rate for a woman with vulvar cancer is 90% if there is no lymph node involvement (ACS). Lymph node involvement and primary lesion size are the two most important prognostic factors. When the regional lymph nodes are involved, one or two involved lymph nodes confer a better prognosis than if three or more lymph nodes are malignant, or if there is bilateral node involvement. Patients who have multiple positive lymph nodes in the groin have a very poor prognosis. The overall 5-year survival rate for patients with lymph node involvement is 50% to 60% (ACS).

Approximately 85% of vulvar cancers occur in women over the age of 50; half of these cases occur in women over the age of 70 years. However, about 15% of new cases of vulvar cancer are diagnosed in women who are under the age of 40 years (Chambers, 2001; Holschneider & Berek, 2002; National Cancer Institute [NCI], 2003a).

ETIOLOGY AND PATHOPHYSIOLOGY

DNA mutations resulting in vulvar cancer are acquired over the course of an individual's life; therefore, the risk for vulvar cancer is not inheritable. Recent research suggests that vulvar cancer evolves as two separate types of cancer. The first type is related to human papillomavirus (HPV) infection. This type of infection frequently leads to vulvar intraepithelial neoplasia (VIN) in younger women. The second type of vulvar cancer is usually diagnosed in women 65–75 years of age and is related to vulvar nonneoplastic epithelial disorders such as lichen sclerosus, squamous cell hyperplasia, and Paget's disease of the vulva (Chambers, 2001; Guarnieri & Klemm, 2000; Holschneider & Berek, 2002; Lee, 2000a).

Human papillomavirus types 16, 18, 31, and others confer a high risk of vulvar cancer and appear to play a role in about 30–50% of diagnosed instances (Chambers, 2001). Women who have HPV as a risk factor tend to be younger and frequently have multiple areas of VIN over their vulvas. Early sexual contact and infection with HPV provides more time for malignant transformation. Women who smoke cigarettes and have HPV also have a higher risk of vulvar cancer. The aforementioned 15% of newly affected women under the age of 40 years often smoke and are infected with HPV (Chambers, 2001; Guarnieri & Klemm, 2000; Lee, 2000a; Holschneider & Berek, 2002).

Vulvar intraepithelial neoplasia (formerly known as Bowen's disease) is a premalignant finding associated with HPV and confers increased risk of vulvar cancer even though most cases do not progress to squamous cell cancer. An estimated 80% of untreated women with warty VIN develop invasive disease (Holschneider & Berek, 2002). The combination of HPV and smoking are known to increase the risk for vulvar and cervical

TABLE 23-1   Cellular Classification of Vulvar Intraepithelial Neoplasia (VIN)

I. Mild dysplasia (formerly mild atypia)

II. Moderate dysplasia (formerly moderate atypia)

III. Severe dysplasia (formerly severe atypia)

IV. Carcinoma in situ

Source: National Cancer Institute, 2003.

cancer (Chambers, 2001; Guarnieri & Klemm, 2000; Lee, 2000a, b). Vulvar intraepithelial neoplasia is classified according to degree of severity (Table 23–1).

Lichen sclerosus (see Chapter 22) slightly increases the risk for vulvar cancer in affected women. Approximately 4% of women with lichen sclerosus will develop vulvar cancer (Tucker Edwards & Saunders-Goldson, 2003). Lichen sclerosus, which causes a severe itch–scratch cycle, is thought to cause squamous hyperplasia, which then progresses to cellular atypia and finally invasive squamous cell carcinoma. Aggressive evaluation and treatment have the potential to decrease the incidence of vulvar cancer in this subgroup of patients (Chambers, 2001; Guarnieri & Klemm, 2000; Lee, 2000b). Older women with lichen sclerosus who are not infected with HPV rarely have VIN, but often will have mutations of the p53 tumor suppressor gene which is diagnosed by DNA testing (Guarnieri & Klemm). The p53 protein stops cell growth and division in DNA-damaged cells, and when the damage cannot be repaired, the p53 protein triggers cell suicide and prevents unregulated cell growth by damaged cells (NCI, 2003d).

Additional risk factors for vulvar cancer include human immunodeficiency virus (HIV), previous gynecologic malignancy, and a history of smoking (Lee, 2000a). HIV causes immunosuppression making tissues susceptible to persistent HPV infections, which in turn increases the risk of vulvar cancer (Lee). Some studies have found that syphilis and other granulomatous diseases are also associated with vulvar cancer, but these findings are controversial because the incidence of syphilis has been declining since 1992 (Centers for Disease Control and Prevention [CDC], 2004).

CLINICAL PRESENTATION

The most common presentation of vulvar cancer is a woman's report of a vulvar lump or mass with a prolonged history of vulvar pruritis; however, up to 50% of women with vulvar cancer are asymptomatic (Chambers, 2001). Symptoms include vulvar bleeding, discharge, dysuria, and pain. On rare occasions, a woman will present with a large, fungating mass or lesion. On physical examination the lesion is usually raised, and may be ulcerated, warty, or fleshy in appearance, or it may appear to be an area of squamous cell hyperplasia (see Chapter 22). Most lesions are solitary and about 50% of the lesions are found on the labia majora. The labia minora, clitoris, and perineum are other possible primary sites (Chambers; Guarnieri & Klemm, 2000; Lee, 2000b; Holschneider & Berek, 2002; Tyring, 2003).

Over 90% of vulvar carcinomas are squamous cell carcinomas and are usually preceded by dysplasia or VIN (Chambers, 2001; Holschneider & Berek, 2002). Malignant melanoma of the vulva accounts for 2–4% of all vulvar cancers and usually occurs on the labia minora and clitoris (Chambers). Adenocarcinomas can develop in Bartholin's glands or with vulvar Paget's disease. A tumor of the Bartholin's gland is easily mistaken for a cyst and delay in accurate diagnosis is common. Less than 2% of vulvar carcinomas are sarcomas; these tumors tend to grow rapidly and can occur at any age (Holschneider & Berek).

ASSESSMENT

Early identification of women at risk is important. Thorough patient education about when and how to perform a vulvar self-examination and visual inspection of the external genitalia is essential to early identification. Annual Papanicolaou (Pap) tests are not always obtained in women after the age of 70 years; however, oncologists recommend an annual Pap test as part of a health promotion and disease prevention plan because it brings the woman in for health care. The incidence of vulvar cancer increases with age. Genital neoplasia in women is often multifocal. Careful examination of the entire vulva, vagina, cervix, perineum, and perianal area, including the anus should be performed on women as part of the routine pelvic examination. The femoral and inguinal lymph nodes should be palpated routinely with pelvic examination.

All women reporting or found to have a vulvar lesion must be thoroughly evaluated to rule out malignancy. Colposcopy may assist in defining the extent of disease. A biopsy (which can be done in the outpatient setting) is required for definitive diagnosis (see Chapter 22).

Both patients and health care providers contribute to the delay in diagnosis of vulvar cancers. Common causes of late-stage diagnosis of vulvar cancer include not seeking treatment when initial symptoms occur and clinicians providing symptomatic treatment for months prior to obtaining a biopsy. Experts recommend that any condyloma not responding to therapy, or any lesion increasing in size, or that has an unusual appearance should be biopsied (Chambers, 2001; Guarnieri & Klemm, 2000; Lee, 2000b; Holschneider & Berek, 2002, Tyring, 2003).

Staging Staging, using the tumor node metastasis (TNM) classification system, identifies vulvar cancer growth with direct extension first, and then by local lymph node involvement (American Joint Committee on Cancer [AJCC], 2002; NCI, 2003d). The TNM classification is a widely used carcinoma classification system that provides a way of describing the size, location, and spread of a tumor. The "T" describes the primary tumor according to its size and location. The "N" refers to the lymph nodes that drain fluid from the area of the tumor and whether or not the cancer has spread to the lymph nodes. The "M" explains whether or not the cancer has spread to distant areas in the body (e.g., from

TABLE 23–2 International Federation of Gynecology and Obstetrics (FIGO) Staging for Cancer of the Vulva

Stage	Characteristics
Stage 0	In situ disease, no lymph node metastases, no distant metastases
Stage I, IA, & IB	Primary tumor confined to vulva, < 2 cm, no lymph node metastases, no distant metastases
Stage II	Primary tumor > 2 cm, no lymph node metastases, no distant metastases
Stage III	Primary tumor of any size with adjacent spread to lower urethra, vagina, perineum, or anus, or unilateral lymph nodes metastases
Stage IVa	Primary tumor of any size with adjacent spread to the upper urethra, bladder mucosa, rectal mucosa, or pelvic bone, and/or bilateral regional lymph node metastases
Stage IVb	Primary tumor of any size, any lymph node metastases, and any distant metastases

Source: American Joint Committee on Cancer, 2002.

the vulva to the lungs). The American Joint Committee on Cancer's TNM categories correspond to the stages accepted by the International Federation of Gynecology and Obstetrics (FIGO). Vulvar cancer staging according to FIGO is presented in Table 23–2.

Well differentiated vulvar cancer lesions tend to be minimally invasive and poorly differentiated; whereas, anaplastic lesions tend to be deeply invasive. Local spread may extend to the urethra, vagina, perineum, and anus. Lymphatic spread usually occurs first in the inguinal lymph nodes, then involves the femoral lymph nodes, and finally spreads to the external iliac chain of the pelvic lymph nodes. The incidence of lymph node involvement is about 30% (ACS, 2004a). The risk of metastasis to the regional lymph nodes increases with increasing size and depth of the primary lesion. Hematogenous spread to distant sites is uncommon but may involve the lungs, liver, and bone (AJCC, 2002; NCI, 2003d).

MANAGEMENT

Prevention Preventive measures for vulvar cancer include the following:

- Avoiding exposure to HPV by limiting the number of sexual partners
- Seeking treatment for vulvar itching caused by chronic vulvar diseases such as lichen sclerosus
- Not smoking
- Routine vulvar self-examination (Guarnieri & Klemm, 2000)

Culturally sensitive interventions are still needed to address the educational needs of diverse communities of women to provide them with accurate prevention and screening information (Cohen & Frank-Stromborg, 2000; Guarnieri & Klemm).

Definitive Treatment   Surgical resection is the standard treatment for patients with vulvar cancer. Patients presenting with symptoms or questionable lesions need to be referred to a gynecologist or gynecologic oncologist who has expertise in cancer surgery (Chambers, 2001). Preoperative work-up may include a chest X-ray, complete blood count (CBC), and imaging studies such as computerized tomography (CT) and magnetic resonance imaging (MRI). The surgery involves removing the tumor and at least a 1 cm margin of normal tissue surrounding the tumor. A wide local excision or a radical vulvectomy are the most commonly performed surgical procedures with radical local excision being performed most often today. The inguinal and femoral lymph nodes are surgically evaluated as part of staging the disease because microscopic metastases may be present in clinically nonsuspicious nodes. Local recurrences are treated with local excision when possible and are followed by postoperative radiation therapy. Chemotherapy is reserved for metastatic disease (Chambers, 2001; NCI, 2003d).

FOLLOW-UP CARE OF THE WOMAN WHO HAS BEEN TREATED FOR VULVAR CANCER

The primary early postoperative complications experienced by women who undergo radical local excision with groin dissection or radical vulvectomy are groin wound infection and tissue breakdown (Holschneider & Berek, 2002). One-third of patients will develop a recurrence within two years of primary treatment (Coulter & Gleeson, 2003). Some recurrences are seen at five or more years after treatment; therefore, lifelong follow-up on a regular schedule is important (Fischer, 1996). Many patients may return to their primary care clinicians for follow-up after surgical recovery and resolution of any postoperative wound healing complications. Typically a woman who has been treated for vulvar cancer is seen for follow-up every three months for the first two years, every six months for the next three years, and annually thereafter (Fischer). A comprehensive annual history and physical examination is a standard part of follow-up. Posttreatment monthly self-examination of the vulva should be taught and emphasized because recurrent disease is always a possibility. Early identification of a recurrence offers the best chance for effective treatment (Chambers, 2001; Guarnieri & Klemm, 2000; Lee, 2000b; Holschneider & Berek). New or persistent symptoms need to be reported promptly and carefully evaluated. Every follow-up visit should focus on the history of any new vulvar lesion, bladder function, bowel function, bone pain, and lower extremity lymphedema. The physical examination should include assessment of the breasts, abdomen, and lymph nodes, as well as a thorough pelvic and rectal examination (Fischer).

Chronic lymphedema of the lower extremities occurs in 20% to 50% of patients who have undergone lymph node dissection and may occur early or late after treatment (Chambers, 2001; Ryan et al., 2003). Lymphedema may cause the urinary stream to change direction causing urine to "spray" rather than "stream." If this occurs, a cone-shaped urinal (sometimes used by women when camping outdoors) may be helpful. Urinary stress incontinence, introital stenosis, altered body image issues, depression, and sexual dysfunction are other late complications associated with the extent of the surgery.

Regular (three times a week) use of vaginal dilators or regular sexual intercourse can help to stretch vaginal tissues and should be initiated before the vaginal introitus becomes stenotic. If introital stenosis occurs, the clinician may need to use a pediatric speculum for vaginal visualization and only a single digit when palpating the vagina. Some degree of sexual dysfunction is almost always present with definitive treatment of vulvar cancer. Problems with arousal, orgasm, vaginal dryness, and sexual relationship issues are common. Vaginal dryness may be helped by the use of vaginal lubricants such as Astroglide or vaginal moisturizers such as Replens. Changing positions for sexual intercourse may reduce discomfort (Holschneider & Berek, 2002).

Counseling that explores relationship issues and discusses possible alternatives to vaginal intercourse allows for the expression of grief over the loss of normal sexual function. It is also important to address the ever-present fear of recurrence or metastasis. Choice of a personal caregiver for these women should be carefully considered; her sexual partner may not always be the best choice. Some women have attributed significant negative change in their sexual relationship to the participation of a sexual partner in postoperative wound care.

CERVICAL CANCER

SCOPE OF THE PROBLEM

An estimated 10,520 new cervical cancer cases and 3900 cervical cancer deaths were projected to occur in the United States in 2004 (ACS, 2004a). Cervical cancer, once the number one cancer killer of women, now ranks 15th in cancer-causing deaths of women in the United States (ACS). As cervical cytology screening becomes more prevalent, precancerous lesions of the cervix are detected significantly more often than invasive cancers. Women with precursor lesions have a 5-year survival rate of nearly 100% (ACS), and when cervical cancers are detected at an early stage, the 5-year survival rate is approximately 92% (ACS). The overall (all stages combined) 5-year survival rate is approximately 71% (ACS). Unfortunately, there is a significant disparity in cervical cancer death rates according to population—with older, poorer, and minority women having the highest mortality (ACS; Snyder, 2003).

ETIOLOGY AND PATHOPHYSIOLOGY

There is overwhelming evidence that HPV is the primary agent in the development of cervical cancer and its precursor, cervical intraepithelial neoplasia (CIN) (NCI, 2004a). An estimated 20 million people in the United States (15% of the population) are currently infected with HPV, and approximately 5.5 million people are infected each year (CDC, 2004). Risk factors for acquiring an HPV infection include the following:

- Early age at first intercourse (age 18 years or younger)
- Multiple sexual partners
- Male partners with multiple previous sexual partners

However, only a small proportion of those infected with HPV go on to develop cervical cancer (CDC). The following cofactors are thought to play a contributing role:

- Smoking—Women who smoke cigarettes are twice as likely as nonsmokers to develop cervical cancer. Smoking exposes the body to many carcinogens that affect more than just the lungs. Carcinogens are absorbed by the lungs and carried in the bloodstream throughout the body. Tobacco by-products have been found in the cervical mucus of women who smoke. It is believed these by-products damage DNA in cervical cells (ACS, 2004b; Gibson & Hainer, 2003; Snyder, 2003).

• Immunosuppression—Patients who are immunocompromised from HIV, AIDS, or other causes have an increased prevalence and persistence of HPV infection. The immune system is important in destroying cancer cells and slowing their growth and spread (ACS; Garcia & Bi, 2002; Snyder).

• Oral contraceptives—Smith et al. (2003) examined the impact of oral contraceptive (OC) use in women with HPV. Data were pooled from 28 eligible studies (four cohort and 24 case-controlled) consisting of 12,531 women with invasive cervical carcinoma (ICC) or carcinoma in situ (CIS). The findings suggest the risk of invasive squamous cervical cancer and carcinoma in situ is increased 3-fold for women who have used OCs for five years or longer. The link between OCs and cervical cancer is unclear. However, OC users are less likely to use barrier protection, thereby increasing their risk of contracting HPV. Findings to date do not warrant discontinuing OC use in the case of an abnormal Pap test.

• High parity—Munoz et al. (2002) examined the impact of parity and the progression of HPV infection to cancer. Data were pooled from eight case-controlled studies on ICC and two studies on CIS. Data were analyzed from 1465 patients with squamous cell ICC, 211 with CIS, 124 with adenocarcinoma or adenosquamous ICC and 265 female controls. The study found that women with one or two full-term pregnancies had a 2.3 times greater risk of developing squamous cell cervical cancer; whereas, those with a history of seven or more full-term pregnancies had a 3.8 times greater risk of developing squamous cell cervical cancer. The link between parity and ICC is unclear. However, women who reported cesarean births showed a reduced risk compared with those who had vaginal births. Although the number of cesarean births in this study was small, the purported influence of cervical trauma during vaginal birth on cancer risk remains uncertain. High parity did not seem to increase the probability of HPV infection in women in the study.

• Genetic predisposition—Studies suggest that women whose mother or sisters have had cervical cancer are more likely to develop the disease. Twin studies also suggest familial susceptibility to cervical cancer. Some researchers suspect this familial tendency is caused by an inherited condition that makes some women more susceptible to HPV infection than others (ACS; Gibson & Hainer).

• Nutritional status—Diets low in fruits and vegetables have been identified as potential contributing factors in the development of cervical cancer. Low levels of vitamin C, E, folate, and carotenoids have been linked to cervical cancer (ACS; Gibson & Hainer; Snyder).

• Diethylstilbestrol—Daughters of women who took diethylstilbestrol (DES) are 40 times more likely to develop clear cell adenocarcinoma (CCA) of the vagina and cervix than women unexposed to DES. Clear cell adenocarcinoma is a rare form of vaginal and cervical cancer. DES was prescribed for some women who were in danger of miscarriage during the years between 1940 and 1971 (CDC, nd).

The most common type of cervical cancer is squamous cell carcinoma which comprises 80% to 90% of cervical cancers (ACS, 2004b). Adenocarcinoma is the second most common cancer type and constitutes about 10% to 20% of cervical cancer cases (ACS). Cervical cancer almost always begins in the transformation zone of the cervix at the squamocolumnar junction. It arises from precursor lesions with atypical cervical cells that gradually progress to invasive cancer. The precursor lesions are referred to as squamous intraepithelial lesions (SIL) or cervical intraepithelial neoplasia (CIN). These early lesions form a continuum that is divided into low-grade or high-grade SIL, or CIN 1, 2, or 3, and reflects the increasingly abnormal changes of the cervical epithelium. The lesions can persist, regress, or progress to invasive malignancy. Low-grade SIL (CIN 1) often regresses spontaneously; whereas, high-grade SIL (CIN 2, 3) is more likely to persist or progress (ACS; NCI 2004a, Porth, 2005). The average time for progression from in situ lesions to invasive cervical cancer is approximately 10–12 years. However, in about 10% of patients, lesions can progress from in situ to invasive in a period of less than one year (NCI, 2003a). Table 23–3 presents the terminology used to describe squamous cell abnormalities.

TABLE 23–3 The 2001 Bethesda Categories of Epithelial Cell Abnormalities

ASC-US	Atypical squamous cells of undetermined significance
	This term is used when the squamous cells do not appear completely normal but it is not possible to determine the cause of the abnormal cells.
ASC-H	Atypical squamous cells—cannot exclude HSIL
LSIL	Low-grade squamous intraepithelial neoplasia
	Encompasses:
	HPV
	CIN 1 (Mild Dysplasia): lesion involves the initial 1/3 of the epithelial layer
HSIL	High-grade squamous intraepithelial neoplasia
	Encompasses:
	CIN 2 (Moderate Dysplasia): lesion involves 1/3 to < 2/3 of the epithelial layer
	CIN 3 (Severe Dysplasia, Carcinoma in situ): Lesion involves 2/3 to full thickness
Squamous Carcinoma	Malignant cells penetrate basement membrane of cervical epithelium and infiltrate stromal tissue (supporting tissue)
	In advanced cases, cancer may spread to adjacent organs such as bladder or rectum, or to distant sites in the body via the blood stream and lymphatic channels.

There are more than 80 distinct types of HPV, approximately 30 of which infect the genital area. HPV types fall into two broad categories based on the risk of oncogenesis. The low-risk types include 6, 11, 42, 43, and 44 (ACS, 2004b; Fey & Beal, 2004; NCI, 2003a; Nuovo, Melnikow, & Howell, 2001). Types 6 and 11 are associated with genital warts and are rarely associated with cervical cancer. Most low-risk infections are transient and regress spontaneously. Types 16, 18, 31, 33, 35, 39, 45, 51, 52, 56, 58, 59, and 68 are considered high-risk types (ACS; Fey & Beal; Garcia & Bi, 2002; NCI; Nuovo et al.). Types 16 and 18 are found in 50% to 80% of squamous intraepithelial lesions (SILs) and in more than 90% of invasive cervical cancer (NCI). Untreated high grade lesions are often associated with cervical carcinoma (ACS 2004b; Canavan, 2000; Garcia & Bi; NCI).

The mechanism that causes certain HPV strains to be more carcinogenic than others is not fully understood. However, characteristic of high-risk types of HPV is DNA integrating itself into the target cell genome and exerting its effect on oncogenes and tumor suppressor genes. Researchers believe the viral protein products (E6 and E7) produced by high-risk HPV types bind and inactivate host tumor suppressor genes p53 and retinoblastoma (Rb). Because E6 binds and inactivates p53, and E7 binds and degrades Rb protein, the mutation and inactivation of these genes prevents DNA repair and apoptosis (programmed cell death). This stimulates cell proliferation and ultimately leads to neoplasia (Fey & Beal, 2004; Garcia & Bi, 2002). The postulated steps in the pathogenesis of cervical cancer are depicted in Figure 23–1.

CLINICAL PRESENTATION

Most women are asymptomatic during the early stage of cervical cancer. Although most precancerous lesions usually occur 10–12 years before the development of invasive carcinoma, some lesions progress more rapidly. The only sign during the early stage of the disease may be the shedding of abnormal cells from the cervix. These abnormal cells can be detected by Pap test. When cancers become clinically overt, they usually produce abnormal vaginal bleeding (e.g., postcoital bleeding, bleeding between menstrual periods, or increased menstrual bleeding), vaginal discharge, and dyspareunia. Late symptoms that herald metastatic spread include bladder outlet obstruction, constipation, back pain, and leg swelling (ACS, 2004b; Garcia & Bi, 2002; Jarvis, 2004; Porth, 2005).

ASSESSMENT

History   Key questions or areas of inquiry that assist health care providers to identify women at high risk for cervical cancer include:

- Abnormal vaginal bleeding (intermenstrual or postcoital bleeding), unusual vaginal discharge, or dyspareunia
- Sexual history—age at first intercourse, number of sexual partners in the past six months, number of lifetime partners, and if there were any lesions in sexual partners.
- Contraceptive history including use of barrier methods
- HPV and other sexually transmitted diseases in the patient and her partners

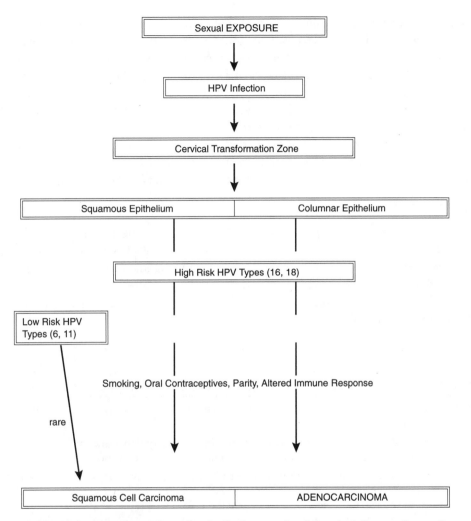

FIGURE 23-I   Postulated Steps in the Pathogenesis of Cervical Cancer. *Source*: Cotran et al., 1999.

- Immunosuppression including HIV
- Prior history of cancer or cancer therapy (e.g., radiation, chemotherapy, surgery)
- In utero diethylstilbestrol (DES) exposure
- The date and result of the most recent Pap test
- Prior abnormal cervical cytology
- Menstrual history including the date of the last menstrual period
- Pregnancy history
- History of tobacco, drug, or alcohol use
- Family history of cervical cancer

Physical examination   Physical examination should include a thorough pelvic, abdominal, inguinal lymph node, and rectal examination. Cervical cancer usually begins around the cervical os. In its earliest stages, a cancerous cervix cannot be distinguished from a normal cervix. As the disease progresses, the cervix may appear abnormal with gross erosion, ulcer, or a mass which bleeds easily on contact. In the late stages, an extensive, irregular, cauliflower-like growth may develop. The cervix may be hard and indurated and its mobility may be restricted or lost. As the tumor enlarges, it grows by extending upward into the endometrial cavity, downward into the vagina, and laterally to the pelvic wall. It can invade the bladder and rectum directly. Common sites for distant metastasis include the pelvic lymph nodes, liver, lungs, and bones (Garcia & Bi, 2002; Jarvis, 2004; Porth, 2005).

DIAGNOSTIC TESTING

Papanicolaou Testing   The Pap test is a screening tool used to detect the presence of abnormal cells on the surface of the cervix or the endocervix. The ACS released revised guidelines for cervical cancer screening in 2002. Data on the natural history of HPV infection suggest that screening can safely be delayed until three years after the onset of sexual activity or until age 21, whichever comes first. The ACS cervical cancer screening recommendations are listed in Table 23–4 (Saslow et al., 2002).

TABLE 23–4   American Cancer Society Cervical Cancer Screening Recommendations

- All women should have a Pap test about three years after they begin having sexual intercourse, but no later than 21 years of age.
- Women under the age of 30 years should have a Pap test every year if the traditional Pap smear is used or every two years if the newer liquid-based Pap test is used.
- Beginning at age 30 years, women who have had three consecutive normal cytology results may be screened every two to three years. Another option for women 30 years and over is to have one of the Pap tests every three years *plus* the HPV DNA test.
- Women who have certain risk factors (HIV infection, immunosuppression, DES exposure before birth) should have a Pap test every year.
- Screening may be discontinued in women 70 years of age or older with three or more consecutive normal Pap test results in the previous 10 years. Continue to screen women with a history of cervical cancer, DES exposure before birth, HIV infection or a weakened immune system.
- Screening is not necessary for women after a total hysterectomy with removal of the cervix for benign gynecologic conditions.
- Continue to screen women who have undergone a hysterectomy for cervical cancer or other precancerous conditions. Screening should continue until three consecutive normal or negative cytology tests with no abnormal tests in an 18–24 month period are achieved.
- Continue to screen women who have had hysterectomies without removal of the cervix according to the guidelines above.

Source: Saslow et al., 2002.

A cervical sample may be prepared for cytology with the conventional Pap test (glass slide) method or by using the newer liquid-based methods (e.g., Thin Prep). See Chapter 6 for more information on obtaining a Pap test. Although the Pap test has been credited with reducing cervical cancer death rates by 70% since its introduction more than 50 years ago, it is associated with high false negative and high false positive rates. Liquid-based methods for cervical cytology screening address some of the limitations of the Pap test. An advantage of liquid-based methods is that they can be combined with a hybrid DNA-capture mechanism for detecting and typing HPV in cervical specimens. The liquid medium preserves specimens for up to three weeks from the date of collection, giving clinicians the opportunity to request reflex HPV testing if a borderline Pap result is received. This eliminates the need for a return visit (ACS, 2004b, d; Fey & Beal, 2004; Nuovo et al., 2001).

Most laboratories use the Bethesda System for reporting the results of cervical cytology. The Bethesda System uses a uniform system of terminology that provides guidance for the clinical management of Pap test results. Table 23–5 provides a description of the 2001 Bethesda System for reporting cervical cytology results (Solomon et al., 2002).

HPV DNA Test   The Hybrid Capture 2 (HC2) assay (Digene Corp., Gaithersburg, MD) can identify 13 of the high-risk types of HPV associated with the development of cervical cancer. HPV DNA typing can help stratify women into follow-up and treatment groups. HPV typing may be particularly helpful in patients with low-grade cytology or cytology of unclear abnormality. The United States Food and Drug Administration (FDA) initially approved the HPV DNA test in March 2000 for testing women who had abnormal Pap test results. In March 2003, the FDA expanded the use of the HC2 test to screening, in conjunction with the Pap test, of women age 30 years and over. The FDA states that the HPV DNA test is not intended as a substitute for regular Pap screening, nor is it intended to screen women under 30 years of age who have normal Pap results (United States Food and Drug Administration [FDA], 2003).

Further Testing   Additional laboratory testing that might be indicated to rule out other causes of vaginal discharge or bleeding includes the following:

- Sexually transmitted Infection (STI) testing—Chlamydia and gonorrhea are common sexually transmitted infections and may produce symptoms similar to those produced when cervical cancer is present. These symptoms include dysuria, urinary frequency, vaginal discharge, and postcoital bleeding. However, most women are asymptomatic. Both infections can be tested using a single cervical swab (Jarvis, 2004) (see Chapter 6).
- Wet mount preparation—Women who have vulvovaginal candidiasis, bacterial vaginosis, or trichonomiasis can present with a variety of symptoms including vaginal discharge, malodor, irritation, burning or itching, dysuria, and dyspareunia. Accurate identification of the pathogen requires microscopic examination of vaginal secretions.

TABLE 23-5 The 2001 Bethesda System for Reporting Cervical Cytologic Diagnoses (Abridged)

Adequacy of Specimen

Satisfactory for evaluation (note presence or absence of endocervical or transformation zone components)

Unsatisfactory for evaluation (specify reason)

General Categorization (optional)

Negative for intraepithelial lesion or malignancy

Epithelial cell abnormality

Other

Interpretation/Result

Negative for intraepithelial lesion or malignancy

Include findings of the following:

- Trichomonas, bacterial, viral, and fungus infection
- Nonneoplastic findings including reactive cellular changes associated with inflammation, radiation, and IUD, glandular cells (posthysterectomy), and atrophy

Epithelial Cell Abnormalities

Squamous Cell

- Atypical squamous cells (ASC) are divided into two categories:
  - o ASC-US: Atypical squamous cells of undetermined significance
  - o ASC-H: Cannot exclude high-grade squamous intraepithelial lesion
- Low-grade squamous intraepithelial lesion (LSIL)
  - o Refers to cervical cancer precursors encompassing the following: human papillomavirus, mild dysplasia, and cervical intraepithelial neoplasia 1 (CIN 1)
- High-grade squamous intraepithelial lesion (HSIL)
  - o Refers to cervical cancer precursors encompassing: moderate and severe dysplasia, carcinoma in situ, and cervical intraepithelial neoplasias 2 and 3 (CIN 2) and (CIN 3)
- Squamous cell carcinoma

Glandular cell

- Atypical glandular cell (AGC)
  - o Specify: Endocervical, Endometrial, or Not otherwise specified (NOS)
- Atypical glandular cells, favor neoplastic
  - o Specify: Endocervical or Not otherwise specified
- Endocervical adenocarcinoma in situ (AIS)
- Adenocarcinoma

Other (List Is Not Comprehensive)

Endometrial cells in a woman 40 years or older

Sources: Solomon et al., 2002; Bethesda System, 2001.

The microscopic examinations include a saline wet mount and a potassium hydroxide (KOH) preparation (Uphold & Graham, 2003).

DIFFERENTIAL DIAGNOSES

Differential diagnoses for cervical cancer include the following, which must be ruled out prior to diagnosing cancer: cervicitis or STI, vaginitis, and cervical polyps.

MANAGEMENT

Prevention   The identification and treatment of early precancerous lesions is critical to the prevention of cervical cancer. Scheduling and keeping appointments for regular gynecologic examinations and Pap tests decreases the incidence and mortality of cervical cancer (NCI, 2004a). Abnormal changes in the cervix are readily detected by the Pap test and are easily cured before cancer develops. Preventive measures should include educating women that the risk of infection can be decreased if the onset of sexual activity is delayed, if the number of sexual partners is decreased, if condoms are used consistently, and if tobacco use is eliminated.

Definitive Treatment   Choice of treatment depends primarily on the stage of disease at the time of diagnosis, but other factors, such as a woman's general health and preferences, should also be considered. Treatment of precancerous lesions and carcinoma in situ may include removal of the lesion by cryosurgery, laser ablation, loop electrosurgical excision procedure (LEEP), and conization (ACS, 2004b). After treatment, patients require lifelong surveillance at regular intervals. The clinician determines the timing and frequency of follow-up based on Pap test results and colposcopy examinations.

Treatment of advanced cervical cancer includes surgery, radiation therapy, and chemotherapy. Usually two or more approaches are used. Surgery can include simple or radical hysterectomy with pelvic lymph node dissection, or pelvic exenteration (removal of all pelvic organs including bladder, rectum, vulva, and vagina). Radiation therapy can involve external beam or intracavitary irradiation. Radiation is often combined with chemotherapy. Recent clinical trial results suggest a combination of radiation therapy and chemotherapy with cisplatin, possibly combined with other drugs, is more effective than radiation alone (NCI, 2003a). The treatment of disseminated cervical cancer is primarily palliative because cure is not possible. Palliative radiation may be used to control bleeding, pelvic pain, or urinary or bowel obstruction from pelvic disease (ACS, 2004b; Canavan, 2000; Garcia & Bi, 2002; Gibson & Hainer, 2003).

Referral   Abnormal Pap test results may require a referral for colposcopic examination. The American Society for Colposcopy and Cervical Pathology (ASCCP) provides algorithms for the management of women with cervical cytologic abnormalities. Algorithms are shown in Figures 23-2 through 23-9.

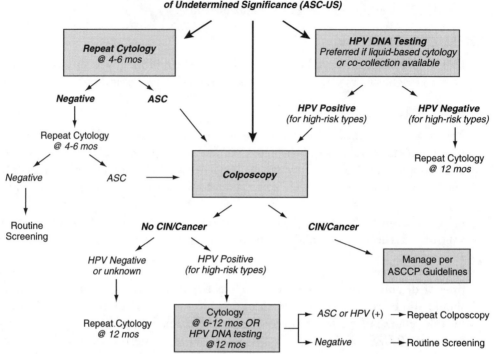

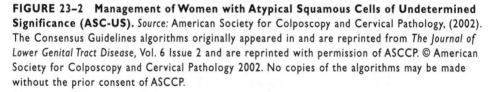

FIGURE 23–2 Management of Women with Atypical Squamous Cells of Undetermined Significance (ASC-US). *Source:* American Society for Colposcopy and Cervical Pathology, (2002). The Consensus Guidelines algorithms originally appeared in and are reprinted from *The Journal of Lower Genital Tract Disease,* Vol. 6 Issue 2 and are reprinted with permission of ASCCP. © American Society for Colposcopy and Cervical Pathology 2002. No copies of the algorithms may be made without the prior consent of ASCCP.

NEW AND EMERGING EVIDENCE FOR THE PRACTICE

HPV Vaccines Vaccines for preventing and treating cervical cancer are being developed and tested. Thus far, one vaccine that protects against HPV-16 has been shown to be effective. In an industry-funded study, a multicenter team in the United States randomized 2392 young women to receive three doses of an intramuscular vaccine that contained HPV-16 virus-like particles (not live virus) or placebo. Sixty-four percent of the women did not have evidence of HPV-16 infection at study entry. After a median follow-up of 17.4 months, significantly more instances of persistent HPV-16 infection were found in the placebo group than in the vaccine group (3.8 cases/100 women-years versus zero cases). A total of nine cases of HPV-16 related cervical intraepithelial neoplasia occurred

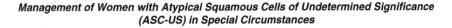

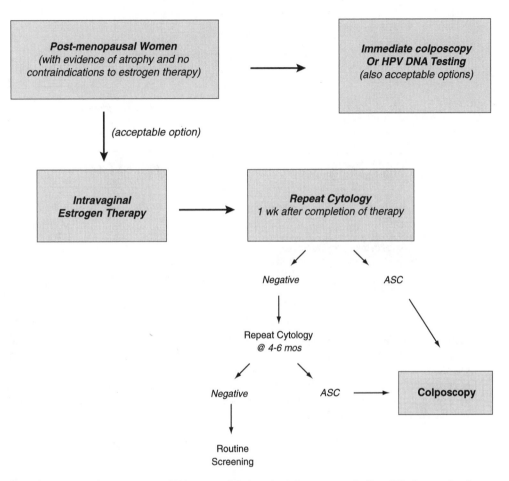

FIGURE 23–3   Management of Women with Atypical Squamous Cells of Undetermined Significance (ASC-US) in Special Circumstances. *Source:* American Society for Colposcopy and Cervical Pathology, (2002). The Consensus Guidelines algorithms originally appeared in and are reprinted from *The Journal of Lower Genital Tract Disease,* Vol. 6 Issue 2 and are reprinted with permission of ASCCP. © American Society for Colposcopy and Cervical Pathology 2002. No copies of the algorithms may be made without the prior consent of ASCCP.

in the placebo group. Among women who were infected with HPV-16 at study entry, rates of persistent HPV-16 infection were 6.3 and 0.6 cases/100 woman-years in the placebo and vaccine groups respectively. No serious vaccine-related adverse events were reported. However, the duration of protection is unknown (Koutsky et al., 2002).

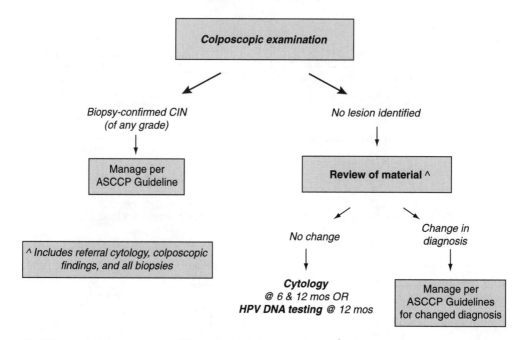

Management of Women with Atypical Squamous Cells: Cannot Exclude High-grade SIL (ASC - H)

Colposcopic examination

Biopsy-confirmed CIN (of any grade)

No lesion identified

Manage per ASCCP Guideline

Review of material ^

^ Includes referral cytology, colposcopic findings, and all biopsies

No change

Change in diagnosis

Cytology
@ 6 & 12 mos OR
HPV DNA testing @ 12 mos

Manage per ASCCP Guidelines for changed diagnosis

FIGURE 23–4 Management of Women with Atypical Squamous Cells: Cannot Exclude High-grade SIL (ASC-H). *Source:* American Society for Colposcopy and Cervical Pathology, (2002). The Consensus Guidelines algorithms originally appeared in and are reprinted from *The Journal of Lower Genital Tract Disease*, Vol. 6 Issue 2 and are reprinted with permission of ASCCP. © American Society for Colposcopy and Cervical Pathology 2002. No copies of the algorithms may be made without the prior consent of ASCCP.

HPV Tests   Researchers are developing new laboratory tests to detect the HPV types that cause cancer. Recent studies indicate the Hybrid Capture HPV test may be useful and cost-effective in determining which women with abnormal cervical cytology results should have a colposcopy (ACS, 2004c).

SPECIAL CONSIDERATIONS

Pregnant Women   A small number of cervical cancers are found in pregnant women. If the cancer is in the early stages, delaying therapy may be an option until fetal viability. However, in more advanced stages, a decision will need to be made about continuing the

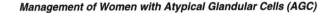

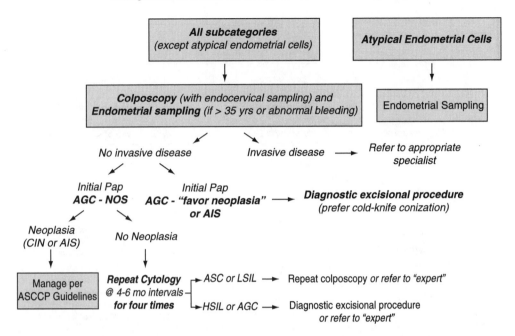

FIGURE 23-5 Management of Women with Atypical Glandular Cells (AGC). *Source:* American Society for Colposcopy and Cervical Pathology, (2002). The Consensus Guidelines algorithms originally appeared in and are reprinted from *The Journal of Lower Genital Tract Disease*, Vol. 6 Issue 2 and are reprinted with permission of ASCCP. © American Society for Colposcopy and Cervical Pathology 2002. No copies of the algorithms may be made without the prior consent of ASCCP.

pregnancy. If the decision is to continue the pregnancy, delivery should be performed as soon as fetal viability is reached. Most experts advocate cesarean birth because the recurrence of the disease at the site of episiotomy is possible (Canavan, 2000).

Talking with the Patient   Many women associate precancerous lesions detected by a Pap test with a diagnosis of cancer. Clinicians should clarify any misperceptions and emphasize the importance of treating these early lesions to *prevent* the development of cancer. Treatment protocols should be reviewed with the patient. The clinician should address STI-prevention strategies and provide guidelines for safer sexual practices. Counseling should include information about the association between HPV infection and cervical cancer. Women should be encouraged to reduce their risk of HPV exposure by delaying

Management of Women with Low-grade Squamous Intraepithelial Lesions (LSIL)*

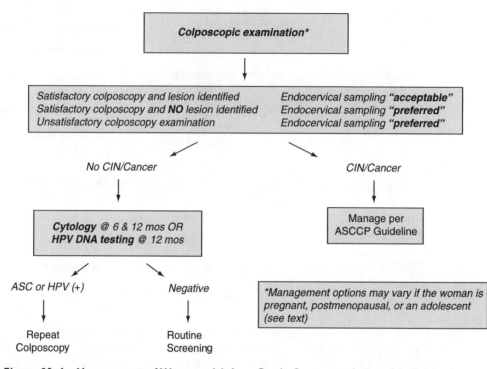

Figure 23–6   Management of Women with Low-Grade Squamous Intraepithelial Lesions (LSIL). *Source:* American Society for Colposcopy and Cervical Pathology, (2002). The Consensus Guidelines algorithms originally appeared in and are reprinted from *The Journal of Lower Genital Tract Disease,* Vol. 6 Issue 2 and are reprinted with permission of ASCCP. © American Society for Colposcopy and Cervical Pathology 2002. No copies of the algorithms may be made without the prior consent of ASCCP.

the onset of sexual activity, decreasing their number of sexual partners, and eliminating tobacco products. Condom use should be encouraged, especially with new, multiple, and nonmonogamous partners.

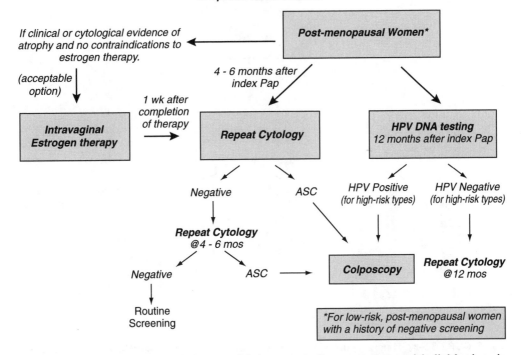

Management of Women with Low-grade Squamous Intraepithelial Lesions in Special Circumstances

FIGURE 23–7 **Management of Women with Low-grade Squamous Intraepithelial Lesions in Special Circumstances: Post-menopausal Women.** *Source:* American Society for Colposcopy and Cervical Pathology, (2002). The Consensus Guidelines algorithms originally appeared in and are reprinted from *The Journal of Lower Genital Tract Disease*, Vol. 6 Issue 2 and are reprinted with permission of ASCCP. © American Society for Colposcopy and Cervical Pathology 2002. No copies of the algorithms may be made without the prior consent of ASCCP.

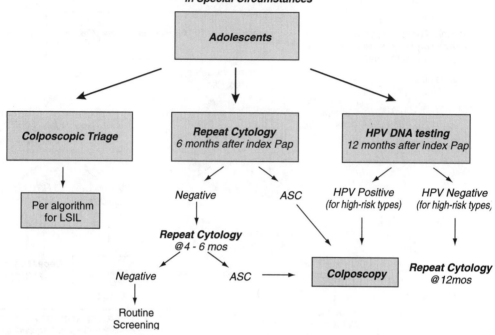

FIGURE 23–8 Management of Women with Low-grade Squamous Intraepithelial Lesions in Special Circumstances: Adolescents. *Source:* American Society for Colposcopy and Cervical Pathology, (2002). The Consensus Guidelines algorithms originally appeared in and are reprinted from *The Journal of Lower Genital Tract Disease,* Vol. 6 Issue 2 and are reprinted with permission of ASCCP. © American Society for Colposcopy and Cervical Pathology 2002. No copies of the algorithms may be made without the prior consent of ASCCP.

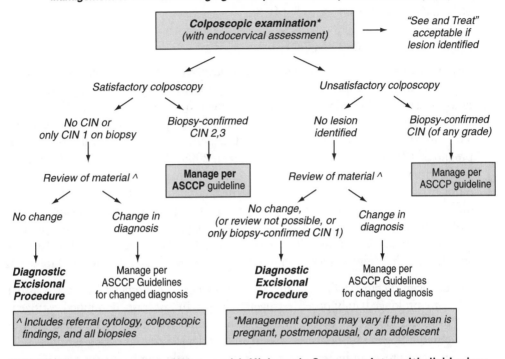

FIGURE 23-9   Management of Women with High-grade Squamous Intraepithelial Lesions (HSIL). *Source:* American Society for Colposcopy and Cervical Pathology, (2002). The Consensus Guidelines algorithms originally appeared in and are reprinted from *The Journal of Lower Genital Tract Disease*, Vol. 6 Issue 2 and are reprinted with permission of ASCCP. © American Society for Colposcopy and Cervical Pathology 2002. No copies of the algorithms may be made without the prior consent of ASCCP.

ENDOMETRIAL CANCER

SCOPE OF THE PROBLEM

Carcinoma of the endometrium is the most prevalent gynecologic malignancy and is the fourth most common malignant neoplasm in women after breast, lung, and colon cancers (ACS, 2004a). An estimated 40,320 new cases of endometrial cancer and approximately 7090 endometrial cancer deaths were projected to occur in 2004 in the United States (ACS). Although the incidence rates are higher in white than in black women, mortality rates in black women are nearly twice as high. A major factor for the increased mortality rate in black women diagnosed with endometrial cancer is the significant occurrence of higher-grade and more aggressive histologies that occur in these black women (ACS;

NCI, 2004c). Five-year survival rates for localized, regional, and metastatic disease are 96%, 64%, and 26% respectively (ACS).

ETIOLOGY AND PATHOPHYSIOLOGY

Two mechanisms are generally believed to be involved in the development of endometrial cancer. A history of exposure to unopposed estrogen, either from endogenous or exogenous sources (Type I endometrial cancer), is the cause in approximately 75% of women. The tumors in these women begin as endometrial hyperplasia and progress to carcinomas. The tumors are usually well-differentiated, superficially invasive, and have a favorable prognosis. (Pazdur, Coia, Hoskins, & Wagman, 2003). In the other 25% of women diagnosed with endometrial cancer, the carcinomas appear spontaneously and are unrelated to estrogen or endometrial hyperplasia. These neoplasms tend to be associated with a poorly differentiated cell type and have a poor prognosis (Type II endometrial cancer). Women with Type II endometrial cancer tend to be thin, multiparous, and are often black (Cotran, Kumar, & Collins, 1999; Creasman, 2002; Pazdur et al., 2003). Risk factors associated with estrogen excess from exogenous estrogen sources include the following:

- Estrogen therapy (ET)—An increased incidence of endometrial cancer is associated with prolonged unopposed estrogen therapy. In contrast, combined estrogen and progestogen therapy decreases the risk of endometrial cancer associated with unopposed estrogen use. However, recent studies demonstrate the long-term use of estrogen and progestin increase a woman's risk of developing breast cancer (ACS, 2004c; Creasman, 2002; NCI, 2004b).
- Tamoxifen (Nolvadex)—Tamoxifen is a drug used for adjuvant therapy in women with early stage breast cancer, as a treatment for recurrent disease, and for reduction of the incidence of breast cancer in women at high risk for the disease. Tamoxifen has site-specific activity in different tissues. It suppresses growth in breast tissue, but stimulates the growth of the endometrial lining (ACS, 2004c; Cotran et al., 1999; Creasman, 2002).

Risk factors associated with endogenous sources of estrogen include the following:

- Early menarche—Starting menstruation before the age of 12 years increases the number of years the endometrium is exposed to estrogen (ACS, 2004c; Cotran et al., 1999; Creasman, 2002).
- Late menopause—Menopause occurring after the age of 55 years of age increases the duration of estrogen exposure (ACS; Cotran et al.; Creasman).
- History of infertility or nulliparity—During pregnancy the hormonal balance shifts toward more progesterone, which protects the uterus; therefore, women who have had many pregnancies have a reduced risk of developing endometrial cancer, and women who are infertile or who have never been pregnant have an increased risk (ACS; Cotran et al.; Creasman).

- Obesity—The majority of women who develop endometrial cancer tend to be obese. Women who are 30 pounds over ideal weight have a 3-fold increased risk of developing endometrial cancer; whereas, those 50 pounds or more over ideal weight have a 10-fold increased risk (Pazdur et al.). Obese women have higher levels of endogenous estrogen as a result of the conversion of androstenedione to estrone and the aromatization of androgens to estradiol, both of which occur in peripheral adipose tissue (ACS; Creasman; Pazdur et al.).
- Chronic anovulation—Anovulation is a common cause of infertility and may be caused by several factors. However, one of the leading causes of chronic anovulation is polycystic ovarian syndrome (PCOS). Women with PCOS are hyperandrogenic, and the androgens may be converted to estrogen in peripheral adipose tissue. Women with PCOS may also have obesity and infertility, further increasing their risk of endometrial cancer (ACS; Creasman; Pazdur et al.).
- Diabetes and hypertension—Endometrial cancer is more common in women with diabetes and hypertension, and is probably related to factors associated with obesity (ACS; Creasman).
- High-fat diet—A high-fat diet may lead to obesity, and obesity is a well-documented risk factor for endometrial cancer. Some researchers believe that fatty foods may also have a direct effect on estrogen metabolism, thereby increasing the risk for endometrial cancer (ACS; Creasman).
- Breast or ovarian cancer—Women who have had breast or ovarian cancer have a higher risk of developing endometrial cancer. The hormonal risk factors associated with breast and ovarian cancers also increase the risk for endometrial cancer (ACS; Creasman).

A risk factor for endometrial cancer that is not associated with estrogen excess is hereditary nonpolyposis colorectal cancer (HNPCC). Most HNPCC is associated with mutations in either of two genes: MSH2 and MLH1. Among women who are HNPCC mutation carriers, the estimated cumulative incidence of endometrial cancer ranges from 20–60% (NCI, 2004b).

The most common endometrial cancer cell type is endometrioid adenocarcinoma, which constitutes 75–80% of endometrial carcinoma cases (NCI, 2004b). Adenocarcinomas arise from glandular cells of the endometrium. Less common types include the following: papillary serous carcinoma (10%), mixed (10%), clear cell carcinoma (4–5%), mucinous (1%), and squamous cell (< 1% [NIC]).

Both papillary serous and clear cell carcinomas tend to be more aggressive than endometrial adenocarcinoma and tend to be detected at advanced stages (ACS, 2004c; NCI; Pazdur et al., 2003).

CLINICAL PRESENTATION

Endometrial cancer occurs more frequently in older women (peak ages 55–65 years), with only a 2–5% incidence among women younger than 40 years (Porth, 2005). The most common early symptom of endometrial cancer is abnormal vaginal bleeding or spotting. In menstruating women this can take the form of bleeding between periods or excessive, prolonged menstrual flow. In postmenopausal women, any bleeding is abnormal and warrants further evaluation. Late signs and symptoms may include cramping, pelvic pain, lower abdominal pressure, enlarged lymph nodes, and weight loss (Creasman, 2002; Pazdur et al., 2003; Porth).

ASSESSMENT

History   Key pieces of information that assist the clinician to identify women at high risk for endometrial cancer include: the character of the bleeding, the pattern of the flow, occurrence and number of pads used when bleeding occurs; inquire about accompanying problems (e.g., dyspareunia, pain, bladder or bowel problems); ask her if she is experiencing any unusual vaginal discharge or if she has ever been diagnosed with an STI. Obtain a menstrual history (see Chapter 6) and inquire if she is taking any hormones. Inquire about the possibility of pregnancy and whether or not she has experienced any symptoms of pregnancy (e.g., missed period, breast tenderness, or nausea and vomiting). If she has previously been pregnant, obtain a pregnancy history in addition to medical and family histories (see Chapter 6). Be sure to ask her if there is personal or family history of breast, ovarian, or colon cancer. Ask her if she has experienced infertility problems or if she has a history of PCOS (Dains, Baumann, & Scheibel, 2003; Jarvis, 2004).

Physical Examination   The physical examination should include a thorough abdominal, inguinal lymph node, pelvic, vaginal, and rectal examination. Abnormal bleeding from the genital tract can occur from the vagina, cervix, uterus, or fallopian tubes. Inspect the external genitalia for lesions or atrophic vaginitis, which may be the cause of the bleeding. Perform a vaginal examination to determine if bleeding is caused by vaginal or cervical infection. Note the amount, color, consistency, and odor of the vaginal discharge; whether or not the cervix is friable or has an unusual discharge; and observe for cervical polyps. Perform a bimanual examination. Palpate the cervix, which normally feels smooth, firm, evenly rounded, and mobile. Note any cervical motion tenderness. Next palpate the uterus, ovaries, and inguinal lymph nodes. Note uterine size and contour. Endometrial cancer seldom causes much uterine enlargement, and any increase in size usually occurs slowly. Uterine fibroids usually feel firm and may make the uterus asymmetrical. Note any enlargement of the ovaries and lymph nodes. Lastly, perform a rectal examination to identify lesions or other abnormalities. Metastatic spread occurs in a characteristic pattern, which is commonly to the pelvic and para-aortic nodes. Common sites for distant metastasis include the lungs, inguinal and supraclavicular lymph nodes, liver, bones, brain, and vagina (Creasman, 2002; Dains et al., 2003; Jarvis, 2004; Porth, 2005).

Screening Tests   There is no screening test currently available to detect endometrial cancer. A Pap test is not effective in detecting endometrial cancer; although, occasionally it does reveal endometrial abnormalities. If endometrial cancer is suspected, or if a woman is at high risk for its development, a gynecologist or gynecologic oncologist should be consulted immediately.

Endometrial Biopsy   Endometrial biopsy is an office procedure in which a sample of endometrial tissue is obtained through a thin, flexible tube inserted into the uterus through the cervix. A small amount of endometrial tissue is removed by suction from negative pressure created within the tube. Most women experience discomfort during the procedure that is similar to severe menstrual cramps. Cramping can be prevented or alleviated by taking ibuprofen 30–60 minutes prior to the procedure. Endometrial biopsy detects 80–90% of endometrial cancers if an adequate tissue sample is obtained (Porth, 2005). However, if the biopsy result fails to provide sufficient diagnostic information or if abnormal bleeding persists, a dilation and curettage (D & C) with or without a hysteroscopy is recommended (Creasman, 2002).

Transvaginal Ultrasound   Transvaginal ultrasound, which uses sound waves to measure endometrial thickness, may be an alternative to endometrial biopsy. An endometrial thickness of less than 4 to 5 mm in postmenopausal women is associated with a low risk of endometrial disease; a thicker lining should be further evaluated by endometrial biopsy (ACS, 2004c; Creasman, 2002).

Dilatation and Curettage   Dilatation and curettage (D & C) is the gold standard for assessing uterine bleeding and diagnosing endometrial cancer. If an endometrial biopsy sample is inadequate or suggests, but does not diagnose, endometrial cancer, a D & C with or without hysteroscopy is recommended. Dilatation and curettage requires anesthesia and is associated with a number of potential complications such as hemorrhage, infection, and perforated uterus (ACS, 2004c; Creasman, 2002). For these reasons, an endometrial biopsy is often used as a first diagnostic measure, and a D & C is used only if the endometrial biopsy is inconclusive. A D & C is usually performed by a physician.

Hysteroscopic-Directed Biopsy   A hysteroscope is a thin telescope that is inserted through the cervix into the uterus. An indication for hysteroscopy is the evaluation of persistent abnormal uterine bleeding in a woman who is premenopausal or postmenopausal when an endometrial biopsy is inconclusive. It allows direct visualization of the endometrial lining. It is used to obtain directed biopsies of abnormal-appearing areas of the endometrium (Creasman, 2002).

DIFFERENTIAL DIAGNOSIS

Differential diagnosis of genital bleeding depends on the clinical picture. Bleeding from the lower genital tract can occur from the vagina (atrophic vaginitis) or cervix (cervicitis, STIs, polyps, or cervical carcinoma). It may also occur from the uterus (carcinoma, fibroids, polyps, pregnancy, or dysfunctional uterine bleeding) or the fallopian tubes (PID, ectopic pregnancy) (Collins, 2003).

MANAGEMENT

Prevention   Although most cases of endometrial cancer cannot be prevented, several factors are associated with a decreased incidence of endometrial cancer. These include the following:

- Combined oral contraceptives (COCs)—A meta-analysis that examined the impact of COCs and endometrial cancer risk included 10 case control studies and one prospective study (NCI, 2004b). Overall, four years of COC use was associated with a reduced risk of endometrial cancer of approximately 58%; eight years of use with a reduced risk of 67%, and 12 years of use with approximately a 72% reduction. The beneficial effect persisted for at least 10 years after COCs were discontinued (NCI).
- Physical activity—Studies investigating the relationship between physical activity and the risk of endometrial cancer have shown a decrease in endometrial cancer risk in women who exercise. It is believed that physical activity modifies the risk of endometrial cancer by reducing obesity, a known risk factor for endometrial cancer (NCI).
- Low-fat diet—A diet low in saturated fats and high in fruit and vegetables is associated with a reduced risk of developing endometrial cancer (NCI).
- Breastfeeding—It is believed that breastfeeding modifies endometrial cancer risk by inhibiting ovulation (NCI).
- Controlling other risk factors—Women with PCOS need appropriate treatment to avoid the effect of unopposed estrogen on the uterus. Menopausal women with an intact uterus should avoid using unopposed estrogen to relieve menopausal symptoms. Women with a history of breast or ovarian cancer or HNPCC need to be closely monitored for endometrial cancer. The American Cancer Society recommends that women with or at increased risk for HNPCC should be offered annual testing for endometrial cancer with endometrial biopsy beginning at the age of 35 years. These women should also be counseled about preventive measures such as the option of prophylactic hysterectomy at the completion of childbearing (ACS, 2004c).

Definitive Treatment   Choice of treatment depends primarily on type and stage of the disease, level of differentiation, the woman's overall health, and her personal preferences. Primary treatment options for endometrial cancer include hysterectomy, radiation therapy, and hormonal therapy. Chemotherapy may be used in recurrent or advanced cases of endometrial cancer. However, there are no standard chemotherapy programs for patients with metastatic disease. Treatment options with single-agent and combination drugs are currently under clinical investigation (NCI, 2003b).

Surgery   The recommended surgery is a total abdominal hysterectomy with bilateral salpingo-oopherectomy. Patients with localized disease are usually cured. However, patients with myometrial invasion are usually treated with a combination of surgery and adjuvant radiation therapy. Lymph node sampling may be done at the same time as surgery. Recovery usually takes about from four to six weeks (NCI, 2003b).

Radiation Therapy Radiation treatments may be given externally (external beam radiation), intracavitary (brachytherapy), or both. Diarrhea and fatigue are common side effects of radiation therapy. Pelvic radiation may also cause vaginal stenosis (narrowing of the vagina from scar tissue) which may make vaginal intercourse painful. The use of a vaginal dilator or having vaginal intercourse several times per week helps prevent scar tissue formation. Use of vaginal lubricants may also be helpful.

Hormone Therapy Patients who are not candidates for surgery or radiation, or who have advanced disease, are treated with hormonal therapy. The most common hormonal agents are progestational drugs such as hydroxyprogesterone (Delalutin), medroxyprogesterone (Provera), and megestrol (Megace). Response to hormones is associated with the presence and level of hormone receptors and the degree of tumor differentiation (NCI, 2003b).

Follow-Up An important part of the treatment plan is a specific schedule of follow-up visits after surgery, chemotherapy, or radiation therapy. Follow-up visits are normally scheduled every three to six months during the first three years after treatment and then reduced to about twice per year after that because the recurrence rate is significantly decreased after three years (Fischer, 1996). Approximately 75% of endometrial cancer recurrences are found within the first three years of follow-up (ACS, 2004c). An examination of the abdomen, pelvis, inguinal lymph nodes, and rectum should be done at every follow-up visit. A Pap smear of the upper vaginal area may also be collected to identify any cancerous cells. History questions should focus on symptoms that might indicate cancer recurrence. If the patient's symptoms or physical examination results suggest recurrent cancer, imaging tests such as a CT scan, ultrasound, CA 125 blood test, or biopsies should be ordered. However, if no symptoms or physical examination abnormalities are identified, routine blood tests and imaging tests are not recommended (ACS).

OVARIAN CANCER

SCOPE OF THE PROBLEM

Ovarian cancer is the fifth most common cause of cancer in the United States and the fourth leading cause of death among women. It is also the most common cause of death from gynecologic cancer (ACS, 2004a). Advancing age is the most significant risk factor for the development of ovarian cancer with the risk increasing at menopause. The average age of women in the United States who are diagnosed with ovarian cancer is 63 years (NCI, 2004h), although primary diagnoses of ovarian cancer occur most commonly in women who are 40–70 years of age. African-American women have a lower lifetime risk of ovarian cancer than Caucasian women but the 5-year survival rates are similar in both groups (ACS).

The prognosis for most women with ovarian cancer continues to be poor primarily because early diagnosis of the disease is infrequent (Berek, 2002; NCI, 2004h). The 5-year survival rates have improved only slightly with advances in surgery and chemotherapy. If the disease is confined to the ovary at the time of diagnosis 5-year survival rates approach 95%; however, only 25% of women have localized disease at the time of diagnosis. The overall 5-year survival rate for all ovarian cancers is less than 50% (NCI). Clinical and technological advances in early detection are urgently needed to decrease the morbidity and mortality associated with ovarian cancer.

ETIOLOGY AND PATHOPHYSIOLOGY

Epithelial ovarian carcinoma is the most common type of ovarian cancer and accounts for about 90% of instances diagnosed. The majority of these cases are diagnosed in postmenopausal women (Ozols, Schwartz, & Eifel, 2001). Epithelial ovarian cancers arise from the epithelial lining of the ovary. As the ovary enlarges with tumor growth, cells from the surface of the ovary are shed into the peritoneal cavity where they implant on the peritoneal surface and omentum and become small tumor sites (Ozols et al.). Invasive spread to the regional para-aortic and pelvic lymph nodes, bowel, and bladder, accompanied by ascites with peritoneal seeding of the liver surface, diaphragm, bladder, and intestines is common (Ozols et al.). Epithelial ovarian cancer can be further subdivided into the following histologic subtypes: serous or mucinous (which are the two most common cell types), endometroid, clear cell, transitional, or undifferentiated carcinomas (NCI, 2004b). Epithelial tumors of low-malignancy potential (borderline ovarian carcinoma) are usually found in younger women and are often confined to the ovary at diagnosis (Ozols et al.). Germ cell and sex cord-stromal tumors account for 5%, of all ovarian cancers (NCI, 2003c; Ozols et al.).

RISK FACTORS

Age is the most significant risk factor for the development of ovarian cancer; however, a personal history of breast, bladder, or colon cancer also increases a woman's risk of developing ovarian cancer (Luce, Hassey Dow, & Holcomb, 2003; O'Rourke & Mahon, 2003). Family history is also an important risk factor of ovarian cancer. Women who have a first- or second-degree relative with ovarian cancer are about three times more likely to develop ovarian cancer than those who do not (Ozols et al., 2001). When a woman carries the BRCA1 and BRCA2 genetic mutations, hereditary ovarian cancer risk is increased to as high as 50%. She is also at significantly increased risk for developing breast cancer (Berek, 2002; NCI, 2004d; Ozol et al.). It is estimated that 5–10% of all ovarian cancers are hereditary and the rest are sporadic (NCI, 2004e; Ozols et al.).

Women who have never been pregnant have a slightly higher risk of developing ovarian cancer than women who have had at least one full-term pregnancy. However, age of menarche and menopause, or the woman's age at the time of her first live birth, appear to be unrelated to the risk of developing ovarian cancer (NCI, 2004h).

Three often suggested, although yet to be proven, risk factors for the development of ovarian cancer include: body weight, use of talcum powder, and hormone therapy. The relationship between body weight and the development of ovarian cancer is unclear. Presently there is no clearly identified relationship between increasing body weight and risk of ovarian cancer (O'Rourke & Mahon, 2003). The use of talcum powder has been suggested as a possible risk factor in the development of ovarian cancer because of its similarity to asbestos; however, recent studies revealed that talcum powder use for more than 20 years conferred no increased risk (Huncharek, Geschwind, & Kupelnick, 2003; O'Rourke & Mahon). Studies evaluating the relationship between hormone therapy and the risk for ovarian cancer also have demonstrated inconsistent results (O'Rourke & Mahon). Hormone therapy in postmenopausal women may be associated with an increased risk of developing ovarian cancer (NCI, 2004c).

Women who have used fertility drugs have also been suggested to be at an increased risk for ovarian cancer; however, an NCI study of 12,000 women found no association between the use of medications that stimulate ovulation and ovarian cancer (Brinton et al., 2004). Clomiphene citrate (Clomid) users actually had slightly fewer ovarian cancers than would be expected in the general population, and gonadotropin users had slightly more cancers. Women who use fertility drugs and then conceive and give birth are not believed to be at an increased risk for ovarian cancer (Brinton et al.; O'Rourke & Mahon, 2003).

CLINICAL PRESENTATION

The majority of cases of ovarian cancer are diagnosed at an advanced stage because symptoms of the disease are vague and offer only subtle signs such as abdominal bloating and discomfort, dyspepsia, and fatigue or weakness, all of which can be caused by many factors (Ozols et al., 2001; Goff, Mandel, Melancon, & Muntz, 2004). Additional symptoms that may or may not accompany ovarian cancer include back pain, changes in bowel or bladder function (e.g. constipation or diarrhea, and a sensation of urinary fullness or urge), urinary incontinence, and unexplained weight gain or loss (Goff et al.; Ozols et al.). Signs of advanced disease include: anorexia, nausea or vomiting, ascites, abdominal or back pain, an abdominal mass or pleural effusion (Ozols et al.; Goff et al.). Effective screening is difficult because of the lack of specific symptoms in the premalignant or very early stages of the disease (Berek, 2002). Table 23–6 identifies the early and late symptoms that may occur with ovarian cancer.

ASSESSMENT

Screening   Routine population-based screening for ovarian cancer is not recommended (NCI, 2004f; US Prevention Services Task Force [USPSTF], 2004). The pelvic examination, tumor-associated antigen CA-125, and transvaginal ultrasound are not sufficiently sensitive or specific enough to be recommended for screening

TABLE 23–6 Clinical Presentation of Ovarian Cancer

Early Symptoms	Later Symptoms
Abdominal bloating/discomfort	Ascites
Early satiety	Anorexia
Indigestion	Nausea or vomiting
Fatigue/weakness	Palpable abdominal or pelvic mass
Vague abdominal pain/painful areas in abdomen on palpation	Distinct abdominal pain
	Back pain
Urinary fullness and/or urge urinary incontinence	Pleural effusion
Diarrhea or constipation	
Unexplained weight gain or loss	

asymptomatic women (NCI). Ovarian cancer is occasionally detected during the pelvic examination and, when detected, it almost always indicates advanced disease. Palpation of the ovaries during pelvic examination has not proven to be useful in identifying ovarian cancer in women who are premenopausal. A palpable pelvic mass in a woman who is postmenopausal is always considered abnormal and should be evaluated further.

CA-125 is a tumor-associated antigen (glycoprotein) that has been used to monitor the clinical status of patients with ovarian cancer (Ozols et al., 2001). It is useful when the CA-125 level is elevated at the time of diagnosis and then drops after definitive primary therapy such as surgical debulking of the primary tumor followed by chemotherapy (Ozols et al.). CA-125 is shed from the surface of the fallopian tubes, endometrium, endocervix, peritoneum, pleura, pericardium, and bronchus. It is not specific for ovarian cancer and may be elevated in women with endometriosis, other nongynecologic malignancies, pelvic inflammatory disease, fibroids, menstruation, and during the first trimester of pregnancy (Ozols et al.). Therefore, CA-125 it is not a recommended screening test. It can be useful as part of the follow-up of treated patients if the CA-125 level was obtained and found to be elevated at the time of diagnosis and then observed to drop significantly after definitive treatment of the ovarian cancer (Berek, 2002; Ozols et al.).

Ultrasound has demonstrated value in the detection of advanced ovarian cancer but accurate detection in the early stage of the disease is poor (O'Rourke & Mahon, 2003). The finding of a palpable pelvic mass combined with a positive transvaginal ultrasound and elevated CA-125 decreases the number of false positives and improves the rate of accurate detection (Berek, 2002; NCI, 2004g, February 20; USPSTF, 2004).

New developments in the screening for ovarian cancer include a search for biomarkers that can be detected by a simple blood test and evaluation of the laparoscopic ovarian Pap test (O'Rourke & Mahon, 2003). Similar to the traditional Pap test used to screen for cervical cancer, the laparoscopic ovarian Pap test obtains a small sample of cells from the surface of the ovaries that are analyzed for malignant changes.

MANAGEMENT

Prevention Factors that inhibit ovulation appear to reduce the risk of developing ovarian cancer. Oral contraceptive use for five or more years reduces the risk of ovarian cancer by 40% to 50%, and the protective effect continues for 10–15 years following discontinuation of their use (Barnes, Grizzle, Grubbs, & Partridge, 2002; NCI 2004g). Pregnancy resulting in at least one full-term birth and breast feeding also reduce ovarian cancer risk (NCI). The more times a woman has been pregnant, the lower her risk of ovarian cancer. (NCI). Tubal ligation and hysterectomy without oophorectomy also appear to reduce the risk of ovarian cancer. Bilateral salpingo-oophorectomy is often recommended to women who have documented mutations in the BRCA1 or BRCA2 genes. Bilateral salpingo-oophorectomy appears to reduce the risk of breast cancer as well as ovarian cancer (Berek, 2002; Hogg & Friedlander, 2004; Martin, 2000). Women considering this option need genetic counseling and testing as well as education regarding the clinical effects of premature menopause so they may make an informed decision.

Staging Persistent ovarian masses in women who are premenopausal, and any palpable pelvic mass in women who are postmenopausal should be evaluated by obtaining a transvaginal ultrasound and CA-125 level (Berek, 2002; Ozols et al., 2001; Martin, 2000). Color flow Doppler ultrasound may also be used to further evaluate a suspicious mass (Berek). Malignancy is suspected if the mass has irregular borders, solid areas with papillary projections, or multiple, dense, irregular septae (Martin). Ascites is present in one third of women at the time of diagnosis (Martin). Referral to a gynecologist with experience in cancer surgery or a gynecologic oncologist is appropriate at this point.

Preoperative work-up prior to surgery includes a CT of the entire abdomen and pelvis with contrast, chest X-ray, and mammogram (Berek, 2002; Ozols et al., 2001). An exploratory laparotomy is required to make a definitive diagnosis of cancer, stage the extent of the disease, and to "debulk" (remove) all of the visible tumor in the abdomen and pelvis. The goal is to leave tumor bulk less than 1 cm in diameter. A total abdominal hysterectomy, bilateral salpingo-oophorectomy, peritoneal cytology, omentectomy, pelvic and para-aortic lymph node sampling, scraping of the undersurface of the diaphragm, multiple peritoneal biopsies, and random biopsies are all part of the standard surgical procedure (Berek; Ozols et al.; NCI, 2004h; National Institutes of Health [NIH], 1995).

Ovarian cancer is surgically staged and the FIGO staging system is used to provide important prognostic information (Table 23–7). The volume of postoperative residual tumor is also of prognostic significance with greater volumes conferring a poorer prognosis.

Postoperative Treatment All women diagnosed with ovarian cancer are possible candidates for clinical trials and should be offered participation if they meet selection criteria. Women with early Stage I disease with well or moderately well-differentiated histologies require no further treatment and have a 5-year survival rate of greater than 90% provided they have undergone total abdominal hysterectomy and bilateral salpingo-oophorectomy with omentectomy, with visualization and biopsy of the undersurface of

TABLE 23–7 FIGO Ovarian Cancer Staging System

Stage	Characteristics
Stage I	Tumor limited to the ovaries
Stage II	Tumor involves one or both ovaries and extends into pelvis
Stage III	Tumor involves one or both ovaries and pelvis; has extended to bowel, peritoneum, or lymph nodes
Stage IV	Tumor involves one or both ovaries with distant metastases to areas such as liver and chest

Source: International Federation of Gynecology and Obstetrics, 2002.

the diaphragm, pelvic and peritoneal biopsies, and peritoneal washings (NCI, 2004h). Standard treatment for women who fall into the unfavorable or high-risk categories includes postoperative chemotherapy with a platinum-based regimen (NCI). Surgery for Stage II disease should include total abdominal hysterectomy, bilateral salpingo-oophorectomy, omentectomy with tumor debulking (to remove as much tumor bulk as possible) followed by combination chemotherapy or total abdominal and pelvic radiation therapy (NCI). Advanced (Stages III and IV) disease is treated with a combination of debulking surgery and postoperative chemotherapy. Standard combination chemotherapy includes the use of platinum-based compounds and the taxanes (NCI; Ozols et al., 2001). After several cycles of chemotherapy have been completed, interval debulking surgery is performed in women who did not have a primary debulking procedure (NCI; Ozols et al.). Secondary debulking surgery is sometimes performed if there is a relapse. Second-look surgery or exploratory surgery at the completion of chemotherapy is an option for women with Stages III and IV disease and who have a normal CA-125 and a negative CT scan. Second-look surgery is controversial because it does not improve survival, and if the patient is found to have residual cancer available treatment is not curative (Berek, 2002; Ozols et al.). Intraperitoneal chemotherapy is the subject of ongoing clinical trials.

FOLLOW-UP CARE OF THE WOMAN WHO HAS BEEN TREATED FOR OVARIAN CANCER

Factors that influence the prognosis of ovarian cancer include diagnosis at a younger age, lower stage of disease, the tumor is well-differentiated, no ascites is present, the tumor has a smaller volume prior to debulking surgery and there is smaller residual volume following debulking surgery, and the cell type is other than mucinous or clear cell (NCI, 2004h).

The annual mortality rate from ovarian cancer is approximately equal to the incidence rate because most patients have widespread disease at the time of diagnosis (ACS). Early stage disease (Stages I and II) have a 5-year survival rate of 90% or more. When ovarian cancer is diagnosed at Stage III or IV, the 5-year survival rate is only 35% (ACS). As more effective treatments have become available, increasing numbers of women with advanced disease at diagnosis are surviving, and they are having remissions of two years or longer.

The majority of recurrences of ovarian cancer happen within the first year after initial treatment. The majority of advanced stage ovarian cancer patients developing recurrent disease do so within two years after treatment (Berek, 2002). Major metastatic sites include the abdomen and pelvis, pelvic and para-aortic lymph nodes, diaphragm, lungs, liver, serosa, pleura, peritoneum overlying the kidneys, adrenal glands, bladder, and spleen. Ascites is present in two thirds of women at the time of their death (Martin, 2000). Intestinal obstruction with tumor or adhesions causing extrinsic compression of the bowel occurs in approximately 25% to 50% of women with ovarian cancer (Martin). Obstruction can be partial or complete, and acute or chronic. The most common presenting symptom is cramping abdominal pain (Martin). Pleural effusion and lymphedema are other possible complications of recurrent disease.

The primary goal of follow-up care is the early identification of recurrence with the hope that additional treatment will offer the possibility of disease control. A therapeutic alliance and partnership between health care provider and patient improves the likelihood that early, subtle signs of recurrence will be promptly reported and evaluated. Lifelong follow-up will be required at regularly scheduled intervals. Follow-up needs to be coordinated with the primary care provider and the gynecologic oncologist, or medical and radiation oncologists. Patients are usually seen for follow-up every three months during the first year with follow-up thereafter determined by the initial stage of their disease and potential for delayed effects of definitive treatment (Fischer, 1996). History taking should include questions about changes in appetite, increase in abdominal size or mass, weight gain or loss, changes in bowel or bladder function, pelvic pain, and leg edema. Physical examination should focus on the breasts, lungs, abdomen, pelvis, and extremities (Ozols et al., 2001). A rising CA-125 level is highly suggestive of recurrent disease. It is important to keep in mind that not all ovarian carcinomas are revealed by CA-125; ovarian cancer may recur without a corresponding rise in the CA-125. Options for treatment of recurrent disease include surgical debulking of gross tumor, additional chemotherapy, and radiation therapy (Ozols et al.).

The fear of recurrence is always present for a woman who has been treated for ovarian cancer. Periods of remission followed by recurrence and the need for retreatment keep women in an ongoing state of uncertainty and anxiety (Ferrell et al., 2003; Steginga & Dunn, 1997). Even in women with a good prognosis, the fear of recurrence commonly persists for years after completion of definitive treatment and may surface at some follow-up appointments and not others. All symptoms should be taken seriously by the woman and her provider because the initial symptoms of ovarian cancer are subtle, vague, and ill defined. She should be seen promptly even though the symptoms may be a result of sometimes minor, transient problems such as indigestion or a muscle strain. Each follow-up assessment must always include the consideration of the possibility of recurrent disease as well as the delayed effects of surgery, chemotherapy, and radiation therapy.

Quality of life and the meaning of life itself are important issues for ovarian cancer survivors. When the diagnosis of ovarian cancer is first received, women commonly feel isolated and wish to avoid others who have the disease, particularly those women whose disease is at an advanced stage. Later, women recently diagnosed with ovarian cancer often will seek relationships with other women who have the disease so that they can share the lived experience and find emotional support. Many women have difficulty coping with the wish that the cancer had been diagnosed sooner. Women with ovarian cancer often will take control of their treatment by seeking out alternative and complementary therapies that they will combine with conventional treatment. Some women worry about passing a genetic predisposition for ovarian cancer on to their daughters (Ferrell et al., 2003; Zebrack, 2000). Relationships are reevaluated and personal beliefs about life and death are examined, as well as one's spirituality (Zebrack). Loss of fertility and the permanent physical changes that accompany total abdominal hysterectomy and bilateral salpingo-oophorectomy followed by chemotherapy add to the stress the cancer diagnosis places on women's personal relationships. Menopausal symptoms such as hot flashes and vaginal dryness, and the side effects of chemotherapy such as peripheral neuropathy and temporary hair loss, often leave women feeling as though they have lost their femininity and sexuality (Ferrell). In spite of these negative aspects of the disease and the treatment process, quality of life is moderately high for most of these women (Ersek, Ferrell, Dow, Melancon, 1997). These women derive great benefit and support from the presence of consistent, sensitive clinicians who take their symptoms and concerns seriously and provide prompt, thorough follow-up that does not offer any false sense of reassurance or undue sense of alarm.

REFERENCES

American Cancer Society. (2004a). *Cancer Facts and Figures.* Retrieved April 20, 2004, from www.cancer.org/dcroot/STT/stt_0.asp.

American Cancer Society. (2004b). *Detailed Guide: Cervical Cancer.* Retrieved April 20, 2004, from www.cancer.org/docroot/CRI/content/CRI_2_4_1X_What_is_cervical_cancer_8.asp.

American Cancer Society. (2004c). *Detailed Guide: Endometrial Cancer..* Retrieved May 16, 2004, from www.cancer.org/docroot/cri/cri_2_3x.asp?dt=11

American Cancer Society. (2004d). Guidelines for the early detection of cervical cancer. *CA: A Cancer Journal for Clinicians, 53*(6), 342–362.

American Joint Committee on Cancer. (2002). *AJCC Cancer Staging Manual and Handbook* (Sixth ed.). New York: Springer.

American Society for Colposcopy and Cervical Pathology. (2002). *The algorithms from the consensus guidelines for the management of women with cervical cytological abnormalities.* Hagerstown, MD: Author.

Barnes, M. N., Grizzle, W. E., Grubbs, C. J., & Partridge, E. E. (2002). Paradigms for the primary prevention of ovarian carcinoma. *CA: Cancer Journal for Clinicians, 52*(4), 216–225.

Berek, J. S. (2002). Ovarian Cancer. In J. S. Berek (Ed.), *Novak's Gynecology* (13th ed., pp. 1245–1319). Philadelphia: Lippincott Williams & Wilkins.

Bethesda System: Terminology for reporting results of cervical cytology. (2002) *Journal of the American Medical Association, 287*(16), 2114–2119.

Brinton, L. A., Lamb, E. J., Moghissi, K. S., Scoccia, B., Althuis, M. D., Mabie, J. E., et al. (2004). Ovarian cancer risk after the use of ovulation-stimulating drugs. *Obstetrics and Gynecology, 103*(6), 1194–1203.

Canavan, T. P. (2000). Cervical cancer. *American Family Physician, 61*(5), 1369–1375.

Centers for Disease Control and Prevention (n.d.). *Facts about DES and vaginal/cervical cancers.* Retrieved July

25, 2004, from http://www.cdc/gov/DES/partners/download/DES&CCAFactSheet.pdf.

Centers for Disease Control and Prevention. (2003, September). *Sexually transmitted disease surveillance, 2002* [Electronic version]. Atlanta, GA: U.S. Department of Health and Human Services. Retrieved July 14, 2004, from http://www.cdc.gov/std/stats/2002pdf/Syphilis.pdf.

Centers for Disease Control and Prevention (2004, January). *Report to Congress: Prevention of genital human papillomavirus infection.* Atlanta, GA: U.S. Department of Health and Human Services. Retrieved July 23, 2004, from http://www.cdc.gov/std/HPV/2004HPV%20Report.pdf.

Chambers, S. K. (2001). Gynecologic cancers. In V. T. DeVita, S. Hellman, & S. A. Rosenberg (Eds.), *Cancer: Principles & practice of oncology* (Vol. 2, pp. 1519–1525). Philadelphia: Lippincott Williams & Wilkins.

Cohen, R. F., & Frank-Stromborg, M. (2000). Assessment and interventions for cancer detection. In S. L. Groenwald, M. H. Frogge, M. Goodman, & C. H. Yarbro (Eds.), *Cancer Nursing: Principles and practice* (5th ed., pp. 150–188). Boston: Jones & Bartlett.

Collins, R. D. (2003). *Differential diagnosis in primary care.* Philadelphia: Lippincott Williams & Wilkins.

Cotran, R. S., Kumar, V., & Collins, T. (1999). *Pathologic basis of disease.* Philadelphia: W. B. Saunders.

Coulter, J. & Gleeson, N. (2003). Local and regional recurrence of vulval cancer: Management dilemmas. *Best practice & research. Clinical obstetrics & gynecology, 17,* 663–681.

Creasman, W. T. (2002). *Endometrial carcinoma.* Retrieved May 10, 2004, from www.emedicine.com/med/topic674.htm.

Dains, J. E., Baumann, L. C., & Scheibel, P. (2003). *Advanced health assessment & clinical diagnosis in primary care.* St. Louis, MO: Mosby.

Ersek, M. Ferrell, B., Dow, K., Melaneon, C. (1997). Quality of life in women with ovarian cancer. *Western Journal of Nursing Research, 19*(3), 334–350.

Ferrell, B. R., Smith, S. L., Ervin, K. S., Itano, J., Melancon, C. (2003). A qualitative analysis of social concerns of women with ovarian cancer. *Psychooncology. 12,* 647–663.

Fey M. C., & Beal, M. W. (2004). The role of human papilloma virus testing in cervical cancer prevention. *Journal of Midwifery and Women's Health, 49*(1), 4–13.

Fischer, D. S. (1996). *Follow-up of cancer: A handbook for physicians.* Philadelphia: Lippincott-Raven.

Garcia, A. A., & Bi, J. (2002). *Cervical cancer.* Retrieved May 10, 2004, from www.emedicine.com/med/topic324.htm.

Gibson, M., & Hainer, B. L. (2003, May 15). Managing abnormal Pap smears. *Patient Care,* 56–67.

Goff, B. A., Mandel, L. S., Melancon, C. H., & Muntz, H. G. (2004). Frequency of symptoms of ovarian cancer in women presenting to primary care clinics. *Journal of the American Medical Association, 291,* 2705–2712.

Guarnieri, C., & Klemm, P. R. (2000). Vulvar and vaginal cancer. In C.H. Yarbro, M. Hansen Frogge, M. Goodman, & S. L. Groenwald (Eds.), *Cancer nursing: Principles and practice.* (5th ed., pp. 1511–1525). Boston: Jones & Bartlett.

Hogg, R., & Friedlander, M. (2004). Biology of epithelial ovarian cancer: Implications for screening women at high genetic risk. *Journal of Clinical Oncology, 22*(7), 1315–1327.

Holschneider, C. H., & Berek, J. S. (2002). Vulvar cancer. In J. S. Berek (Ed.), *Novak's Gynecology* (13th ed., pp. 1321–1351). Philadelphia: Lippincott Williams & Wilkins.

Huncharek, M., Geschwind, J. F., & Kupelnick, B. (2003). Perineal application of cosmetic talc and the risk of invasive epithelial ovarian cancer: A meta-analysis of 11,933 subjects from sixteen observational studies. *Anticancer Research, 23*(2C), 1995–1960.

International Federation of Gynecology and Obstetrics. (2002). Ovarian Cancer Staging System. In F. L. Green, D. L. Page, I. D. Fleming, A. Fritz, C. M. Balch, D. G. Haller, et al. (Eds.), *American Joint Committee on Cancer Staging Manual and Handbook* (6th ed.). New York: Springer.

Jarvis, C. (2004). *Physical Examination and Health Assessment.* Philadelphia: W. B. Saunders.

Koutsky, L. A., Ault, K. A., Wheeler, C. M., Brown, D. R., Barr, E. Alvarez, F. B., et al., (2002). A controlled trial of human papillomavirus type 16 vaccine. *New England Journal of Medicine, 347*(21), 1645–1651.

Lee, C. O. (2000a). Gynecologic cancers: Part I—risk factors. *Clinical Journal of Oncology Nursing 4*(2), 67–71.

Lee, C. O. (2000b). Gynecologic cancers: Part II—risk assessment and screening. *Clinical Journal of Oncology Nursing 4*(2), 73–77.

Luce, T. L., Hassey Dow, K., & Holcomb, L. (2003). Early diagnosis for epithelial ovarian cancer. *The Nurse Clinician: The American Journal of Primary Health Care, 28*(12), 41–49.

Martin, V. R. (2000). Ovarian cancer. In C. H. Yarbro, M. Hansen Frogge, M. Goodman, & S. L. Groenwald (Eds.), *Cancer nursing: Principles and practice.* (5th ed., pp. 1371–1399). Boston: Jones & Bartlett.

Munoz, N., Franceschi, S., Bosetti, C., Moreno, V., Herrero, R., Smith, J. S., et al. (2002). The role of parity and human papilloma virus in cervical cancer: The International Agency for Research on Cancer (IARC) multicentric case-control study. *Lancet, 359,* 1093–1101.

National Cancer Institute. (2003a). *Cervical cancer (PDQ): Treatment, health professional version.* Retrieved July 1, 2004, from http://www.cancer/gov/cancertopics/pdq/treatment/cervical/healthprofessional/print.

National Cancer Institute. (2003b). *Endometrial cancer PDQ): Treatment, health professional version.* Retrieved June 29, 2004, from http://www.nci.nih.gov/cancertopics/pdq treatment/endometrial/HealthProfessional.

National Cancer Institute. (2003c). *Ovarian low malignant potential tumors (PDQ): Treatment, Health professional version.* Retrieved May 29, 2004, from http://www.nci.nih.gov/cancertopics/pdq/screening/ovarian/healthprofessional.

National Cancer Institute. (2003d). *Vulvar cancer (PDQ): Treatment, health professional version.* Retrieved November 5, 2004, from http://www.nci.nih.gov/cancertopics/pdq/treatment/vulvar/Health-Professional/page2.

National Cancer Institute. (2004a). *Cervical cancer (PDQ): Prevention, health professional version.* Retrieved July 1, 2004, from http://www.cancer.gov/cancertopics/pdq/prevention/cervical/healthprofessional/print.

National Cancer Institute. (2004b). *Endometrial cancer (PDQ): Prevention, health professional version.* Retrieved June 29, 2004, from http://www.cancer.gov/cancertopics/pdq/prevention/endometrial/healthprofessional/print.

National Cancer Institute. (2004c*). Endometrial cancer (PDQ): Screening, health, professional version.* Retrieved February 19, 2005, from http://www.nci.nih.gov/cancertopics/pdq/screening/endometrial/healthprofessional.

National Cancer Institute. (2004d). *Genetics of breast and ovarian cancer (PDQ), health professional version.* Retrieved May 29, 2004, from http://www.cancer.gov/cancerinfo/pdq/genetics/breast-and-ovarian/HealthProfessional.

National Cancer Institute. (2004e). *Hormone replacement therapy and breast cancer relapse.* Retrieved July 26, 2004, from http://www. cancer.gov/clinicaltrials/results/hrt-and-breast-cancer0204.

National Cancer Institute. (2004f). *Ovarian cancer (PDQ): Prevention, health professional version.* Retrieved May 29, 2004, from http://www.nci.nih.gov/cancertopics/pdq/screening/ovarian/healthprofessional.

National Cancer Institute. (2004g). *Ovarian cancer (PDQ): Screening, health professional version.* Retrieved May 29, 2004, from http://www.nci.nih.gov/cancertopics/pdq/screening/ovarian/healthprofessional.

National Cancer Institute. (2004h). *Ovarian epithelial cancer (PDQ): Treatment, health professional version.* Retrieved May 29, 2004, from http://www.nci.nih.gov/cancerinfo/pdq/treatment/ovarianepithelial/healthprofessional/.

NIH consensus conference. (1995). Ovarian cancer: Screening, treatment, and follow-up. NIH Consensus Development Panel on Ovarian Cancer. *Journal of the American Medical Association, 273*(8), 491–497.

NIH Consensus Development Statement. (1994). *Gynecologic Oncology, 55*(Suppl.), S4–S14.

Nuovo, J., Melnikow, J., & Howell, L. (2001). New tests for cervical cancer screening. *American Family Physician, 64*(5),780–786.

O'Rourke, J., & Mahon, S. (2003). A comprehensive look at the early detection of ovarian cancer. *Clinical Journal of Oncology Nursing, 7*(1), 41–47.

Ozols, R. F., Schwartz, P. E., & Eifel, P. J. (2001). Ovarian cancer, fallopian tube carcinoma, and peritoneal carcinoma. In V. T. DeVita, S. Hellman, & S. A. Rosenberg (Eds.), *Cancer: Principles & practice of oncology* (Vol. 2). Philadelphia: Lippincott Williams & Wilkins.

Pazdur, R., Coia, L. R., Hoskins, W. J., & Wagman, L. D. (2003). *Cancer management: A multidisciplinary approach: Medical, surgical and radiation oncology* (7th ed.). Philadelphia: F. A. Davis.

Porth, C. M. (2005). *Essentials of pathophysiology: Concepts of altered health states.* Philadelphia: Lippincott, Williams & Wilkins.

Ryan, M., Stainton, M. C., Jaconelli, C., Watts, S., MacKenzie, P., & Mansberg, T. (2003). The experience of lower limb lymphedema for women after treatment for gynecologic cancer. *Oncology Nursing Forum, 30*(3), 417–423.

Saslow, D., Runowicz. D., Solomon, D., Moscicki, A., Smith, R. A., Eyre, H. J., et al. (2002). American Cancer Society guideline for the early detection of cervical cancer. *CA: A Cancer Journal for Clinician, 52*(6), 342–362.

Sherman, M. E. (2000). Theories of endometrial carcinogenesis: A multidisciplinary approach. *Modern Pathology, 13*(3), 295–308.

Smith, J. S., Green, J., de Gonzalez, A. B., Appleby P., Peto J., Plummer, M., et al. (2003). Cervical cancer and use of hormonal contraceptives: A systematic review. *Lancet, 361,* 1159–1167.

Snyder, U. (2003). A look at cervical cancer. Retrieved April 24, 2004, from www.medscape.com/ viewarticle/ 452727.

Solomon, D., Davey, D., Kurman, R., Moriarty, A., O'Connor, D., Prey, M., et al. (2002). The 2001 Bethesda System: Terminology for reporting results of cervical cytology. *Journal of the American Medical Association, 287*(16), 2114–2119.

Steginga, S. K., & Dunn, J. (1997). Women's experiences following treatment for gynecologic cancer. *Oncology Nursing Forum, 24*(8), 1403–1408.

Tucker Edwards, Q., & Saunders-Goldson, S. (2003). Lichen sclerosus of the vulva in women: Assessment, diagnosis, and management for the nurse clinician. *Journal of the American Academy of Nurse Clinicians, 15*(3), 115–119.

Tyring, S. K. (2003). Vulvar squamous cell carcinoma: Guidelines for early diagnosis and treatment. *American Journal of Obstetrics and Gynecology, 189*(Suppl. 3), S17–S23.

U.S. Food and Drug Administration (2003, March 31). *FDA approves expanded use of HPV test.* Retrieved July 24, 2004, from http://www.fda.gov/bbs/topics/NEWS/ 2003/NEW00890.html.

U.S. Preventive Services Task Force (2004, May). *Recommendation statement: Screening for ovarian cancer.* Retrieved May 29, 2004, from http://www.ahrq. gov/clinic/uspstf/uspsovar.htm.

Uphold, C. R., & Graham, M. V. (2003). *Clinical guidelines in family practice.* Gainesville, FL: Barmarrae Book.

Wilbur, D., Wright, T., & Young, N. (2002). The 2001 Bethesda System: Terminology for reporting results of cervical cytology. *Journal of the American Medical Association, 287*(16), 2114–2119.

Zebrack, B.J. (2000). Cancer survivor identity and quality of life. *Cancer Practice, 8,* 238–242.

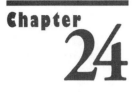

URINARY INCONTINENCE

SANDRA H. HINES
JANIS M. MILLER

The International Continence Society defines urinary incontinence (UI) as "the complaint of any involuntary leakage of urine" (Abrams et al., 2002, p. 168). As many as 58% of premenopausal women (42–50 years of age) report they have experienced symptoms of UI (Burgio, Matthews, & Engel, 1991), and 21% of working women age 18 years and older report experiencing UI at least once a month (Fitzgerald, Palmer, Berry, & Hart, 2000). However, the condition may actually be underreported to providers because of the belief that UI is not a socially acceptable health problem, and women may be too embarrassed to discuss their concerns with their health care provider. Many women mistakenly view UI as a normal occurrence that accompanies increasing age or occurs as a result of childbirth. The development of chronic UI may occur gradually over time, and this probably contributes to women normalizing it. This normalization may be supported by well-meaning comments from health care providers as well as friends and family.

The experience of UI may also be associated with feelings of anxiety and social withdrawal. It is important for health care providers to routinely inquire about UI in women of all ages because women may not initiate the discussion unless prompted. Early case finding may thwart the negative impacts UI has on women's lives. Urinary incontinence might be accurately viewed as a concern or symptom rather than a specific pathophysiology. It is important for health care providers to elucidate from the woman which type of leakage is of greatest concern, for instance, urgency symptoms versus the occasional leakage with a sneeze, as well as her desire for treatment.

ANATOMY

Understanding UI requires an understanding of the pelvic structures and their relationship to each other. For continence to be assured, bladder pressure must be lower than ure-

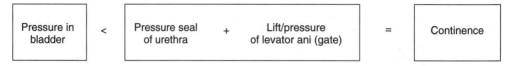

FIGURE 24–1 Continence Equation

thral pressure. In simple terms, the bladder is a reservoir, functioning as a low-pressure holding tank nearly 24 hours per day, with reversal to high pressure emptying during only a few minutes of each day. The urethra forms a tight seal of high pressure against the urine-filled reservoir. The seal formed by the urethra relaxes for only a few minutes out of each day which occurs during voiding. There is also a reinforcing gate system—the levator ani muscles, which provide holding pressure against the outflow of urine by supporting the urethra and bladder neck from below. When conditions of high load or intra-abdominal pressure occur, the levator ani form a resistive plate onto which the urethra compresses and thereby closes in response to downward forces. The interrelationship among these structures is represented in the continence equation presented in Figure 24–1 and detailed in the anatomic sketch in Figure 24–2.

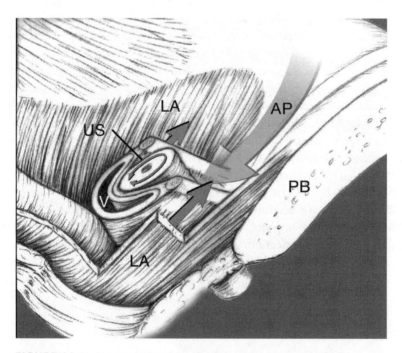

FIGURE 24–2 Interrelationship of pelvic structures to achieve continence. LA = levator ani, US = urethral sphincter, V = vagina, PB = pubic bone, AP = abdominal pressure.
Source: © DeLancey, 2004. Used with permission.

THE URINARY BLADDER OR RESERVOIR

The urinary bladder is a muscular reservoir located within the pelvic cavity and situated in women posterior to the symphysis pubis and anterior to the uterus and vagina. The urinary bladder, as it fills, expands toward the surrounding organs. Basically, the urinary bladder takes on the shape created by the pressure of surrounding structures; therefore, an enlarged uterus (as during pregnancy) or feces in the rectum impact the shape of and pressure on the urinary bladder. The wall of the urinary bladder contains the detrusor muscle, which is composed of smooth muscle fibers. The urinary bladder floor contains a funnel-shaped opening called the bladder neck, which opens into the urethra (Shier, Butler, & Lewis, 2004). The detrusor muscle surrounds the bladder neck and contraction of the detrusor muscle increases pressure within the bladder, reduces its size, and forces urine into the urethra prior to expelling it from the body. This neck of the bladder is referred to as the internal urethral sphincter/proximal sphincteric mechanism, and must be narrow to adequately hold urine in the bladder.

THE URETHRA OR THE SEAL

The urethra is a small tube beginning at the urinary bladder and ending at the urinary meatus. In adult women, the urethra is approximately 3.0 to 3.6 cm in length (Krantz, 1950). Closure of the proximal 20% of the urethra within the bladder wall (the internal urethral sphincter/proximal sphincteric mechanism) is achieved by smooth, involuntary muscles. The next 60% of the urethra includes circumferential, striated muscle under voluntary control. It is also surrounded by the urethrovaginal sphincter and compressor urethra muscles. These striated muscle structures, all under voluntary control, make up the distal sphincteric mechanism/external urethral sphincter. The most distal 20% of the urethra, ending at the urinary meatus, has minimal impact on continence. For adequate resistant urethral closure pressure to occur there must be coaptation ability (stickiness) of the mucosal inner lining, adequate tissue fullness from intravascular pressure, and both smooth and striated functional muscle structures.

PELVIC FLOOR STRUCTURE OR THE GATE

The urethra is supported by muscle and by attachment to both bony and fibrous tissues, all of which contribute to the continence mechanism (Sampselle & DeLancey, 1998; DeLancey, 1990; Ashton-Miller, Howard, & DeLancey, 2001). The levator ani muscle is part of the pelvic floor structure. The pelvic floor consists of three layers contributing to support of the internal organs located therein. The innermost layer, the endopelvic fascia, anchors the pelvic organs to the bony structure. The middle layer, the levator ani muscle, is known as the Kegel muscle. This muscle actually consists of a group of muscles that work together when contracted to lift the rectum, vagina, and urethra in an anterior direction, compressing the lumen of these structures closed. The arcus tendineus is a fibrous band extending from the pubic bone ventrally to the ischial spines dorsally and is a source of attachment for muscles making up the levator ani. With firm attachment, this complex of muscle provides a shelf of support preventing excessive descent of the pelvic organs. The most superficial layer of the pelvic floor is made up of the anal sphincter and the perineal membrane, a triangular fibrous complex that attaches the perineal body to the pubic symphysis anteriorly and serves to support the pelvic organs during defecation, urination, and birth when the levator ani muscle must relax.

To achieve urinary continence, the body must maintain support of the vesicle neck and also use the closure pressure of the sphincteric mechanisms. The closure pressure within the urethra must exceed the intra-abdominal pressure during events such as a cough, sneeze, or laugh to avoid leakage of urine. Maintaining the high position of the bladder neck is important during a cough or sneeze because the increase in intra-abdominal pressure exerted actually helps compress the urethra and maintain continence when there is a firm shelf of support. When the bladder is allowed to descend, the internal sphincter is pulled open and closure pressure to the urethra during a cough or sneeze is compromised. An additional component of the continence mechanism involves the innervation of the muscles. Without adequate innervation, the strength or speed of the contraction in the sphincter muscles may be inadequate to avoid urine leakage. Although stronger components of the continence mechanism may compensate for weaker ones, the continence mechanism is most effective when all components are functioning effectively.

CONTRIBUTING FACTORS IN URINARY INCONTINENCE

Urinary incontinence occurs for a number of reasons and is classified according to the precipitating event or mechanism. The International Continence Society emphasizes the importance of fully assessing UI relative to "type, frequency, severity, precipitating factors, social impact, effect on hygiene and quality of life, the measures used to contain the leakage, and whether or not the individual seeks or desires help" (Abrams et al., 2002, p. 168). The following sections identify factors that are important to consider when managing care of patients with UI.

FLUID INTAKE

Fluid intake, both amount and type, may contribute to UI. Some women will limit fluids when UI is a concern; however, limiting fluids may cause bladder irritation with increased urge to urinate accompanied by incontinence. Drinking large amounts of fluids also is provocative as it places an unnecessary overload on the bladder that results in either frequency or leakage.

High intake of particular types of fluids, such as caffeinated beverages, may worsen symptoms of UI. Women who experience UI are advised to eliminate caffeine intake to determine its effect on their symptoms (Gray, 2000). Similarly, alcoholic beverages, decaffeinated coffee or tea, carbonated beverages, and artificial sweeteners may play a role in urgency and frequency symptoms.

CONSTIPATION

The accumulation of stool in the rectum alters the position of the pelvic organs and presses on the bladder, thereby reducing its capacity to hold urine. Severe limitation of fluids may contribute to constipation. Fiber in the diet helps prevent constipation and decreases symptoms of UI caused by constipation.

HABITUAL PREVENTATIVE EMPTYING

Habitual preventative emptying of the bladder may result in training the bladder to hold only small amounts of urine. Some women empty their bladders on initial urge or any time a toilet is available. This practice can lead to urge sensations at increasingly lower bladder volumes. A desirable interval between urinations is three to four hours (Sampselle et al., 1997). Women who drink very large amounts of fluid may need to reduce their fluid intake to achieve this interval. Women who have habitually emptied more frequently may have to gradually retrain their bladders. Bladder retraining is covered in more detail later in this chapter.

FAMILIAL OR RACIAL INCIDENCE

Women reporting UI have a greater likelihood of having at least one immediate family member who also has UI (Giovanni, Bergman, & Dye, 2002). Sze, Jones, Ferguson, Barker, and Dolezal (2002) found Caucasian women reported UI at a significantly higher rate than black or Hispanic women (41% compared to 31% and 30% respectively).

AGE

Age-related anatomic changes may be a factor in the development of UI. Striated muscle takes longer to develop force and attains a lower maximum force as an individual ages (Ashton-Miller et al., 2001), and a significant decline in the number and density of urethral striated muscle fibers is observed with increasing age (Perucchini, DeLancey, Ashton-Miller, Peschers, & Kataria, 2002).

PREGNANCY AND CHILDBIRTH

Pregnancy, childbirth, and increased parity have long been associated with UI. Studies demonstrate the prevalence of UI in nulliparous women is lower than in parous women (Jolleys, 1988; Hunskaar et al., 2000; Sampselle, Harlow, Skurnick, Brubaker, & Bondarenko, 2002). The strength of the pelvic muscle contraction is decreased following a vaginal birth (Sampselle, 1990; Sampselle, Miller, et al., 1998). Urinary incontinence associated with pregnancy rises as the fetal size increases; however, following birth most women experience resolution of UI symptoms over the postpartum year (Chaliha, Kalia, Stanton, Monga, & Sultan, 1999; Sampselle, Miller, et al., 1998). The role of childbirth as a predisposing factor may be related to loss of support to pelvic structures or damage to structures during the birthing process.

COMORBIDITIES

Childhood enuresis, fecal incontinence, and other bowel problems are associated with UI. As body mass index (BMI) increases, UI also increases. Women who smoke cigarettes, whether currently or in the past, have a higher risk of experiencing incontinence. Many medications are associated with UI such as diuretics, estrogen, benzodiazepines, tranquilizers, antidepressants, hypnotics, laxatives, and antibiotics. Specific diseases associated with UI include diabetes, stroke, hypertension, cognitive impairment, Parkinson's, arthritis, back problems, and hearing and visual impairments. Functional impairment is also associated with UI (Holroyd-Leduc & Straus, 2004).

ASSESSMENT

Full assessment and therapeutic plans for urinary incontinence may require collaboration with numerous health care professionals. Scope and standards of practice for nurses and other health care providers working with patients diagnosed with UI are defined by the Society of Urological Nurses and Associates (SUNA, 1997).

An excellent screening questionnaire has just two questions: "How often do you experience urinary leakage?" and "How much urine do you lose each time?" (Sandvik et al., 1993). These questions help women identify and begin the discussion about UI. Answers indicating UI concerns can be followed by the 8-item Leakage Index Questionnaire developed by Antonakos, Miller, and Sampselle (2003) to specify and quantify the subjective experience of UI (Figure 24–3). In addition to the presence of symptoms, assessment of bother to the individual should be determined. A simple question about "bother" used in one study asked a question such as, "On a scale of one to five, with one being very little bother and five being very much bother, how much does this leakage bother you?" (Sampselle et al., 2000).

The most common types of urinary incontinence (Table 24–1) in women are stress urinary incontinence, urge urinary incontinence, and mixed urinary incontinence. Less common forms are continuous urinary incontinence, extraurethral urinary incontinence, uncategorized incontinence, and functional urinary incontinence (Abrams et al., 2002).

The assessment process for incontinence involves targeting the specific problem underlying an individual woman's symptoms. Once the etiology is identified, treatment follows logically in the direction of correcting the causative pathology. The equation for continence (Figure 24–1) can be used as a diagnostic guideline. The variables that contribute to the continence equation are multifactorial, with each factor potentially altering the delicate balance between bladder pressure and urethral pressure.

THE URINARY BLADDER OR RESERVOIR

High Intra-Abdominal Pressure   There are many situations that can result in high intra-abdominal pressure, which acts on the bladder and affects the continence equation. Women with asthma, bronchitis, a history of heavy smoking, or use of angiotensin-con-

Leakage Index Questionnaire

Other than the few drops right after urinating, have you involuntarily lost or leaked any amount of urine or been unable to hold your water and wet yourself?

	YES	NO
	1	0

Next is a list of things that some people say can cause them to leak urine and wet themselves. Tell me whether each one has caused you to lose urine since we last saw you [date of last visit].

	YES	NO
Coughing hard	1	0
Laughing...	1	0
Sneezing..	1	0
Not being able to wait at least 5 minutes until it is convenient to go to the toilet..................	1	0
Arriving at your door or putting your key in the lock	1	0
Suddenly finding that you are losing or about to lose urine with very little warning.................	1	0

Imagine that you are standing in the check-out line at the grocery store with a full bladder that you would like to empty as soon as possible. Now imagine that you have to sneeze or cough several times very hard. What is most likely to happen about urine leakage?

Check One

0   Stay dry

1   Leak a few drops, *or*
                 Wet underpants but not soak through, *or*
                 Possibly drip onto the floor

TOTAL SCORE
(Sum All Items)

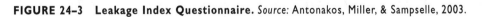

FIGURE 24-3   Leakage Index Questionnaire. *Source:* Antonakos, Miller, & Sampselle, 2003.

TABLE 24–1 Classification of Urinary Incontinence

Type of Incontinence	Definition	Description	Associated Conditions or Findings
Stress urinary incontinence	Involuntary leakage with effort or exertion, sneezing, or coughing	Involuntary leakage with effort or exertion, sneezing, or coughing	Hypermobility of bladder neck or insufficient urethral closure pressure
Urge urinary incontinence	A strong desire to urinate that is difficult to postpone	Involuntary leakage accompanied by or immediately preceded by urgency	Uninhibited contractions of the detrusor muscle, frequency
Mixed urinary incontinence	Involuntary urine leakage associated with symptoms of both stress and urge urinary incontinence	Involuntary leakage with symptoms of both stress and urge incontinence	
Continuous urinary incontinence	Continuous urine leakage	Continuous urine leakage	Extremely low urethral closure pressure
Extra-urethral urinary incontinence	Leakage of urine from areas other than the urethral meatus	Leakage of urine from areas other than the urethral meatus	Fistula
Functional urinary incontinence	Urine loss related to physical conditions outside of the urinary tract or cognitive impairment	Involuntary urine leakage related to physical conditions outside the urinary tract or by cognitive impairment	Immobility, often diagnosis of exclusion
Uncategorized urinary incontinence	Involuntary urine leakage that cannot be classified by signs and symptoms	Involuntary urine leakage that cannot be classified by signs and symptoms	

Sources: Abrams et al., 2002; Fantl, Newman, Colling, et al., 1996.

verting enzyme (ACE) inhibitors, may experience frequent episodes of coughing. Women who are trained for particular occupations such as operatic singing, lifting heavy loads, aerobic exercise, or other high-impact activities, or women who are overweight, also have high intra-abdominal pressure. Women with otherwise healthy bladders may experience leakage of urine because of their inability to compensate for such exceptionally high abdominal loads. Ultimately, there is a threshold of load beyond which all women will leak urine. Assessment to determine the underlying cause of incontinence includes identifying situations of high intra-abdominal pressure as potential causative factors. For this, the primary assessment tool is the targeted history, which includes inquiry about occupation, physical activity, smoking or other respiratory factors, and a physical assessment indicating both BMI and body habitus proportions.

For those clinicians who have specialized equipment available to them, precise measurement of intra-abdominal pressure transferred to the bladder is possible. The most common test used establishes how high the intra-abdominal pressure must be to produce leakage in an individual woman. This is known as the leak point pressure test. It is commonly accepted that leakage occurring only when pressures reach greater than 150 cm H_2O on coughing suggests that high intra-abdominal pressures are a key contributing factor to urinary leakage. It is important for the woman to validate the finding as important to her experience of symptoms. That is, following a cough test with leakage, the clinician asks, "Do you routinely cough this hard outside of the clinic setting, or undertake activities that would impose an equal level of pressure?" And, "Is this the type of leakage that you experience, and that you find bothersome?" If not, further assessment should be undertaken to determine if additional causative factors account for the leakage or bother. With treatment prioritized according to the symptom of highest concern to the woman, the goal of assessment is to mimic a natural situation that instigates leakage.

High Within-Bladder Pressure   Several situations can account for greater pressures within the bladder that act to change the balance of the continence equation. For some women, situations such as occupational restrictions beyond their control can lead to habitual overfilling of the bladder. This situation is so common that in certain occupations the bladder problem is known by the occupation itself, such as "teacher's bladder," "nurse's bladder," or "factory worker's bladder." Women who are restricted in their access to toilets can, over long intervals, train their bladders to be unresponsive to normal urge sensations. Instead of receiving mild and then progressively stronger urge sensations as the bladder fills, these women receive only a late and very strong urge sensation without adequate warning to make it to the bathroom in time. Subjectively these women present with descriptions such as unable to delay despite having a strong bladder.

A similar scenario occurs in women who drink excessive amounts of fluid. Typically, these women are acting on inappropriate information by which they believe pushing fluids is good for them and without adverse consequences. In reality, women who drink excessive amounts of fluids will also need excessive numbers of voids per day or risk suffering the consequences of incontinence from an overly full bladder.

Paradoxically, women can also suffer consequences from habitually avoiding a filled bladder. These are women with voiding intervals of every hour, who "map the bathrooms" across the city, and who live in fear of being unable to reach one in time. These women with low bladder capacity demonstrate an imbalance in the continence equation because their bladders are trained toward detrusor activation at low volumes. Known as detrusor instability, this overtriggering of the detrusor muscle results in high within-bladder pressure at unfortunate times and with accompanying leakage.

A 3-day voiding diary (Figure 24–4) is a simple and valuable tool in illuminating situations that might be responsible for increased pressure within the bladder. Although a

Instructions: Please record each time you drink fluids, you empty your bladder, you lose urine accidentally, and you perform pelvic muscle contractions for 3 consecutive days.
- "Time" columns: Be sure to write AM or PM.
- "Type" column: Write caffeinated or decaf for beverages such as coffee, tea, and cola. Other examples of beverage types include milk, juice, water, alcohol, milkshakes, etc.
- "Amount" column: Write one of the following numbers to indicate the amount of accidental urine loss:
  - 1 – leak a few drops
  - 2 – wet underpants, but not soak through
  - 3 – soak all the way through to outer clothes
  - 4 – possibly drip onto the floor
- "Urge" column: Write 'yes' if you had a sudden urge and couldn't get to the bathroom in time.
- "Activity" column: Please describe what you were doing when you accidentally lost urine (i.e., coughing, sneezing, laughing, reaching, jumping, lifting a heavy object, rising from chair, heard running water, etc.).

DATE BEGUN

_____/_____/_____

Day 1 Awakening Time: _____ Bedtime: _____

Fluids I Drank Today:			Urinated in Toilet:			
Time (AM/PM)	Type	Amount oz or ml	Time (AM/PM)	Time (AM/PM)	Time (AM/PM)	Time (AM/PM)

			Accidental Leakage of Urine:			
			Time (AM/PM)	Amount	Urge (yes/no)	Activity

FIGURE 24–4 Voiding Diary Example.

diary can be inconvenient for women to fill out, willingness is typically improved when women understand the value of the tool in providing a picture to the clinician of the daily struggles caused by bladder problems. A clinic visit devoted entirely to a review of the diary helps reinforce the message from the clinician that the diary data is truly needed and drives treatment. The following four columns of data are critical to record:

1. How often voiding occurs and of what amount
2. How often incontinence occurs and at what time of day
3. A comments section that offers a brief description of incontinence episodes and associated events
4. A column for recording type and amount of fluid intake

The diary, although certainly an assessment tool, can equally be viewed as an intervention in and of itself. A woman may not be fully aware of her own patterns and can find the self-monitoring experience to be illuminating. "I had no idea I was drinking this much coffee in a day" can be a comment frequently heard from first-time diary keepers. The diary also serves to monitor progress over time when a repeat diary is recorded later in treatment.

THE URETHRA OR THE SEAL

The factor that is perhaps most critical to maintaining a high margin of continence (urethral pressure greater than bladder pressure) is the urethra itself. This small structure is responsible for holding back a load in the bladder that several times daily reaches 300–400 ml, and can under occasional situations reach 600–700 ml of urine.

A weak urethra is highly suspected if a woman not only describes leakage with coughing, but also with bending or reaching, or says, "I just find myself wet," and is in an older age bracket. This symptom is often associated with women aged 60 years or older (Perucchini et al., 2002). Numeric quantification of urethral closure pressures can be obtained by performing a urethral pressure profilometry. However, the equipment involved is not readily accessible in general practice environments and is expensive. An estimate of urethral pressure adequacy can be made indirectly by using a simple and inexpensive paper towel to quantify urine loss during a full bladder standing stress test (Miller, Ashton-Miller, & DeLancey, 1998a). With the woman in a standing position and with a full bladder (150–450 cc), she is asked to hold a trifold brown paper towel lightly against the perineum while coughing hard. The resulting wetted area (from a few drops to saturation) of the paper towel provides an indicator of relative functional urethral closure pressure (Figure 24–5). A weak urethra is particularly suspected if the wetted area of the paper towel test cannot be reduced through intentional contraction of the pelvic floor muscles during coughing. Volitional contraction of the urethral striated muscle is possible, as it is with other striated muscle of the body. Thus, an increase in circular contractile force should occur, and does when there is adequate functional striated urethral muscle available.

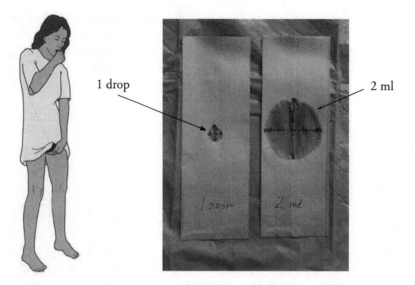

1 drop

2 ml

FIGURE 24–5   Use of a Paper Towel to Quantify Volume of Urine Loss Upon Coughing.

PELVIC FLOOR STRUCTURE OR THE GATE

Two muscles act to increase urethral closure pressure when women are asked to volitionally contract their pelvic floor muscles: the striated portion of the urethral muscles and the striated levator ani support muscles. In a healthy state, these muscles shorten under volitional contraction effort, compressing and closing the rectal, vaginal, and urethral orifices. When the levator ani is fully relaxed, the orifices are allowed to open, allowing urine, feces, and birthing babies to pass through.

Babies, by nature of their size, impose a great deal of stretching and compression force onto the levators during vaginal birth. Approximately 1 in 10 women sustain injury to the levators during childbirth that persists over time. An additional unknown portion of women sustain what is known as a paravaginal defect during childbirth that disrupts the fascial tethers to the pelvic sidewalls (Richardson, Edmonds, & Williams, 1981). In both types of injury, the muscles lose their ability to dynamically alter their stiffness in response to varying loads which results in poor support and hypermobility of the urethra and bladder, with a loss of compression on the urethra during increases in intra-abdominal pressure. This occurs at the very moment the urethral seal is most essential to preventing UI.

Women who leak urine only during a hard cough or high-impact exercise activities may have injured their levator ani muscles causing hypermobility of the urethra and resultant UI. This cause of UI is suspected when adequate urethral pressures are demonstrated. Hypermobility of the urethra can be documented with dynamic magnetic resonance imaging (MRI) or perineal ultrasound, but availability and cost of imaging equipment limits its feasibility. The cotton swab (Q-tip) measure of hypermobility can also be used. This measure of hypermobility is easy and inexpensive. The swab end is placed in the bladder, and the angle of the stick portion remaining externally is measured at rest and during straining down. A straining angle anteriorly of greater than 35° has traditionally been considered an indicator of hypermobility (Bergman, McCarthy, Ballard, & Yanai, 1987); however, more recent data suggests that strain angles up to 60° may be normative (Fenner, Miller, Morgan, Hsu, & DeLancey, 2004).

Additional evidence that hypermobility may be the causative factor includes a weak, thin, or absent pubococcygeus portion of the levator ani muscle on palpation. The levator muscles are readily palpated by placing the index finger laterally in the lower one-third of the vagina, so that the middle of the distal phalanx is hooked to right or left 2–3 cm beyond the hymen. Upon asking a woman to contract, a gross assessment of function can be obtained by estimating the response of the muscle beneath the palpating finger. A second method of assessing a weak or injured levator ani muscle is accomplished by measuring the genital hiatus or introitus while the woman strains down. The genital hiatus is measured from the middle of the external urethral meatus to the posterior midline hymen border (or perineal body if the hymen is not clearly evident). This measurement of the vagina is typically less than 4 cm in women with healthy levators. A larger measurement indicates a weakened levator support system.

A weak or overly elongated levator muscle in combination with high intra-abdominal pressure is an indication of leakage consistent with hypermobilty. The resulting leakage might be of smaller volume and again, it is important to ask the question, "Is this the type of leakage that you find most bothersome?" For some women, leakage that is of smaller volume, perhaps transient or with predictable exacerbations (for instance during a cold) and which can readily be contained by a pad may be of less consequence than the unpredictable, larger-volume leakage associated with detrusor instability.

Pelvic organ prolapse may also cause UI and therefore should be ruled out as a cause. The woman should be asked to strain down fully so that the clinician can observe the presence or absence of prolapse. The type of prolapse is not always immediately evident. If anterior vaginal wall descent is evident, it is important to determine that leakage is not resulting from a cystocele that is causing inadequate emptying. A postvoid residual should be obtained to rule out large residuals (greater than 100 cc) that may be indicative of overflow-related leakage. If a rectocele or uterine prolapse is evident, then the anatomical misalignment may get in the way of the levators' active support to the urethra. It is important to note that in some women, prolapse of the bladder may actually support continence because the urethra is kinked, comparable to bending a garden hose to reduce flow. Correcting the cystocele (surgically or with a pessary), unkinks the urethra and may worsen incontinence in selected women.

In sum, adequate treatment relies on careful elucidation of the underlying factors that cause an imbalance in the continence equation. Treatment is aimed at education about normal anatomy and correction of the underlying causative factors of the incontinence. The woman's indication of which symptom is most bothersome is critically important in the prioritization of treatment.

DIFFERENTIAL DIAGNOSIS

Urinary incontinence can be a presenting symptom of broader system pathology. Bacterial urinary tract infection, diabetes mellitus, neurological disorders (multiple sclerosis, dementia or Alzheimer's, stroke), and traumatic injury (back injury, pelvic trauma, surgical trauma) can all present initially as UI. Newer studies are demonstrating an association between depression and UI, with a possible common underlying physiologic mechanism (Melville, 2004; Nygaard, Turvey, Burns, Crischilles, & Wallace, 2003).

Urine loss should be differentiated by assessment from sweating or vaginal discharge. If there is doubt, a Pyridium test can be performed. After taking Pyridium (available without prescription) urine becomes orange or red. The woman is instructed to wear an absorbent pad and note if the wetness is red or orange which indicates the leakage is urine. If the leakage is urine, then appropriate laboratory testing, such as urinalysis or fasting blood glucose, neurologic assessment, and diagnostic testing or referral for specialized evaluation assists in ruling out underlying factors.

MANAGEMENT OF URINARY INCONTINENCE

Management of UI is aimed at reducing the factors that allow bladder pressure to exceed urethral pressure resulting in urine leakage. The impact of lifestyle, diet, fluid habits, toilet habits, constipation, coexisting disease states, and medications form the basis for initial treatment.

BEHAVIORAL INTERVENTIONS

Behavioral interventions for UI are effective alone or in combination with pharmaceuticals. Behavioral interventions are recommended as a first consideration for treatment of UI because these interventions are less invasive and lower in risk than other treatments. "Pelvic muscle training, along with education on good bladder habits in general, provides . . . women with the needed wellness intervention for a lifelong sense of control" (Miller, 2002, p. 307).

The Knack   The Knack is a pelvic muscle contraction (incorporating the levator ani and urethral striated muscle) strategically timed to increase intraurethral pressure just before and during an event that would potentially increase intra-abdominal pressure. The maneuver is taught to women as a self-help technique to intentionally increase the margin of continence enough to decrease urine leakage at any moment (for example, with a cough, sneeze, or when lifting a heavy object). The Knack can be used to reduce incontinent episodes that occur during a woman's day-to-day routine (Miller, Ashton-Miller, & DeLancey, 1998b). Steps for teaching the Knack are described in Box 24–1. Women can practice the Knack during planned maneuvers such as blowing the nose, during voluntary coughs, prior to turning on the water faucet, or upon arriving home to suppress latchkey

BOX 24–1   STEPS IN TEACHING THE KNACK

1. Confirm voluntary control: Palpate the body of the muscle bilaterally through the vaginal wall while the woman attempts a pelvic muscle contraction. You should feel a bulking up of the muscle. If not, or if she bears down (Valsalva maneuver), instruct her in an easy flick of the muscles, the same maneuver she would use to hold back gas, to see if this elicits correct isolation.
2. Maximize the contraction: The woman should be taught to contract the pelvic muscles as deeply into the vagina as she is able. In some women, this is most easily accomplished by learning a stacking contraction. Start with a small flick-and-release maneuver, then build into stacking two to three small flicks. This is commonly known as the "elevator" technique (imagined as moving from one floor to the next).
3. Begin to coordinate: Teach her to maintain a steady hold of the pelvic muscle contraction while inhaling and exhaling. Remind her to avoid the tendency to incorrectly hold her breath during the pelvic muscle contraction. The coordination maneuver eventually required is to be able to hold a contraction steadily throughout a secondary activity, such as diaphragm movement. She can practice by talking while holding, or blowing her nose while holding. As soon as she is ready, she is taught to hold the contraction during a voluntary cough, or other activity that she expects to cause leakage.
4. The final goal is habit establishment. With practice she should nearly reflexively contract the pelvic muscles just prior to any event known to increase intra-abdominal pressure or cause an unwanted urge sensation. The contraction should be held until the abdominal wall relaxes or upon completion of the event.

urgency. As skill develops, women will be ready to handle the surprise cough, sneeze, or urge sensation. An additional Knack habit is to contract the pelvic floor muscles after voiding, to reset the continence mechanism into holding mode. Women who are unable to achieve a voluntary pelvic muscle contraction or who have pelvic organ prolapse below the hymenal ring will probably be unable to acquire the skill to perform the Knack (Miller et al., 1998b).

Pelvic Floor Muscle Exercise   Pelvic muscle exercise, commonly known as Kegels, is accomplished by repetitive contraction and relaxation of the pelvic floor muscles. The goal is to increase muscle mass and strength. Kegel exercises offer rehabilitation for women with weak or injured pelvic muscles, enabling them to employ the muscles for Knack skill development. Assessment of a woman's ability to contract the levator ani muscles must be completed prior to recommending pelvic muscle training or Knack for UI. Recommending either will likely be ineffective if a woman is unable to voluntarily contract her levator ani muscles. Describing the muscle as the same one used to prevent passing gas is helpful in teaching women to correctly identify the levator ani muscles. It is important to assess that women are not bearing down (e.g., Valsalva maneuver) during the exercise practice. Sampselle et al. (1997) recommend 30 contractions of moderate to near maximum intensity each day; each contraction should be followed by at least 10 seconds of rest. Most women will notice improvement in strength and control within one month; although, three months or more may be needed to see full results that incorporate the Knack habit spontaneously.

Biofeedback is sometimes added to pelvic muscle training to facilitate skill development, particularly in the early stages. Although studies demonstrate no statistically significant difference in reduction of urine leakage between groups undertaking pelvic muscle training with or without biofeedback (Morkved, Bo, & Fjortoft, 2002), some women find the visual feedback to be motivating and reassuring. Vaginal cones may be used to help women train the pelvic floor muscles and are a form of biofeedback. Cones of increasingly heavier weights are placed into the vagina and the pelvic floor muscles must contract to prevent the cones from falling out. The effectiveness of cones appears to be similar to pelvic floor exercises performed without cone assistance (Herbison, Plevnik, & Mantle, 2002).

Bladder Training Bladder training (also known as retraining) is recommended for women experiencing urge UI ("overactive bladder" or detrusor instability). It is designed to reduce urgency and frequency of urination and treat urge UI. Bladder training may be taught to women who report urinary frequency without UI. A voiding diary should be kept and evaluated prior to recommending bladder training. It is important to consider fluid and caffeine intake because simply scaling back on the consumption of these may reduce urinary frequency.

Simple bladder retraining involves educating women to delay the first urge sensation and reassuring her that it is healthy to do so. She should be taught to contract the pelvic floor muscles as a Knack urge suppression technique and to use distraction strategies (such as counting backward) to ignore the urge. Women who do not respond to simple bladder retraining can advance to strict bladder retraining. Strict bladder retraining is thought to work by reducing frequent urges to urinate by emptying the bladder before there is an urge. The voiding diary helps to determine voiding frequency before bladder training is started. The initial interval should be one that is comfortable for the woman, which may mean voiding every 30 minutes. That interval should be followed for one week. The following week, she should increase the interval by 15–30 minutes, and empty on that schedule for a week or until that interval becomes comfortable. If the urge to urinate occurs prior to the scheduled time, the woman should attempt to delay emptying until the scheduled time (or at least delay past the initial urge). Each week (or longer if necessary to become comfortable with the new interval) she should try to increase the interval by 15–30 minutes until the interval is, on average, three to four hours between voiding. For most women, an average interval of three to four hours between voids means two to three hours in the morning, four to five hours in the afternoon, and three to four hours in the evening, assuming normal fluid intake. The scheduled voiding is only followed during waking hours. The purpose of this training is to regain control over the bladder so voiding can occur on the individual woman's schedule.

Women who take diuretics or have a high fluid intake may have to adjust their voiding to a realistic level that accommodates an increased voiding frequency. As a rule of thumb, women should aim for about one cup of urine every three to four hours and a yellow color to the urine, neither dark nor nearly colorless. Providing women with a container that fits into their toilet for urine collection to monitor color and amount of output is a valuable tool. This guideline helps monitor both intake and voiding intervals, adjusting for healthy levels.

Reverse Bladder Retraining   For selected women with urge incontinence experienced as late signaling (no urge sensation until the bladder is excessively full and signals a strong and uncontrollable urge), reverse bladder retraining is appropriate. These women show intervals of five to eight hours or more between voids, routinely report high volumes per void (greater than 300 cc), and describe themselves as having no early warning of bladder filling. Bladder training for these women involves voiding by the clock every two to three hours until normalized urge sensations can be relied upon.

ELECTRICAL STIMULATION FOR URINARY INCONTINENCE

Electrical stimulation has demonstrated efficacy in patients with stress UI and detrusor instability. It offers an additional nonsurgical treatment modality. The electrical stimulation treatments can be administered in the clinician's office or using a home unit. The units should not be used during pregnancy or in individuals with a heart pacemaker. Electrical stimulation causes the same muscles to contract as in pelvic muscle exercises. An investigation of home-managed electrical stimulation found this management routine to be practical and well accepted (Indrekvam & Hunskaar, 2002). A wide range of side effects including pain, psychological distress, and local irritation were reported, but none were deemed serious. In a randomized trial comparing intravaginal stimulation to standard therapy for stress UI and detrusor instability, electrical stimulation was found to be safe and as effective as standard therapy, but not statistically better (Smith, 1996).

Other treatments similar to electrical stimulation are available. A surgically implanted sacral nerve stimulator is available for select individuals experiencing urge urinary incontinence. Also, a chair has been developed to deliver magnetic pulses that cause pelvic muscle contractions similar to those induced by electrical stimulation.

BARRIER DEVICES FOR URINARY INCONTINENCE

Vaginal Devices for Urinary Incontinence   Vaginal pessaries are designed to support the pelvic organs as a space-filling device, replacing normal pressure on the vaginal walls when levator ani support is unreliable. Pessaries come in many forms and fitting may require a number of visits to find the correct size and type. Some women with mild stress UI may get satisfactory relief from the use of tampons with the same principle of a space-filling supportive device. Tampons should be worn for short periods to decrease the risk of infection, and they can be quite effective for exercise-related incontinence (Nygaard, 1995).

Urethral Inserts Urethral inserts designed for self-insertion and made of a soft material such as silicone are designed to provide a barrier that prevents stress UI. The insert is removed to allow voiding and a new insert is then inserted for continued protection.

PHARMACOLOGIC TREATMENT

Pharmacologic treatment for UI varies according to underlying incontinence etiology. Currently, the most effective pharmacologic treatments are available for urge UI. The main limitation in efficacy is associated with lack of selectivity for the tissues in the urinary tract.

Urge Urinary Incontinence The drugs prescribed for urge UI (also referred to as overactive bladder) belong to the class known as anticholinergic antimuscarinic agents. They target the parasympathetic muscarinic cholinergic receptor sites of smooth muscle in the bladder. The action of these drugs reduces the involuntary contractions of the detrusor muscle of the urinary bladder and increases the bladder capacity. They do not reliably increase the time between urge and emptying or the ability to suppress the urge, and are therefore most effective when combined with behavioral therapies. The most common side effects of the antimuscarinic agents include dry mouth, blurred vision, constipation, nausea, dizziness, and headaches. The drugs approved for treatment of urge UI are oxybutynin (Ditropan) and tolterodine (Detrol) with various forms including extended-release oral and patch products (Oxytrol). Flavoxate hydrochloride (Urispas) has a spasmolytic effect and was thought to be an anticholinergic, but has been shown to have no anticholinergic effect. Propantheline bromide (Probanthine) is an anticholinergic prescribed for UI as off label use (Wein & Rovner, 2002). Immediate release oxybutynin is considered the gold standard of treatment based on its long-time use, but newer formulations are reported to be as effective with a lower incidence of dry mouth, which is the most frequently reported side effect of these agents (Appell, 2002). Tricyclic antidepressants, usually imipramine (Tofranil), have been effectively used off label to decrease bladder contractions and increase bladder outlet resistance. The mechanism for this is unknown, but it is suggested that serotonin activity is increased through blockage of reuptake in the central nervous system, which may reduce bladder contractions (Wein & Rovner). Information about dosing is in Table 24–2.

Stress Urinary Incontinence Drugs used to treat stress UI are selected for ability to increase outlet resistance (urethral pressure). The drugs are prescribed for off label use. Alpha-adrenergic agonists act on the alpha1-receptor sites in the bladder neck and proximal urethra. Ephedrine and pseudoephedrine (Sudafed) are most often prescribed. Potential side effects include elevated blood pressure, headaches, dry mouth, insomnia, anxiety, nervousness, tachycardia, and palpitations (Wein & Rovner, 2002). Information about dosing is in Table 24–2. Duloxetine is an investigational oral agent acting as a dual serotonin and norepinephrine reuptake inhibitor. At the time of this writing, it has completed phase

TABLE 24-2 Pharmacologic Treatments for Urinary Incontinence

Name	Dose	Action	Side Effects	Notes
Oxybutynin chloride (*Ditropan, Oxytrol*)	5 mg tid or qid 10 mg qd (extended release) patch 2 X weekly	Decreases detrusor contractions and increases bladder capacity	Dry mouth, constipation, blurred vision, heat intolerance	Extended release formulation may have lower incidence of dry mouth.
Tolterodine tartrate (Detrol)	1–2 mg bid 2 or 4 mg qd (extended release)	Decreases detrusor contractions and increases bladder capacity	Dry mouth, constipation, blurred vision, heat intolerance	Favorable side effect profile with dry mouth, bowel, and CNS symptoms. Start lower dosing rate in elderly.
Flavoxate hydrochloride (Urispas)	100–200 mg tid or qid	Reduces spasms of smooth muscle in urinary tract, also analgesic and anesthetic properties	Blurred vision, confusion (especially in elderly)	When symptoms improve, the dosage may sometimes be reduced.
Propantheline bromide (Probanthine)	15–30 mg tid	Decreases detrusor contractions and increases bladder capacity	Dry mouth, blurred vision, constipation, confusion	
Imipramine (Tofranil)	25–75mg qd	Decreases detrusor contractions and increases outlet resistance	Dry mouth (rarely: postural hypotension, cardiac toxicity, weakness, fatigue)	Begin at lowest dose and increase 25 mg every 7–10 days as needed. Use caution in doses > 50 mg in elderly. Do not use with MAO inhibitors.
Pseudoephedrine (Sudafed)	30–60 mg tid	Increases bladder outlet resistance	Palpitations, anxiety, nervousness, hypertension, headaches, dry mouth, insomnia	Use caution in the presence of hypertension, cardiovascular disease, or hyperthyroidism. Available OTC
Ephedrine sulphate	25–50 mg qid	Increases bladder outlet resistance	Same as pseudoephedrine	Same as pseudoephedrine Not available OTC

Note: Prior to prescribing above drugs, contraindications, allergies, and drug interactions should be checked.

III trials and is under FDA consideration for treatment of UI and depression. This investigational agent has shown promise in reducing stress UI across all levels of severity (Norton, Zinner, Yalcin, & Bump, 2002).

SURGICAL INTERVENTIONS FOR URINARY INCONTINENCE

There are a number of surgical treatments for stress UI. Urge incontinence can be exacerbated by surgical intervention or may occur as a result of a surgical procedure. Surgery for stress incontinence of primarily poor urethral closure pressure without hypermobility includes bulking agents. Bulking agents are injected under local anesthesia by direct vision into the proximal urethra. Although the means by which bulking agents improve incontinence is not fully understood, they are believed to reduce incontinence by adding bulk to the periurethral tissue, which increases urethral closure pressure and improves resistance to urine outflow (Kershen, Dmochowski, & Appell, 2002). Bovine collagen is an approved injectable agent with studies demonstrating variable results. Carbon-coated zirconium beads suspended in a water-based carrier gel are also approved as a bulking agent, similar in efficacy to collagen (Dmochowski & Appell, 2003). There has been some concern about migration of bulking agents after injection. The efficacy of bulking agents may be transient, but the procedure is repeatable.

Surgical treatment for stress incontinence includes a number of variations on surgical suspensions and slings. The aim of these procedures is to support and stabilize the urethra. The tension-free vaginal tape (TVT) sling procedure is the least invasive and is typically an outpatient procedure. The current trend is to perform either a TVT, a pubovaginal sling, or retropubic urethropexy. More traditional surgeries include the Marshall-Marchetti-Krantz or Burch procedure or transvaginal bladder neck suspensions such as the Stamey-Raz or Gittes surgical approach.

REFERRAL

Many women will respond to behavioral, barrier, or pharmacologic treatments, and some may be satisfied with education about UI alone, even if their symptoms remain. A woman should be referred to an incontinence specialist or incontinence specialty clinic if management is ineffective in meeting her expectations for improvement, or if complicating factors are suspected. Some women find it difficult to identify and contract the targeted pelvic muscles and should be referred for physical therapy when the muscles are functional but very weak. Referral for electrical stimulation might be appropriate for some individuals in this population. If the muscles have clearly been injured beyond functional capacity, and stress incontinence is the dominant symptom of bother, then referral for surgical evaluation should be considered.

If at all possible, referral to an urogynecologist (a subspecialty in gynecology), or urologist with specialty practice in correcting female UI should be the priority. Education about the full scope of treatment modalities is important in the evaluation of UI and some women will choose an intervention because the results are more immediate and require less personal involvement; others prefer to exhaust the full complement of behavioral approaches before considering pharmaceutical or surgical options. It is important to recognize each individual's self-knowledge in her choice of treatment modalities.

EVIDENCE FOR PRACTICE

Urinary incontinence receives much attention from the research community, probably because it affects a large number of women. Evidence for treatment, diagnosis, and prevention continues to evolve.

PREVENTION OF URINARY INCONTINENCE

Behavioral practices have been recommended to prevent UI without evidence to support this recommendation. Diokno et al. (2004) recently reported the results of the test of a behavioral modification program using pelvic muscle training, bladder training, and education about UI. In their sample of postmenopausal women who reported zero to five days of incontinence in the year prior to entering the study, the women in the treatment group were twice as likely to have experienced no incontinence in the year of the study as those women in the control group. The women were instructed in the behavior modification program in a group setting. In addition to demonstrating the efficacy of this program in preventing UI, it demonstrates that the information can be disseminated in a group setting.

EMERGING KNOWLEDGE

New instrumentation, particularly imaging technologies of ultrasound and magnetic resonance, along with histologic and anatomic studies, are rapidly advancing understanding about the continence mechanism, pathologic factors involved, predictive variables for dysfunction, and hopes for developing improved prevention and treatment modalities. The research findings are accumulating daily and compose an arena where the literature should be reviewed routinely to keep abreast of the rapidly unfolding advancements. Along with the advancing knowledge about the physiologic and mechanical factors are new understandings of women's lived experiences of incontinence. Further development of a language and public knowledge of UI and continence-mechanism understanding is still needed. There is only beginning knowledge of how to answer the postpartum woman's question, "Why do I feel different down there, is this degree of change normal, and must I live with it?" There is even less certainty in answering, "Why does my bladder trigger unexpectedly, and will this ever completely go away?" New advances are bringing new hope and a larger body of knowledge to draw from to reduce or cure incontinence.

SPECIAL CONSIDERATIONS

ADOLESCENTS

Women of all ages should receive information about healthy bladder practices. Learning pelvic muscle exercises and the Knack (Figure 24–6) provide adolescents with tools that can allow those participating in high-impact sports to concentrate on their performance rather than potential urine leakage. These are tools they can use their entire adult lives.

PREGNANCY AND THE POSTNATAL PERIOD

Childbirth classes frequently emphasize the importance of practicing pelvic muscle exercises during pregnancy. Sampselle, Miller, et al. (1998) report that primiparous women who practiced pelvic muscle exercises during pregnancy experience reduced and early recovery from symptoms of UI during late pregnancy and postpartum over those in the control group.

CULTURE

In some religious groups, women are required to perform ritual cleansing before prayer. An episode of UI renders a woman who has cleansed to be unclean and she must cleanse again before she can pray (Wilkinson, 2001). These same women may hesitate to discuss incontinence outside of their family for concern they may be perceived as unclean. In one study, Jewish and Muslim women experienced the greatest restrictions as a result of UI (Chaliha & Stanton, 1999).

CONCLUSION

Urinary incontinence detracts from a woman's quality of life and may direct her concentration to how well her body is behaving. Women who experience incontinence become vigilant about hiding evidence on clothes and odors, and may experience a sense of losing control. Health care providers, through assessment and education, can provide the opportunity for women to discuss UI, weigh options for treatment, and make informed judgments about the basic bodily function of urine storage and emptying.

INTERNET RESOURCES:*

Collaborative to Support Urinary Incontinence and Women's Health
http://stressui.org/clinicaltools. htm

National Institute of Diabetes & Digestive & Kidney Diseases
http://www.niddk.nih.gov

American Foundation for Urologic Disease
http://www.afud.org or http://www.incontinence.org

Association of Women's Health Obstetric & Neonatal Nurses
http://www.awhonn.org

Medicine Specialties
http://www.emedicine.com/med/toppic3084.htm

American Urogynecologic Society (Information for Women)
http://www.augs.org

Some may be corporately sponsored

REFERENCES

Abrams, P., Cardozo, L., Fall, M., Griffiths, D., Rosier, P., Ulf, U., et al. (2002). The standardization of terminology of lower urinary tract function: Report from the standardization sub-committee of the International Continence Society. *Neurourology and Urodynamics, 21*, 167–178.

Antonakos, C. L., Miller, J. M., & Sampselle, C. M. (2003). Indices for studying urinary incontinence and levator ani function in primiparous women. *Journal of Clinical Nursing, 12*, 554–561.

Appell, R. A. (2002). The newer antimuscarinic drugs: Bladder control with less dry mouth. *Cleveland Clinic Journal of Medicine, 69*(10), 761–769.

Ashton-Miller, J. A., Howard, D., & DeLancey, J. O. L. (2001). The functional anatomy of the female pelvic floor and stress continence control system. *Scandinavian Journal of Urological Nephrology,* (Suppl. 207), 1–7.

Bergman, A., McCarthy, T. A., Ballard, C. A., & Yanai, J. (1987). Role of the Q-tip test in evaluating stress urinary incontinence. *The Journal of Reproductive Medicine, 32*(4), 273–275.

Burgio, K. L., Matthews, K. A. & Engel, B. T. (1991). Prevalence, incidence and correlates of urinary incontinence in healthy, middle-aged women. *The Journal of Urology, 146*, 1255–1259.

Chaliha, C., Kalia, V., Stanton, S. L., Monga, A., & Sultan, A. H. (1999). Antenatal prediction of postpartum urinary and fecal incontinence. *Obstetrics and Gynecology, 94*, 689–694.

Chaliha, C. & Stanton, S. L. (1999). The ethnic cultural and social aspects of incontinence: A pilot study. *International Urogynecology Journal, 10*, 166–170.

DeLancey, J. O. L. (1990). Anatomy and physiology of urinary continence. *Clinical Obstetrics and Gynecology, 33*(2), 298–307.

Diokno, A. C., Sampselle, C. M., Herzog, A. R., Raghunathan, T. E., Hines, S., Messer, K. L., et al. (2004). Prevention of urinary incontinence by behavioral modification program: A randomized, controlled trial among older women in the community. *The Journal of Urology, 171*, 1165–1171.

Dmochowski, R., & Appell, R. A. (2003). Advancements in minimally invasive treatments for female stress urinary incontinence: Radio frequency and bulking agents. *Current Urology Reports, 4*, 350–55.

Fantl, J. A., Newman, D. K., Colling, J., et al. (1996). *Urinary incontinence in adults: Acute and chronic management* (AHCPR Publication No. 96-0682). Rockville, MD: U.S. Department of Health and Human Services, Public Health Service, Agency for Health Care Policy and Research.

Fenner, D. E., Miller, J. M., Morgan, D. M., Hsu, Y. & DeLancey, J. O. L. (2004). What is normal? Values of pelvic floor testing in asymptomatic research volunteers. *Journal of Pelvic Medicine & Surgery, 10*(Suppl. 1), S22–S23.

Fitzgerald, S. T., Palmer, M. G., Berry, S. J., & Hart, K. H. (2000). Urinary incontinence: Impact on working women. *American Association of Occupational Health Nurses Journal, 48*(3), 112–118.

Giovanni, E., Bergman, J., & Dye, T. D. (2002). Familial incidence of urinary incontinence. *American Journal of Obstetrics and Gynecology, 187*, 53–55.

Gray, M. (2000). Caffeine and urinary continence. *Journal of Wound, Ostomy, and Continence Nursing, 28*(2), 66–69.

Herbison, P., Plevnik, S., & Mantle, J. (2002). Weighted vaginal cones for urinary incontinence [Database]. *Cochrane Database of Systematic Reviews, 1*(No. CD002114).

Holroyd-Leduc, J. M., & Straus, S. E. (2004). Management of urinary incontinence in women: Scientific review. *Journal of the American Medical Association, 291*(8), 986–995.

Hunskaar, S., Arnold, E. P., Burgio, K., Diokno, A. C., Herzog, A. R., & Mallett, V. T. (2000). Epidemiology and natural history of urinary incontinence. *International Urogynecological Journal, 11*, 301–319.

Indrekvam, S., & Hunskaar, S. (2002). Side effects, feasibility, and adherence to treatment during home-managed electrical stimulation for urinary incontinence: A Norwegian national cohort of 3,198 women. *Neurourology and Urodynamics, 21*, 546–552.

Jolleys, J. V. (1988). Reported prevalence of urinary incontinence in women in a general practice. *British Medical Journal, 296*, 1300–1302.

Kershen, R. T., Dmochowski, R. R., & Appell, R A. (2002). Beyond collagen: Injectable therapies for the treatment of female stress urinary incontinence in the new millennium. *Urologic Clinics of North America, 29*(3), 559–574.

Krantz, K. E. (1950). The anatomy of the urethra and anterior vaginal wall. *American Journal of Obstetrics and Gynecology, 62*(2), 374–386.

Melville, J. (2004, August). *Urinary incontinence in U.S. women: A population-based study.* Paper presented at the International Continence Society Annual Meeting, Paris, France.

Miller, J. M. (2002). Criteria for the therapeutic use of pelvic floor muscle training in women. *Journal of Wound, Ostomy, and Continence Nursing, 29*(6), 301–311.

Miller, J. M., Ashton-Miller, J. A., & DeLancey, J. O. L. (1998a). Quantification of cough-related urine loss using the paper towel test. *Obstetrics and Gynecology, 91*, 705–709.

Miller, J. M., Ashton-Miller, J. A., & DeLancey, J. O. L. (1998b). A pelvic muscle precontraction can reduce cough-related urine loss in selected women with mild SUI. *Journal of the American Geriatrics Society, 46*(7), 870–874.

Morkved, S., Bo, K., & Fjortoft, T. (2002). Effect of adding biofeedback to pelvic floor muscle training to treat urodynamic stress incontinence. *Obstetrics & Gynecology, 100*(4), 730–739.

Norton, P. A., Zinner, N. R., Yalcin, I., & Bump, R. C. (2002). Duloxetine versus placebo in the treatment of stress urinary incontinence. *American Journal of Obstetrics and Gynecology, 187*, 40–48.

Nygaard, I. (1995). Prevention of exercise incontinence with mechanical devices. *Journal of Reproductive Medicine. 40*(2), 89–94.

Nygaard, I., Turvey, C., Burns, T. L., Crischilles, E., & Wallace, R. (2003). Urinary incontinence and depression in middle-aged United States women. *Obstetrics and Gynecology, 101*, 149–156.

Perucchini, D., DeLancey, J. O. L., Ashton-Miller, J. A., Peschers, U., & Kataria, T. (2002). Age effects on urethral striated muscle. *American Journal of Obstetrics and Gynecology, 186*, 351–355.

Richardson, A. C., Edmonds, P. B., & Williams, N. L. (1981). Treatment of stress urinary incontinence due to paravaginal fascial defect. *Obstetrics & Gynecology, 57*, 357–362.

Sampselle, C. M. (1990). Changes in pelvic muscle strength and stress urinary incontinence associated with childbirth. *Journal of Obstetric, Gynecologic and Neonatal Nursing, 19*(5), 371–377.

Sampselle, C. M., Burns, P. A., Dougherty, M. C., Newman, D .K., Thomas, K. K., & Wyman, J. F. (1997). Continence for women: Evidence-based practice. *Journal of Obstetric, Gynecologic and Neonatal Nursing, 26*, 375–385.

Sampselle, C. M., & DeLancey, J. O. L. (1998). Anatomy of female continence. *Journal of Wound, Ostomy, and Continence Nursing, 25*, 63–74.

Sampselle, C. M., Harlow, S. D., Skurnick, J., Brubaker, L., & Bondarenko, I. (2002). Urinary incontinence predictors and life impact in ethnically diverse perimenopausal women. *Obstetrics and Gynecology, 100*(6), 1230–1238.

Sampselle, C. M., Miller, J. M., Mims, B. L., DeLancey, J. O. L, Ashton-Miller, J. A., & Antonakos, C. L. (1998). Effect of pelvic muscle exercise on transient incontinence during pregnancy and after birth. *Obstetrics and Gynecology, 91*, 406–412.

Sampselle, C. M., Wyman, J. F., Thomas, K. K., Newman, D. K., Gray, M., Dougherty, et al. (2000). Continence for women: A test of AWHONN's evidence-based protocol in clinical practice. *Journal of Obstetric, Gynecologic, and Neonatal Nursing, 29*, 18–26.

Sandvik, H., Junskaar, S., Seim, A., Hermstad, R., Vanvik, A., & Bratt, H. (1993). Validation of a severity index in female urinary incontinence and its implementation in an epidemiological survey. *Journal of Epidemiology and Community Health 47*(6), 497–499.

Shier, D., Butler, J., & Lewis, R. (2004) *Hole's human anatomy & physiology* (10th ed.). Boston: McGraw Hill.

Smith, J. J., III. (1996). Intravaginal stimulation randomized trial. *The Journal of Urology, 155*(1), 127–30.

Society of Urologic Nurses and Associates (SUNA). (1997). *Scope and standards of urologic nursing practice.* Pitman, NJ: Author.

Sze, E. H., Jones, W. P., Ferguson, J. L., Barker, C. D., & Dolezal, J. M. (2002). Prevalence of urinary incontinence symptoms among black, white, and Hispanic women. *Obstetrics & Gynecology, 99*, 572–575.

Wein, A. J., & Rovner, E. S. (2002). Pharmacologic management of urinary incontinence in women. *Urologic Clinics of North America, 29*(3), 537–550.

Wilkinson, K. (2001). Pakistani women's perceptions and experiences of incontinence. *Nursing Standard, 16*(5), 33–39.

Chapter 25

CHRONIC PELVIC PAIN

LINELL DEHLIN
KERRI DURNELL SCHUILING

Pelvic pain affects many women and is one of the more common reasons for women to seek health care (Shulman & Winer, 2004). Historically, when a woman presented with pelvic pain, the clinician automatically focused only on the reproductive organs, assuming they were the cause of the problem. This clinical "gynevision"' promoted treatment modalities that encouraged the use of a surgical approach in which organ pathology was a priority (Ling, 1995; Martin & Ling, 1999). A narrow clinical view assumes pathology and risks categorizing normal female physiologic processes as abnormal. Additionally, a number of the causes of pelvic pain in women are unrelated to the reproductive organs. Often pelvic pain is caused by multiple factors requiring clinicians to take a multidisciplinary, holistic approach to assessment and management. An appreciation for the intertwining influence of the mind and body during assessment and in planning intervention is also paramount. This approach places the woman at the center of her management plan, and respects her credibility as the authoritative "knower."

Pain in the pelvic region concerns many women because of its significance to both sexuality and reproduction (Fogel, 1995). Much of the pelvic pain experienced by women is associated with normal physiologic functions such as menstruation and childbearing; although, there are other common causes that include pathologic processes such as endometriosis and infection (Fogel). The focus of this chapter is on pelvic pain that is chronic in nature and gynecologic in origin, although some acute and nongynecologic causes, such as irritable bowel syndrome (IBS) and interstitial cystitis, will be discussed because of their significant association with pelvic pain (Rosenfeld, 2001).

DESCRIPTION AND DEFINITION

Pelvic pain is a broad term encompassing a number of etiologies, within or across body systems. Pelvic pain can be acute, chronic, cyclic, or noncyclic. Chronic pelvic pain is often so severe it adversely affects a woman's normal functioning, prohibiting her from participating in her normal lifestyle.

There is no universally accepted definition of chronic pelvic pain. For the purpose of this chapter, chronic pelvic pain is defined as "noncyclic pain of six or more months duration that localizes to the anatomic pelvis, anterior abdominal wall at or below the umbilicus, the lumbosacral back, or the buttocks, and is of sufficient severity to cause functional disability or lead to medical care" (American College of Obstetricians and Gynecologists [ACOG], 2004). It is important to note there are other widely accepted definitions of chronic pelvic pain, and a consistent definition has not been used in research (Williams, Hartmann, & Steege, 2004).

SCOPE AND INCIDENCE OF THE PROBLEM

Chronic pelvic pain is probably far more common than data from incidence reports suggest because there are various definitions for the term and because many women will not seek health care until the pain is unrelenting and debilitating, thus causing underreporting (Williams, Hartmann, & Steege, 2004; Zondervan et al., 1999). Estimates of women of reproductive age who live in the United States or the United Kingdom experiencing either acute or chronic pelvic pain range from 12–39% (Gunter, 2003; Williams, Hartmann, Sandler, Miller, & Steege, 2004). This range represents more than 9 million women living in developed countries who suffer from pelvic pain (Gunter). Of women aged 18–50, 15% to 20% have chronic pelvic pain that lasts longer than one year (ACOG, 2004). Women experiencing chronic pelvic pain are reported to use significantly more medication, have nongynecologic operations much more often, and are more likely to have a hysterectomy and reduced quality of life than women who do not have pelvic pain (Williams, Hartmann, Sandler, et al.). Clearly, chronic pelvic pain is a serious health problem for women.

Clinical data from the United Kingdom reveal that causes of pelvic pain related to the urinary and gastrointestinal tract are far more common than those caused by gynecologic disease (Zondervan et al., 1999). In fact, many women with pelvic pain have more than one diagnosis as the possible cause of their pain, and women who have multiple diagnoses related to pelvic pain have been shown to suffer greater pain than those women who have one diagnostic cause (ACOG, 2004).

Pain is an intimate experience that only the woman experiencing it can comprehend. Because pain is a subjective phenomenon it should be able to be reliably assessed from the woman's personal perspective. However, much of the literature on pain is based on the response of males to pain, and when a comparison is made between the responses of men and women, women's ability to verbalize the emotions they associate with their pain causes their responses to be viewed psychologically, and treated accordingly (Vallerand, 1995). Despite findings that identify either no differences in the experience of pain between men and women, or an increased sensitivity to pain in women, women's responses to pain are often viewed with suspicion and treated less aggressively (Vallerand).

Pain can also have a negative economic impact on a woman's life. Estimates are in the millions of health care dollars spent each year in the United States by women who have pelvic pain (Beckman et al., 2002). Many women with chronic pelvic pain are unable to work and therefore unable to contribute to their family's household income. The loss of daily functioning creates increased psychosocial stressors including hopelessness, loss of interest in sexual intimacy, and despair compounded by financial stress, all of which can lead to depression (Hornyak & Green, 2000).

ETIOLOGY

Pelvic pain generally arises from either a visceral source such as the reproductive, genitourinary, or gastrointestinal tracts, or from a somatic source like the pelvic bones, ligaments, muscles, and fascia (ACOG, 2004). Somatic pain may be superficial or deep. Superficial pain occurs when the body surface is stimulated, and deep pain originates in muscles, joints, bones, or connective tissue. Somatic pain is often described as being either sharp or dull and is usually localized. Chronic pelvic pain is often sensed as deep pain.

Visceral pain arises from internal organs and is often associated with strong contractions of visceral muscles. Visceral pain is transmitted through the sympathetic tracts of the autonomic nervous system, and is usually described as being dull or poorly localized. Nausea, vomiting, and diaphoresis are typical visceral pain phenomena (Gunter, 2003).

It is also common to classify pelvic pain as either gynecologic or nongynecologic (Carter, 2000). Gynecologic causes of chronic pelvic pain include the following:

- Endometriosis
- Pelvic inflammatory disease (PID)
- Pelvic adhesions
- Tumors (benign or malignant)
- Uterovaginal prolapse
- Physiologic causes such as mittelschmerz or menstrual cramps (Shulman & Winer, 2004)

Nongynecologic causes of chronic pelvic pain are numerous and include the following:

- Musculoskeletal
- Neurologic
- Gastrointestinal (GI)
- Urinary
- Psychiatric and psychosocial (Shulman & Winer)

Chronic pelvic pain may also result from psychologic disorders and neurogenic diseases (ACOG, 2004).

Clearly the approach to health care for the woman with pelvic pain needs to be multi-faceted. Determining the cause of pelvic pain and developing a successful treatment plan is often difficult, time consuming, and costly for the woman, and difficult and confusing, at best, for even the most experienced clinician. Many of the diseases believed to cause pelvic pain do not meet epidemiologic criteria for causality; that is, the evidence may strongly suggest such criteria as the cause, but there is not enough research yet for definitive support. This ambiguity increases the difficulty in assessment, diagnosis, and treatment of pelvic pain (ACOG, 2004). Although the causes of many disorders relating to pelvic pain are not well established, the majority of clinicians treat the condition empirically.

CLINICAL PRESENTATION

Chronic pelvic pain, as previously mentioned, has many causes and is often classified as either gynecologic or nongynecologic. Gynecologic causes of pelvic pain can be further subdivided into cyclic and noncyclic categories. Categorizing the pain into cyclic or noncyclic categories assists the clinician to assess whether or not the pain may be related to the woman's menstrual cycle. It is important to understand, however, that some cyclic pain has no relationship to the menstrual cycle and may be totally unrelated to the pelvic organs.

Women presenting with pelvic pain often have had the pain for some time and do not come for treatment until they are so negatively impacted by the pain they can no longer perform activities of daily living. Often they will describe an inability to work or function at home and describe a pain that is unrelenting.

ASSESSMENT

HISTORY

The approach to assessment and diagnosis of pelvic pain needs to be systematic and detailed for the cause to be identified and an appropriate treatment plan developed. Care must be taken during the first visit to validate the woman's symptoms and acknowledge her agency in the health care process. The importance of a meticulous health history cannot be overemphasized.

Areas of inquiry that will accurately detail a woman's health history may include the following:

- Ask her when the pain first began.
- Ask her to identify the pattern of the pain, and activities that precipitate or mitigate the pain.
- If she is of reproductive age, inquire if the pain is affected by ovulation or her menstrual cycle.
- If she is sexually active, ascertain if she has pain during intercourse.
- If pain occurs during intercourse, ask her if the pain is experienced with penile insertion, or if the pain occurs with thrusting.
- Asking her to track her pain over a period of days, weeks, or even a month may also be helpful.

Focused questioning is important for an accurate history; however, actively *listening* is absolutely essential. Valuing the woman's description of her pain and validating her feelings is paramount in developing trust and rapport. A holistic approach considers how the pain a woman describes is affecting every facet of her life. The multiple roles most women play are all impacted by pain, and obtaining information about how the pain affects her physically and emotionally, how it impacts her activities of daily living, and how it changes her relationships is important.

Pain is the common symptom shared by both acute and chronic causes of pelvic pain. The patient may describe the pain as a dull ache, sharp, stabbing, or a burning sensation depending on whether or not the pain is visceral, somatic, or neuropathic in origin. Differentiating the exact type of pain the patient is experiencing is paramount in sound clinical decision making.

The use of a pain-rating scale may assist clinicians to comprehend the intensity of the woman's pain. Subjective measurement tools are more reliable and accurate than empirically observing the quality of a patient's pain (Ignatavicius & Workman, 2002). Pain-rating scales, such as the numeric-ranking scale, visual-analog scales, and verbal-descriptive scales, allow the patient to determine the severity of the pain she experiences. If there is a language barrier related to culture or mental ability, the Wong-Baker FACES pain-rating scale (smile to frown) may be helpful (Ignatavicius & Workman). For additional information on pain-rating scales readers are referred to the general reading references listed at the end of this chapter.

Women presenting with chronic pelvic pain often do not appear to be experiencing the amount of distress that individuals with severe pain often display. This may be because they have lived with the pain for so long they have normalized it, and therefore do not present as the typical patient suffering from significant pain. Attention to posture, gait, affect, mood, and cognition are important. Substance abuse, as a pain mitigator, is unfortunately higher in women with chronic pelvic pain (Gunter, 2003). Always inquire about the use of narcotics, alcohol, and recreational drugs when assessing clients who have chronic pelvic pain. It is important to recall that pain, particularly chronic pain, can lead to depression, which should always be considered when assessing a woman who presents with pelvic pain. Depression is not the cause of pelvic pain, but it may be the result of undiagnosed, long-standing pain.

An accurate and nonjudgmental sexual history is very important. Clinicians should not allow heterosexism to blind their objectivity; a woman's partner may be female. Keep in mind that although a woman may believe she is monogamous with one partner, her partner may have other partners. Additionally, a woman may report a monogamous relationship, but fail to mention that this is her third monogamous relationship in the past year. Therefore, it is important to ask about her number of sexual partners and the possibility of her partner having multiple partners. A thorough menstrual and reproductive history also need to be obtained (see Chapter 6). Always assess for sexual abuse including intimate partner violence. Additionally, assess how this pain affects her public and private lifestyles. Pertinent family history and medical history also need to be obtained.

PHYSICAL EXAMINATION

Always obtain baseline vital signs, including blood pressure, temperature, pulse, and respirations prior to performing the physical examination. Abnormalities can signal an infection as the cause of her pelvic pain. If the woman has not had a complete physical examination in the last year, one should be performed during the first visit (see Chapter 6). Begin by examining the head, neck, cardiac, and respiratory systems to rule out abnormalities. A brief, but succinct neurologic examination, including inspection, palpation, and percussion of the spinal column can be helpful in ruling out radiculopathy. Inspection of the abdomen includes noting any scars, auscultating for bowel sounds, percussing, and palpating for organomegaly. Palpating over the area the woman identifies as the origin of the pain and pain mapping may also aid diagnosis and can be accomplished during this part of the physical examination.

Pain mapping enables clients who feel like they "hurt all over" to identify the location of their pain. Pain mapping is done by asking the client to point or specify the exact location of the pain or painful areas. Sometimes it is useful to have the client use a diagram of the body to identify the locations. It may be necessary to focus on one area at a time and move methodically to be sure all areas that hurt are identified or mapped. Clients who feel like they hurt all over are often relieved to realize their pain is localized and that other areas are not painful.

The external genitalia are inspected next. Palpate the external structures and note any edema or tenderness of the Bartholin's glands. Next palpate the pelvic floor musculature to assess for normality and to see if palpation elicits pain. A speculum examination follows inspection of the external genitalia. Be sure to visualize the vaginal wall, cervix, and if hysterectomy has been performed, the vaginal cuff. After completing the speculum examination, a bimanual examination should be performed on all patients who present with pelvic pain except for very young children (Gunter, 2003). During the bimanual examination, assess the mobility of the uterus, its position and size, and whether or not there is nodularity of the cul-de-sac. Palpate the ovaries and assess their size and if abnormal cysts are present. Finally, assess for coccygeal tenderness. A rectal examination should also be performed, noting tightness of the anal sphincter, presence of stool, fissure formation, and whether or not there is tenderness.

GENERAL SCREENING AND DIAGNOSTIC TESTING

The screening and diagnostic tests selected are based on the findings of the history and physical examination. Therefore, not all women will need the same screening and diagnostic tests. Common screening tests include the following:

- Complete blood count (CBC)
- Erythrocyte sedimentation rate (ESR)
- Urinalysis
- Pregnancy testing (if appropriate)
- Vaginal smears or cultures to rule out infection

- Stool guaiac to evaluate gastrointestinal (GI) pathology
- Abdominal or vaginal ultrasound

A laparoscopy may be needed when pelvic pathology is unable to be detected by physical examination or other testing.

DIFFERENTIAL DIAGNOSES

Pathology within systems (nongynecologic and gynecologic) needs to be considered when developing a list of differential diagnoses for pelvic pain. It is important to recall there may be more than one cause of pelvic pain, and there may be involvement of more than one body system (Table 25–1). Evaluation of the pain must differentiate between acute and chronic etiologies as well as gynecologic and nongynecologic causes (Forrest, 2004).

After all other causes of pelvic pain are ruled out, psychogenic pain needs to be considered as a possibility. Psychiatric and psychosocial disorders include substance abuse, depression, physical and emotional abuse, somatization, and hypochondriasis (Shulman & Winer, 2004).

TABLE 25–1   Differential Diagnoses of Pelvic Pain

Diagnoses of Gynecologic Origin	Nongynecologic Diagnoses
Endometriosis	**Gastrointestinal**
Chronic pelvic inflammatory disease (PID)	Irritable bowel syndrome (IBS)
Dysmenorrhea	Diverticulitis
Pelvic adhesions	Constipation
Pelvic congestion	Bowel obstruction
Mittelschmerz	Appendicitis
Vulvodynia	Colon cancer
Uterine prolapse	
Ovarian cyst	**Genitourinary**
Adenomyosis	Interstitial cystitis
Fibroids	Urinary tract infection
Ovarian cancer	Urinary retention
Cervical cancer	Renal calculi
	Musculoskeletal
	Scoliosis
	Radiculopathy
	Arthritis
	Herniated disk

COMMON GYNECOLOGIC CAUSES OF CHRONIC PELVIC PAIN

Endometriosis is the leading cause of chronic pelvic pain that is gynecologic in origin. The following are additional common gynecologic causes of pelvic pain:

- Vulvodynia
- Ovarian cysts
- Uterine fibroids
- Dysmenorrhea
- Female reproductive cancers
- Pelvic inflammatory disease (PID)
- Dyspareunia
- Some sexually transmitted infections (STIs) (Bossard & Knapp, 2004)

Testing for STIs should always be considered when assessing a woman with pelvic pain (see Chapter 18 for specific testing procedures). Another cause of gynecologic pelvic pain may be a varicosity of the ovarian vein which causes pooling of blood and subsequent pelvic congestion (Stone & Mountfield, 2003).

COMMON NONGYNECOLOGIC CAUSES OF CHRONIC PELVIC PAIN

Irritable bowel syndrome (IBS) is the leading cause of pelvic pain originating in the gastrointestinal system (Talley & Spiller, 2002). Incidence of IBS is reported to be as high as 48% in women with chronic pelvic pain (Williams, Hartmann, Sandler, et al., 2004). IBS is characterized by a chronic, relapsing pattern of abdominal and pelvic pain, and is usually accompanied by constipation or diarrhea (ACOG, 2004). During physical examination of the abdomen, areas of hard feces may be felt in the transverse and descending colon, and the rectal examination may yield the presence of a hard, lumpy stool if constipation is one of the symptoms. Women with IBS often experience bloating and general intestinal irritability. Passage of mucus rectally is common. Less frequently, women with IBS may experience blood in their stools, thus guaiac testing is important. Additional gastrointestinal causes of pelvic pain to keep in mind (although not as common as IBS) include chronic appendicitis, adhesions from previous bowel surgery, and abdominal wall hernia, including umbilical hernias.

Interstitial cystitis is the leading urinary system-related cause of chronic pelvic pain (Walling, 2002). Anterior pain that occurs when palpating the vaginal wall over the border of the bladder is suggestive of interstitial cystitis. Cystoscopy findings of petechiae or decreased bladder capacity (under 350 ml) are diagnostic (ACOG, 2004).

GENERAL TREATMENT MODALITIES

Treatment options discussed in this section will focus on gynecologic causes of pelvic pain. Enlisting the women's input in developing a treatment plan, and encouraging her to take an active role and feel ownership of the plan, is encouraged and often critical to the success of the management plan. Treatment needs to be comprehensive and may include pharmacologic as well as complementary approaches.

Exercise has been shown to be helpful with some, but not all, women who experience pelvic pain related to dysmenorrhea (Bolton, Del Mar, & O'Connor, 2003). Aerobic exercises as well as nonaerobic exercises, such as weight lifting, have shown positive results. Determining what type of exercise a woman is likely to do and encouraging that activity may be helpful in reducing the severity of the pain, especially in cases where no known cause can be found.

A number of treatments are used for pelvic pain of gynecologic origin, although not all have evidence to support their use. Tender points (areas where pain is elicited when pressure is applied) and trigger points (areas associated with pain located in deep muscles of the pelvic floor) can often be identified during physical examination. Medical treatment of these areas may include injection of a local anesthetic (ACOG, 2004). If injection at the trigger points with an anesthetic (such as lidocaine) is being considered, marking the area with a pen during the physical examination is appropriate (Gunter, 2003). Some benefit has been reported with physical therapy and the use of electrotherapy of the striated muscles of the pelvic floor combined with massage of the myofascial trigger points also located in the pelvic floor (ACOG). Sacral nerve stimulation has been found to be helpful in treating women with pelvic pain caused by voiding dysfunction.

Hormonal treatment offers another alternative and several options are available. Oral contraceptives are useful in providing relief from primary dysmenorrhea and endometriosis (ACOG, 2004). The gonadotropin-releasing hormone (GnRH) agonist goserelin may be helpful in reducing pelvic pain from endometriosis and dyspareunia (ACOG). Progestin therapy can be useful in treating chronic pelvic pain that results from endometriosis and pelvic congestion syndrome (ACOG). Nonsteroidal anti-inflammatory drugs (NSAIDs), both nonselective and the cyclo-oxygenase 2 (COX-2) inhibitors, have been shown to be useful in relieving pain from dysmenorrhea (ACOG).

Surgical intervention may be necessary and has been shown to be helpful in reducing chronic pelvic pain that is unrelieved by any other measure. When endometriosis is present, excision or laser ablation of the endometrial tissue is performed with varying success rates (ACOG, 2004). Presacral neurectomy has been useful in treating chronic pelvic pain associated with dysmenorrhea after other treatment methods have failed. Hysterectomy is, of course, a last resort, and should only be considered after other methods have failed. If the woman is of reproductive age every attempt should be made to treat her pain with nonsurgical methods before considering hysterectomy.

Psychotherapy should always be considered for a woman with chronic pelvic pain. Physical and sexual abuse is a significant cause of pelvic pain, and as many as 50% of chronic pelvic pain sufferers have experienced either physical or sexual abuse or both (ACOG, 2004). Psychotherapies found to be useful include cognitive therapy, operant conditioning, and behavioral modification (ACOG).

ALTERNATIVE AND COMPLEMENTARY TREATMENT

Alternative and complementary therapies are now much more widely accepted and available within developed countries. It is not unusual for even small towns to hold yoga and Tai Chi classes. Additionally, women have increased access to massage, therapeutic touch, acupressure, acupuncture, and reikki therapies (Blonna, 2000). Techniques such as biofeedback, hypnosis, relaxation, and desensitization have all been used to treat pelvic pain with varying degrees of success (Proctor & Farquhar, 2003). Pain causes muscular contraction; therefore, techniques that relax muscles may help to reduce some types of chronic pelvic pain. Often these relaxation techniques can be used adjunctively with a combination of pharmaceutical agents and alternative therapies (Blonna). Hypnosis has been shown to be helpful for women who are experiencing chronic pelvic pain, particularly that caused by vaginismus and endometriosis (Hornyak & Green, 2000). Knowing what is available in the community and talking with the patient to gain an understanding of what she would favor are important parts of the multifaceted approach needed to resolve symptomatology. The patient needs to be receptive to trying these measures to obtain any degree of effectiveness.

Some practitioners have used herbal, nutritional, and other forms of complementary therapy for the treatment of pelvic pain; however, the evidence base for their use is lacking (ACOG, 2004). Although these alternatives to allopathic procedures may hold promise in the future, there are no current evidence-based recommendations for their use.

CURRENT AND EMERGENT EVIDENCE FOR PRACTICE

There is strong scientific evidence (Level A) supporting the use of oral contraceptives in the treatment of primary dysmenorrhea. Progestins and gonadotropin-releasing hormone (GnRH) agonists are documented to be effective in treating pain from endometriosis and IBS. NSAIDs have been shown to be successful in treating pain related to dysmenorrhea by reducing the level of prostaglandin production (ACOG, 2004). Additionally, presacral neurectomy may be considered for treating centrally located dysmenorrhea, although its efficacy is limited in relieving chronic pelvic pain or pain that is not centrally located (ACOG).

Recommendations based on limited or inconsistent scientific evidence (Level B) include using GnRH agonists to treat chronic pelvic pain that is not caused by endometriosis or IBS. These are often tried only because they have been shown to be effective in treating pelvic pain associated with endometriosis; there is no scientific evidence to support their use for long-standing chronic pelvic pain. Other Level B treatments ACOG (2004) suggests for consideration include the following:

- Surgical adhesiolysis for adhesions other than bowel adhesions
- Hysterectomy to treat chronic pelvic pain associated with reproductive tract symptoms
- Sacral nerve stimulation
- Various physical therapies

- Nutritional supplementation with vitamin B$_1$ or magnesium for pain associated with dysmenorrhea
- Injection of trigger points of the abdominal wall, vagina, and sacrum with local anesthetic
- Treatment of abdominal trigger points by application of magnets to the trigger points
- Acupuncture, acupressure, and transcutaneous nerve stimulation for treatment of pain related to primary dysmenorrhea (ACOG, p. 11)

Recommendations identified by ACOG (2004), which are based primarily on consensus and expert opinion (Level C), include the following:

- A detailed history and physical examination as the basis for differential diagnoses
- Antidepressants
- Opioid analgesics (ACOG, p. 11)

SPECIAL CONSIDERATIONS

ADOLESCENTS

Pelvic pain in adolescents is almost always gynecologic in origin, cyclic, and not as uncommon as one would think (Hewitt & Brown, 2000). Common causes of pelvic pain in adolescents, listed in order of frequency, include those of gynecologic, urologic, gastrointestinal, musculoskeletal, and psychosocial origins (Hewitt & Brown). Interestingly, pelvic pain of gynecologic origin supersedes gastrointestinal causes, specifically IBS, within this age group. PID is important to rule out as a cause of pelvic pain in adolescents because it is so commonly diagnosed in this age group. Rarely do adolescents present with pelvic pain that is chronic. Estimates of the percentage of adolescent women presenting with chronic pelvic pain are absent from the literature.

Adolescents, because of their emotional and physical development, pose challenges to clinicians that are different from that of women in their twenties and beyond. Developing a rapport with any teenager may be the biggest challenge facing the clinician working with this age group. Suggestions for developing a rapport include maintaining eye contact, using a nonjudgmental attitude, treating her with respect, and giving her undivided attention. It is important to validate her symptoms and the feelings she associates with them.

It is important to be familiar with state and local statutes regarding health care for minors. Many states have parental consent laws. Each practice needs to have its own policy that must follow the legal parameters already in place.

CULTURE

Knowing and appreciating the cultural background of a patient is significant. Cultural and social stratification influences decision making for both patient and clinician, as well as treatment options. Should the clinician be shaking hands, making eye contact, or addressing the patient directly? Or if her husband is present, does the couple's culture dictate that the clinician include him in the conversation as well? How close should the clinician stand or sit when taking a history? These are all culturally significant questions to consider. Also, women of different cultures express pain differently. The expression of pain may vary from stoicism to wailing (Luckmann, 1999). Validating a patient's feelings, and recognizing and appreciating her cultural and ethnic background is important, not only to gaining her trust and establishing rapport, but also in helping the clinician understand the scope of the problem the woman presents.

REFERENCES

American College of Obstetricians and Gynecologists. (2004, March). *Chronic pelvic pain: Clinical management guidelines for obstetrician-gynecologists.* Practice bulletin 51. Washington, DC: Author.

Beckman, C. R., Ling, F. W., Laube, D. W., Smith, R. P., Barzansky, B. M., & Herbert, W. N. (2002). *Obstetrics and gynecology* (4th Ed.). Philadelphia: Lippincott, Williams & Wilkins.

Blonna, R. (2000). *Coping with stress in a changing world* (2nd ed.), New York: McGraw Hill.

Bolton, P., Del Mar, C., & O'Connor, V. (2003). *Exercise for primary dysmenorrhea.* (The Cochrane Library). Retrieved February 28, 2004, from http://www.gateway2.ovid.com.

Bossard, S., & Knapp, B. (2004). When to suspect pelvic inflammatory disease. *Emergency Medicine, 36,* 45–50.

Carter, J. F. (2000). Nongynecologic causes of chronic pelvic pain. *Female Patient, 25,* 33–37.

Fogel, C. I., & Woods, N. F. (1995). *Women's health care.* Thousand Oaks, CA: Sage.

Fogel, C. I. (1995). Common symptoms. In C. I. Fogel & N. F. Woods (Eds.), *Women's health care. A comprehensive handbook (pp. 517-570).* Thousand Oaks, CA: Sage.

Forrest, D. E. (2004). Common gynecologic pelvic disorders. In E. Youngkin & M. Davis (Eds.), *Women's health* (3rd. ed., pp. 303–350). Upper Saddle River, NJ: Pearson Prentice Hall.

Gunter, J. (2003). Chronic pelvic pain: An integrated approach to diagnosis and treatment. *Obstetrical & Gynecological Survey, 58,* 615–623.

Hewitt, G. D., & Brown, R. T. (2000). Chronic pelvic pain in the adolescent. *The Female Patient, 84*(4), 1009–1025.

Hornyak, L. M., & Green, J. P. (Eds.). (2000). *Healing from within: The use of hypnosis in women's health care,* Washington, DC: American Psychological Association.

Ignatavicius, D., & Workman, M. (2002). *Medical-surgical nursing: Critical thinking for collaborative care.* Philadelphia: W. B. Saunders.

Ling, F. (1995). Pelvic pain. In D. Nichols & P. Sweeney (Eds.), *Ambulatory gynecology* (pp. 200–212). Philadelphia: JB Lippincott.

Luckmann, J. (1999). *Transcultural communication in nursing.* New York: Delmar.

Martin, D., & Ling, F. (1999). Endometriosis and pain. *Clinical Obstetrics and Gynecology, 42*(3), 664–86.

Proctor, M. L., & Farquhar, C. M. (2003 June). Dysmenorrhea. *Clinical evidence* (9): 1994–2013.

Rosenfeld, J. A. (2001). Chronic pelvic pain, dysmenorrhea, and dyspareunia. In J. A. Rosenfeld (Ed.), *Handbook of women's health* (pp. 292–305). UK: Cambridge University Press.

Shulman, L. P., & Winer, S. (2004). Chronic pelvic pain. *The Forum 1,* 12–17.

Stone, R. W., & Mountfield, J. (2000). Interventions for treating chronic pelvic pain in women [Database]. *Cochrane Database of Systematic Reviews, 4*(No. CD000387).

Talley, N. J., & Spiller, R. (2002). Irritable bowel syndrome: A little understood organic bowel disease? *Lancet, 360,* 555–564.

Vallerand, A. (1995). Gender differences in pain. *Image: Journal of Nursing Scholarship, 27,* 235–237.

Walling, A. D. (2002). Chronic pelvic pain? Think interstitial cystitis. *American Family Physician, 66,* 1976.

Williams, R., Hartmann, K., Sandler, R., Miller, W., & Steege, J. (2004). Prevalence and characteristics of irritable bowel syndrome among women with chronic pelvic pain. *The American College of Obstetrics & Gynecology, 104*, 452–458.

Williams, R., Hartmann, K., & Steege, J. (2004). Documenting the current definitions of chronic pelvic pain: Implications for research. *The American College of Obstetrics and Gynecology, 103*, 686–691.

Zondervan, K., Yudkin, P., Vessey, M., Dawes, M., Barlow, D., & Kennedy, S. (1999). Prevalence and incidence of chronic pelvic pain in primary care: Evidence from a national general practice database. *British Journal of Obstetrics & Gynecology, 106*(11), 1149–55.

GENERAL REFERENCES FOR FURTHER READING

Bolton, R. J., & Wilkinson, R. (1998). Responsiveness of pain scales: A comparison of three pain intensity measures in chiropractic patients. *Journal of Manipulative & Physiological Therapeutics, 21*, 1–7.

Brown, C., Ling, F., Wan, J., & Pilla, A. (2002). Efficacy of static magnetic field therapy in chronic pelvic pain: A double-blind study. *American Journal of Obstetrics & Gynecology, 187*, 1581–7.

Haggerty, C., Schulz, R., & Ness, R. (2003). Lower quality of life among women with chronic pelvic pain after pelvic inflammatory disease. *American Journal of Obstetrics & Gynecology, 102*, 934–939.

Larroy, C. (2002). Comparing visual-analog scales and numeric scales for assessing menstrual pain. *Behavioral Medicine, 27*, 179–81.

Morgan, M. (2002). Pain: The fifth vital sign. In D. Ignatavicius & M. Workman (Eds.), *Medical-surgical nursing: Critical thinking for collaborative practice* (pp. 61–94). Philadelphia: W. B. Saunders.

Index

About the Contributors

Alida D. Alden received her BSN from Aurora University and is a master's student at Johns Hopkins University School of Nursing. She is certified as a sexual assault nurse examiner-adult/adolescent (SANE-A) and works in emergency and critical care.

Ivy M. Alexander is an associate professor at the Yale University School of Nursing and director of the Adult, Family, Gerontological, and Women's Health Primary Care Specialty. She is also a practicing clinician in the Internal Medicine Department of the Yale University Health Services. Dr. Alexander received her bachelor of science in nursing from Pennsylvania State University, her master of science degree from Northeastern University, a post-master's certificate in teaching from the University of Pennsylvania, and her PhD from the University of Connecticut. She has practiced as a nurse practitioner in internal medicine with a focus on women's health since 1992. Dr. Alexander has published numerous articles concerning women's health, is active in several state and national organizations, and is regularly invited to speak at national meetings. Her primary interest is menopause and midlife health issues, and she is currently conducting research focusing on menopause experiences and midlife health perceptions among black women.

Heather M. Aliotta obtained her master's degree in nursing from the MGH Institute of Health Professions in Boston, Massachusetts. She is a member of the multidisciplinary team of breast oncology specialists at the Gillette Center for Women's Cancers of the Massachusetts General Hospital. Her collaborating physician is a breast surgeon. Ms. Aliotta's research interests include menopausal symptom management, breast cancer risk reduction, and breast cancer screening test evaluation. She is an item writer for the NCC Women's Health Care Nurse Practitioner Certification Examination.

Christine L. Anderson received her undergraduate education at Penn State University in University Park, Pennsylvania, with a bachelor of science in human development and family studies. In 2000, she graduated from the MGH Institute of Health Professions in Boston, Massachusetts, where she received her master of science in nursing. She is dually certified by NCC and ANCC as both a women's health care nurse practitioner and an adult nurse practitioner. She has been employed by Planned Parenthood League of Massachusetts in Boston, Massachusetts, and Planned Parenthood of the Rochester/Syracuse Region in Rochester, New York. Her clinical interests focus on women's reproductive health care and women's reproductive endocrinology. A new mother, she plans to take a short break from clinical practice to focus on her family.

Linda C. Andrist received her PhD in sociology at Brandeis University, her WHNP from the University of Colorado Health Sciences Center, her MS from Russell Sage College, her BSN from the University of Maryland, and her diploma from Johns Hopkins School of Nursing. She has over 25 years of experience in women's health nursing. She has done research and published on women's decisions about taking hormone therapy. Her current area of scholarship is focused on the media, body image disturbance, chronic dieting, and overeating. She practices as an NP in a reproductive health clinic.

Linda A. Bernhard received her nursing education in Minnesota, Iowa, California, and Illinois. She has been teaching nursing for nearly 30 years. Currently she holds a joint appointment in nursing and women's studies at The Ohio State University, where she teaches courses in women's health, sexuality, lesbian studies, adult health nursing, and nursing research. Her principal research interest has been women's experiences of hysterectomy and menopause, as well as understanding conditions that often result in hysterectomy. She has also conducted research on lesbian health.

Jacquelyn C. Campbell received her BSN from Duke University, her MSN from Wright State University, and her PhD from the University of Rochester. Dr. Campbell's overall research and policy initiatives are in the area of family violence and violence against women, with continuous research funding since 1984 from NIH (NINR, NIDA, NIMH), NIJ, CDC, and DOD. Dr. Campbell was principal investigator on many studies of battering, including three funded by NIH, two by the CDC, one by the Department of Defense, and one by the National Institute of Justice. Specific research areas include risk factors and assessment for intimate partner homicide, abuse during pregnancy, marital rape, physical and mental health effects of intimate partner violence, prevention of dating violence, and interventions to prevent and address domestic violence. Her research results are used as the basis of health policy recommendations to state, national, and international organizations. Dr. Campbell's awards include Fellowship in the American Academy of Nursing, the Kellogg National Leadership Program, a Robert Wood Johnson Urban Health Fellowship, three honorary doctorates, the Simon Visiting Scholar at the University of Manchester in the UK, and elected membership in the Institute of Medicine. She has authored or co-authored more than 125 articles and chapters, mainly about battered women and family violence. She is author, co-author, or editor of 5 books: *Nursing Care of Survivors of Family Violence; Sanctions and Sanctuary: Cultural Perspectives on the Beating of Wives,* which has been updated with the new title *To Have and To Hit; Assessing Dangerousness: Violence by Sexual Offenders, Batterers and Child Abusers; Ending Domestic Violence: Changing Public Perceptions/Halting the Epidemic;* and *Empowering Survivors of Abuse: Health Care for Battered Women and their Children,* as well as the forthcoming *Family Violence in Nursing Practice.* Dr. Campbell also has been working with wife abuse shelters and advocacy organizations for the last 25 years, including leading support groups and serving on four shelter boards. Currently, she is on the board of directors of the Family Violence Prevention Fund in San Francisco, the House of Ruth in Baltimore, and has served on the congressionally appointed Department of Defense Task Force on Domestic Violence.

Katherine Camacho Carr is an associate professor at Seattle University College of Nursing, where she teaches in the graduate Master of Science in Nursing Program. She also works as a nurse-midwife at Highline Midwifery and Women's Health, providing care to a diverse and primarily low income group of women. Additionally, Dr. Carr serves as the current ACNM president. Dr. Carr received her BSN (1971) from Loyola University, her MS and CNM from the University of Illinois (1974), and her PhD from the University of Washington (1989). Dr. Carr has served as faculty, teaching research in the midwifery education program at the State University of New York, Health Science Center at Brooklyn, Institute of Midwifery, Women and Health (IMWAH), and the Frontier School of Midwifery and Family Nursing, Community-based Nurse-midwifery Education Program. Dr. Carr is a noted expert in curriculum design/evaluation and is frequently a curriculum consultant for distance education. Dr. Carr's research focus is barriers to midwifery education.

Susan Chasson completed her MSN and midwifery education at the University of Utah in 1991 and a family nurse practitioner certificate program at the State University of New York, Stony Brook in 2001. She practiced full-scope nurse-midwifery for 13 years and is presently providing primary care to women at the Utah Valley Family Practice Center in Provo, Utah. Ms. Chasson received a Juris Doctorate from Brigham Young University in 1996. She lectures in both J. Reuben Clark Law School and the College of Nursing at Brigham Young University. This combination of nursing and law resulted from a desire to advocate for women and children who are victims of violence. She is a sexual assault nurse examiner and has worked to create programs to serve victims of interpersonal violence throughout Utah. In 2001 she received the Robert Wood Johnson Community Health Leadership Award for her efforts to develop health care services for women and children who are victims of sexual abuse and assault.

Linell Dehlin is a full-time nurse educator at Bay de Noc Community College, where she teaches didactic and clinical nursing courses along with pharmacology to students pursuing their associate degree in nursing. Ms. Dehlin received her diploma in nursing from Harper Hospital School of Nursing (1973), and her BSN and MSN from Northern Michigan University (1992 and 1996). Additionally, she received her certificate in women's health from Planned Parenthood of Wisconsin (1994). Prior to her current position, Ms. Dehlin worked in the capacity of a nurse practitioner for many years at her local health department, serving women ranging in age from 14–80. Her experience also includes pre- and postnatal care in a private clinic setting. Her mission is to encourage her students to feel empowered through education and their own personal growth to make healthy lifestyle choices.

Mary Ann Faucher is a certified nurse-midwife who has been practicing midwifery in the Dallas community for the last 15 years. Dr. Faucher received two master's degrees from Columbia University in New York City, a master of science and a master of public health. Her doctorate is in health behavior and health education from Texas Women's University. She has taught in graduate education for 15 years, specifically teaching in nurse-midwifery and women's health at U.T. Southwestern Medical Center and Parkland Hospital in Dallas. Dr. Faucher recently joined the faculty in the School of Nursing at Baylor in Dallas, Texas. Mary Ann is a nationally sought after speaker and is widely published. Her research interests include evidence-based practice; adolescent risk behaviors, specifically smoking in young women; cardiovascular health and prevention in women; and environmental exposures and implications for women's health. As a member of the Association of Women's Health, Obstetric, and Neonatal Nurses (AWHONN), Dr. Faucher was the team leader and lead author of an evidence-based practice guideline for the primary prevention of cardiovascular disease in women. She is also an associate editor of the *Journal of Midwifery and Women's Health.*

Linda A. Fernandes received her BSN from the University of Pittsburgh and is currently a master's student at Johns Hopkins University School of Nursing. She is a sexual assault forensic examiner at Howard County General Hospital in Columbia, Maryland.

Catherine Ingram Fogel received her BSN and MS from the University of North Carolina at Chapel Hill, and a PhD in sociology with a minor in women's studies from North Carolina State University. Her clinical practice experience includes conducting a prenatal clinic for women at high risk for preterm delivery for 14 years. She is currently conducting socio-behavioral preventive research at a major women's prison in the Southeast, which is also her clinical practice site. She is the author of several books on women's health care and is the author of numerous chapters and refereed articles.

Sandra H. Hines is a doctoral candidate at the University of Michigan School of Nursing, specializing in women's health. She received her BSN from Eastern Michigan University School of Nursing and her MS from the University of Michigan School of Nursing. Her clinical practice experience includes inpatient surgery, labor and delivery, postpartum and gynecology, and outpatient work as a nurse practitioner in women's health. Her research in urinary incontinence includes prevention in post-menopausal women and the psychosocial aspects of seeking treatment for urinary incontinence.

Nancy J. Hughes received her master of science degree in nurse-midwifery from Case Western Reserve University. Currently she is serving in the US Army Nurse Corps as the director of nursing for OB/GYN, pediatrics, and family medicine at Tripler Army Medical Center (TAMC), Hawaii. She also serves as the consultant to the Army Surgeon General for women's health advanced practice nursing issues. While working as the nursing director, Lieutenant Colonel (LTC) Hughes continues to practice midwifery, is adjunct faculty for the army medical department's OB/GYN nursing course, and stays actively involved in research. LTC Hughes has spent 20 years as an active duty officer serving as an OB/GYN nurse at Ft. Knox, Kentucky; Ft. Leavenworth, Kansas; and Supreme Headquarters Allied Powers Europe, Belgium. After completing her masters degree in nurse-midwifery, she served as a certified nurse-midwife at Ft. Hood, Texas; Ft. Belvoir, Virginia; and TAMC, Hawaii. LTC Hughes has been active in many projects throughout her years in obstetrics and women's health, including childbirth education, implementing uncomplicated pregnancy clinical practice guidelines and a family centered care curriculum, teaching in several general medical education programs, pursuing a multimillion-dollar renovation project for LDRs at TAMC, and doing research in the area of family violence.

Holly Powell Kennedy obtained her master's degree as a family nurse practitioner at the Medical College of Georgia, her certificate in midwifery from the Frontier School of Midwifery and Family Nursing, and her doctoral degree from the University of Rhode Island. She is currently the co-director of the UCSF/SFGH Interdepartmental Nurse-Midwifery Education Program. She chairs the ACNM Division of Research and is the co-chair of the Research Standing Committee of the International Confederation of Midwives. Dr. Kennedy is a well known researcher and international speaker on the processes and outcomes of midwifery care. She is currently conducting a clinical trial on Centering Pregnancy, a model of group prenatal care, funded by the TriService Nursing Research Program at two military community hospitals. She has published and presented on evidence-based practice.

Suzanne M. Leclaire received her master of science degree in nursing from Grand Valley State University, Michigan; and master in health care systems from Denver University, Colorado. She retired from the United States Army Reserves in 1997 as a Lieutenant Colonel after serving more than 29 years in the military's Nurse Corps, following numerous overseas deployments to Viet Nam, Saudi Arabia, and Germany. Her civilian career has encompassed research, administrative, and clinical roles in the fields of obstetrics and gynecology, pediatrics, psychiatry, adult medical and surgical nursing, health care contract administration, case management, and home health care. She was an assistant professor at Ferris State University in Michigan, where she taught nursing. Currently, Ms. Leclaire is a case manager at Tripler Army Medical Center and manages predominately head and neck oncology patients. Her research interests have been in the fields of women's health and osteoporosis prevention. An avid traveler and humanitarian, Ms. Leclaire has been involved in health care missions to Miraflor, Nicaragua, as part of a Nursing Center for Global Health Program.

Frances E. Likis received her BS and MSN from Vanderbilt University, and her nurse-midwifery and women's health care nurse practitioner certificates from the Frontier School of Midwifery and Family Nursing. She is certified as a family nurse practitioner, nurse-midwife, and women's health care nurse practitioner. Her clinical experience includes family practice in community health and urgent care centers, performing sexual assault examinations, and midwifery practice in a freestanding birth center and a large obstetrics and gynecology group practice. She is currently the women's health course coordinator at the Frontier School of Midwifery and Family Nursing. She is also a doctoral student at the University of North Carolina at Chapel Hill School of Public Health, where she is the recipient of a Caroline H. and Thomas S. Royster, Jr. Fellowship awarded for academic potential and record of achievement. She is an associate editor of the *Journal of Midwifery and Women's Health* and a reviewer for *Obstetrics and Gynecology.* She has authored articles in the *Journal of Midwifery and Women's Health, The Nurse Practitioner,* and the *Journal of Obstetric, Gynecologic, and Neonatal Nursing* as well as book chapters. She is a frequent speaker both locally and nationally and is an active participant in professional organizations. Her primary areas of interest are contraception and the challenges of implementing evidence-based clinical practice.

Lisa Kane Low received her BSN in nursing from the University of Michigan, her master's degree from the University of Illinois at Chicago in midwifery, and her doctoral degree in women's health from the University of Michigan with a graduate certificate in women's studies. She was also a NIH-BIRCWH (Building Interdisciplinary Research Centers in Women's Health) scholar from 2001–2003. Lisa has worked in full scope clinical practice at Hutzel Hospital in Detroit, Michigan, and more recently at the University of Michigan Nurse-Midwifery Service. She teaches in the women's studies program and conducts research within the School of Nursing at the University of Michigan. Her research focus has been on the role of social support and selected care practices during labor on the optimal perinatal outcomes, including the social and emotional experience of childbirth. She has focused on the experience of childbirth for women from vulnerable populations, including adolescents. She has also conducted international work exploring the transitions in models of maternity care including the use of traditional birth attendants, birth centers, and combined systems of care.

Janis M. Miller is an assistant research scientist in the School of Medicine, Department of Obstetrics and Gynecology, and the School of Nursing at the University of Michigan, Ann Arbor. Dr. Miller is also a nurse practitioner at Taubman OB/GYN Incontinence Clinic at the University of Michigan. She received her MSN from Loyola University in Chicago, Illinois, and a PhD (nursing) and a gerontology postdoctoral fellowship from the University of Michigan. Her professional research interests include the structure and function of the levator ani muscle group in women with pelvic organ prolapse, the prevention of urinary incontinence (UI) during childbirth, and the epidemiology and biology of female UI. She has been a principal investigator or co-investigator in many research projects. A noted authority on UI, Dr. Miller has published works in several journals, including *Journal of Obstetrics and Gynecology, Journal of the American Geriatrics Society, Urologic Nursing, Journal of Women's Health,* and *Journal of Wound, Ostomy and Continence Nursing (JWOCN).* In 2003, she was the recipient of the *JWOCN* Publisher's Manuscript of the Year Award and the International Continence Society's Best Clinical Abstract Award. An accomplished speaker, Dr. Miller has been an invited lecturer and presenter at many conferences and special university courses, and has authored refereed papers presented throughout the United States and abroad.

Katherine Morgan received her BS and MSN from the University of Utah. She is also a graduate of the Harbor-UCLA Nurse Practitioner Program. She practices at Birthcare-Healthcare in Salt Lake City, Utah and at Planned Parenthood, where she was formerly the assistant medical director.

Patricia Aikins Murphy is a graduate of the Pace University School of Nursing. She received her nurse-midwifery education at Columbia University, and holds a doctorate in public health (epidemiology) from the Mailman School of Public Health at Columbia University. Dr. Murphy was on the faculty of the Columbia University School of Nursing from 1991 through 1997, where she taught in the nurse-midwifery and doctoral programs. She was a research scientist in the Department of Obstetrics & Gynecology of Columbia's College of Physicians and Surgeons from 1997 through 2004, where she practiced in the family planning clinic and conducted research about contraception. Her research background includes clinical trials of new contraceptive methods, as well as investigator-initiated studies of contraceptive management options. She is an active member of ACNM, ARHP, and APHA, and speaks frequently on topics related to contraception and women's health. Currently she is an associate professor in the University of Utah College of Nursing, where she is the first recipient of the Annette Poulson Cumming Presidential Endowed Chair in Women's and Reproductive Health.

Deborah Narrigan completed the University of Kentucky's Graduate Program in Nurse-Midwifery in 1980 and since then has practiced midwifery with underserved women in Nashville, Tennessee, in a variety of public sector positions. She has held several educational positions, including directing the Perinatal Clinical Nurse Specialist Program at Vanderbilt University; coordinating the newborn courses for the Community-based Nurse-midwifery Education Program in Hyden, Kentucky; and acting as a short term advisor on curriculum development for the American College of Nurse-Midwives in the PRIME Project in Indonesia. Most recently she has taught the Introduction to Health Policy Course for the distance education Graduate Program in Midwifery at Philadelphia University. She is currently a member of the Center for Reducing Asthma Disparities at Meharry Medical College in Nashville, Tennessee, where she is working on a National Institutes of Health clinical study examining interventions to improve health outcomes during pregnancy for women of color with asthma.

Ellen Olshansky is chair of the Department of Health and Community Systems at the University of Pittsburgh School of Nursing. She earned a BA from the University of California, Berkeley, and a BSN, MSN, and DNSc from the University of California, San Francisco. Her research focuses on emotional aspects of infertility, with a recent emphasis on the co-morbidity of infertility and depression in women. She counsels infertile individuals and couples. Dr. Olshansky is currently developing a group psychotherapy intervention for depressed infertile women. She is also interested in pregnancy and parenting after infertility, and menopause after infertility. She has expertise in qualitative research, specifically grounded theory and dimensional analysis. She teaches a doctoral level qualitative methods course, which is open to students in nursing and other disciplines. She was a member of the executive board of the American Orthopsychiatric Association. She participated in the Relational Research Group of the Jean Baker Miller Training Institute at the Stone Center at Wellesley College, as well as the Practitioners Program at that Institute. She is active in the Eastern Nursing Research Society; Association of Women's Health, Obstetrics, and Neonatal Nurses; and Sigma Theta Tau International. Dr. Olshansky is editor of the *Journal of Professional Nursing*, the official journal of the American Association of Colleges of Nursing (AACN).

Kathryn Osborne received her master of science in nursing from Case Western Reserve University and her midwifery certificate from the Frontier School of Midwifery and Family Nursing (FSMFN). She is noted for her outstanding teaching acumen and has been the recipient on more than one occasion of the Faculty Excellence in Teaching Award from the FSMFN. In addition to holding a faculty appointment with the FSMFN, she is in full scope nurse-midwifery practice with the Aurora UW Nurse-Midwifery Center in Milwaukee, Wisconsin. Clinical interests include public health and health promotion for women throughout the lifespan.

Anna Sanford received her BSN and MSN from Wayne State University. She is an adult nurse practitioner certified as an advanced oncology certified nurse with 25 years of experience in oncology nursing in medical and radiation oncology. She is now a full-time faculty member at Northern Michigan University, where she teaches in both the undergraduate BSN program and the graduate FNP program and maintains a part-time clinical practice in an outpatient community clinic for uninsured adults. Her current clinical interests include gerontology and palliative care.

Nancy J. Schaeffer received her BSN from Salem State College and her MSN and NP education from the Massachusetts General Hospital (MGH) Institute of Health Professions. Her clinical interest is breast cancer. She was the first nurse practitioner in oncology at MGH and established a practice model with her supervising physician. There are now 25 nurse practitioners in the MGH Cancer Center. She is currently co-chair of the Advanced Practice Oncology Group. Her experience in oncology includes 13 years in surgical oncology and 12 years in medical oncology, 9 of which have been as a nurse practitioner. She is the co-author of articles on enteral nutrition, Hickman catheter, hepatic artery infusion pumps, and early discharge post modified mastectomy. Her video productions include patient information for port-a-cath and implantable infusion pump refill procedure.

Kerri Durnell Schuiling has been an advanced practice nurse and educator for over 27 years. She holds a master's degree in advanced maternity nursing from Wayne State

University, and a PhD in nursing and graduate certificate in women's studies from the University of Michigan. Kerri received her nurse practitioner education from Planned Parenthood Association of Milwaukee, Wisconsin, and her nurse-midwifery education from the Frontier School of Midwifery and Family Nursing. She is dually certified as a WHCNP and CNM. She has presented nationally on the subject of abnormal uterine bleeding, and as a member of the American College of Nurse-Midwives (ACNM) Clinical Practice Committee, assisted in the development of two clinical bulletins related to abnormal uterine bleeding. She has been an item writer for the NCC certification examination for women's health care nurse practitioners and currently is a peer reviewer for the *Journal of Midwifery and Women's Health* and the *Journal of Professional Nursing*. She has received numerous awards for her work including a Clinical Merit Award from the University of Michigan for outstanding clinical practice, the Kitty Ernst Award from the ACNM for recognition of innovative, creative endeavors in midwifery and women's health, and was inducted as a Fellow of the ACNM. Currently she is professor and associate dean for nursing education at Northern Michigan University and works with the ACNM as a senior researcher.

Beth A. Collins Sharp is a health scientist administrator at the DHHS Agency for Healthcare Research and Quality. In the Center for Outcomes and Evidence, she is a project officer and task order officer with interests in the areas of workforce issues, nursing research and practice, and evidence-based practice and outcomes. She received an associate degree in nursing and BS (psychology) from Shenandoah College and Conservatory, a BS (nursing) and MS (nursing) from Medical of Virginia/Virginia Commonwealth University, and a PhD (nursing) from the University of Texas at Austin. She has taught at three large university schools of nursing; served as nurse coordinator in a national research network; and practiced in a community hospital's general medicine and postpartum units, an obstetric emergency room, and a university mother-baby inpatient unit. Most recently, she served on the faculty of the Medical University of South Carolina College of Medicine and as director of research for the Department of Obstetrics and Gynecology. Along the way, she has served as a member of a university institutional review board, chair of a university general clinical research center scientific research committee, reviewer for university intramural funding, president of the Southern Nursing Research Society, and science team leader for the Evidence-Based Guideline on Cyclic Perimenstrual Pain and Discomfort, Association for Women's Health, Obstetric and Neonatal Nurses.

Daniel J. Sheridan has a dual appointment as an assistant professor in the Johns Hopkins University School of Nursing, where he has developed a Forensic Nursing Clinical Specialist Master's Program; and as a forensic clinical nurse specialist in the Johns Hopkins Hospital Department of Emergency Medicine. Dr. Sheridan also works for the Oregon Department of Human Resources Mental Health and Developmental Disabilities Division, where he serves as a consultant and expert witness for both abused institutionalized people with profound cognitive and physical disabilities and the elderly. Dr. Sheridan owns and operates a home-based consulting and educational practice as a family violence consultant and forensic nurse clinical specialist. Dr. Sheridan has over 20 years' experience working with survivors of domestic and family violence and has created and managed two hospital-based family violence intervention programs, the first in Chicago, Illinois, and the second in Portland, Oregon. Dr. Sheridan has published more than 20 clinical and research articles on nursing's role in abuse and forensics and has given over 500 invited lectures on these topics nationally and internationally. Dr. Sheridan is the president-elect of the International Association of Forensic Nurses. He is the former chair of the Emergency Nurses Association's Forensic Nursing Special Interest Group. He served on the Board of the Nursing Network on Violence Against Women, International, for over six years and is a founding member of the Nursing Research Consortium on Violence and Abuse.

Katherine Simmonds graduated with a BA from Cornell University, an MSN from the MGH Institute of Health Professions (1993), and an MPH from Harvard University (2001). She joined the faculty at the MGH Institute of Health Professions in 2000 as clinical instructor in women's health and community health. She currently teaches in both the advanced practice and the generalist levels of the nursing program. Her areas of expertise include women's health, and family and community health. She has a particular interest in reproductive health. In addition to teaching, Ms. Simmonds is active in clinical practice in family planning/gynecology/obstetrics and is a clinical preceptor for students. She is the founder and director of the Reproductive Options Education Consortium for Nursing, an initiative to bring training and curricula on reproductive options to nurse educators in New England and across the United States. She also serves as a consultant to the Abortion Access Project, and to the Action for Boston Community Development/ Boston Family Planning Program. Ms. Simmonds has been involved in research including a current study of women's experiences with medical abortion, and a 1997 study of the inclusion of content on reproductive choice into Massachusetts nursing schools.

Nancy M. Steele received a PhD in nursing from the University of Michigan, a master of science in nursing from Grand Valley State University in Michigan, and has two post-graduate certifications as a women's health nurse practitioner and perinatal clinical nurse specialist. Currently, she is serving in the US Army Nurse Corps as a nurse manager for an antepartum/gynecology unit at Tripler Army Medical Center, Hawaii. She is also part of the military research team and serves as an adjunct faculty member for the Army Medical Department's Obstetrics Course for Nurses. Major Steele spent 12 years with the Army Reserve Nurse Corps prior to her active duty appointment, where she served on deployments for Joint Endeavor Bosnia, humanitarian missions to Honduras and El Salvador, and a health aid clinic in Japan. Her civilian career has encompassed education, research, administration, and nurse practitioner roles in the fields of obstetrics, gynecology, and women's health. For the past 10 years, prior to military active duty, she was an assistant professor at Grand Valley State University, a research assistant for the University of Michigan, and a women's health nurse practitioner for a private office. Her research has dealt extensively with promoting health in women. She has completed research studies involving the use of acupressure for the prevention of nausea and vomiting during pregnancy, exercise promotion during pregnancy, and the empowerment of women in Nicaragua as part of a health relief brigade.

Diana Taylor, nurse practitioner, educator, and researcher, is professor emeritus in the University of California, San Francisco School of Nursing, and formerly the director of the Women's Primary Care Program, the first women's health training program in California (founded in 1970). Another first, she was appointed co-director of the Center for Collaborative Primary Care to advance interprofessional collaboration and innovation related to primary care education, practice, and research at UCSF. With over 30 years of experience in providing women's health care, Dr. Taylor proposed new models of women's health to guide research efforts and provide a curriculum for educating women's health care providers that include capacity building in social/community responsibility and advocacy along with clinical competency and care management knowledge and skill. She has received awards for the advancement of primary care practice and research: the Loretta Ford Nurse Practitioner Advancement Award, the Achievement in Research Award from the National Organization of Nurse Practitioner Faculties, and a fellowship from the Bellagio Center, Rockefeller Foundation. Dr. Taylor has focused much of her clinical and research work on the understanding of the biopsychosocial and lifespan factors that affect the health and illness of women with the context of their daily lives including the structural conditions (racism, sexism, classism) that negatively impact health. She has recently published a science-based consumer health book for women to assist them in managing symptoms and promoting their health.

Dawn M. Van Pelt received her BSN from Pennsylvania State University in 1998. She is currently pursuing a master's degree as a clinical forensic nurse specialist at Johns Hopkins University.

Carol A. Verga graduated from Sacred Heart School of Nursing in Eugene, Oregon, in 1964. With her RN obtained, she received a BSN from Seattle University in Seattle, Washington, in 1969. She earned her MSN from the University of Washington in 1975 with a minor in physiology and biophysics. An MS in nurse-midwifery and maternal health followed from Columbia University in 1976. As the first licensed nurse-midwife in Alaska, Ms. Verga also served on the Alaskan Board of Nursing. In 1979 she established the Virginia Mason Nurse-Midwifery practice and, with the excellent work of many skilled CNMs, the service was open for 21 years. Ms. Verga also served on the Washington State Board of Nursing. Since 1991, Ms. Verga has focused on women's health, most recently on cervical and vulvar disease.

Mary Wallace received her BSN degree from the University of Florida and master's degree from the University of Wisconsin. She is a certified family nurse practitioner and is the coordinator of the Family Nurse Practitioner Program at Northern Michigan University. She has been an educator and practitioner for more than 20 years. Her teaching responsibilities include courses in the graduate and undergraduate programs, including pathophysiology, health assessment, and community health nursing. She has practiced in a variety of clinical settings including NMU University Health Center, Planned Parenthood, and Marquette County Health Department. She was one of two faculty recently recognized across the university with a teaching excellence award. She is a member of the American Academy of Nurse Practitioners and National Organization of Nurse Practitioner Faculties. She is president of the Xi Sigma chapter of Sigma Theta Tau.